Pocket Companion to

Robbins

PATHOLOGIC
BASIS *of*
DISEASE

Pocket Companion to

Robbins

PATHOLOGIC BASIS *of* DISEASE ● Sixth Edition

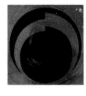

Stanley L. Robbins, M.D.
Consultant in Pathology
Brigham and Women's Hospital
Boston, Massachusetts

Ramzi S. Cotran, M.D.
Frank Burr Mallory Professor of Pathology
Harvard Medical School
Chairman, Department of Pathology
Brigham and Women's Hospital
The Children's Hospital
Boston, Massachusetts

Vinay Kumar, M.D.
Vernie A. Stembridge Chair in Pathology
Department of Pathology
The University of Texas
Southwestern Medical School
Dallas, Texas

Tucker Collins, M.D., Ph.D.
Professor of Pathology
Harvard Medical School
Pathologist
Brigham and Women's Hospital
Boston, Massachusetts

W.B. SAUNDERS COMPANY
An Imprint of Elsevier Science

W.B. SAUNDERS COMPANY
An Imprint of Elsevier Science

The Curtis Center
Independence Square West
Philadelphia, Pennsylvania 19106

Library of Congress Cataloging-in-Publication Data

Pocket companion to Robbins pathologic basis of disease /
Stanley L. Robbins . . . [et al.]—6th edition

p.   cm.

Companion v. to: Robbins pathologic basis of disease. 6th
ed. / Ramzi S. Cotran, Vinay Kumar, Tucker Collins. c1999.

Includes index.

ISBN 0–7216–7859—9

1. Pathology—Handbooks, manuals, etc.   I. Robbins,
   Stanley L. (Stanley Leonard)   II. Cotran, Ramzi S.
   Robbins pathologic basis of disease.
   [DNLM: 1. Pathology handbooks. QZ 39 P7392 1999]

RB111.R62 1999 Suppl.   616.07—dc21

DNLM/DLC   98–32245

Pocket Companion to Robbins

PATHOLOGIC BASIS OF DISEASE   ISBN 0–7216–7859–9

Printed in China

Last digit is the print number: 9   8   7   6

Contributors

Daniel M. Albert, M.D.
F.A. Davis Professor and Chair, Department of Ophthalmology
and Visual Sciences, University of Wisconsin Medical School,
Madison, Wisconsin
Diseases of the Eye

Douglas C. Anthony, M.D., Ph.D.
Associate Professor of Pathology, Harvard Medical School;
Director of Neuropathology, Children's Hospital,
Boston, Massachusetts
*Diseases of Peripheral Nerves and Muscle, Diseases of the Central
Nervous System*

Jon Aster, M.D., Ph.D.
Assistant Professor of Pathology, Harvard Medical School;
Pathologist, Brigham and Women's Hospital,
Boston, Massachusetts
Diseases of White Cells

James M. Crawford, M.D., Ph.D.
Associate Professor of Pathology, Director, Program in
Gastrointestinal Pathology, Yale University School of Medicine,
New Haven, Connecticut
*Diseases of the Gastrointestinal Tract, Diseases of the Liver, Biliary
System, and Pancreas*

Christopher P. Crum, M.D.
Professor of Pathology, Harvard Medical School; Director
Women's and Perinatal Pathology, Brigham and Women's
Hospital, Boston, Massachusetts
Diseases of the Female Genital Tract

Umberto De Girolami, M.D.
Associate Professor of Pathology, Harvard Medical School;
Director of Neuropathology, Brigham and Women's Hospital,
Boston, Massachusetts
*Diseases of Peripheral Nerves and Muscle, Diseases of the Central
Nervous System*

Thaddeus P. Dryja, M.D.
David Glen Denning Cogan Professor, Department of
Ophthalmology, Massachusetts Eye and Ear Infirmary,
Harvard Medical School, Boston, Massachusetts
  Diseases of the Eye

Matthew P. Frosch, M.D., Ph.D.
Assistant Professor of Pathology, Harvard Medical School;
Neuropathologist, Brigham and Women's Hospital,
Boston, Massachusetts
  *Diseases of Peripheral Nerves and Muscle, Diseases of the Central
  Nervous System*

Lester Kobzik, M.D.
Associate Professor of Pathology, Harvard Medical School;
Pathologist, Brigham and Women's Hospital,
Boston, Massachusetts
  Diseases of the Respiratory System

Susan C. Lester, M.D., Ph.D.
Assistant Professor of Pathology, Harvard Medical School,
Pathologist, Brigham and Women's Hospital,
Boston, Massachusetts
  Diseases of the Breast

Richard N. Mitchell, M.D., Ph.D.
Assistant Professor of Pathology, Harvard Medical School;
Pathologist, Brigham and Women's Hospital,
Boston, Massachusetts
  Hemodynamic Disorders, Thrombosis, and Shock

George F. Murphy, M.D.
Professor of Pathology, Jefferson Medical College; Director of
Cutaneous Pathology and Medical Education, Department of
Pathology, Thomas Jefferson University Hospital,
Philadelphia, Pennsylvania
  Diseases of the Skin

Andrew E. Rosenberg, M.D.
Associate Professor of Pathology, Harvard Medical School;
Associate Pathologist, Massachusetts General Hospital,
Boston, Massachusetts
  Diseases of the Skeletal System, and Soft Tissue Tumors

John Samuelson, M.D., Ph.D.
Associate Professor, Department of Immunology and Infectious
Diseases, Harvard School of Public Health,
Boston, Massachusetts
  Infectious Diseases

Frederick J. Schoen, M.D., Ph.D.
Professor of Pathology, Harvard Medical School; Director,
Cardiac Pathology, Brigham and Women's Hospital,
Boston, Massachusetts
Diseases of the Blood Vessels, Diseases of the Heart

Deborah Schofield, M.D., M.B.A.
Associate Professor of Pathology, University of Southern
California; Attending Pathologist, Children's Hospital of Los
Angeles, Los Angeles, California
Diseases of Infancy and Childhood

Preface

The publication of yet another new edition of *Robbins Pathologic Basis of Disease* has made necessary a parallel revision of its *Pocket Companion*. Despite strenuous effort to contain its size, the *Pocket Companion* has lamentably gained somewhat in the number of pages. In part, this is caused by the expanding body of knowledge presented in the parent book and by its increasing complexity. In addition, new chapters have been written. The subjects of cellular injury and cellular death, acute and chronic inflammation and repair, formerly presented in three chapters, have in the present edition been reordered and expanded into four chapters. The disorders of the female genital tract and breast, formerly discussed in one chapter, have now been divided into separate chapters. The coverage of white cells and their disorders has been necessarily expanded greatly as dictated by the increased knowledge about lymphomas and leukemias. An entirely new chapter on diseases of the eye has also been added. These changes have made the *Pocket Companion* and its parent—The Big Book—entirely concordant. It has been made easier to cross reference from one to the other. This has been done by cross-referencing page numbers throughout the *Pocket Companion* to the *Robbins Pathologic Basis of Disease,* sixth edition.

The Pocket Companion is more than a topical outline. The goals continue to be as follows:

- To facilitate the reading and comprehension of the more detailed presentations in the parent book by providing introductory overviews along with relevant page numbers to *Robbins Pathologic Basis of Disease,* sixth edition.
- To help students identify the core material that requires their primary attention.
- To serve as a useful tool for the review of a large body of information.

Although in this present world, and particularly in medical education, there is too much to do and too little time to do it, and although much can be said for an abbreviated guide such as this, we must caution against the use of the *Pocket Companion* as the sole source of information in the study of pathology. It does contain the salient facts, but it omits the discussions and expositions that enrich the fuller presentations. We hope, therefore, that this abbreviated overview of pathology will be referred to as a companion to the parent book, enhancing the pleasure to be derived from and the value of both.

STANLEY L. ROBBINS
RAMZI S. COTRAN
VINAY KUMAR
TUCKER COLLINS

Preface

Contents

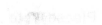

Cellular Injury and Death

INTRODUCTION (p. 1)

Pathology is the study of the structural and functional causes of human disease. The four aspects of a disease process that form the core of pathology are

- Its cause.
- The pathogenesis or sequence of events that give rise to the manifestations of the disease.
- The morphologic changes or structural alterations induced in cells and tissues by the disease.
- The functional consequences of the morphologic changes, as observed clinically.

DEFINITIONS (p. 2)

Normal cellular function requires a balance between the physiologic demands imposed on it and the constraints of the cell's structure and metabolic capability. This delicate balance creates a homeostatic steady state. Cells can alter their functional state in response to modest stress and maintain their homeostasis. They react to more excessive physiologic stresses, or adverse pathologic stimuli, by (1) adapting, (2) sustaining reversible injury, or (3) suffering irreversible injury and dying.

Cellular adaptation occurs when excessive physiologic stresses, or some pathologic stimuli, result in a new but altered state that preserves the viability of the cell. Examples are *hypertrophy* (increase in mass of the cell) or *atrophy* (decrease in mass of the cell). *Reversible cell injury* denotes pathologic changes that can be reversed when the stimulus is removed or if the cause of injury is mild. *Irreversible injury* denotes pathologic changes that are permanent and cause cellular death.

There are two morphologic patterns of cellular death, necrosis and apoptosis:

- *Necrosis* is the more common type of cellular death after exogenous stimuli and is manifested by severe cell swelling, denaturation and coagulation of proteins, breakdown of cellular organelles, and cell rupture.
- *Apoptosis* occurs when a cell dies through the activation of an internal suicide program. It is a carefully orchestrated disassembly of cellular components designed to eliminate unwanted cells with minimal disruption of the surrounding tissue. It is characterized morphologically by chromatin condensation and fragmentation. Apoptosis occurs in single or small clusters of

cells and results in the elimination of unwanted cells during embryogenesis and in various physiologic and pathologic states.

CAUSES OF CELLULAR INJURY (p. 4)

The adverse effects can be grouped into broad categories, as follows:

1. *Oxygen deprivation (hypoxia),* which occurs as a result of
   • *Ischemia* (loss of blood supply)
   • Inadequate oxygenation (e.g., cardiorespiratory failure)
   • Loss of oxygen-carrying capacity of the blood (e.g., anemia, carbon monoxide poisoning)
2. *Physical agents,* including trauma, heat, cold, radiation, and electric shock
3. *Chemical agents and drugs,* including therapeutic drugs (e.g., acetaminophen [Tylenol]) and nontherapeutic agents (e.g., lead, alcohol)
4. *Infectious agents,* including viruses, rickettsiae, bacteria, fungi, and parasites
5. *Immunologic reactions,* which can cause cell injury as well as serve in the defense against biologic agents
6. *Genetic derangements,* such as chromosomal alterations or specific mutations in genes
7. *Nutritional imbalances,* including protein-calorie deficiency and lack of specific vitamins as well as nutritional excesses. Additionally the composition of the diet can make a significant contribution to disease.

CELLULAR INJURY AND NECROSIS (pp. 5–18)

General Mechanisms (p. 5)

The molecular mechanisms responsible for cellular injury are complex, although there are some helpful general considerations, such as the following:

■ The cellular response to injurious stimuli depends on the type of injury, its duration, and its severity.
■ The consequences of cell injury depend on the type, state, and adaptability of the injured cell.
■ Four intracellular systems are particularly vulnerable to injury: (1) *aerobic respiration* involving mitochondrial oxidative phosphorylation and production of adenosine triphosphate (ATP); (2) *maintenance of the integrity of cell membranes,* on which the ionic and osmotic homeostasis of the cell and its organelles depends; (3) *protein synthesis;* and (4) *preservation of the integrity of the genetic apparatus* of the cell.
■ The structural and biochemical elements of the cell are so closely interrelated that whatever the precise point of initial attack, injury at one locus leads to wide-ranging secondary effects.
■ The morphologic changes of cellular injury become apparent only some time after a critical biochemical system within the cell has been deranged.

Five general biochemical themes are important in mediating cellular injury and death, *whatever the inciting agent:*

1. *Decreased ATP synthesis and ATP depletion.* ATP is generated by oxidative phosphorylation in the mitochondria and through

the glycolytic pathway. ATP is required for such important processes as membrane transport, protein synthesis, and phospholipid turnover. *Decreased ATP synthesis and ATP depletion are common consequences of both ischemic and toxic injury.*

2. *Oxygen-derived free radicals.* Oxygen-derived free radicals are partially reduced reactive oxygen forms that are produced as a byproduct of mitochondrial respiration. These reactive species can damage lipids, proteins, and nucleic acids. An imbalance between free radical–generating and free radical–scavenging systems results in *oxidative stress,* a condition that has been associated with many types of cellular injury.

3. *Loss of calcium homeostasis* and *increased intracellular calcium.* Cytosolic calcium is maintained at extremely low levels by an energy-dependent transport system. Ischemia and certain toxins cause net influx of Ca^{2+} across the plasma membrane and release of Ca^{2+} from mitochondria and endoplasmic reticulum. Increased cytosolic calcium activates *phospholipases,* which degrade membrane phospholipids; *proteases,* which break down membrane and cytoskeletal proteins; *ATPases,* which hasten ATP depletion; and *endonucleases,* which are associated with chromatin fragmentation.

4. *Defects in membrane permeability.* Membranes can be damaged directly by toxins, physical and chemical agents, lytic complement components, and perforins or indirectly as described by the preceding events.

5. *Irreversible mitochondrial damage.* Mitochondria are important targets for virtually all types of injurious stimuli. They can be damaged by increases of cytosolic Ca^{2+}; oxidative stress; and breakdown of phospholipids by the phospholipase A_2 and sphingomyelin pathways and lipid breakdown products derived therefrom, such as free fatty acids and ceramide. Commonly the damage is expressed as the formation of a high conductance channel—the so-called *mitochondrial permeability transition* (MPT)—in the inner mitochondrial membrane. Although reversible in its early stages, this nonselective pore becomes permanent if the inciting stimuli persist. Mitochondrial damage causes leakage of *cytochrome c* into the cytosol and activation of the apoptotic death pathways.

Ischemic and Hypoxic Injury (p. 7)

Ischemic and hypoxic injury is the most common type of cellular injury in clinical medicine. Reasonable scenarios concerning the mechanisms underlying the morphologic changes have emerged. During ischemia, there is progressive compromise of multiple biochemical and structural components. Up to a certain point, this injury is amenable to repair, and the affected cells can recover if oxygen is made available. Pathologic changes characteristic of ischemic cells that can recover are described as *reversible injury.* With further progression of the ischemia, the cells' energy-generating machinery becomes irreparably damaged, and the cells pass a "point of no return" after which they cannot be rescued. Pathologic changes characteristic of permanent ischemic damage are designated *irreversible injury.* When blood flow is restored to cells that have been previously ischemic, injury can be exacerbated. This additional damage is called *reperfusion injury.* Cellular injury that occurs after blood flow is restored is a clinically important process that contributes to tissue damage during myocardial infarction and stroke.

CELL CHANGES DURING ISCHEMIA/HYPOXIA

Reversible Cellular Injury

Hypoxia first causes loss of oxidative phosphorylation and ATP generation by mitochondria. The resulting depletion in ATP has multiple effects (Fig. 1–1), as follows:

- Failure of ouabain-sensitive Na^+, K^+-ATPase active membrane transport causes sodium to enter the cell and potassium to diffuse out of the cell. The net gain of solute is accompanied by an isosmotic gain of water, *cell swelling,* and dilation of the endoplasmic reticulum. A second mechanism for cell swelling in ischemia is the increased intracellular *osmotic load* generated by the accumulation of metabolic breakdown products, such as lactate.
- *Cellular energy metabolism* is altered. When oxygen levels are low, cells rely on glycolysis for energy production. This results in an increased rate of *anaerobic glycolysis* designed to maintain the cell's energy sources by generating ATP via metabolism of glucose derived from glycogen. Consequently, *glycogen stores are rapidly depleted.* Glycolysis results in the accumulation of lactic acid, which *reduces the intracellular pH.*
- Reduced protein synthesis results from detachment of ribosomes from the granular (rough) endoplasmic reticulum.
- Hypoxic cells can sense diminishing oxygen levels and increase the production of a select set of proteins in an austerity program that is designated the *hypoxic response.*
- Functional consequences can occur in reversible cellular injury.

Continued hypoxia causes further morphologic deterioration. *All of the aforementioned changes are reversible if oxygenation is restored.*

Irreversible Cellular Injury

If ischemia persists, irreversible injury ensues.

Mechanisms of Irreversible Cellular Injury. Two critical events are involved in irreversible injury:

- *ATP depletion.* ATP depletion is an early event in cellular injury that contributes to the functional and structural consequences of ischemic hypoxia and to cell membrane damage.
- *Membrane dysfunction.* The earliest phase of irreversible injury is associated with functional and structural defects of cell membranes, particularly mitochondrial membranes.
  1. *Mitochondrial membrane damage* is generated in two ways:
     - ATP depletion causes changes in the *inner* mitochondrial membrane, designated the MPT. The formation of pores within the inner mitochondrial membrane results in a reduction in the membrane potential and diffusion of solutes.
     - ATP depletion induced by hypoxia also causes increased permeability of the *outer* mitochondrial membrane and *release of cytochrome c,* a soluble but integral component of the electron transport chain that is a key regulator in determining the susceptibility to cellular death, as discussed in more detail later.
  2. *Progressive loss of phospholipids* damages membranes as a result of
     - Activation of membrane phospholipases by the increased

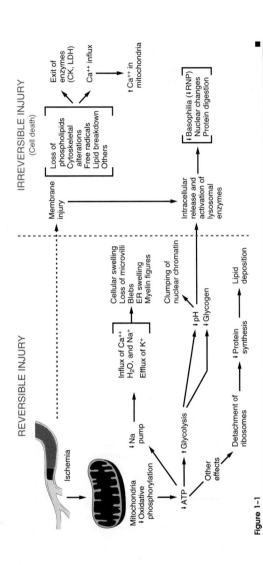

Figure 1-1

Postulated sequence of events in ischemic injury. Note that although reduced oxidative phosphorylation and ATP levels have a central role, ischemia can cause direct membrane damage. (From Kumar V, Cotran RS, Robbins SL: Basic Pathology, 6th ed. Philadelphia, WB Saunders, 1997.)

REVERSIBLE INJURY

IRREVERSIBLE INJURY
(Cell death)

Ischemia

Mitochondria
↓Oxidative phosphorylation

↓ATP

↓Na pump

Other effects

↑Glycolysis

Detachment of ribosomes

Influx of Ca⁺⁺, H₂O, and Na⁺
Efflux of K⁺

Cellular swelling
Loss of microvilli
Blebs
ER swelling
Myelin figures

Clumping of nuclear chromatin

↓pH
↓Glycogen

↓Protein synthesis

Lipid deposition

Membrane injury

Loss of phospholipids
Cytoskeletal alterations
Free radicals
Lipid breakdown
Others

Exit of enzymes (CK, LDH)

Ca⁺⁺ influx

↑Ca⁺⁺ in mitochondria

Intracellular release and activation of lysosomal enzymes

↓Basophilia (↓RNP)
Nuclear changes
Protein digestion

5

cytosolic calcium, leading to phospholipid degradation and phospholipid loss
  - Decreased phospholipid reacylation and synthesis, possibly related to loss of ATP
3. *Cytoskeletal abnormalities.* Activation of intracellular proteases, induced by increased cytosolic calcium, may cause degradation of intermediate cytoskeletal elements, rendering the cell membrane susceptible to stretching and rupture, particularly in the presence of cell swelling.
4. *Reactive oxygen species.* Partially reduced oxygen free radicals are highly toxic molecules that cause injury to many cellular components, including cell membranes.
5. *Lipid breakdown products.* Free fatty acids and lysophospholipids accumulate in ischemic cells as a result of phospholipid degradation and are directly toxic to membranes.
6. *Loss of intracellular amino acids,* such as glycine, predisposes cells to irreversible membrane damage.

Whatever the mechanism of membrane injury, the resultant loss of membrane integrity causes massive influx of calcium from the extracellular space. The increased level of intracellular calcium results in inhibition of cellular enzymes, denaturation of proteins, and cytologic alterations characteristic of coagulative necrosis.

Summary

Hypoxia affects oxidative phosphorylation and hence the synthesis of vital ATP supplies; membrane damage is critical to the development of lethal cellular injury; and calcium is an important mediator of the biochemical and morphologic alterations leading to cellular death.

ISCHEMIA-REPERFUSION INJURY

Ischemia-reperfusion refers to a cessation in blood flow followed by restoration of the circulation. As we have seen, restoration of blood flow to ischemic tissues can result in recovery of cells if they are reversibly injured. Depending on the intensity and duration of the ischemic insult, however, cells may die after blood flow resumes, by necrosis as well as apoptosis. This additional damage has been designated *reperfusion injury,* and it is typically associated with a neutrophilic infiltrate. Reperfusion injury contributes to tissue damage during myocardial infarction, acute renal failure, and stroke. Several mechanisms have been proposed to explain how reperfusion causes this pattern of injury; including the following:

- ATP depletion during ischemia or hypoxia causes increased cytosolic calcium and elevated mitochondrial phospholipase activity. Collectively, these events induce the MPT, outlined previously. During reoxygenation, production of reactive oxygen species can promote the MPT, which precludes mitochondrial recovery and leads to cellular death.
- Hypoxia-induced *release of cytochrome c* triggers *apoptosis* if ATP production by glycolysis is high during reoxygenation because activation of the suicide program requires cellular energy. If ATP production is limited during reoxygenation, necrosis of the parenchymal cell results.
- Lack of oxygen also leads to the accumulation of metabolic intermediates. Reactive oxygen species in postischemic tissue can be derived from incomplete reduction of oxygen by mito-

chondria or due to the action of oxidases derived from leukocytes, endothelial cells, or parenchymal cells. Accumulation of
these products may overwhelm the cell's antioxidant defense
mechanisms leading to inappropriate oxidation of vital cell
components.

- Cellular death is associated with the production of cytokines
  and adhesion molecules by adjacent parenchymal and endothelial cells. These agents recruit circulating polymorphonuclear
  neutrophils to the reperfused tissue, and the ensuing inflammatory response causes additional injury.

Free Radical–Induced Cellular Injury (p. 12)

Free radicals are highly reactive, unstable species that can interact with proteins, lipids, and carbohydrates and are involved in
cellular injury induced by a variety of chemical and biologic
events. Free radical generation occurs by

- Absorption of radiant energy (e.g., ultraviolet light, x-rays). For
  example, ionizing radiation can hydrolyze water into hydroxyl
  (OH·) and hydrogen (H·) free radicals.
- Enzymatic metabolism of exogenous chemicals or drugs, such
  as carbon tetrachloride (CCl_4 can generate CCl_3·).
- The reduction-oxidation reactions that occur during normal metabolic processes. For example, during normal respiration, molecular oxygen is sequentially reduced by the addition of four
  electrons to generate water. In this process, small amounts of
  toxic intermediates are produced; these include *superoxide
  anion radical (O_2^-·), hydrogen peroxide (H_2O_2), and hydroxyl
  ions (OH·).*
- *Transition metals,* such as iron and copper, which donate or
  accept free electrons during intracellular reactions and catalyze
  free radical formation, as in the Fenton reaction ($H_2O_2 + Fe^{++}$
  $\rightarrow$ $Fe^{+++} + OH· + OH^-$). Because most of the intracellular
  free iron is in the ferric (Fe^{+++}) state, it must be first reduced
  to the ferrous (Fe^{++}) form to participate in the Fenton reaction.
  This reduction can be enhanced by superoxide, and *thus sources
  of iron and superoxide are required for maximal oxidative
  cellular damage.*
- *Nitric oxide* (NO), an important chemical mediator, which can
  act as a free radical and can also be converted to highly reactive
  peroxynitrite anion ($ONOO^-$) as well as NO_2· and NO_3^-.

The effects of these reactive species are wide ranging, but three
reactions are particularly relevant to cellular injury, as follows:

1. *Lipid peroxidation of membranes.* Free radicals in the presence of oxygen may cause peroxidation of lipids within plasma
and organellar membranes. Oxidative damage is *initiated* when
the double bonds in unsaturated fatty acids of membrane lipids
are attacked by oxygen-derived free radicals, particularly by OH·.
The lipid-radical interactions yield peroxides, which are themselves unstable and reactive, and an autocatalytic chain reaction
ensues (called *propagation*), which can result in extensive membrane, organellar, and cellular damage. Other more favorable *termination* options take place when the free radical is captured by a
scavenger, such as vitamin E, embedded in the cell membrane.

2. *Oxidative modification of proteins.* Free radicals promote
oxidation of amino acid residue side chains, the formation of
protein-protein cross-linkages (e.g., sulfhydryl-mediated), and the
oxidation and fragmentation of the protein backbone. Oxidative

modification enhances degradation of critical enzymes by the multicatalytic proteasome complex.

3. *Damage to deoxyribonucleic acid (DNA).* Reactions with thymidine in nuclear and mitochondrial DNA produce single-strand breaks in DNA. This DNA damage has been implicated in cellular aging (see Chapter 2) and in malignant transformation of cells.

Multiple mechanisms remove free radicals and thereby minimize cellular injury, as follows:

- Free radicals are *inherently unstable and generally decay spontaneously.* Superoxide, for example, is unstable and decays spontaneously into oxygen and hydrogen peroxide.
- Several systems contribute to inactivation of free radical reactions:

  1. *Antioxidants* either block the initiation of free radical formation or inactivate (e.g., scavenge) free radicals and terminate radical damage. These include the lipid-soluble vitamins E and A as well as ascorbic acid and glutathione in the cytosol.
  2. The levels of the reactive forms generated by iron and copper (as noted previously) are minimized by binding of the ions to storage and transport proteins (e.g., *transferrin, ferritin, lactoferrin,* and *ceruloplasmin*).
  3. A series of *enzymes* act as free radical–scavenging systems and break down hydrogen peroxide and superoxide anion. These enzymes are located near the sites of generation of these oxidants and include the following:
     - *Catalase,* present in peroxisomes, decomposes H_2O_2 (2 $H_2O_2 \rightarrow O_2 + 2 H_2O$).
     - *Superoxide dismutases* are found in many cell types and convert superoxide to H_2O_2 ($2O_2 \cdot^- + 2H \rightarrow H_2O_2 + O_2$). This group includes both Mn-superoxide dismutase (MnSOD), which is localized in mitochondria, and Cu-Zn-superoxide dismutase, which is found in the cytosol.
     - *Glutathione peroxidase* also protects against injury by catalyzing free radical breakdown ($H_2O_2 + 2 GSH \rightarrow GSSG$ [glutathione homodimer] $+ 2 H_2O$, or $2 OH\cdot + 2 GSH \rightarrow GSSG + 2 H_2O$).

Chemical Injury (p. 14)

Chemicals cause cellular injury by two general mechanisms:

- *Directly,* by binding to some critical molecular component (e.g., mercury of mercuric chloride binds to SH groups of cell membrane proteins, causing increased permeability and inhibition of ATPase-dependent transport).
- *Indirectly,* by conversion to reactive toxic metabolites. Toxic metabolites, in turn, cause cellular injury either by direct covalent binding to membrane protein and lipids or, more commonly, by the formation of reactive free radicals. Two examples are carbon tetrachloride and acetaminophen.
  - *Carbon tetrachloride* (CCl_4), widely used in the dry-cleaning industry, is converted to $CCl_3\cdot$ in the smooth endoplasmic reticulum in the liver by the enzyme complex P-450. $CCl_3\cdot$ initiates lipid peroxidation and autocatalytic reactions that cause swelling and breakdown of the endoplasmic reticulum, dissociation of ribosomes, and decreased hepatic protein synthesis. There is reduced lipid export from hepatocytes because of their inability to synthesize apoprotein to complex with triglycerides and thereby facilitate lipoprotein secretion. This

reduced lipid export leads to lipid accumulation and fatty change in the liver. This is followed by progressive cellular swelling, plasma membrane damage, and cellular death.

- *Acetaminophen* is a commonly used analgesic drug that is metabolized in the liver by sulfation and glucuronidation. Small amounts of the agent are also converted to a toxic metabolite by cytochrome P-450, which is detoxified by interaction with reduced glutathione (GSH). When large doses are ingested, the reactive metabolites accumulate in the cell owing to GSH depletion. These reactive forms covalently bind proteins and nucleic acids, thus increasing drug toxicity and resulting in massive liver cell necrosis.

Morphology of Reversible and Irreversible Cellular Injury and Necrosis (p. 15)

REVERSIBLE INJURY

Cellular swelling dominates the pattern of reversible cellular injury recognized by the light microscope. The ultrastructural changes in reversible cellular injury are presented in Figure 1–2.

IRREVERSIBLE CELLULAR INJURY AND NECROSIS

Irreversible injury is marked by severe mitochondrial vacuolization; extensive damage to plasma membranes; swelling of lysosomes; and the appearance of large, amorphous densities in mitochondria. Injury to lysosomal membranes leads to leakage of the enzymes into the cytoplasm and, by their activation, to enzymatic digestion of cell and nuclear components.

Leakage of intracellular enzymes or proteins across the abnormally permeable plasma membrane and into the plasma provides important clinical parameters of cellular death. Cardiac muscle, for example, contains glutamic-oxaloacetic transaminase (GOT), lactic dehydrogenase (LDH), and creatine kinase (CK). Elevated serum levels of such enzymes, and particularly the isoenzymes specific for heart muscle (e. g., CK-MB), were at one time widely used as markers of myocardial infarction (a locus of cellular death). Today, serum levels of troponins I or T, proteins of the myofibrils, are more widely used.

Necrosis is the sum of the morphologic changes that follow cellular death in living tissue or organs. Two processes cause the basic morphologic changes of necrosis:

- Denaturation of proteins
- Enzymatic digestion of organelles and other cytosolic components

The morphology of necrosis has several distinctive features: The necrotic cell is *eosinophilic* (pink) and glassy and may be vacuolated. The cell membranes are fragmented. Nuclear changes in necrotic cells include *pyknosis* (small, dense nucleus), *karyolysis* (faint, dissolved nucleus), and *karyorrhexis* (nucleus broken up into many clumps). *Autolysis* may follow owing to digestion by lysosomal enzymes of the dead cells themselves. *Heterolysis* is digestion by lysosomal enzymes of immigrant leukocytes. Necrotic cells may attract calcium salts in the form of granular basophilic deposits, referred to as *dystrophic calcification* (see Chapter 2). This is particularly true of necrotic fat cells.

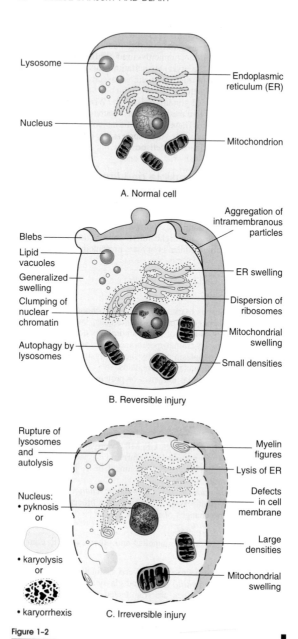

A. Normal cell

B. Reversible injury

C. Irreversible injury

Figure 1-2 ■

Schematic representation of a normal cell *(A)* and the ultrastructural changes in reversible *(B)* and irreversible *(C)* cellular injury (see text). (From Kumar V, Cotran RS, Robbins SL: Basic Pathology, 6th ed. Philadelphia, WB Saunders, 1997.)

Types of Necrosis (p. 15)

- *Coagulation necrosis* is the most common pattern of necrosis and is characterized by denaturation of cytoplasmic proteins with preservation of the framework of the coagulated cell. This pattern of ischemic necrosis occurs in the myocardium, kidney, liver, and other organs.
- *Liquefaction necrosis* occurs when autolysis and heterolysis prevail over protein denaturation. The necrotic area is soft and filled with fluid. This type of necrosis is most frequently seen in localized bacterial infections (abscesses) and in the brain.
- *Caseous necrosis* is characteristic of tuberculous lesions and appears grossly as soft, friable, "cheesy" material and microscopically as amorphous eosinophilic material with cell debris.
- *Fat necrosis* refers to necrosis in adipose tissue, induced by the action of lipases (derived from injured pancreatic cells or macrophages) that catalyze enzymatic release of fatty acids from triglycerides, which then complex with calcium to create calcium soaps. These generate chalky white areas (fat saponification), which can be identified by inspection. Histologically the necrotic fat shows shadowy outlines of cells and basophilic stippling as a result of calcium deposition-dystrophic calcification.

APOPTOSIS (pp. 18–25)

Physiologic (or programmed) cellular death occurs when a cell within an organism dies through activation of an internal suicide program. The function of this process is to eliminate unwanted cells selectively, with minimal disturbance to surrounding cells and the host. This morphologic pattern of death has been designated *apoptosis,* and it is thought to be responsible for numerous physiologic and pathologic events, including the following:

- Programmed destruction of cells during embryogenesis
- Hormone-dependent involution of tissues (e.g., endometrium, prostate) in the adult
- Cell deletion in proliferating cell populations (e.g., intestinal crypt epithelium), tumors, and lymphoid organs as well as pathologic atrophy in parenchymal organs after duct obstruction
- Cellular death in tumors
- Cellular death by cytotoxic T cells
- Death of immune cells (T and B cells) after cytokine depletion
- Death of neutrophils during an acute inflammatory response
- Cellular injury and death in certain viral diseases
- Cellular death produced by a variety of injurious stimuli that are capable of producing necrosis but when given in low doses induce apoptosis (e.g., radiation, mild thermal injury, cytotoxic anticancer drugs)

The *morphologic features* of apoptosis include

- Cell shrinkage
- Chromatin condensation and fragmentation
- Cellular blebbing and fragmentation into apoptotic bodies
- Phagocytosis of apoptotic bodies by adjacent healthy cells or macrophages; lack of inflammation

In contrast to apoptosis during development, secondary necrosis as well as apoptosis can occur after some injurious stimuli. The severity of the injury, rather than the specificity of stimulus, determines the form in which death is expressed. Because apoptosis occurs in single or small clusters of cells and does not cause inflammation, it may be difficult to demonstrate histologically.

The distinctive biochemical features of apoptosis include the following:

- Protein cleavage by cysteine proteases, called *caspases*
- Protein cross-linking by transglutaminase, which converts cytoplasmic proteins into a linked meshwork
- Internucleosomal cleavage of DNA into a characteristic ladder pattern of oligonucleosomal multiples of about 200 base pairs
- Plasma membrane alterations, such as flipping of phosphatidylserine from the inner to the outer layer of the plasma membrane.

The last-mentioned change and expression of other cell surface molecules permit recognition of dead cells by macrophages, allowing the apoptotic response to dispose of cells swiftly and specifically with minimal damage to surrounding tissues.

Mechanisms (p. 20)

Apoptosis can be activated by a variety of death-triggering signals, ranging from a lack of growth factor or hormone, to a positive ligand-receptor interaction, to specific injurious agents. Studies in the nematode *Caenorhabditis elegans,* which undergoes a programmed pattern of cellular death, have allowed the identification of specific genes (the so-called *ced genes*—for *C. elegans* death), which can either initiate or inhibit cellular death. Apoptosis is the end point of a cascade of energy-dependent molecular events, consisting of separable but overlapping stages (Fig. 1–3).

SIGNALING PATHWAYS

Apoptotic stimuli generate signals that are either transmitted across the plasma membrane to intracellular regulatory molecules or addressed more directly at targets present within the cell. Some stimuli, such as growth factors, cytokines, and hormones, generate signals that suppress preexisting death programs and are thus normal survival stimuli. Conversely, absence of survival factors (e.g., growth factor withdrawal) leads to failure of suppression of such programs and triggers apoptosis.

CONTROL OR INTEGRATION

In the control or integration stage, the death signals are connected to the execution program. There are two general schemes for such regulation:

1. *Adapter proteins.* This involves transmission of death signals by specific adapter proteins to the execution mechanism, as described subsequently.

2. *bcl-2 family members.* This family affects the outcome of cellular death by regulating mitochondrial function.

Death agonists can generate signals that affect mitochondria in two general ways (Fig. 1–4).

- *Mitochondrial permeability transitions.* Some apoptotic stimuli induce pores in the inner mitochondrial membrane and disrupt mitochondrial homeostasis.
- The death signals cause increased permeability of the outer

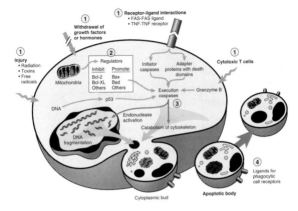

Figure 1-3   ■

Schematic representation of apoptic events. *(1)* Labeled are mutiple stimuli of apoptosis.
These include specific death ligands (tumor necrosis factor [TNF] and Fas-ligand),
withdrawal of growth factors or hormones, or injurious agents (e.g., radiation). Some
stimuli (such as cytotoxic cells) directly activate execution caspases *(right)*. Others act
by way of adapter proteins and initiator caspases, or by mitochondrial events involving
cytochrome *c.* *(2)* Control and regulation are influenced by members of the *bcl-2* family
of proteins, which can either inhibit or promote the cell's death. *(3)* Execution caspases
activate latent cytoplasmic endonuclease and proteases that degrade cytoskteleal and
nuclear proteins. This activation results in a cascade of intracellular degradation, including fragmentation of the nuclear chromatin and breakdown of the cytoskeleton. Not
shown is transglutaminase-induced cross-linking of proteins. *(4)* The end result is
formation of apoptotic bodies containing various intracellular organelles and other
cytosolic components; these bodies also express new ligands for binding and uptake by
phagocytic cells.

mitochondrial membrane, releasing an apoptotic trigger, cytochrome *c,* into the cytosol. Cytochrome *c* release precedes the
morphologic changes of apoptosis, showing that it occurs early,
consistent with a regulatory function.

Members of the *bcl-2* family regulate mitochondrial permeability
and control cellular death. *bcl-2* suppresses apoptosis in two ways:

- *Direct actions on mitochondria to prevent increased permeability.* bcl-2, the mammalian homolog of the antiapoptotic *ced 9*
  gene in *C. elegans,* is situated primarily in the outer mitochondrial membrane. Its function is regulated by other members of
  the *bcl-2* family. Mitochondrial permeability is determined by
  the ratio of proapoptotic and antiapoptotic members of the
  bcl-2 family in the membrane.
- *Effects mediated by interactions with other proteins.* bcl-2 can
  also function as a *docking protein* by binding proteins from the
  cytosol and sequestering them on the mitochondrial membrane.
  When cytochrome *c* is released from mitochondria, it binds
  proapoptotic protease activating factor (Apaf-1), the mammalian homolog of the nematode gene CED-4, and activates it,
  triggering the caspases (see subsequently) and setting in motion
  the proteolytic events that eventually kill the cell.

EXECUTION PHASE

The heterogeneous signaling and regulatory mechanisms converge on a final proteolytic cascade, which exhibits common

Possible modes of action of Bcl-2

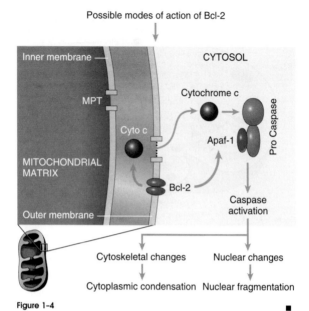

Figure 1–4 ∎

Mitochondrial events and the effects of *bcl-2* in apoptosis. Death agonists cause changes in the inner mitochondrial membrane, resulting in the mitochondrial permeability transition (MPT) and release of cytochrome *c* into the cytosol by currently unclear mechanisms. Released cytochrome *c* disrupts the binding between *bcl-2* and proapoptotic protease activating factor (Apaf). The latter activates an initiator caspase, which begins the proteolytic events that eventually kill the cell. *Bcl-2* thus suppresses apoptosis by inhibition of cytochrome *c* release and by binding and thus inactivating Apaf-1.

themes found in all forms of apoptosis. The proteases that trigger and mediate the execution phase are highly conserved and belong to the *caspase* family. These enzymes exist as zymogens that must undergo an activating cleavage for apoptosis to be initiated. Caspases can be divided into *initiators* and *executors,* depending on the order by which they are activated before cellular death. The execution caspases are responsible for the morphologic changes characteristic of apoptosis.

REMOVAL OF DEAD CELLS

Apoptotic cells and their fragments have marker molecules on their surfaces that facilitate early recognition by phagocytes or adjacent cells for phagocytic uptake and disposal. We review some specific examples of apoptosis that illustrate some of the stages involved in cellular death.

Signaling by Tumor Necrosis Factor Family of Receptors

Members of the tumor necrosis factor (TNF) family of receptors (TNFR) initiate apoptosis, some initiate cell proliferation, and others initiate both. A subfamily of TNFR, such as Fas and

TNFRI, have a cytoplasmic 80 amino acid *death recognition domain.* Death signaling involves clustering of the receptors by ligand and binding of the receptor to cytoplasmic adapter proteins via interactions between death domains found in both the receptor and the adapter. In turn, the *death effector domains* in the adapter proteins and initiator caspases interact, and autocatalytic activation triggers the execution step. Examples of cellular death mediated by this subfamily include the following:

- *Fas-mediated and Fas ligand (FasL)–mediated apoptosis.* Fas-FasL (or CD95L) is one of the best-defined signaling pathways activating apoptosis. FasL is a cytokine produced by cells of the immune system that binds to a specific receptor, designated *Fas,* and activates a death program in lymphocytes. This system eliminates activated cells from an immune response, thereby limiting the host response. The receptor interacts with an adapter protein (FADD) and activates an *initiator caspase,* which triggers the subsequent proteolytic signaling cascade that results in cellular death (Fig. 1–5).
- *TNF-induced apoptosis.* Activation of one of the TNF receptors (TNFRI) by the cytokine TNF can lead to apoptosis by inducing the association of the receptor with the adapter protein *TRADD* (TNFR-adapter protein with a death domain). As with the Fas-FasL system, TRADD, in turn, binds to FADD and leads to apoptosis via caspase activation. In contrast to Fas, however, under certain conditions TNFRI binding to TRADD is followed by binding not to FADD but to different adapters called *TRAF2 (TNFR-associated factor)* and *RIP (rest in peace),* a death domain kinase. This binding leads to activation of the important transcription factor nuclear factor-κB (NF-κB), by stimulating

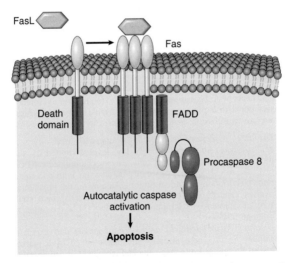

Figure 1-5   ∎

A model of Fas-mediated signaling, caspase activation, and induction of a death signal. Fas ligand interacts with Fas, trimerizing the receptor, resulting in the binding of the cytoplasmic adapter protein FADD via a death domain. The adapter protein then activates procaspase 8 triggering the execution phase of cellular death.

degradation of its inhibitor (IκB). This transcriptional regulatory system is important for *cell survival* and for increasing expression of a number of genes (e.g., cytokines, adhesion molecules) important in inflammatory responses (Fig. 1–6).

Cytotoxic T-Lymphocyte–Stimulated Apoptosis

Cytotoxic T lymphocytes (CTLs) recognize foreign antigens presented on the surface of infected host cells. CTLs induce apoptosis through the action of *perforin,* a transmembrane pore-forming molecule, and the exocytotic release of cytoplasmic granules from the CTL into target cells. The serine protease *granzyme B* is the critical cytotoxic component in this process. Granzyme B has the ability to cleave proteins at aspartate residues and is able to activate a variety of cellular caspases. In this way, the CTL kills target cells by bypassing the upstream signaling events and directly induces the effector phase of apoptosis.

DNA Damage–Mediated Apoptosis

Exposure of cells to radiation or chemotherapeutic agents induces apoptosis by a mechanism that is initiated by DNA damage (genotoxic stress) and that involves the tumor-suppressor gene, *p53*. *p53* accumulates when DNA is damaged and arrests the cell cycle (at the G_1 phase) to allow additional time for repair (see Chapter 8). If the repair process fails, however, *p53* triggers apoptosis through a mechanism that engages the distal death effector machinery—the caspases. Thus, *p53* normally stimulates apoptosis, but when mutated or absent (as it is in certain cancers), it favors cell survival. Thus, *p53* seems to serve as a critical "life or death" switch in the case of *genotoxic* stress. The mechanism by which DNA damage leads to cellular death is complex but seems to involve *p53*'s well-characterized function in transcriptional regulation.

Dysregulation of Apoptosis in Disease States

The concept of *dysregulated apoptosis* ("too little or too much") has emerged to explain components of a wide range of diseases. There are two possible general scenarios for dysregulation:

- *Disorders associated with inhibited apoptosis and increased cell survival.* An inappropriately low level of apoptosis may prolong survival of abnormal cells. These accumulated cells can give rise to (1) *cancers,* especially carcinomas with *p53* mutations or hormone-dependent tumors, such as breast, prostate, or ovarian cancers, and (2) *autoimmune disorders,* which could arise if autoreactive lymphocytes are not removed after an immune response.
- *Disorders associated with increased apoptosis and excessive cellular death.* These diseases are characterized by a marked loss of normal or protective cells and include (1) *neurodegenerative diseases,* manifested by loss of specific sets of neurons, such as in the spinal muscular atrophies, (2) *ischemic injury,* discussed previously, such as in myocardial infarction and stroke; and (3) *virus-induced lymphocyte depletion,* such as occurs in acquired immunodeficiency syndrome (AIDS).

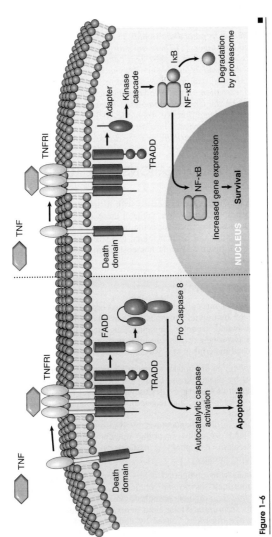

Figure 1-6

A model of tumor necrosis factor receptor (TNFRI)–mediated signaling and the induction of apoptosis or nuclear factor-κB (NF-κB) and cell survival signals (see text).

Summary

Apoptosis is a distinctive form of cellular death manifested by characteristic chromatin condensation and DNA fragmentation, whose function is the deletion of cells in normal development, organogenesis, immune function, and tissue growth but that can also be induced by pathologic stimuli. The mechanism of apoptosis has several key stages: (1) There are multiple pathways of commitment to cellular death; (2) there is a control stage, in which the apoptotic threshold is established by the relative abundance of different positive and negative regulators; and (3) there is a conserved execution stage, involving the activation of caspases, which perform the terminal proteolysis. There are multiple inhibitors of this regulated process. Apoptotic bodies are then engulfed by macrophages by receptor-mediated phagocytosis. Dysregulation of this process may contribute to some disease states.

SUBCELLULAR ALTERATIONS IN CELLULAR INJURY (pp. 25–28)

Certain conditions are associated with distinctive alterations in cell organelles or cytoskeleton. Some of these alterations are found along with those described for acute lethal injury, others occur in more chronic forms of cellular injury, and still others are adaptive responses that involve specific homeostatic mechanisms or cellular organelles.

Lysosomes (p. 25)

Primary lysosomes are membrane-bound organelles that contain a variety of hydrolytic enzymes. Primary lysosomes fuse with membrane-bound vacuoles containing ingested material forming *secondary lysosomes* or phagolysosomes. Lysosomes break down phagocytosed material in two ways:

■ *Heterophagy* is the uptake of materials from the external environment by phagocytosis. Examples include phagocytosis and degradation of bacteria by leukocytes, removal of necrotic debris by macrophages, and reabsorption of protein by the proximal tubules.

■ *Autophagy* is the phagocytosis by lysosomes of deteriorating intracellular organelles, including mitochondria and endoplasmic reticulum. Autophagy is particularly pronounced in cells undergoing atrophy.

Lysosomes with undigested debris (autophagic vacuoles) may persist within cells as *residual bodies* or may be extruded from the cell. *Lipofuscin* pigment granules represent undigested material that results from intracellular lipid peroxidation. Hereditary *lysosomal storage disorders,* caused by deficiencies of enzymes that degrade various macromolecules, result in the accumulation of abnormal amounts of these compounds in lysosomes throughout the body (see Chapter 6).

Induction: Hypertrophy of Smooth Endoplasmic Reticulum (p. 26)

Prolonged forms of stress (stimulation of cells) may induce hypertrophy of the endoplasmic reticulum. For example, chronic ingestion of certain drugs (e.g., phenobarbital) stimulates hypertrophy of the smooth endoplasmic reticulum, the site of detoxification of these drugs by the mixed-function oxidase electron transport pathway (P-450). This hypertrophy results in increased tolerance to the drug and increased capacity to detoxify other drugs handled by the same system.

Mitochondrial Alterations (p. 26)

We have seen that mitochondrial dysfunction plays an important role in acute cellular injury and apoptosis. In addition, various alterations in the number, size, and shape of mitochondria occur in some pathologic conditions, as follows:

- In *cell hypertrophy and atrophy,* there is an increase or a decrease in the number of mitochondria in cells (see Chapter 2).
- Mitochondria may assume extremely *large and abnormal shapes* (megamitochondria), as can be seen in the liver in alcoholic liver disease and in certain nutritional deficiencies.
- In the *mitochondrial myopathies,* or inherited metabolic diseases of skeletal muscle, defects in mitochondrial metabolism are associated with increased numbers of mitochondria that often are unusually large, have abnormal cristae, and contain crystalloids.
- *Oncocytomas,* benign tumors found in salivary glands, thyroid, parathyroids, and kidneys, consist of cells with abundant enlarged mitochondria, giving the cell a distinctly eosinophilic appearance.

Cytoskeletal Abnormalities (p. 27)

The cytoskeleton consists of microtubules, thin filaments that are composed of actin and myosin, and various classes of intermediate filaments. Cytoskeletal abnormalities may be responsible for defects in cell function, such as cell locomotion and intracellular organelle movements (e.g., defects in the organization of microtubules cause immotile cilia or Kartagener's syndrome), or may be caused by cellular injury (e.g., intracellular accumulations of fibrillar material producing eosinophilic intracytoplasmic inclusions in alcoholic liver disease—Mallory bodies—derived from intermediate filaments).

Adaptations in Cellular Growth and Differentiation, Intracellular Accumulations, and Cellular Aging

In Chapter 1, we outlined the morphologic expression and mechanisms of irreversible cell injury and cell death. As was noted, however, cells can respond to excessive physiologic stresses or pathologic stimuli by undergoing physiologic and morphologic *cellular adaptations*, in which a new steady-state is achieved preserving the viability of the cell. Adaptive responses also include the *intracellular accumulation* and storage of products in abnormal amounts.

CELLULAR ADAPTATIONS OF GROWTH AND DIFFERENTIATION (pp. 32–38)

Hyperplasia (p. 32)

Hyperplasia constitutes an increase in the number of cells in an organ or tissue. It is usually accompanied by hypertrophy (see later). Hyperplasia can occur only with cells capable of synthesizing DNA (such as epithelial, hematopoietic, and connective tissue cells). Nerve, cardiac, and skeletal muscle cells have little or no capacity for hyperplastic growth, and so muscle cells undergo almost pure hypertrophy when stimulated by increased functional load or hormones. Hyperplasia can be physiologic or pathologic.

PHYSIOLOGIC HYPERPLASIA

Examples of physiologic hyperplasia include

- *Hormonal* hyperplasia (e.g., endometrial proliferation after estrogen stimulation).

- *Compensatory* hyperplasia (e.g., hyperplasia of the liver after partial hepatectomy).

Mechanisms of Physiologic Hyperplasia: Lessons from Hepatic Regeneration

After partial hepatectomy, all the remaining cellular populations of the liver proliferate to rebuild the lost hepatic tissue. The increase in cell proliferation is due to the combined actions of *growth factors*, such as hepatocyte growth factor, transforming growth factor-α (TGF-α), and epidermal growth factor as well as *cytokines*, such as tumor necrosis factor-α and interleukin-6. None of the growth factors or cytokines is sufficient to induce proliferation in the remnant hepatic cells, which apparently must be *primed* for the action of the mitogens. Certain hormones, such as norepinephrine and insulin, potentiate the growth factor and cytokine effects. Eventual cessation of cell growth is caused by growth inhibitors (e.g., transforming growth factor-β), produced in the liver itself.

PATHOLOGIC HYPERPLASIA

Examples of pathologic hyperplasia are *excessive hormonal stimulation* (e.g., hyperestrinism and atypical endometrial hyperplasia) and *locally produced growth factors on target cells* (e.g., proliferation of connective tissue cells in wound healing or squamous epithelium induced by viruses). In pathologic hyperplasia, if the stimulus abates, the hyperplasia disappears. Thus, cells respond to regular growth control, differentiating the process from neoplasia. Pathologic hyperplasia, however, constitutes a fertile soil in which cancerous proliferation may eventually arise. Examples are endometrial and cervical hyperplasia (Chapter 24), which are precursors of cancers of the endometrium and cervix.

Hypertrophy (p. 33)

Hypertrophy is an increase in the number of organelles (e.g., myofilaments) and size of cells and, with such changes, an increase in the size of the organ. Hypertrophy can be *physiologic* or *pathologic* and is caused by

1. *Increased functional demand* (e.g., hypertrophy of striated muscles in muscle builders [physiologic] or of cardiac muscle cells in cardiac diseases that induce volume overload [pathologic])
2. Specific *hormonal stimulation* (e.g., uterine hypertrophy or breast enlargement during pregnancy)

Hypertrophy is triggered by cell membrane interactions, which in the myocardium include *mechanical forces* (stretch) and *trophic factors* (growth factors and vasoactive agents) (Fig. 2–1). These interactions lead to intracellular signal transduction events that include not only an increase in the size of the cell, but also phenotypic alterations of the hypertrophied cell. In the heart, for example, genes are induced that are normally expressed only during early cardiac development, including atrial natriuretic factor and β-myosin heavy chain. These changes and others are associated with a salutary slowing of the velocity of contraction of hypertrophied muscle fibers. Hypertrophy eventually reaches a limit, at which time degenerative changes occur in cells. In the heart, cardiac failure ensues.

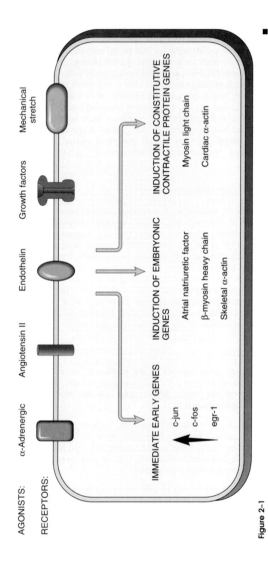

AGONISTS: α-Adrenergic Angiotensin II Endothelin Growth factors Mechanical stretch

RECEPTORS:

IMMEDIATE EARLY GENES

c-jun
c-fos
egr-1

INDUCTION OF EMBRYONIC GENES

Atrial natriuretic factor
β-myosin heavy chain
Skeletal α-actin

INDUCTION OF CONSTITUTIVE CONTRACTILE PROTEIN GENES

Myosin light chain
Cardiac α-actin

Figure 2–1

Schematic diagram of the phenotypic changes in hypertrophy, shown here in a myocardial fiber subjected to hemodynamic overload.

Atrophy (p. 35)

Atrophy is shrinkage in the size of the cell and in the size of the organ as a result of loss of cell substance. Atrophic cells have diminished function but are not dead. Causes of atrophy are

- Decreased workload (atrophy of disuse)
- Loss of innervation (denervation atrophy)
- Diminished blood supply
- Inadequate nutrition
- Loss of endocrine stimulation
- Aging (senile atrophy)
- Pressure

The reduction in the structural components in atrophy occurs through several mechanisms:

- *Decreased synthesis*: The balance between synthesis and degradation has been altered.
- *Endocytic mechanisms*: Atrophic cells exhibit autophagy with a reduction in the number of cell organelles and often a marked increase in the number of *autophagic vacuoles.* Components resisting digestion are converted to *lipofuscin* granules, which, in sufficient numbers, make the organ brown (*brown atrophy*).
- *Proteasomal pathway*: The ubiquitin-proteasome pathway is thought to be responsible for the accelerated proteolysis seen in a variety of catabolic conditions as well as in the degradation of abnormal or aggregated proteins.

Metaplasia (p. 36)

Metaplasia is a reversible change in which one adult cell type is replaced by another (epithelial or mesenchymal). The most common example is a change from *columnar* to *squamous* epithelium, as occurs in the squamous metaplasia of respiratory epithelium in response to chronic irritation (as with protracted cigarette smoking). Although metaplastic epithelium is benign, the influences that predispose to such metaplasia, if persistent, may induce atypical metaplasia, which may progress to cancer. Metaplasia can also occur in mesenchymal cells by which fibroblasts may become transformed to osteoblasts or chondroblasts to produce bone or cartilage.

Metaplasia is thought to occur from genetic reprogramming of stem cells that are known to exist in most epithelia and in undifferentiated mesenchymal cells. This genetic reprogramming is brought about by changes in signals generated by mixtures of cytokines, growth factors, and extracellular matrix components in the cells' environment. The external signals induce specific transcription factors that lead the cascade of phenotype-specific genes toward a fully differentiated cell. When the underlying stimulus abates, the metaplastic changes reverse.

INTRACELLULAR ACCUMULATIONS (p. 38)

Metabolic alterations in cells may result in the accumulation of abnormal amounts of various substances, as follows:

- A *normal* cellular constituent accumulating in excess, such as water, protein, or carbohydrate
- An *abnormal* substance, either exogenous, such as a product of

an infectious agent, or endogenous, such as a product of abnormal metabolism
- A *pigment*, which can also be either exogenous, such as coal dust, or endogenous, such as melanin or hemosiderin

Processes that result in abnormal intracellular accumulations are of three general types:

- A *normal* endogenous substance is produced at a normal or increased rate, but the rate of metabolism is inadequate to remove it (e.g., the accumulation of fat in liver cells).
- A *normal or abnormal* endogenous substance accumulates because of genetic or acquired defects in the *metabolism, packaging, transport, or secretion* of these substances. Examples include accumulations found in the following types of disorders:
  1. *Genetic defects* generating proteins that fold improperly and accumulate, such as in
     - α_1-antitrypsin disease (α_1-antitrypsin accumulates in the endoplasmic recticulum of liver cells that produce it)
     - Sickle cell disease (hemoglobin S aggregates into polymers resulting in distortion of the red cell)
  2. *Lysosomal storage diseases* (accumulation of various types of complex lipids and carbohydrates [Chapter 6])
  3. *Cytoskeletal abnormalities* (accumulation of keratin intermediate filaments as Mallory bodies [*alcoholic hyalin*] in alcoholic liver disease)
- *Deposition of abnormal exogenous substances* (e.g., macrophages laden with carbon dust from the air).

Lipids (p. 39)

Triglycerides, cholesterol and cholesterol esters, and phospholipids can accumulate in cells. The most common form of accumulation involves triglycerides.

STEATOSIS (FATTY CHANGE)

Steatosis (fatty change) represents a normal constituent (triglycerides) accumulating in excess and leading to an absolute increase in intracellular lipids. It results in the formation of intracellular fat vacuoles. It occurs occasionally in almost all organs but is most common in the liver. Fatty change in the liver is reversible, but when excessive it may lead to cirrhosis.

Pathogenesis of Fatty Liver

Causes of fatty liver include alcohol abuse, protein malnutrition, diabetes mellitus, obesity, hepatotoxins, and drugs. Fatty livers are enlarged, yellow, and greasy, and the fat is seen microscopically as small, fatty, cytoplasmic droplets or as large vacuoles. The condition is caused by one of the following mechanisms, as illustrated in Figure 2–2:

- Excessive entry of free fatty acids into the liver (e.g., starvation, corticosteroid therapy)
- Enhanced fatty acid synthesis
- Decreased fatty acid oxidation
- Increased esterification of fatty acids to triglycerides as a result of an increase in α-glycerophosphate (alcohol)
- Decreased apoprotein synthesis (carbon tetrachloride poisoning)

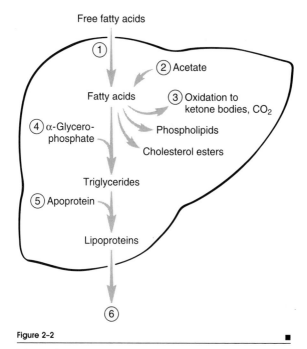

Free fatty acids

Figure 2–2   ■

Schematic diagram of the possible mechanisms leading to accumulation of triglycerides in fatty liver. Depicted are the uptake and metabolism of fatty acids by the liver, formation of triglycerides, and secretion of lipoproteins. Defects in any of the six steps can lead to accumulation of triglycerides and fatty liver. (From Kumar V, Cotran RS, Robbins SL: Basic Pathology, 6th ed. Philadelphia, WB Saunders, 1997.)

■ Impaired lipoprotein secretion from the liver (alcohol, orotic acid administration)

Acute fatty liver of pregnancy and *Reye's syndrome* are rare but sometimes fatal conditions in which a defect in mitochondrial oxidation is suspected.

CHOLESTEROL AND CHOLESTEROL ESTERS

Cholesterol is used for the synthesis of cell membranes. Accumulations, manifested by intracellular vacuoles, are seen in several pathologic processes, as follows:

■ In *atherosclerosis*, these lipids accumulate in smooth muscle cells and macrophages in the walls of arteries, owing to mechanisms discussed on p. 508. Intracellular cholesterol accumulates in the form of small cytoplasmic vacuoles. Extracellular cholesterol gives characteristic rhomboid cleftlike cavities formed by the dissolved cholesterol crystals.
■ In acquired and hereditary *hyperlipidemia*, lipid accumulates in macrophages and mesenchymal cells, forming *xanthomas*.
■ In *inflammation and necrosis*, lipid-laden macrophages result from phagocytosis of membrane lipids derived from injured cells (*foamy macrophages*).

Proteins (p. 40)

Excesses of proteins within cells may cause morphologically visible accumulations, which appear as rounded eosinophilic droplets or masses in the cytoplasm. They occur because of excessive synthesis, absorption, or defects in cellular transport.

Classic examples of protein deposits include the following: With protracted proteinuria, reabsorption of protein forms droplets in proximal convoluted tubules. Another form of protein accumulation is seen in plasma cells. When filled with immunoglobulin within distended cisternae of the endoplasmic reticulum, the protein creates *Russell bodies.*

Defects in *protein folding* may underlie some protein depositions in a variety of unrelated diseases. After protein synthesis, partially folded intermediates arise, which are vulnerable to form intracellular aggregates among themselves or by entangling other proteins. Under normal conditions, these intermediates are stabilized by direct interactions with a number of molecular *chaperones.* Altered protein folding can cause intracellular accumulations by different mechanisms, as follows:

- *Defective intracellular transport and secretion of critical proteins.* Examples include α_1-antitrypsin deficiency, in which mutations slow protein folding, resulting in accumulation of partially folded intermediates in the endoplasmic reticulum of hepatocytes. In *cystic fibrosis,* the most common mutation delays dissociation of the protein from one of its chaperones, resulting in abnormal folding and loss of function.
- *Toxicity of aggregated, abnormally folded proteins.* Aggregation of abnormally folded proteins, caused by genetic mutations, aging, or unknown environmental factors, is a recognized feature of *neurodegenerative disorders,* including the Alzheimer, Huntington, and Parkinson diseases as well as certain forms of amyloidosis.

Glycogen and Other Intracellular Accumulations (p. 41)

Glycogen is a readily available energy store that is present in the cytoplasm. Excessive intracellular deposits are seen in abnormalities of glycogen and glucose metabolism, as follows:

- Glycogen, as in the genetic storage diseases (p. 160).
- *Complex lipids and polysaccharides* (e.g., Gaucher disease, Niemann-Pick disease) (pp. 156–159).
- *Exogenous pigments*:
  - *Anthracosis* (accumulation of carbon in the macrophages of the lungs and lymph nodes from air pollution).
  - *Tattooing* (injected pigment is taken up by macrophages and persists forever in the cells and extracellularly).
- *Endogenous pigments*:
  - *Lipofuscin* (the *wear-and-tear* pigment, seen microscopically as yellow-brown, fine, intracytoplasmic granules, usually associated with atrophy [*brown atrophy*]). The pigment is composed of complex lipids, phospholipids, and protein, suggesting that it is derived from peroxidation of polyunsaturated lipids of cellular membranes.
  - *Melanin* (an endogenous, non–hemoglobin-derived, brown-black pigment formed when the enzyme tyrosinase catalyzes

the oxidation of tyrosine to dihydroxyphenylalanine in melanocytes).
- *Hemosiderin* (a hemoglobin-derived, golden yellow-to-brown, granular pigment composed of aggregates of ferritin micelles). Intracellular accumulation occurs as a localized process or a systemic derangement.

Local hemosiderosis results from gross hemorrhage or rupture of small vessels because of vascular congestion. Macrophages take up hemoglobin, and lysosomal enzymes convert it to hemosiderin, a ferritin-containing pigment.

Systemic hemosiderosis occurs with

- Increased absorption of dietary iron (primary hemochromatosis)
- Impaired utilization of iron (e.g., thalassemia)
- Hemolytic anemias, causing excessive breakdown of red cells
- Transfusions, increasing the exogenous load of iron

PATHOLOGIC CALCIFICATION (p. 43)

Pathologic calcification implies the abnormal deposition of calcium salts in soft tissues. *Dystrophic calcification* occurs in nonviable or dying tissues in the presence of normal calcium serum levels. In *metastatic calcification,* deposition of calcium salts is in vital tissues and is always associated with hypercalcemia. Calcification involves two general phases:

- *Initiation* occurs extracellularly or intracellularly. *Extracellular* initiation occurs in membrane-bound vesicles derived from dead or dying cells (200 nm) that concentrate calcium by their affinity for acidic phospholipids; phosphates accumulate as a result of the action of membrane-bound phosphatases; the cycle of calcium and phosphate binding is repeated, eventually producing a deposit. Initiation of *intracellular* calcification occurs in mitochondria of dead or dying cells.
- *Propagation* of crystal formation depends on the concentration of calcium and phosphates, the presence of inhibitors, structural components of the extracellular matrix (e.g., collagen) as well as other matrix proteins such as osteonectin (SPARC) and γ-carboxyglutamic acid (GLA)–containing proteins, such as matrix GLA protein (Mpg).

Dystrophic Calcification (p. 43)

Dystrophic calcification occurs in arteries in atherosclerosis, in damaged heart valves, and in areas of necrosis (coagulative, caseous, and liquefactive). Calcium can be intracellular, extracellular, or in both locations.

Metastatic Calcification (p. 45)

Metastatic calcification results from hypercalcemia, which has four principal causes:

1. *Increased secretion of parathyroid hormone*, as occurs in hyperparathyroidism resulting from parathyroid tumors and in ectopic secretion of parathyroid hormone by malignant tumors (e.g., certain forms of lung carcinoma)
2. *Destruction of bone tissue*, as occurs with primary tumors of

bone marrow components (e.g., multiple myeloma) or by diffuse skeletal metastasis (e.g., breast cancer)

   3. *Vitamin D–related causes*, including vitamin D intoxication and systemic sarcoidosis

   4. *Associated with renal failure*, which causes secondary hyperparathyroidism

Calcium deposits are seen as amorphous basophilic densities that may occur widely throughout the body, affecting the interstitial tissues of blood vessels, kidneys, lungs, and stomach.

HYALINE CHANGE (p. 45)

   Hyaline change refers to any alteration within cells or in the extracellular spaces or structures that gives a homogeneous, glassy pink appearance in routine histologic sections stained with hematoxylin and eosin. Examples of *intracellular hyaline change* include the following:

- With proteinuria, absorption of protein causing hyaline droplets in proximal epithelial cells of the kidney
- Russell bodies in plasma cells
- Viral inclusions in the cytoplasm or the nucleus
- Masses of altered intermediate filaments (such as alcoholic hyalin, p. 27)

   Extracellular hyaline change occurs in hyaline arteriolosclerosis, in atherosclerosis, and in damaged glomeruli. *Amyloid* (p. 251) also has a hyaline appearance but is a fibrillar protein with specific biochemical characteristics. Amyloid can be differentiated from hyaline connective tissue by its characteristic staining with *Congo red*, with which it appears red and shows apple-green bipolar refringence.

CELLULAR AGING (p. 45)

   With age, physiologic and structural alterations occur in almost all organ systems. Aging in individuals is affected by genetic factors; diet; social conditions; and the occurrence of age-related diseases, such as arteriosclerosis, diabetes, and arthritis. In addition, age-induced alterations in cells, which could represent the progressive accumulation over the years of sublethal injury, are thought to be important components of aging.

   A number of functional and morphologic alterations occur in aging cells, including

- *Diminished metabolic functions*:
  - Reduced oxidative phosphorylation by mitochondria
  - Diminished synthesis of structural, enzymatic, and regulatory proteins
  - Decreased capacity for uptake of nutrients
  - Increased DNA damage and diminished repair of chromosomal damage
  - Accumulation of oxidative damage in proteins and lipids (e.g., lipofuscin pigment)
  - Accumulation of advanced glycosylation end products, which cause cross-linking of adjacent proteins and are important in the pathogenesis of diabetes (Chapter 17)
- *Morphologic alterations*:
  - Irregular and abnormally lobed nuclei

- Pleomorphic and vacuolated mitochondria
- Decreased endoplasmic reticulum
- Distorted Golgi apparatus

Although several mechanisms have been proposed to account for cellular aging, more recent concepts center on two interrelated processes: (1) existence of a genetically determined clock that times aging and (2) the effects of continuous exposure to exogenous influences, which result in the progressive accumulation of cellular and molecular damage.

Timing of the Aging Process—the Concept of a Clock (p. 46)

Cellular senescence can be inferred from in vitro studies showing that normal human diploid fibroblasts in culture have finite life spans and population doublings that are age dependent (i.e., they have *clocks* [the Hayflick theory]). Many changes in gene expression accompany cellular senescence. Possible causes of the process are the activation of genes that inhibit progression of the

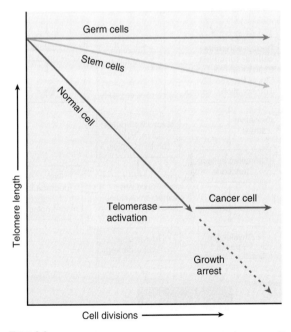

Figure 2–3   ∎

The telomere-telomerase hypothesis and proliferative capacity. Telomere length is plotted against the number of cell divisions. In normal somatic cells, there is no telomerase activity, and telomeres progressively shorten with increasing cell divisions until growth arrest, or senescence, occurs. Germ cells and stem cells both contain telomerase activity, but only the germ cells have levels of the enzyme that are sufficient to stabilize telomere length completely. Telomerase activation in cancer cells inactivates the telomeric clock that limits the proliferative capacity of normal somatic cells. (Modified and redrawn from Holt SE, et al: Refining the telomere-telomerase hypothesis of aging and cancer. Nat Biotech 14:836–839, 1996.)

cell cycle (e.g., cyclin-dependent kinase inhibitors, such as p21) as well as other mechanisms. Two phenomena may be involved in timing the aging process:

■ *Telomere shortening or incomplete replication of chromosome ends.* Telomeres are short repeated sequences of DNA that compose the linear ends of chromosomes and are important in (1) ensuring the complete replication of chromosome ends and (2) protecting chromosomal termini from fusion and degrada-

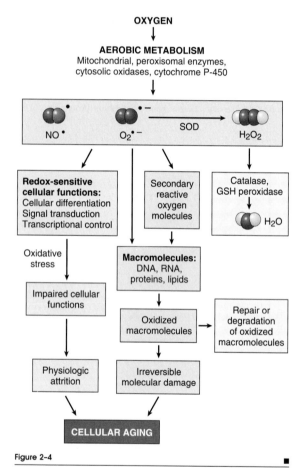

Figure 2–4   ■

Oxidative stress and aging. Aerobic metabolism generates reactive oxygen metabolites (free radicals), such as hydrogen peroxide, superoxide anion, and nitric oxide. These reactive species can be inactivated by antioxidant defense mechanisms or give rise to a variety of secondary reactive oxygen metabolites (e.g., peroxynitrite). Interactions between the reactive species and macromolecules may cause both reversible and irreversible oxidative modifications. The accumulation of irreversible oxidative damage may be a causal factor in aging and certain diseases. A bullet indicates control by an antioxidant defense mechanism (e.g., glutathione, vitamin E, vitamin C, and urate). SOD, superoxide dismutase. (Modified and redrawn from Weindruch R, Sohal RS: Caloric intake and aging. N Engl J Med 337:986, 1997.)

tion. When cells replicate, a small section of the telomere is not replicated. As these cells divide further, telomeres become progressively shortened, which signals a growth checkpoint causing the cells to become senescent. In some cancer cells, telomerase seems to be activated, suggesting that telomere elongation might be important in conferring immortality on cells, thus giving rise to tumor formation (Fig. 2–3).

- *Clock genes.* The identification of genes in animal models that control the rate and timing of aging supports the concept of a clock.

Metabolic Events, Genetic Damage, and Aging (p. 47)

Cellular aging may also be determined by the balance between *cellular damage* resulting from metabolic events occurring within the cell and a counterbalancing *genetic response* that can repair the damage. Reactive oxygen metabolites are byproducts of oxidative phosphorylation and can cause covalent modifications of proteins, lipids, and nucleic acids, found throughout the cell but particularly in mitochondria. The amount of oxidative damage increases with age and may be an important component of senescence. Increased production of these reactive species (e.g., because of a high caloric diet or exposure to ionizing radiation) correlates with a shortened life span. A model outlining the role of oxidative stress in aging is illustrated in Figure 2–4.

Protective cellular responses counterbalance the progressive damage. These systems include the following:

- *Antioxidant defense mechanisms.* A reduction in antioxidant defense mechanisms (e.g., vitamin E) correlates with a shortened life span.
- *Recognition and repair of damaged DNA.* The importance of DNA repair in the aging process is illustrated by patients with *Werner syndrome*, who show premature aging. A defect in the *DNA helicase* causing this syndrome results in rapid accumulation of chromosomal damage that mimics the injury that normally accumulates during cellular aging. Genetic instability is also characteristic of other disorders associated with premature aging, such as Cockayne syndrome and ataxia telangiectasia.

Much more could be said about the mechanisms of cellular aging, but it probably involves both programmed events in cell proliferation and the consequences of progressive oxidative damage overwhelming the cell's defense mechanisms.

Acute and Chronic Inflammation

Inflammation is the reaction of vascularized living tissue to local injury. It is evoked by microbial infections, physical agents, chemicals, necrotic tissue, and immunologic reactions. The roles of inflammation are to contain and isolate injury, to destroy invading microorganisms and inactivate toxins, and to prepare the tissue or organ for healing and repair (Chapter 4). Inflammation and repair may be potentially harmful, however, causing life-threatening hypersensitivity reactions and progressive organ damage with chronic inflammation, and may lead to permanent scarring.

ACUTE INFLAMMATION (p. 52)

Major Events in Inflammation (p. 52)

Acute inflammation has three major components:

- Alterations in vascular caliber that lead to an increase in blood flow
- Structural changes in the microvasculature that permit the plasma proteins and leukocytes to leave the circulation to produce an inflammatory exudate
- Emigration of the leukocytes from the microcirculation and their accumulation in the focus of injury

These changes produce the *classic clinical signs* of inflammation. There are four cardinal signs of inflammation:

- Heat (calor)
- Redness (rubor)
- Edema (tumor)
- Pain (dolor)

Loss of function (functio laesa) has been added as a classic sign.

DEFINITIONS

Exudation The escape of fluid, proteins, and blood cells from the vascular system into the interstitial tissue or body cavities.

Exudate An inflammatory extravascular fluid that has a high protein concentration, much cellular debris, and a specific gravity above 1.020.

Transudate   A fluid with low protein content and a specific gravity of less than 1.012. It is essentially an ultrafiltrate of blood plasma and results from hydrostatic imbalance across the vascular endothelium.

Edema   Denotes an excess of fluid in the interstitial tissue or serous cavities; it can be either an exudate or a transudate.

Pus   A purulent inflammatory exudate rich in leukocytes and parenchymal cell debris.

CHANGES IN VASCULAR FLOW AND CALIBER

Changes in vascular flow and caliber constitute one of the three major components of the inflammatory response. They begin immediately after injury and develop at various rates depending on the severity of the injury.

- Initially, transient vasoconstriction of arterioles occurs.
- Vasodilation follows, causing increased flow; it accounts for the heat and redness.
- Eventual slowing of the circulation occurs as a result of increased vascular permeability (see later), leading to *stasis*. The increased permeability is the cause of edema.
- With slowing, the larger white cells fall out of the axial stream, and leukocytic *margination* appears, a prelude to the cellular events (see later).

INCREASED VASCULAR PERMEABILITY

Increased vascular permeability leads to the escape of protein-rich fluid into the interstitium.

- Normal fluid exchange depends on Starling's law and an intact endothelium. Starling's law maintains that normal fluid balance is modulated mainly by two opposing forces: (1) hydrostatic pressure causing fluid to move out of the circulation and (2) plasma colloid osmotic pressure causing fluid to move into the capillaries (Fig. 3–1A).
- In inflammation, there is increased hydrostatic pressure, caused by vasodilation, and decreased osmotic pressure, caused by leakage of high-protein fluid across a hyperpermeable endothelium—resulting in marked net outflow of fluid and edema formation (Fig. 3–1B).

There are six possible mechanisms of increased endothelial permeability:

1. *Endothelial cell contraction in venules*, leading to the formation of widened intercellular junctions, or intercellular gaps. This is the most common form elicited by chemical mediators (e.g., histamine); occurs immediately after injection of the mediator; is short-lived (*immediate-transient response*); and classically involves only venules 20 to 60 mM in diameter, leaving capillaries and arterioles unaffected.

2. *Endothelial retraction* owing to cytoskeletal and junctional reorganization, also resulting in widened interendothelial junctions. This results in a somewhat delayed response that can be long-lived and is induced by cytokine mediators, such as interleukin-1 (IL-1) and tumor necrosis factor (TNF).

A. NORMAL

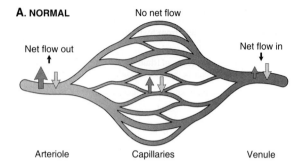

B. ACUTE INFLAMMATION

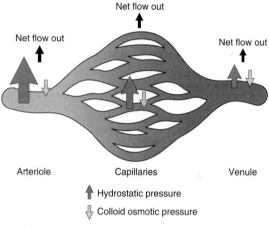

Figure 3–1 ■

Blood pressure and plasma colloid osmotic forces in normal and inflamed microcirculation. *A,* Normal hydrostatic pressure is about 32 mm Hg *(open upward arrows)* at the
arterial end of the capillary and 12 mm Hg at the venous end *(open downward arrows).*
The mean colloid osmotic pressure of tissues is approximately 25 mm Hg. Although
fluid tends to leave the precapillary arteriole, it is returned in equal amounts via the
postcapillary venule. Under these conditions, net flow *(black arrows)* in or out of the
vessel is zero. *B,* Acute inflammation. Mean capillary pressure is increased to 50 mm
Hg. The mean capillary pressure is increased because of arteriolar dilation. The venous
pressure increases to approximately 30 mm Hg. At the same time, osmotic pressure is
reduced (averaging 20 mm Hg) because of protein leakage across the venule. The net
result is an excess of extravasated fluid. (From Kumar V, Cotran RS, Robbins SL: Basic
Pathology, 6th ed. Philadelphia, WB Saunders, 1997.)

3. *Direct endothelial injury,* resulting in endothelial cell necrosis and detachment. This is caused by severe necrotizing injuries
and affects all levels of the microcirculation, including venules,
capillaries, and arterioles. The damage usually evokes an *immediate* and *sustained endothelial leakage.*
4. *Leukocyte-mediated endothelial injury* resulting from leukocyte aggregation, adhesion, and emigration across the endothelium.
These leukocytes release toxic oxygen species and proteolytic

enzymes, which cause endothelial injury or detachment, resulting in increased permeability.

5. *Increased transcytosis* across the endothelial cytoplasm via vesicles and vacuoles of the vesiculovacuolar organelle. Some growth factors (e.g., vascular endothelial growth factor) may cause vascular leakage by increasing the number and size of these channels.

6. *Leakage from regenerating capillaries*, during healing. This occurs when new capillary sprouts are leaky.

CELLULAR EVENTS: LEUKOCYTE EXTRAVASATION AND PHAGOCYTOSIS

A critical function of inflammation is the delivery of leukocytes to the site of injury. The sequence of events in this journey, called *extravasation*, can be divided into the following steps:

- *Margination, rolling, and adhesion of leukocytes* in the lumen
- *Transmigration* across the endothelium (also called *diapedesis*)
- *Migration* in interstitial tissues toward a chemotactic stimulus (Fig. 3–2)

Adhesion and Transmigration

Adhesion and transmigration occur largely as a result of interactions between complementary adhesion molecules on the leukocytes and on the endothelium. Chemoattractants and some cytokines affect these processes by modulating the surface expression or avidity of the adhesion molecules. The major ligand-receptor adhesion pairs are shown in Table 3–1 and include

- *The selectins (E, P, and L)*, which bind through their lectin (sugar binding) domains to oligosaccharides (e.g., sialylated Lewis X), which themselves are covalently bound to cell surface glycoproteins.
- The *immunoglobulin family*, which includes the endothelial *ICAM-1* (intercellular adhesion molecule 1) and *VCAM-1* (vascular cell adhesion molecule 1).
- The *integrins*, which function as receptors for some of the members of the immunoglobulin family and the extracellular matrix. The principal integrin receptors for ICAM-1 are the β_2 integrins LFA-1 and MAC-1 (CD11a/CD18 and CD11b/CD18), and those for VCAM-1 are the integrins $\alpha_4\beta_1$ (VLA4) and $\alpha_4\beta_7$.

These molecules induce leukocyte adhesion in inflammation by three mechanisms:

1. *Redistribution of preformed adhesion molecules to the cell surface.* For example, after exposure to histamine or thrombin, P-selectin is rapidly translocated from the endothelial Weibel-Palade body membranes to the cell surface, where it can bind leukocytes.

2. *Induction of adhesion molecules on endothelium.* For example, IL-1 and TNF induce the synthesis and surface expression of E-selectin and increase expression of ICAM-1 and VCAM-1, rendering such *activated* endothelial cells more adherent to leukocytes.

3. *Increased avidity of binding.* This is most relevant to the binding of *integrins* (LFA-1 and MAC-1), which are normally

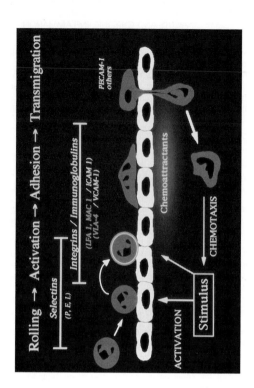

Figure 3-2

Sequence of leukocytic events in inflammation. The leukocytes first roll; then arrest and adhere to endothelium; and then transmigrate through an intercellular junction, pierce the basement membrane, and migrate toward chemoattractants emanating from the source of injury. The roles of selectins, activating agents, and integrins are also shown.

Table 3–1. LEUKOCYTE-ENDOTHELIAL ADHESION MOLECULES

Endothelial Molecule	Leukocyte Receptor	Major Role
P-selectin	Sialyl-Lewis X PSGL-1	Rolling (neutrophils, monocytes, lymphoytes)
E-selectin	Sialyl-Lewis X ESL-1, PSGL-1	Rolling, adhesion to activated endothelium (neutrophils, monocytes, T cells)
ICAM-1	CD11/CD18 (integrins) (LFA-1, Mac-1)	Adhesion, arrest, transmigration (all leukocytes)
VCAM-1	α4β1 (VLA4) (integrins) α4 β7 (LPAM-1)	Adhesion (eosinophils, monocytes, lymphocytes)
GlyCam-1 CD34	L-selectin	Lymphocyte homing to high endothelial venules Neutrophil, monocyte rolling

ICAM-1 and VCAM-1 belong to the immunoglobulin family of proteins: ESL-1, E-selectin ligand 1; PSGL-1, P-selectin glycoprotein ligand 1.

present on leukocytes but can be converted from a state of low-affinity binding to high-affinity binding toward their ligand ICAM-1 by chemical mediators. Such activation causes firm adhesion of the leukocytes to the endothelium and is also necessary for subsequent transmigration across endothelial cells.

It is now thought that neutrophil adhesion and transmigration in acute inflammation occur by a series of overlapping steps:

- *Endothelial activation*: Mediators present at the inflammatory sites increase the expression of E-selectin and P-selectin by endothelial cells.
- *Leukocyte rolling*: There is an initial rapid and relatively loose adhesion, resulting from interactions between the selectins and their carbohydrate ligands.
- *Firm adhesion*: The leukocytes are then activated by chemokines or other agents to increase the avidity of their integrins.
- *Transmigration*: This is mediated by interactions between platelet-endothelial cell adhesion molecule-1 (PECAM-1 or CD31) on leukocytes and endothelial cells.

The importance of adhesion molecules is emphasized by the clinical genetic deficiencies in adhesion molecules: In *leukocyte adhesion deficiency type I*, there is a defect in the synthesis of β_2 integrins. In *leukocyte adhesion deficiency type II*, a defect in fucose metabolism results in the absence of sialyl Lewis X, the ligand for E-selectin and P-selectin. Both deficiencies result in impaired leukocyte adhesion and recurrent bacterial infections.

Chemotaxis and Leukocyte Activation

Adherent leukocytes emigrate through interendothelial junctions, traverse the basement membrane, and move toward the site of injury along a gradient of chemotactic agents. Neutrophils emigrate first, and monocytes and lymphocytes follow. Chemotactic agents for neutrophils include bacterial products, complement fragments (e.g., C5a), arachidonic acid metabolites (e.g., leukotriene B_4), and chemokines (e.g., IL-8).

Chemotaxis involves binding of chemotactic agents to specific receptors on leukocytes and production of second messengers (Chapter 4). This signal transduction process results in activation of phospholipase C and protein kinase C, increased intracellular calcium, and assembly of the contractile elements responsible for cell movement. The leukocyte moves by extending a pseudopod that pulls the remainder of the cell in the direction of the extension. Locomotion is controlled by the effects of *calcium* ions and *phosphoinositols* on *actin regulatory proteins*, such as *gelsolin*, *filamin*, and *calmodulin*.

Chemotactic agents also cause *leukocyte activation*, characterized by:

- Degranulation and secretion of enzymes
- Activation of an oxidative burst
- Production of arachidonic acid metabolites
- Modulation of leukocyte adhesion molecules

Phagocytosis

Phagocytosis and the release of enzymes by neutrophils and macrophages constitute two of the major benefits derived from the accumulation of leukocytes at the inflammatory focus. Phagocytosis involves three steps:

- *Recognition and attachment* of the particle to be ingested by the leukocyte. Many microorganisms are coated with specific factors, called *opsonins*, which enhance the efficiency of phagocytosis because they are recognized by receptors on the leukocytes. The two major opsonins are the Fc fragment of immunoglobulin G and a product of complement, C3b.
- Engulfment by pseudopods encircling the phagocytosed particle, with subsequent formation of a phagocytic vacuole or *phagosome*. The membrane of the phagocytic vacuole then fuses with the membrane of a lysosomal granule, resulting in discharge of the granule's content into the phagolysosome.
- *Killing and degradation of bacteria.* Phagocytosis stimulates a burst of oxygen consumption and production of reactive oxygen metabolites. There are two types of bactericidal mechanisms:

  1. *Oxygen-dependent mechanisms.* Bacterial killing is accomplished largely by oxygen-dependent mechanisms. This is triggered by activation of *nicotinamide-adenine dinucleotide phosphate (reduced form) (NADPH) oxidase*, in the process reducing oxygen (O_2) to superoxide anion (O_2^-) and hence to hydrogen peroxide (H_2O_2) (Fig. 3–3). *Myeloperoxidase* (MPO) from lysosomal granules then converts H_2O_2, in the presence of a halide such as Cl^-, to the highly bactericidal $HOCl\cdot$. Although the H_2O_2-MPO-halide system is the most efficient bactericidal mechanism, the reactive oxygen species produced during an oxidative burst can kill bacteria directly.
  2. *Oxygen-independent mechanisms.* These include bactericidal permeability increasing protein, lysozyme, lactoferrin, major basic protein (MBP) of eosinophils, and arginine-rich *defen-*

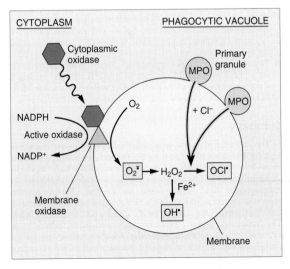

Figure 3–3   ■

Summary of oxygen-dependent bactericidal mechanisms within phagocytic vacuole, as described in text.

sins. Killed organisms are then degraded by hydrolases and other enzymes in lysosomes.

Release of Leukocyte Products and Leukocyte-Induced Tissue Injury

During phagocytosis, leukocytes release products not only within the phagolysosome, but also potentially into the extracellular space. These released products include

- *Lysosomal enzymes,* by regurgitation during feeding, reverse endocytosis, or cytotoxic release
- *Oxygen-derived active metabolites*
- *Products of arachidonic acid metabolism,* including prostaglandins and leukotrienes

These products are powerful mediators of tissue damage and amplify the effects of the initial inflammatory stimulus. If persistent, the leukocyte-dependent tissue injury can cause chronic inflammation.

Defects in Leukocyte Function

Defects in leukocyte function interfere with inflammation and increase susceptibility to infections. They include both genetic and acquired defects, such as a deficiency in the number of circulating cells (neutropenia). Clinical genetic deficiencies have been identified in most phases of leukocyte function, from adherence to vascular endothelium to microbicidal activity, and include the following:

- *Defects in leukocyte adhesion,* such as leukocyte adhesion deficiency type I and type II.
- *Defects in phagocytosis,* such as *Chédiak-Higashi syndrome.* Neutrophils in patients with this syndrome have giant granules because of aberrant organelle fusion and reduced transfer of lysosomal enzymes to phagocytic vacuoles (causing susceptibility to infections).
- *Defects in microbicidal activity.* In *chronic granulomatous disease,* there are inherited defects in NADPH oxidase, leading to a defect in the respiratory burst, H_2O_2 production, and the MPO-H_2O_2-halide bactericidal mechanism.

Summary

The vascular phenomena in acute inflammation are characterized by increased blood flow to the injured area, resulting mainly from arteriolar dilation and opening of capillary beds. Increased vascular permeability results in the accumulation of protein-rich extravascular fluid, which forms the exudate. Plasma proteins leave the vessels most commonly through widened interendothelial cell junctions of the venules or by direct endothelial cell injury. The leukocytes, initially predominantly neutrophils, adhere to the endothelium via adhesion molecules, transmigrate across the endothelium, and migrate to the site of injury under the influence of chemotactic agents. Phagocytosis of the offending agent follows, which may lead to the death of the microorganism. During chemotaxis and phagocytosis, activated leukocytes may release toxic metabolites and proteases extracellularly, potentially causing tissue damage.

CHEMICAL MEDIATORS OF INFLAMMATION (p. 65)

The vascular and white cell events described previously are brought about by a variety of chemical mediators, derived *either from plasma or from cells* (Fig. 3–4). Most perform their biologic activity by binding initially to specific receptors on target cells, although some have direct enzymatic activity (e.g., proteases), and others mediate oxidative damage (e.g., oxygen metabolites). One mediator can *stimulate the release of other mediators by the target cells* themselves, providing a mechanism for amplification or in certain instances counteracting the initial mediator action. Once activated and released, most *mediators are short-lived*, either quickly decaying or becoming inactivated by enzymes or inhibited by inhibitors. Thus, a system of checks and balances exists in the regulation of mediator action because *most mediators also have potentially harmful effects.*

Vasoactive Amines (p. 66)

Histamine and serotonin are available from preformed cellular stores and are among the first mediators to be released during inflammation. They are found in mast cells, basophils, and platelets and cause vasodilation and increased vascular permeability. Release from mast cells is caused by

- Physical agents (e.g., trauma, heat)
- Immunologic reactions involving binding of IgE antibodies to mast cells
- Complement fragments C3a and C5a (anaphylatoxins)
- Neuropeptides (substance P)
- Cytokines (IL-1 and IL-8)
- Histamine-releasing factors derived from leukocytes

Release from platelets is stimulated by contact with collagen, thrombin, adenosine diphosphate (ADP), and antigen-antibody complexes and by platelet-activating factor (PAF).

Plasma Proteases (p. 67)

There are three interrelated plasma-derived mediators that play key roles in inflammatory responses:

- Complement system
- Kinin system
- Clotting factor system

COMPLEMENT SYSTEM

Activation of complement functions in host defense against microbial agents, culminating in the assembly of the *membrane attack complex* (MAC) and lysis of the offending agent. In the process, complement components are generated that cause increased vascular permeability, chemotaxis, and opsonization. Activation of complement (Fig. 3–5) occurs via two general mechanisms:

1. The classic pathway, initiated by antigen-antibody complexes.
2. The alternate complement pathway, activated by endotoxin, complex polysaccharides, and aggregated globulins.

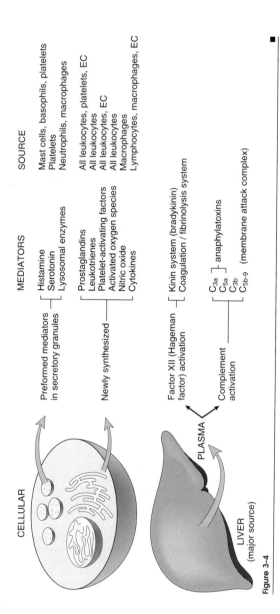

Figure 3-4

Chemical mediators of inflammation. (From Kumar V, Cotran RS, Robbins SL: Basic Pathology, 6th ed. Philadelphia, WB Saunders, 1997.)

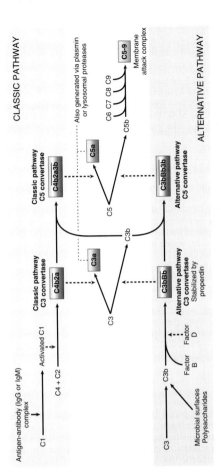

CLASSIC PATHWAY

Antigen-antibody (IgG or IgM) complex

C1 → Activated C1

C4 + C2

Classic pathway C3 convertase
C4b2a

C3a

Classic pathway C5 convertase
C4b2a3b

C5a

Also generated via plasmin or lysosomal proteases

C5b

C6 C7 C8 C9

C5-9
Membrane attack complex

C3

C3b

C5

Alternative pathway C5 convertase
C3bBb3b

Alternative pathway C3 convertase Stabilized by properdin
C3bBb

Factor B   Factor D

C3b

Microbial surfaces
Polysaccharides

C3

ALTERNATIVE PATHWAY

Figure 3-5

Overview of complement activation pathways. The classic pathway is initiated by C1 binding to antigen-antibody complexes, and the alternative pathway is initiated by C3b. Alternative pathway initiation may be generated in several ways, including spontaneously, by the classic pathway, or by the alternative pathway itself (see text). Both pathways converge and lead to the formation of inflammatory complement mediators (C3a and C5a) and the membrane attack complex. In this figure, bars over the letter designations of complement components indicate enzymatically active forms, and dashed lines indicate proteolytic activities of various components. (Modified from Abbas AK, et al: Cellular and Molecular Immunology, 3rd ed. Philadelphia, WB Saunders, 1997.)

43

Complement components with inflammatory activity include

- C3a, which increases vascular permeability
- C5a, which increases vascular permeability and is highly chemotactic to most leukocytes
- C3b and C3bi—the opsonins—important in phagocytosis
- C5b-9, the MAC that lyses cells and stimulates arachidonic acid metabolism and production of reactive oxygen metabolites by leukocytes.

The complement system is closely controlled by protein inhibitors including the following:

- Regulation of C3 and C5 convertases, by *decay-accelerating factor*. *Paroxysmal nocturnal hemoglobinuria* is a disease in which cells lack the ability to express phosphatidylinositol-linked membrane proteins, including decay-accelerating factor. Paroxysmal nocturnal hemoglobinuria is characterized by recurrent bouts of intravascular hemolysis resulting from complement-mediated lysis of red blood cells, leading to chronic hemolytic anemia (Chapter 14).
- Binding of active complement components by specific proteins in the plasma, such as by *C1 inhibitor*. Deficiency of C1 inhibitor is associated with the syndrome of *hereditary angioneurotic edema*, characterized by episodic edema accumulation in the skin and extremities as well as in the laryngeal and intestinal mucosa, provoked by emotional stress or trauma.

KININ SYSTEM

The kinin system generates vasoactive peptides from plasma proteins called *kininogens* by specific proteases called *kallikreins*, ultimately resulting in the production of *bradykinin*. Surface activation of Hageman factor (factor XII) produces clotting factor XIIa, which converts plasma prekallikrein into kallikrein; the latter cleaves high-molecular-weight kininogen to produce bradykinin, a potent stimulator of increased vascular permeability. Kallikrein in an autocatalytic loop is a potent activator of Hageman factor, has chemotactic activity, and causes neutrophil aggregation. Thus, kallikrein can, by feedback, activate Hageman factor, resulting in profound amplification of the effects of the initial contact.

CLOTTING SYSTEM

The clotting system is divided into two interrelated systems, designated the intrinsic and extrinsic pathways, that converge to activate a primary hemostatic mechanism (Chapter 5).

- The *intrinsic pathway* consists of a series of plasma proenzymes that can be activated by Hageman factor, resulting in the activation of *thrombin*, cleavage of *fibrinogen*, and generation of a fibrin clot. During this process, *fibrinopeptides* are formed that induce vascular permeability and are chemotactic for leukocytes. Thrombin also has inflammatory properties, causing increased leukocyte adhesion to endothelium.
- At the same time that factor XIIa is inducing clotting, it can also activate the *fibrinolytic system*, which produces *plasmin* and degrades fibrin, thereby solubilizing the clot. Plasmin can contribute to inflammation in several ways:

1. Cleave C3 to produce C3 fragments

2. Form fibrin *split* products, which may increase vascular permeability
3. Activate Hageman factor, amplifying the response

Arachidonic Acid Metabolites (p. 70)

Cells respond to activating stimuli by remodeling their cellular membranes to generate biologically active lipid mediators that serve as short-range signaling agents. *Eicosanoids* are synthesized from arachidonic acids by two major classes of enzymes: Cyclo-oxygenases generate *prostaglandins* and *thromboxanes*; lipoxygenases produce *leukotrienes* and *lipoxins* (Fig. 3–6). The inflammatory prostaglandins and leukotrienes include the following:

- Prostaglandin I_2 (prostacyclin) and prostaglandin E_2 cause vasodilation.
- Prostaglandin E_2 is hyperalgesic in that it makes the skin hypersensitive to painful stimuli.
- Thromboxane A_2 causes vasoconstriction.
- Leukotrienes C_4, D_4, and E_4 increase vascular permeability and cause vasoconstriction.
- Leukotriene B_4 is a powerful chemotactic agent.
- Lipoxins may be endogenous negative regulators of leukotriene action.

Cell-cell interactions are important in the biosynthesis of both the leukotrienes and the lipoxins. Arachidonic acid products can pass from one cell to another to generate these classes of eicosanoids. This *transcellular biosynthesis* allows cells that are not capable of generating specific eicosanoids to produce these mediators from intermediates generated in other cells.

Platelet-Activating Factor (p. 72)

PAF is a bioactive phospholipid-derived mediator. It is produced by mast cells and other leukocytes after a number of stimuli, including IgE-mediated reactions. PAF causes platelet aggregation and release, bronchoconstriction, vasodilation, increased vascular permeability, increased leukocyte adhesion, and leukocyte chemotaxis. Thus, PAF can elicit most of the cardinal features of inflammation.

Cytokines (p. 73)

Cytokines are proteins produced principally by activated lymphocytes and macrophages that modulate the function of other cell types. Many classic *growth factors* (Chapter 4) act as cytokines, and conversely many cytokines have growth-promoting properties.

DEFINITIONS

Monokines   Cytokines generated by mononuclear phagocytes.
Lymphokines   Cytokines generated by activated lymphocytes.
Colony-stimulating factors   Cytokines produced by monocytes and macrophages that stimulate the growth of immature leukocytes in the bone marrow.
Interleukins   Broad family of cytokines that are made by hematopoietic cells and act primarily on leukocytes.

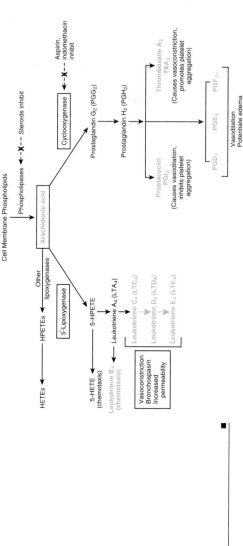

Figure 3-6

Arachidonic acid metabolites in inflammation.

Chemokines   Cytokines that share the ability to stimulate leukocyte movement (chemokinesis) and directed movement (chemotaxis) and are particularly important in inflammation.

GENERAL PROPERTIES AND CLASSES OF CYTOKINES

General properties and classes of cytokines are as follows:

- Cytokines are produced during immune and inflammatory responses, and secretion of these mediators is transient and closely regulated.
- Many cell types produce multiple cytokines.
- The proteins are pleiotropic in that they can act on different cell types.
- Cytokine effects are often redundant, and these proteins can influence the synthesis or action of other cytokines.
- Cytokines are multifunctional in that an individual cytokine may have both positive and negative regulatory actions.
- Cytokines mediate their effects by binding to specific receptors on target cells, and the expression of cytokine receptors can be regulated by a variety of exogenous and endogenous signals.

FUNCTIONS OF CYTOKINES

Cytokines can be grouped into five classes, depending on their major function or on the nature of the target cell:

- *Cytokines that regulate lymphocyte function.* These cytokines regulate lymphocyte activation, growth, and differentiation (e.g., IL-2 and IL-4, which favor lymphocyte growth; IL-10 and transforming growth factor-β, which are negative regulators of immune responses).
- *Cytokines involved with natural immunity.* This group includes the inflammatory cytokines (e.g., TNF-α and IL-1β), the type I interferons (IFN-α and IFN-β), and IL-6.
- *Cytokines that activate inflammatory cells.* These cytokines activate macrophages during cell-mediated immune responses (e.g., IFN-γ, TNF-α, IL-5, IL-10, and IL-12).
- *Chemokines.* This group of cytokines is characterized by chemotactic activity for various leukocytes (e.g., IL-8; see later).
- *Cytokines that stimulate hematopoiesis.* These cytokines mediate immature leukocyte growth and differentiation (e.g., IL-3, IL-7, c-kit ligand, granulocyte-macrophage colony stimulating factor [GM-CSF], macrophage-CSF [M-CSF], granulocyte-CSF [G-CSF], and stem cell factor).

IL-1 and TNF-α are the major cytokines that mediate inflammation and are produced by activated macrophages. Their most important actions in inflammation are their effects on endothelium, leukocytes, and induction of the systemic acute-phase reactions (Fig. 3–7).

- Secretion is stimulated by endotoxin, immune complexes, toxins, physical injury, and a variety of inflammatory products.
- TNF and IL-1 induce *endothelial activation*, which includes induction of endothelial adhesion molecules and chemical mediators (e.g., other cytokines [IL-6], chemokines [IL-8], growth factors, eicosanoids [prostaglandin I_2 and PAF], and nitric oxide), production of enzymes associated with matrix remodeling, and increases in the surface thrombogenicity of the endothelium.

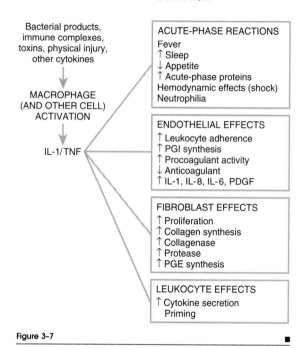

Figure 3–7   ■

Major effects of interleukin-1 (IL-1) and tumor necrosis factor (TNF) in inflammation.

- IL-1 and TNF also induce the systemic *acute-phase responses* associated with infection or injury, including fever; loss of appetite; production of sleep; release of neutrophils into the circulation; release of adrenocorticotropic hormone and corticosteroids; and, particularly with regard to TNF, hemodynamic effects of septic shock—hypotension, decreased vascular resistance, increased heart rate, and decreased blood pH (Chapter 5).
- TNF-α has a key role in the normal *control of body mass*. In *obesity*, the physiologic actions of TNF-α as a signal to control food intake are impaired (Chapter 10). In *cachexia*, a pathologic state characterized by weight loss and anorexia that accompanies some infections and neoplastic diseases, there is an overproduction of TNF-α.

Chemokines (p. 74)

Chemokines are a superfamily of small (8 to 10 kD) proteins that act primarily as activators and chemoattractants for specific types of leukocytes. They are expressed by a wide range of cell types. Chemokines are classified into four major classes, which have relatively distinct biologic activities, according to the arrangement of the conserved cysteine (C) residues:

- *C-X-C or α chemokines* have one amino acid residue separating the first two conserved cysteine residues. The C-X-C chemokines act primarily on neutrophils, and *IL-8* is typical of this group.
- *C-C or β chemokines* have the first two conserved cysteine

residues adjacent. The C-C chemokines, such as *monocyte chemoattractant protein* (MCP-1), generally attract monocytes, eosinophils, basophils, and lymphocytes but not neutrophils. Although most of the chemokines in this class have overlapping properties, *eotaxin* selectively recruits eosinophils.

- *C or γ chemokines* lack two (the first and third) of the four conserved cysteines. The C chemokines are relatively specific for lymphocytes (e.g., lymphotactin).
- *CX₃C chemokines* include *fractalkine*. They exist in two forms:
  1. A cell surface–bound protein can be induced in endothelial cells that promotes adhesion of leukocytes.
  2. A soluble form, derived by proteolysis of membrane-bound protein, has chemoattractant activity.

Chemokines mediate their activities by binding to G-protein-linked receptors, designated CXCR (1–4) for the C-X-C chemokines, and CCR (1–5) for the C-C chemokines.

Nitric Oxide (p. 75)

Also known as *endothelium-derived relaxation factor*, nitric oxide acts in a paracrine manner and causes vasodilation; inhibits platelet aggregation and adhesion; and may act as a free radical, becoming cytotoxic to certain microbes, tumor cells, and also possibly other tissue cells. Nitric oxide is synthesized from arginine, molecular oxygen, NADPH, and other cofactors by the enzyme *nitric oxide synthase* (NOS). There are three types of NOS (endothelial [eNOS], neuronal [nNOS], and cytokine inducible [iNOS]), which exhibit two patterns of expression: (1) eNOS and nNOS are present constitutively and are rapidly activated by an increase in cytoplasmic calcium. (2) iNOS is present in macrophages and is induced by cytokines, such as IFN-γ, without an increase in intracellular calcium. Nitric oxide has many properties; notable are the following:

- Nitric oxide plays an important role in vascular function during an inflammatory response. eNOS is important in maintaining *vascular tone*. Increased production of nitric oxide from iNOS is an endogenous compensatory mechanism that reduces leukocyte recruitment in inflammatory responses. iNOS production of nitric oxide by activated macrophages is also important in the pathogenesis of *septic shock.*
- Nitric oxide acts in the host response to infection. *Interactions occur between nitric oxide and reactive oxygen species,* leading to the formation of multiple antimicrobial metabolites (e.g., peroxynitrite [OONO⁻], S-nitrosothiols [RSNO], and nitrogen dioxide [NO₂·]). Each reactive form is distinct, but they share the ability to damage microbes, at the *potential cost of inflammatory damage* to host cells and tissues.

Lysosomal Constituents of Leukocytes (p. 76)

Neutrophils and monocytes contain lysosomal granules, which when released may contribute to the inflammatory response and to tissue injury. ·

- *Neutrophils* have two main types of granules. The smaller *specific (or secondary) granules* contain lysozyme, collagenase, gelatinase, lactoferrin, plasminogen activator, histaminase, and alkaline phosphatase. The large *azurophil (or primary)* granules contain myeloperoxidase, bactericidal factors (lysozyme, defensins), acid hydrolases, and a variety of neutral proteases (elastase, cathepsin G, nonspecific collagenases, proteinase 3).

■ *Both specific and azurophil granules can empty into phagocytic vacuoles that form around engulfed material, or the contents can be secreted extracellularly as well as released after cell death.* Acid proteases degrade proteins, bacteria, and debris within the acidic environment of the phagolysosome. Neutral proteases can degrade extracellular components. *Monocytes* and *macrophages* also contain hydrolases (collagenase, elastase, phospholipase, and plasminogen activator), which may be particularly active in chronic inflammatory reactions.

■ Lysosomal constituents can potentiate further increases in vascular permeability and chemotaxis and cause tissue damage. These harmful proteases, however, are held in check by a system of *antiproteases* in the serum and tissue fluids. α_1-antitrypsin is the major inhibitor of neutrophilic elastase. A deficiency of these inhibitors may lead to sustained action of leukocyte proteases, as is the case in patients with α_1-antitrypsin deficiency (Chapter 19).

Oxygen-Derived Free Radicals (p. 76)

Oxygen-derived free radicals are metabolites that may be released extracellularly from leukocytes after exposure to chemotactic agents, immune complexes, or a phagocytic challenge. These include O_2^-, H_2O_2, and hydroxyl radical (OH^-), and these metabolites can combine with nitric oxide to form other reactive nitrogen intermediates, which cause

■ Endothelial cell damage with resultant increased vascular permeability
■ Inactivation of antiproteases, thus leading to unopposed protease activity
■ Injury to a variety of cell types (e.g., tumor cells, red cells, parenchymal cells)

Oxygen metabolites are detoxified by antioxidants, which include the serum proteins ceruloplasmin and transferrin and enzymes such as superoxide dismutase, catalase, and glutathione peroxidase. The net effects on tissue injury of oxygen metabolites depend on the balance between their production and inactivation.

Neuropeptides (p. 77)

Neuropeptides play a role in the initiation of an inflammatory response. The small peptides, such as *substance P*, belong to a family of tachykinin neuropeptides in the central and peripheral nervous systems. Substance P has many biologic functions, including the transmission of pain signals, regulation of blood pressure, and stimulation of secretion by immune and endocrine cells, but is notable as a powerful mediator of vascular permeability. Release of substance P alters vascular permeability leading to influx of plasma components at the site of injury and amplification of the initial inflammatory stimulus.

Summary

During the early course of inflammation, increased vascular permeability is mediated by histamine; the anaphylatoxins (C3a

and C5a); the kinins; leukotrienes C, D, and E; PAF; and substance P (Table 3–2). For chemotaxis, complement fragment C5a, lipoxygenase products (leukotriene B_4), other chemotactic lipids, and chemokines are the most likely protagonists. Additionally, prostaglandins play an important role in vasodilation, pain, and fever and in potentiating edema. IL-1 and TNF are involved with endothelial-leukocyte interactions and with acute-phase reactions. Lysosomal products and oxygen-derived radicals are the most likely candidates as causes of the ensuing tissue destruction. Nitric oxide is involved in vasodilation and cytotoxicity.

OUTCOME OF ACUTE INFLAMMATION
(p. 78)

The process of acute inflammation can be altered by the nature and intensity of the injury, the site and tissue affected, and the responsiveness of the host, but generally the process has one of four outcomes:

- *Complete resolution*, with regeneration of native cells and restoration of the site of acute inflammation to normal
- *Abscess formation*, particularly in infections with pyogenic organisms
- *Healing by connective tissue replacement (fibrosis) and scarring*, which occurs after substantial tissue destruction, when the inflammation occurs in tissues that do not regenerate or when there is abundant fibrin exudation
- *Progression to chronic inflammation*, as is outlined in more detail subsequently.

CHRONIC INFLAMMATION (p. 79)

Chronic inflammation can be defined as *inflammation of prolonged duration (weeks or months) in which active inflammation, tissue destruction, and attempts at healing may all be proceeding simultaneously.* It arises in several ways:

- It may follow acute inflammation, either because of the persistence of the inciting stimulus or because of some interference in the normal process of healing.
- It may result from repeated bouts of acute inflammation.
- Most commonly, it begins insidiously as a low-grade, smoldering response that does not follow classic acute inflammation, in one of the following settings:
  1. Persistent infection by intracellular microbes (e.g., tubercle bacilli, viral infection), which are of low toxicity but evoke an immunologic reaction
  2. Prolonged exposure to potentially toxic exogenous (e.g., silica and silicosis in the lung) or endogenous substances (e.g., plasma lipid components and atherosclerosis)
  3. Immune reactions, particularly those perpetuated against the individual's own tissues (e.g., autoimmune diseases)

In contrast to acute inflammation, which is manifested by vascular changes, edema, and largely neutrophilic infiltration, chronic inflammation is characterized by

- *Infiltration with mononuclear cells*, which include macrophages,

Table 3-2. SUMMARY OF MEDIATORS OF ACUTE INFLAMMATION

Mediator	Source	Action		
		Vascular Leakage	Chemotaxis	Other
Histamine and serotonin	Mast cells, platelets	+	—	
Bradykinin	Plasma substrate	+	—	Pain
C3a	Plasma protein via liver	+	—	Opsonic fragment (C3b)
C5a	Macrophages	—	+	Leukocyte adhesion, activation
Prostaglandins	Mast cells, from membrane phospholipids	Potentiate other mediators	—	Vasodilation, pain, fever
Leukotriene B₄	Leukocytes	—	+	Leukocyte adhesion, activation
Leukotriene C₄, D₄, E₄	Leukocytes, mast cells	+	—	Bronchoconstriction, vasoconstriction
Oxygen metabolites	Leukocytes	+	—	Endothelial damage, tissue damage
PAF	Leukocytes, mast cells	—	+	Bronchoconstriction, leukocyte priming
IL-1 and TNF	Macrophages, other	—	+	Acute-phase reactions, endothelial activation
Chemokines	Leukocytes, other	—	+	Leukocyte activation
Nitric oxide	Macrophages, endothelium	+	+	Vasodilation, cytotoxicity

PAF, platelet-activating factor; IL, interleukin; TNF, tumor necrosis factor.

52

lymphocytes, and plasma cells, a reflection of a persistent reaction to injury
- *Tissue destruction,* largely induced by the inflammatory cells
- Attempts at *repair by connective tissue replacement—* proliferation of small blood vessels *(angiogenesis)* and, in particular, *fibrosis.*

Mononuclear Infiltration: Cells and Mechanisms (p. 79)

MACROPHAGES

Macrophages are the major cellular players in chronic inflammation.

- They are derived from peripheral blood monocytes that have been induced to emigrate across the endothelium by chemokines (e.g., MCP-1) as well as other chemotactic agents. When the monocyte reaches the extravascular tissue, it transforms into a larger phagocytic cell, the macrophage.
- Macrophages are central figures in chronic inflammation because of the great number of biologically active products they can secrete (Fig. 3–8). They can be *activated* by cytokines (e.g. IFN-γ) produced by immune activated T cells or by nonimmune factors (e.g., endotoxin) to secrete numerous factors, including

1. Neutral proteases
2. Chemotactic factors
3. Arachidonic acid metabolites
4. Reactive oxygen and nitrogen species
5. Complement components
6. Coagulation factors
7. Growth factors
8. Cytokines (such as IL-1 and TNF)
9. Other factors (e.g., PAF and α-IFN)

- Although macrophage products are important components in host defense, some of these mediators induce the *tissue damage characteristic of chronic inflammation.* The secretory products can be toxic to cells (reactive oxygen and nitric oxide metabolites) or extracellular matrix (proteases); other products cause fibroblast proliferation, connective tissue production, and angiogenesis (cytokines and growth factors).
- In chronic inflammation, macrophage accumulation persists primarily through *continued recruitment of monocytes from the circulation,* which results from the steady expression of adhesion molecules and chemotactic factors.

OTHER CELLS IN CHRONIC INFLAMMATION

Other cells involved in chronic inflammation are *lymphocytes, mast cells,* and *eosinophils.*

- *Lymphocytes* are mobilized by antibody- and cell-mediated immune reactions and by nonimmunologic reactions. They have a unique reciprocal relationship to macrophages in chronic inflammation (Fig. 3–9). They can be activated by contact with antigen and nonspecifically by bacterial endotoxin. Activated lymphocytes produce *lymphokines,* and these (particularly IFN-γ) are major stimulators of monocytes and macrophages. Activated macrophages produce *monokines,* which, in turn, influence B-cell and T-cell function. *Plasma cells* produce antibodies

Activated T cell

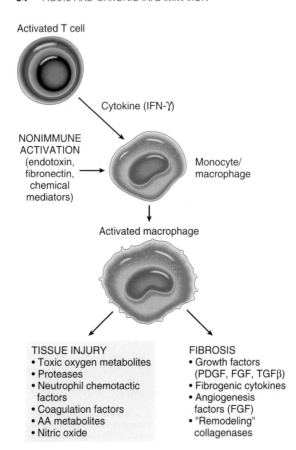

Cytokine (IFN-γ)

NONIMMUNE
ACTIVATION
(endotoxin,
fibronectin,
chemical
mediators)

Monocyte/
macrophage

Activated macrophage

TISSUE INJURY
• Toxic oxygen metabolites
• Proteases
• Neutrophil chemotactic
  factors
• Coagulation factors
• AA metabolites
• Nitric oxide

FIBROSIS
• Growth factors
  (PDGF, FGF, TGFβ)
• Fibrogenic cytokines
• Angiogenesis
  factors (FGF)
• "Remodeling"
  collagenases

Figure 3–8   ∎

Macrophage products involved in tissue destruction and fibrosis. The products made by activated macrophages that also mediate tissue injury and fibrosis are indicated.

directed against either foreign antigen or altered tissue components.

■ *Mast cells* are widely distributed in connective tissues and participate in both acute and persistent inflammatory reactions. Mast cells express on their surface the receptor that binds the Fc portion of the IgE antibody. In acute reactions, IgE antibodies bound to the cells' Fc receptors specifically recognize antigen, and the cells degranulate and release mediators, such as histamine. This type of response occurs during anaphylactic reactions to foods, insect venom, or drugs, frequently with catastrophic results. Specific types of parasite infections are also associated with increased levels of IgE and activation of mast cells.

■ *Eosinophils* are also characteristic of immune reactions mediated by IgE and of parasitic infections. The recruitment of eosinophils depends on *eotaxin*, a member of the C-C family

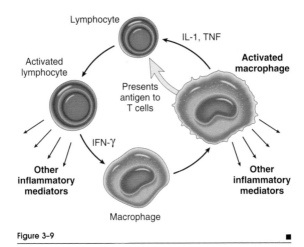

Figure 3-9   ■

Macrophage-lymphocyte interactions in chronic inflammation. Activated lymphocytes and macrophages influence each other, and both cell types release inflammatory mediators that affect other cells. (From Kumar V, Cotran RS, Robbins SL: Basic Pathology, 6th ed. Philadelphia, WB Saunders, 1997.)

of chemokines. Eosinophils have granules that contain MBP, a highly cationic protein that is toxic to parasites but also causes lysis of mammalian epithelial cells. They may thus be of benefit in parasitic infections but contribute to tissue damage in immune reactions.

Granulomatous Inflammation (p. 83)

Granulomatous inflammation is a distinctive chronic inflammatory reaction in which the *predominant cell type is an activated macrophage with a modified epithelial-like (epithelioid) appearance.*

■ Granulomatous inflammation is encountered in a relatively few but widespread chronic immune and infectious diseases, such as tuberculosis, sarcoidosis, and syphilis. Table 3–3 lists the features of the major immune granulomatous diseases.
■ Granulomatous inflammation is characterized by *granulomas—focal collections of epithelioid macrophages that are surrounded by a collar of mononuclear leukocytes, principally lymphocytes and occasionally plasma cells.* Epithelioid cells may coalesce to form multinucleate giant cells. Central necrosis may also be present in some granulomas.
■ There are two types of granulomas:
  1. *Foreign body granulomas,* incited by relatively inert foreign bodies.
  2. *Immune granulomas,* formed by immune T cell–mediated reactions to poorly degradable antigens. *Lymphokines,* principally IFN-γ from activated T cells, cause transformation of macrophages to epithelioid cells and multinucleate giant cells. The prototype for the immune granuloma is that caused by the bacillus of tuberculosis. In this disease, the granuloma

Table 3-3. EXAMPLES OF GRANULOMATOUS INFLAMMATIONS

Disease	Cause	Tissue Reaction
Bacterial		
Tuberculosis	*Mycobacterium tuberculosis*	*Noncaseating tubercle (granuloma prototype)*: a focus of epithelioid cells, rimmed by fibroblasts, lymphocytes, histiocytes, occasional Langhans' giant cell *Caseating tubercle*: central amorphous granular debris, loss of all cellular detail, acid-fast bacilli
Leprosy (tuberculoid form)	*Mycobacterium leprae*	Acid-fast bacilli in macrophages; granulomas and epithelioid types
Syphilis	*Treponema pallidum*	*Gumma*: Microscopic to grossly visible lesion, enclosing wall of histiocytes; plasma cell infiltrate; center cells are necrotic without loss of cellular outline
Cat-scratch disease	Gram-negative bacillius	Rounded or stellate granuloma containing central granular debris and recognizable neutrophils; giant cells uncommon
Parasitic		
Schistosomiasis	*Schistosoma mansoni, S. haematobium, S. japonicum*	Egg emboli; eosinophils
Fungal		
	Cryptococcus neoformans	Organism is yeastlike, sometimes budding; 5–10 mm; large, clear capsule
	Coccidioides immitis	Organism appears as spherical (30–80 mm) cyst containing endospores of 3–5 mm each
Inorganic Metals and Dusts		
Silicosis, berylliosis		Lung involvement; fibrosis
Unknown		
Sarcoidosis		*Noncaseating granuloma*: giant cells (Langhans' and foreign-body types); asteroids in giant cells; occasional Schaumann body (concentric calcific concretion); no organisms

is referred to as a *tubercle* and is *classically characterized by the presence of central caseous necrosis.*

MORPHOLOGIC PATTERNS IN ACUTE AND CHRONIC INFLAMMATION (p. 84)

Inflammatory responses often have certain features that point to their possible cause and create distinctive morphologic patterns:

- *Serous inflammation* implies a modest increase in vascular permeability. It is marked by an accumulation of fluid, which, when it occurs in the peritoneal, pleural, and pericardial cavities, is called an *effusion* but can occur elsewhere (e.g., skin burn blisters).
- *Fibrinous inflammation* occurs when the injury causes a more marked increase in vascular permeability. The exudate contains large amounts of fibrinogen, which is converted to fibrin as a result of activation of the coagulation system. When a serosal surface is involved, such as the pericardium or pleura, it is referred to as *fibrinous pericarditis* or *pleuritis*.
- *Suppurative or purulent inflammation* is characterized by the production of purulent exudate or pus consisting of white cells and necrotic cells. An *abscess* refers to a localized collection of purulent inflammatory tissue that is accompanied by liquefactive necrosis (e.g., pyogenic staphylococcal abscesses).
- *Ulcers are local defects, or excavations, of the surface of an organ or tissue that are produced by the sloughing (shedding) of inflammatory necrotic tissue.*
- *Granulomatous inflammation* is a distinctive inflammatory reaction as noted and has relatively few possible causes, cited in Table 3–3.

SYSTEMIC EFFECTS OF INFLAMMATION

(p. 85)

The major systemic manifestations of acute inflammation involve a wide range of endocrine, autonomic, and behavioral responses, as follows:

- *Endocrine and metabolic*: Secretion of acute-phase proteins by the liver (including C-reactive protein, serum amyloid A, complement, and coagulation proteins)
- *Autonomic*: A redirection in blood flow from cutaneous to deep vascular beds, to minimize heat loss through the skin; increased pulse and blood pressure; and decreased sweating
- *Behavioral*: Rigors (shivering), chills (search for warmth), anorexia, somnolence, and malaise.

Other major systemic manifestations are as follows:

- The principal manifestation of fever is an elevation of body temperature, usually by 1 to 4°C.
- *Cytokines play a key role in signaling a fever. IL-1, IL-6, and TNF-α, produced by leukocytes in response to infectious agents or immunologic reactions, are released into the circulation. IL-1 acts directly and also by inducing IL-6,* which has essentially similar effects in producing the acute-phase responses. IL-1 and TNF interact with vascular receptors in the thermoregulatory centers of the hypothalamus, inducing local prostaglandin E_2 production, resulting in sympathetic nerve stimulation, vasoconstriction of skin vessels, and fever.
- *Leukocytosis* (elevation in total white blood cell count) is a common feature of inflammatory reactions, especially those induced by bacterial infection. Extreme elevations are referred to as *leukemoid reactions*. The leukocytosis occurs because of the proliferation of precursors in the bone marrow and the accelerated release of cells from the bone marrow, induced by CSFs.

- Most bacterial infections induce *neutrophilia (an increased number of polymorphonuclear leukocytes in the blood)*, but some viral infections (e.g., mononucleosis, mumps, and German measles) produce a leukocytosis because of an absolute increase in the number of lymphocytes *(lymphocytosis)*. In other disorders, there is an absolute increase in the number of eosinophils creating an *eosinophilia* (e.g., bronchial asthma, hay fever, and parasitic infestations). Certain infections (typhoid fever and infections caused by viruses, rickettsiae, and certain protozoa) are associated with a decreased number of circulating white cells *(leukopenia)*. Leukopenia is also encountered in infections that overwhelm patients debilitated by disseminated cancer.

Thus, the major systemic effects of a significant inflammatory reaction are fever, leukocytosis (most often owing to an increased number of circulating neutrophils, sometimes lymphocytes), and chills, well known to all who have had a respiratory infection.

Tissue Repair: Cellular Growth, Fibrosis, and Wound Healing

Replacement of injured or dead cells is critical to survival. Repair of tissues involves two distinct processes: (1) *regeneration,* denoting replacement of dead cells by proliferation of cells of the same type, and (2) *replacement by connective tissue* or fibroplasia. In most cases, both processes contribute to repair. Both regeneration and fibroplasia are determined by largely similar mechanisms involving *cell growth and differentiation* and cell-matrix interactions.

CONTROL OF NORMAL CELL GROWTH
(p. 90)

The size of a population of cells in adult tissues is determined by the rates of cell proliferation, differentiation, and death by apoptosis. Cell proliferation can be stimulated by injury, mechanical forces acting on tissues, or cell death. The most important factors that regulate cell proliferation are those that recruit quiescent cells into the cell cycle.

Cell Cycle and Proliferative Potential
(p. 91)

Cells are divided into three groups based on their proliferative capacity and their relationship to the cell cycle:

1. *Continuously dividing cells (labile cells)*, such as surface epithelia and cells of the bone marrow and hematopoietic cells
2. *Quiescent (or stable) cells*, normally with slow turnover but capable of rapid division in response to stimuli—such as liver, kidney, fibroblasts, smooth muscle, and endothelial cells
3. *Nondividing (permanent) cells*, which cannot undergo division in postnatal life—for example, neurons, skeletal muscle, and cardiac muscle

Molecular Events in Cell Proliferation
(p. 92)

The explosion in understanding of the molecular events controlling cell growth comes largely from the discovery that growth factors induce cell proliferation by affecting the expression of genes involved in normal growth control pathways, the *protooncogenes*. Alterations in the structure or expression of these genes can convert them into *oncogenes*, which contribute to the uncontrolled growth characteristic of cancer (Chapter 8).

There are three general schemes of intercellular signaling important in the regulation of cell proliferation:

1. *Autocrine signaling*: Cells respond to signaling substances that they themselves secrete.
2. *Paracrine signaling*: A cell produces substances that affect only a target cell in close proximity.
3. *Endocrine signaling*: Hormones are synthesized by cells of endocrine organs and act on target cells distant from their site of synthesis.

The chain of molecular events induced by growth factors includes the following components.

CELL SURFACE RECEPTORS

Cell growth is initiated by binding of a signaling agent, most commonly a growth factor, to a specific receptor frequently located on the plasma membrane. Some of these receptors are illustrated in Figure 4–1:

- *Receptors with intrinsic kinase activity*: Most growth factor (e.g. platelet-derived growth factor [PDGF], epidermal growth factor [EGF], and fibroblast growth factor [FGF]) receptors have intrinsic tyrosine kinase activity, which is activated by ligand binding. Receptor activation creates binding sites for a series of cytosolic proteins, which couple the receptor to the Ras signaling pathway, the phosphoinositide 3-kinase pathway, phospholipase Cγ in the protein kinase C pathway, and members of the Src family of kinases. Collectively, these signaling sys-

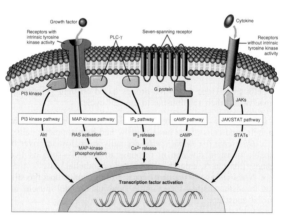

Figure 4–1

A simplified overview of the major types of cell surface receptors and the principal signal transduction pathways (see text). Signaling events from tyrosine kinase receptors, G protein–coupled receptors, and cytokine receptors are outlined.

tems generate a cascade of responses that commit the cell to enter the cell cycle.

- *Receptors without intrinsic kinase activity*: Other growth factor receptors associate with and activate cytosolic protein kinases. Receptors for *cytokines* frequently fall into this category.

- *G protein–linked receptors*: G protein–linked receptors *all contain seven transmembrane loops and are frequently called seven-spanning (or serpentine) receptors. Although not closely linked to growth, this class of receptors is associated with a variety of important functions and includes the chemokine receptors (Chapter 3) as well as the receptors for epinephrine and glucagon. Ligand binding activates a signal transducing G protein complex, which, in turn, activates an effector system that generates intracellular second messengers.*

SIGNAL TRANSDUCTION SYSTEMS

Signal transduction is the process by which extracellular signals are detected and converted into intracellular signals. These systems are typically arranged as networks of sequential protein kinases (Fig. 4–1).

- *Mitogen-activated protein (MAP) kinase pathway*: This signaling system is particularly relevant to signaling by growth factors. The activated tyrosine kinase receptor binds to adapter proteins, which activate Ras. Activated Ras binds to Raf, which phosphorylates a family of kinases collectively called *MAP*. The net result of this pathway is the activation of a protein phosphorylation cascade, which amplifies the signal and stimulates the quiescent cells to enter the growth cycle.

- *Other signaling systems* are also outlined in Figure 4–1:
  1. *Phosphoinositide 3-kinase pathway*: Growth factors that bind to tyrosine kinases do not all convey the same signals. This pathway activates a series of kinases including Akt that eventually leads to cell survival.
  2. *Inositol-lipid pathway*: This signaling system can be coupled to either tyrosine kinase or seven-spanning G protein–linked receptors and results in phospholipase Cγ activation, inositol 1,4,5-triphosphate production, diacylglycerol formation, protein kinase C activation, release of calcium ions and phosphorylation of a variety of components important in cell metabolism.
  3. *Cyclic adenosine monophosphate (cAMP) pathway*: Binding of some hormones (epinephrine or glucagon) or chemokines to seven-spanning receptors is coupled to G proteins, activation of adenylate cyclase, and generation of cAMP. This second messenger then activates protein kinase A, which through a series of intermediate steps stimulates expression of specific target genes.
  4. *JAK/STAT pathway*: Cytokine receptors associate with protein kinases (Janus kinases [JAKs]), which phosphorylate downstream STATs (for *s*ignal *t*ransducers and *a*ctivators of *t*ranscription), which change functional as opposed to proliferative responses.

TRANSCRIPTION FACTORS AND THE REGULATION OF GENE EXPRESSION

The signal transduction systems described previously transfer information to the nucleus, where specific changes occur in the regulation of gene expression. This regulation is largely achieved at the level of transcription of genes, a process controlled by transcription factors. Transcription factors are phosphorylated and activated by specific signaling kinases. Among the transcription factors regulating cell proliferation are a number of protooncogenes, in which mutations may be associated with tumors, and various types of tumor-suppressor genes (or antioncogenes), such as *p53* and the retinoblastoma gene.

Cell Cycle and the Regulation of Cell Proliferation (p. 95)

The cell growth cycle consists of G_1 (presynthetic), S (DNA synthesis), G_2 (premitotic), and M (mitotic) phases. Quiescent cells are in a physiologic state called G_0. Two types of molecular controls regulate the passage of cells through specific phases of the cell cycle:

- A cascade of *protein phosphorylation pathways* involving cyclins and cyclin-dependent kinases
- A set of *checkpoints* that monitor completion of the molecular events and, if necessary, delay progression to the next phase of the cell cycle

CYCLINS AND CYCLIN-DEPENDENT KINASES

The cell cycle itself is controlled by a series of regulatory proteins, called *cyclins*, whose concentrations rise and fall during the cell cycle and which form complexes with constitutively present protein kinases called *cyclin-dependent kinases (CDKs)*. Different combinations of cyclins and CDKs are associated with each of the important transitions in the cell cycle. For example, as the cell moves into the G_2 phase of the cell cycle, cyclin B binds to constitutive CDK1, creating a cyclin B/CDK1 complex. The activity of this complex is necessary for the transition from G_2 to M. The cyclin-kinase complexes generated during each phase of the cell cycle phosphorylate multiple proteins, including those involved in initiation of DNA replication and formation of mitotic spindles. The active CDK complexes can be regulated by binding of *CDK inhibitors* (p. 284).

CHECKPOINTS

Checkpoints provide a *surveillance mechanism* for ensuring that critical transitions in the cell cycle occur in the correct order and that important events are completed with fidelity. For example, the tumor-suppressor gene *p53* is activated in response to DNA damage and inhibits further progression through the cell cycle by increasing expression of a CDK inhibitor.

Growth Inhibition (p. 96)

Growth inhibition, in addition to growth stimulation, regulates cell growth. Inhibitors are also largely polypeptide factors that use receptors, signal transduction, second messengers, and transcriptional factors. The best-studied is transforming growth factor-β (TGF-β), although interferon-γ also inhibits cell growth.

Growth Factors (p. 97)

Growth factors act by endocrine, paracrine, or autocrine signaling and, in addition to their growth effects, influence cell movement, contractility, and differentiation—all important processes in wound healing (see later). The major growth factors (Table 4–1) include the following:

■ *EGF* and *TGF-α* have extensive homology and bind to an identical cell receptor, c-*erb-B1*. They are mitogenic for epithelial cells and fibroblasts.
■ *PDGF* is found in platelets but is also made by endothelial cells, macrophages, and smooth muscle cells. PDGF causes migration and proliferation of fibroblasts and smooth muscle cells and is important in angiogenesis.
■ *FGFs* are a family of growth factors that include acidic and basic FGF. FGFs have been implicated in
   1. Angiogenesis (growth of new blood vessels) (basic FGF causes endothelial cell migration, proliferation, and differentiation—steps necessary for angiogenesis)
   2. Wound repair
   3. Development
   4. Hematopoiesis
■ *Vascular endothelial cell growth factor (VEGF)*, is a family of proteins that promotes blood vessel formation in early development (vasculogenesis) and plays a role in angiogenesis. Members of the family have distinct functions. VEGF promotes angiogenesis in chronic inflammatory states and in healing wounds. VEGF-C induces specific lymphatic endothelial proliferation.
■ *TGF-β* belongs to a large family of growth factors with wide-

---

Table 4-1.   GROWTH FACTORS

Epidermal Growth Factor (EGF) Family
   EGF
   Transforming Growth Factor-α (TGF-α)
Platelet-Derived Growth Factor (PDGF)
Fibroblast Growth Factor (FGF)
   Basic
   Acidic
Transforming Growth Factor-β (TGF-β) Family
   TGF isoforms
   Insulin-Like Growth Factors (IGFs)
   IGF-1
   IGF-2
Vascular Endothelial Growth Factor (VEGF)
Hepatic Growth Factor (HGF)
   (Scatter factor)
Myeloid Colony-Stimulating Factors (CSFs)
   Granulocyte-macrophage CSF (GM-CSF)
   Granulocyte CSF (G-CSF)
   Macrophage CSF (M-CSF)
Erythropoietin
Cytokines
   Interleukins
   Tumor Necrosis Factor (TNF)
   Interferons
Nerve Growth Factor (NGF)

ranging functions. It is produced by a variety of cell types, including platelets, endothelial cells, T cells, and macrophages. TGF-β is a growth inhibitor to most epithelial cells. Most importantly, it induces fibrosis by
1. Stimulating fibroblast chemotaxis
2. Stimulating collagen and fibronectin synthesis
3. Inhibiting collagen degradation.

■ *Cytokines* have important functions as mediators of immune and inflammatory responses and can be considered growth factors because many of them have growth-promoting activities for a variety of cells (p. 73, Chapter 3).

EXTRACELLULAR MATRIX AND CELL-MATRIX INTERACTIONS (p. 98)

The extracellular matrix (ECM) markedly influences cell growth and function. The ECM consists of *fibrous structural proteins* (e.g., collagen) and *adhesive glycoproteins* embedded in a gel of *proteoglycans and hyaluronan.* These macromolecules assemble into an *interstitial matrix*, present in the spaces between cells, or into a *basement membrane*, located close to the plasma membrane of some cells.

Collagen and Fiber Assembly (p. 98)

Collagens are divided into 14 types: Types I, II, and III are the fibrillar collagens, and types IV, V, and VI are amorphous and present in interstitial tissue and basement membranes. Adult skin collagen is mostly type I. Collagen synthesis involves first synthesis of α chains on ribosomes, followed by a number of enzymatic hydroxylations, which are necessary to hold the three α chains together. Proteolytic processing of a C-terminal fragment of the procollagen molecule during or shortly after secretion from fibroblasts and smooth muscle cells results in the formation of fibrils. Extracellular lysyl hydroxylysyl oxidation results in cross-linkages between α chains of adjacent molecules, which contribute to the tensile strength of collagen (dependent on vitamin C).

Elastin, Fibrillin, and the Microfibrillar Network (p. 99)

Elastin provides tissues with elasticity or the ability to stretch and recoil. Elastic fibers consist of a central core of *elastin*, a 70-kD protein, and a surrounding peripheral network consisting of fibrillin, a 350-kD glycoprotein. Inherited defects in fibrillin result in formation of abnormal elastic fibers in Marfan's syndrome (Chapter 6).

Adhesive Matrix Glycoproteins and Integrins (p. 100)

Adhesive matrix glycoproteins and integrins link the ECM with specific integral cell membrane proteins.

FIBRONECTIN

Fibronectin, a 400-kD adhesion glycoprotein, binds to several ECM components (collagen, heparin, fibrin, proteoglycans) on the one hand and to cell membranes on the other. Binding to ECM is mediated by recognition of a specific amino acid sequence, RGD (arginine, glycine, aspartic acid), present in the matrix protein. Binding to cells is via *integrins* or receptors that span the cell surface membrane and interact with the cytoskeleton at points of *focal adhesion*. Thus, fibronectin is directly involved in cell attachment, spreading, and locomotion and interacts with growth factors to affect growth and differentiation.

LAMININ

Laminin, a cross-shaped glycoprotein spanning basement membranes, also binds to cells through specific receptors and to collagen type IV and heparin and is involved in cell attachment, locomotion, and growth.

INTEGRINS

Integrins are the major family of cell surface receptors that mediate cellular attachment to the ECM. Many integrins are widely expressed, and most cells have more than one integrin on the cell surface. Integrin receptors span the cell membrane and bind to many components (e.g., fibronectin, laminin, and some collagens) of the ECM by recognizing the RGD sequence. Integrin receptors are important both in organizing the actin cytoskeleton of cells at points of *focal adhesion* and in transduction of signals from the ECM to the cell interior. The mechanical linkage between the integrin receptors and the cytoskeletal signaling system may be a mechanism by which cells convert mechanical force into biochemical signals.

MATRICELLULAR PROTEINS

Matricellular proteins are secreted proteins that do not function as structural components of the ECM. These proteins interact with matrix components, cell surface receptors, or other molecules (e.g., growth factors, cytokines, or proteases), which interact, in turn, with the cell surface. The group shares the ability to disrupt cell-matrix interactions. This family of versatile adapter proteins includes *SPARC* (*s*ecreted *p*rotein *a*cidic and *r*ich in *c*ysteine, also known as *osteonectin*), the *thrombospondins*, *osteopontin*, and the *tenascin* family members.

PROTEOGLYCANS AND HYALURONAN

Proteoglycans are ECM components that consist of a core protein linked to one or more polysaccharides called *glycosaminoglycans*. Glycosaminoglycans are long repeating polymers of modified disaccharides (e.g., heparan sulfate). Proteoglycans can also be integral membrane proteins, as in the *syndecan* family, in which the core protein spans the plasma membrane. *Hyaluronan* is a huge molecule consisting of many repeats of a disaccharide. It serves as a ligand for core proteins and cell surface receptors. Hyaluronan binds large amounts of water, which helps give connective tissue turgor pressure and the ability to resist compression forces.

Summary

Cell growth and differentiation involve the cellular integration of multiple signals. Some of these signals are derived from growth

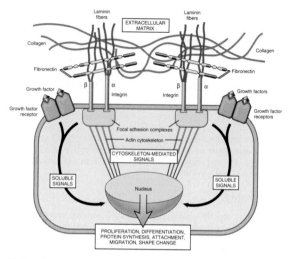

Figure 4-2 ∎

Schematic showing the mechanisms by which extracellular matrix (ECM) (e.g., fibronectin and laminin) and growth factors can influence cell growth, motility, differentiation, and protein synthesis. Integrins bind ECM and interact with the cytoskeleton at focal adhesion complexes (protein aggregates that include vinculin, α-actinin and talin). This can initiate the production of intracellular messengers or can directly mediate nuclear signals. Cell surface receptors for growth factors also initiate second signals. Collectively, these are integrated by the cell to yield various responses, including changes in cell growth, locomotion, and differentiation. (From Kumar V, Cotran RS, and Robbins SL: Basic Pathology, 6th ed. Philadelphia, WB Saunders, 1997, p 53.)

factors and growth inhibitors. Others are derived from components in the extracellular matrix and proceed through integrin-dependent signaling pathways. Figure 4–2 is a model of the interactions between growth factors, ECM, and cell responses.

REPAIR BY CONNECTIVE TISSUE (FIBROSIS)

Because tissue destruction in wound healing and chronic inflammation involves both parenchymal cells and the stromal framework, repair cannot be accomplished solely by regeneration of parenchymal cells. Repair thus involves in large part the replacement of lost cells and tissues by connective tissue, which, in time, produces *fibrosis* and *scarring*. Connective tissue repair is then the systematic processes by which unregenerated damage is replaced by fibrosis and scarring. The initial response to a wound consists of the formation of *granulation tissue*, which consists of a richly vascular connective tissue, containing new capillaries, proliferating fibroblasts, and variable numbers of inflammatory cells.

There are four components to this orderly process:

1. Formation of new blood vessels (angiogenesis), spanning the wound

2. Migration and proliferation of fibroblasts filling and bridging the wound

3. Deposition of ECM
4. Maturation and reorganization of the fibrous tissue into a scar, also known as *remodeling*

Angiogenesis (p. 103)

Angiogenesis is critical for chronic inflammation, formation of collateral circulation, and tumor growth. Blood vessels are assembled by two processes: *vasculogenesis*, in which a primitive vascular network is assembled during development, and *angiogenesis* (or neovascularization), in which preexisting blood vessels give rise to capillary buds to produce new vessels.

Multiple steps underlie *angiogenesis*: proteolytic degradation of the basement membrane of the parent vessel basement membrane; endothelial cell migration and formation of a capillary sprout; proliferation and maturation of endothelial cells, which includes remodeling into capillary tubes; and recruitment of periendothelial cells, including pericytes for small capillaries and vascular smooth muscle cells for larger vessels to support the endothelial tubes.

The formation, maintenance, and remodeling of blood vessels are controlled by the following:

- *Growth factors and receptors*: Many growth factors have angiogenic activity, but *VEGF and the angiopoietins (Ang)* are particularly important in establishing and maintaining new blood vessels. They interact with the corresponding tyrosine kinase receptors (VEGF-R and Tie) uniquely expressed by endothelial cells. PDGF and its receptors are important in recruiting periendothelial cells.
- *ECM proteins, as regulators of angiogenesis*: The cell motility and directed migration of endothelial cells that occurs during angiogenesis is regulated by *integrins* (e.g., $\alpha v\beta 3$), *matricellular proteins* (e.g., SPARC), and *proteases* (e.g., plasminogen activators and matrix metalloproteases).
- *Angiogenesis inhibitors*: These act to down-regulate new vessel growth and include certain *cytokines* (e.g., interferon-α); *tissue inhibitors of metalloproteinases*; certain *matricellular proteins* (e.g., thrombospondin); and tumor-derived factors, such as *angiostatin* (a fragment of plasminogen) and *endostatin* (a fragment of collagen).

Fibrosis (Fibroplasia) (p. 106)

Fibrosis occurs within the granulation tissue framework formed at the site of repair and involves two processes:

- *Fibroblast migration and proliferation*: Increased vascular permeability leads to the deposition of plasma proteins, such as fibronectin and fibrinogen, which provide a provisional stroma for ingrowth of fibroblasts. Migration of fibroblasts and their subsequent proliferation is also mediated by growth factors such as PDGF, EGF, FGF, and TGF-β and the fibrogenic cytokines IL-1 and TNF-α.
- *ECM deposition*: As repair progresses, the number of proliferating endothelial cells and fibroblasts decreases. The fibroblasts become more synthetic and deposit increased amounts of collagen and other components of the ECM. Collagen synthesis is stimulated by growth factors (e.g., PDGF, FGF) and by cytokines (e.g., IL-1) secreted by fibroblasts and leukocytes in healing wounds. TGF-β is thought to play a particularly important role in chronic inflammatory fibrosis. Eventually the

granulation tissue scaffolding is converted into a scar composed of fibroblasts and collagen.

Tissue Remodeling (p. 106)

The replacement of granulation tissue with a scar involves transitions in the composition of the ECM. Some of the growth factors that stimulate synthesis of collagen and other connective tissue molecules modulate the synthesis and activation of *matrix metalloproteinases* (MMPs), enzymes that serve to degrade these ECM components. MMPs consist of *interstitial collagenases*, which cleave the fibrillar collagen types I, II, and III; *gelatinases (or type IV collagenases)*, which degrade amorphous collagen as well as fibronectin; *stromelysins*, which act on a variety of ECM components, including proteoglycans, laminin, fibronectin, and amorphous collagens; and the family of *membrane-bound MMPs*, which are cell surface–associated proteases. Secretion of MMPs by fibroblasts and leukocytes is induced by growth factors and cytokines and inhibited by TGF-β. The enzymes are secreted as proenzymes, which are activated extracellularly. Activated MMPs can be rapidly inhibited by a family of specific *tissue inhibitors of metalloproteinase*. The net effect of ECM *synthesis* versus *degradation* results in debridement of injured sites and *remodeling* of the connective tissues framework—important features of both chronic inflammation and wound repair.

WOUND HEALING (p. 107)

Wound healing is a complex but orderly phenomenon involving many of the processes just described:

- Induction of an acute inflammatory process by the initial injury
- Regeneration of parenchymal cells
- Migration and proliferation of both parenchymal and connective tissue cells
- Synthesis of ECM proteins
- Remodeling of connective tissue and parenchymal components
- Collagenizaton and acquisition of wound strength

Healing by First Intention (p. 107)

Healing of a clean surgical approximated incision (first intention) involves an orchestrated sequence of events, as follows:

- *0 hours*: The incision is filled with clot.
- *3 to 24 hours*: Neutrophils from the margins infiltrate the clot. Mitoses begin to appear in epithelial basal cells; epithelial closure takes place by 24 to 48 hours.
- *Day 3*: Neutrophils are replaced by macrophages. Granulation tissue begins to appear.
- *Day 5*: The incision space is filled with granulation tissue, neovascularization is maximal, collagen fibrils begin to appear, and epithelial proliferation is now maximal.
- *Week 2*: There is proliferation of fibroblasts and continued collagen accumulation to produce a scar. Collagen deposited early in granulation tissue is type III, which is then replaced by adult type I collagen. Collagen fibers account in large part for wound strength. Inflammation and newly formed vessels have largely disappeared.

■ *Month 2*: Scar now consists of connective tissue devoid of inflammation covered by intact epidermis.

Healing by Second Intention (p. 109)

Healing by second intention occurs when there is more extensive loss of tissue, such as infarction, ulceration, abscess formation, and large wounds. Abundant granulation tissue grows in from the margins to fill the defect, but at the same time the wound *contracts*; that is, the defect is markedly reduced from its original size. *Myofibroblasts* contribute to wound contraction.

SUMMARY

Wound healing involves orchestrated events of early inflammation; followed by a stage of fibroplasia characterized by granulation tissue; followed by ECM deposition, tissue remodeling, and scarring.

Wound Strength (p. 109)

Wound strength at the end of the first week is approximately 10% of normal; it is largely dependent on surgical suturing and tissue adhesion. The progressive recovery of tensile strength to 70% to 80% of normal by the third month (which may persist for life) is associated first with increased collagen synthesis exceeding collagen degradation and subsequently with the cross-linking and increased fiber size of collagen fibers.

Systemic and Local Factors That Influence Wound Healing (p. 109)

A number of systemic and local factors modify the severity of the inflammatory response and the quality of repair. The *systemic* influences include the following:

■ Nutritional status of the host (e.g., protein nutrition and vitamin C intake)
■ Metabolic status (diabetes mellitus delays healing)
■ Circulatory status or the adequacy of the blood supply
■ Hormones, concurrent glucocorticoid therapy, which hinders the inflammatory-reparative process

Local factors that influence healing include the following:

■ Infection, which can delay healing
■ Mechanical factors, such as motion directly affecting the wound, which can delay healing
■ Foreign bodies, which impede healing
■ Size, location, and type of the wound

Pathologic Aspects of Wound Healing (p. 110)

Complications in wound healing can arise from abnormalities in any of the basic repair processes. These aberrations can be grouped into three general categories:

■ *Deficient scar formation*: This can lead to two types of complications:
  1. *Wound dehiscence*
  2. *Ulceration*

- *Excessive formation of the repair components*: The formation of excessive amounts of granulation tissue, which protrudes above the level of the surrounding skin and blocks reepithelialization, has been called *exuberant granulation* or *proud flesh*. The accumulation of excessive amounts of collagen may give rise to a raised tumorous scar known as a *keloid,* or *hypertrophic scar.*

- *Formation of contractures*: As we have seen, *contraction* in the size of a wound is an important part in the normal healing process. An exaggeration of this process, as, for example, in the hand or face, is designated a *contracture* and results in deformities of the wound and the surrounding tissues, producing in the hand *claw* deformities or limiting the mobility of a joint.

Hemodynamic Disorders, Thrombosis, and Shock

EDEMA (p. 113)

Edema refers to increased fluid in the interstitial tissue spaces or body cavities (e.g., *hydrothorax, hydropericardium,* and *hydroperitoneum* [*ascites*]). Edema may be localized (e.g., secondary to isolated venous or lymphatic obstruction) or systemic (as in heart failure), called *anasarca* when severe.

Table 5–1 lists the pathophysiologic categories of edema, which may be broadly grouped into *noninflammatory* (yields protein-poor *transudate*) and *inflammatory* (yields protein-rich *exudate*; Chapter 3). Noninflammatory causes of edema are as follows:

- *Increased hydrostatic pressure* forces fluid *out of* the vessels. *Congestive heart failure* (CHF) (p. 546) falls in this category and *is the most common cause of systemic edema.* Edema in CHF is due, in part, to increased venous hydrostatic pressure, but reduced cardiac output with renal hypoperfusion and resulting sodium and water retention also contributes.

- *Decreased osmotic pressure* reduces movement of fluid *into* vessels. This occurs with loss of albumin (most important cause is proteinuria in the *nephrotic syndrome*, p. 952) or reduced albumin synthesis (occurs with liver pathology [e.g., cirrhosis, p. 853] or as a consequence of protein malnutrition). In either case, reduced plasma osmotic pressure leads to a net movement of fluid into the interstitium and plasma volume contraction. As with CHF, edema precipitated by *hypoproteinemia* is exacerbated by secondary salt and fluid retention.

- *Primary sodium retention*, with its obligatory associated water, causes *both* increased hydrostatic pressure and reduced osmotic pressure. This occurs with excessive salt intake and renal dysfunction, such as acute renal failure or poststreptococcal glomerulonephritis (p. 949).

- *Lymphatic obstruction* blocks removal of interstitial fluid. Obstruction is usually localized and most often related to inflammatory or neoplastic processes.

Table 5–1. PATHOPHYSIOLOGIC CATEGORIES OF EDEMA

Increased Hydrostatic Pressure

Impaired venous return
   Congestive heart failure
   Constrictive pericarditis
   Ascites (liver cirrhosis)
   Venous obstruction or compression
      Thrombosis
      External pressure (e.g., mass)
      Lower extremity inactivity with prolonged dependency
Arteriolar dilation
   Heat
   Neurohumoral dysregulation

Reduced Plasma Osmotic Pressure (Hypoproteinemia)

Protein-losing glomerulopathies (nephrotic syndrome)
Liver cirrhosis (ascites)
Malnutrition
Protein-losing gastroenteropathy

Lymphatic Obstruction

Inflammatory
Neoplastic
Postsurgical
Postirradiation

Sodium Retention

Excessive salt intake with renal insufficiency
Increased tubular reabsorption of sodium
   Renal hypoperfusion
   Increased renin-angiotensin-aldosterone secretion

Inflammation

   Acute inflammation
   Chronic inflammation
   Angiogenesis

Modified from Leaf A, Cotran RS: Renal Pathophysiology, 3rd ed. New York, Oxford University Press, 1985, p 146.

Morphology (p. 116)

Edema is most easily recognized grossly; microscopically, edema manifests only as subtle cell swelling, with separation of the extracellular matrix.

- *Subcutaneous edema* may be diffuse or occur primarily at the sites of highest hydrostatic pressures (e.g., influenced by gravity, so-called *dependent edema* [legs when standing, sacrum when recumbent]). Dependent edema is typical of CHF. Edema resulting from hypoproteinemia is generally more severe and affects all parts of the body; it is often prominent in loose connective tissue matrix, such as the eyelids, causing *periorbital edema*.
- *Edema of solid organs* results in an increase in size and weight. Separation of parenchymal elements occurs.

- *Pulmonary edema* (p. 700) is typical in left ventricular failure but is also seen with renal failure, adult respiratory distress syndrome (p. 700), infections, and hypersensitivity reactions. The lungs are two to three times normal weight; sectioning reveals a frothy, blood-tinged mixture of air, edema fluid, and erythrocytes.
- *Brain edema* may be localized to sites of injury (e.g., abscess or neoplasm) or may be generalized, as in encephalitis, hypertensive crises, or obstruction to venous outflow. When generalized, the brain is grossly swollen with narrowed sulci and distended gyri flattened against the skull.

HYPEREMIA AND CONGESTION
(p. 116)

The terms *hyperemia* and *congestion* both mean increased volume of blood in a particular site. *Hyperemia* is an *active process* with augmented blood inflow caused by arteriolar dilation (e.g., skeletal muscle during exercise or at sites of inflammation). Tissues are redder owing to engorgement with oxygenated blood. *Congestion* is a *passive process* caused by impaired outflow from a tissue. Isolated venous obstruction may cause local congestion; systemic venous obstruction occurs in CHF (p. 546). Tissues acquire a blue-red color (*cyanosis*), particularly as worsening congestion leads to accumulated deoxygenated hemoglobin. Longstanding stasis of deoxygenated blood can result in hypoxia severe enough to cause cell death.

Morphology (p. 116)

In *acute congestion*, vessels are distended, and organs are grossly hyperemic. *Capillary bed congestion is also commonly associated with interstitial edema.* In *chronic congestion*, capillary rupture may cause focal hemorrhage; breakdown of erythrocytes at these sites leaves residua of hemosiderin-laden macrophages. Parenchymal cell atrophy or death (with scarring) may also be present. Grossly, tissues may appear brown, with contraction and fibrosis. Commonly affected organs include the lungs and liver.

- The *lungs* are typically involved in left ventricular failure (i.e., myocardial infarction, cardiomyopathy, mitral valve disease). Acutely, engorged capillaries and septal edema are seen, with transudate in the airspaces. Chronically, hemosiderin-laden macrophages *(heart failure cells)* are seen, with edematous to fibrotic septa *(brown induration)*.
- The *liver* is typically involved in right heart failure or rarely with hepatic vein or superior vena cava obstruction. Acutely, there is distention of central veins and sinusoids; central hepatocyte degeneration may also be present. Chronically the central regions of the hepatic lobules are grossly red-brown and slightly depressed (loss of cells) relative to the surrounding uncongested tan liver (so-called *nutmeg liver*). Microscopically, there is *centrilobular necrosis* with hepatocyte drop-out and hemorrhage including hemosiderin-laden macrophages. In severe, longstanding congestion, there may even be hepatic fibrosis *(cardiac cirrhosis)*. Because the central portion of the hepatic lobule is the last to receive blood, centrilobular necrosis can occur whenever hepatic perfusion is reduced; previous hepatic congestion is not a prerequisite.

HEMORRHAGE (p. 117)

Hemorrhage refers to extravasation of blood because of vessel rupture. Rupture of a large artery or vein is usually due to vascular injury, such as from trauma, atherosclerosis, or inflammatory or neoplastic erosion of the vessel. Capillary bleeding can occur with chronic congestion. A tendency to hemorrhage from insignificant injury is seen in a variety of disorders called *hemorrhagic diatheses* (p. 633). Hemorrhage may be external or enclosed within a tissue; the latter is called a *hematoma*. Hematomas may be trivial (e.g., a bruise) or may accumulate sufficient blood to cause death (e.g., a massive retroperitoneal hematoma resulting from rupture of an aortic aneurysm). Hemorrhage is grouped roughly according to size:

- *Petechiae*: Minute 1- to 2-mm hemorrhages in skin, mucous membranes, or serosal surfaces. Petechiae occur with increased intravascular pressure, low platelet counts *(thrombocytopenia)*, defective platelet function, and clotting factor deficits.
- *Purpura*: Larger ($\geq$ 3 mm) hemorrhages. Purpuric lesions are associated with similar pathologies as well as trauma, local vascular inflammation *(vasculitis)*, and increased vascular fragility (e.g., in amyloidosis).
- *Ecchymoses*: Larger (> 1 to 2 cm) subcutaneous hematomas (commonly called *bruises*). Ecchymoses typically follow trauma but may be exacerbated by any of the aforementioned conditions.
- Large accumulations of blood in body cavities are called *hemothorax, hemopericardium, hemoperitoneum*, or *hemarthrosis*, depending on the location.

Erythrocytes in these lesions are degraded by macrophages. The hemoglobin (red-blue color) is converted to bilirubin and biliverdin (blue-green color) and eventually to hemosiderin (golden brown), accounting for the characteristic color changes in a bruise. Patients with extensive hemorrhages occasionally develop jaundice from the massive red cell breakdown and systemic release of bilirubin.

The clinical significance of hemorrhage depends on the volume and rate of blood loss. Rapid loss of up to 20% of the blood or slow losses of even larger amounts may have little impact; greater losses result in *hemorrhagic (hypovolemic) shock*. Location is also important: Bleeding that would be trivial in the subcutaneous tissues may cause death when present in the brain.

HEMOSTASIS AND THROMBOSIS

(p. 119)

Hemostasis and thrombosis are closely related processes, both dependent on three components: *the vascular endothelium, platelets, and the coagulation cascade. Hemostasis is a normal physiologic process* maintaining blood in a fluid, clot-free state in normal vessels and inducing a rapid and localized hemostatic plug at sites of vascular injury. *Thrombosis represents a pathologic state*; it is inappropriate activation of hemostatic mechanisms in uninjured vasculature or thrombotic occlusion of a vessel after relatively minor injury.

Normal Hemostasis (p. 119)

The general sequence of events in hemostasis after injury is as follows:

1. Transient reflex neurogenic arteriolar vasoconstriction occurs, augmented by *endothelin* (a potent endothelium-derived vasoconstrictor).

2. In *primary hemostasis*, exposed subendothelial extracellular matrix allows platelet adhesion and *activation* (shape change and secretory granule release). Secreted products recruit other platelets to form a *temporary hemostatic plug*.

3. In *secondary hemostasis*, injury also exposes *tissue factor*, a membrane-bound procoagulant factor synthesized by endothelium. Tissue factor activates the coagulation cascade (p. 122), resulting in *thrombin* generation and conversion of circulating fibrinogen to insoluble *fibrin*. Thrombin induces further platelet recruitment and granule release. Polymerized fibrin and platelet aggregates form a solid, *permanent plug*.

4. At this stage, counter-regulatory mechanisms (e.g., tissue plasminogen activator [t-PA]) are set into motion to restrict the hemostatic plug to the site of injury.

ENDOTHELIUM

Endothelium modulates several, frequently opposing, aspects of hemostasis. Endothelial cells normally exhibit antiplatelet, anticoagulant, and fibrinolytic properties, yet after injury or activation, these cells can exhibit *procoagulant function* (Fig. 5–1). The balance between endothelial antithrombotic and prothrombotic ac-

ANTITHROMBOTIC	PROTHROMBOTIC
Inhibition of Platelet Aggregation	Stimulation of Platelet Aggregation Adhesion
• PGI_2 • NO • ADPase	• von Willebrand's factor • Platelet-activating factor (PAF)
Anticoagulant—Binding and Inhibition of Thrombin	Procoagulation Factors
• Antithrombin III acceleration by heparin-like molecules • Thrombomodulin activation of protein C/S • alpha$_2$-macroglobulin	• Tissue factor • Binding factors IXa, Xa • Factor V
Fibrinolysis	Inhibition of Fibrinolysis
• Tissue plasminogen activator (t-PA)	• (t-PA) inhibitor

Figure 5–1   ∎

The endothelial thrombotic-antithrombotic balance. Major factors favoring and inhibiting thrombosis are shown. (From Cotran RS, Kumar V, Collins T: Robbins Pathologic Basis of Disease, 5th ed. Philadelphia, WB Saunders, 1994, p 100.)

tivities determines whether thrombus formation, propagation, or dissolution occurs.

PLATELETS

Platelets play a central role in normal hemostasis and thrombosis. With vascular injury, platelets encounter extracellular matrix constituents (collagen, proteoglycans, fibronectin, and other adhesive glycoproteins) normally sequestered beneath an intact endothelium. Platelets then undergo *activation* involving adhesion and shape change, secretion (release reaction), and aggregation.

- *Adhesion* to extracellular matrix is mediated largely by von Willebrand factor, which acts as a bridge between platelet surface receptors (mostly glycoprotein Ib) and exposed collagen. Genetic deficiencies of von Willebrand factor (von Willebrand disease) or of its glycoprotein-Ib receptor (Bernard-Soulier syndrome) result in bleeding disorders.
- *Secretion* of the contents of platelet granules occurs soon after adhesion. Platelets have two granule types: *Alpha granules* express the adhesion molecule P-selectin and contain coagulation and growth factors; *dense bodies* or *delta granules* contain adenosine nucleotides (adenosine diphosphate [ADP] and adenosine triphosphate [ATP]), calcium, and vasoactive amines (e.g., histamine). Calcium is an important cofactor in the coagulation cascade, and ADP is a potent mediator of *platelet aggregation*. The release reaction also results in surface expression of *phospholipid complex*, providing a site for calcium and coagulation factor binding in the *intrinsic clotting cascade*.
- *Platelet aggregation* (platelets adhering to other platelets) is promoted by ADP and the platelet vasoconstrictor product thromboxane A_2 (p. 70). Platelet aggregation creates the *primary hemostatic plug*, which is reversible. Activation of the coagulation cascade generates *thrombin* and *fibrin*, which act to form an irreversibly fused mass of platelets and fibrin constituting the definitive *secondary hemostatic plug*. Erythrocytes and leukocytes are also found in hemostatic plugs. Leukocytes adhere to platelets via P-selectin and to endothelium using a number of adhesion receptors; they contribute to the inflammatory response that accompanies thrombosis.

Note: The endothelial-derived prostaglandin I_2 (p. 70) inhibits platelet aggregation and is a potent vasodilator; the platelet-derived prostaglandin thromboxane A_2 activates platelet aggregation and is a potent vasoconstrictor. The interplay of prostaglandin I_2 and thromboxane A_2 is therefore an exquisitely balanced mechanism for modulating human platelet function.

COAGULATION CASCADE

The coagulation cascade is a sequence of conversions of inactive proenzymes into activated enzymes, culminating in the generation of insoluble *fibrin* from the soluble plasma protein *fibrinogen*. Traditionally, coagulation has been divided into *extrinsic* and *intrinsic* pathways, converging where factor X is activated (Fig. 5–2). The intrinsic cascade is classically initiated by activation of Hageman factor (factor XII), whereas the extrinsic cascade is activated by *tissue factor*, a cellular lipoprotein exposed at sites of tissue injury. This division is largely an artifact of in vitro testing, and there is a rather broad overlap between the two pathways.

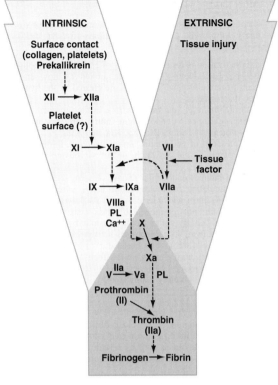

Figure 5–2   ■

The coagulation cascade. Note the common link between the intrinsic and extrinsic pathways at the level of factor IX activation. Activated factors are indicated with a lower case *a*. The anticoagulant inhibitory pathways are not shown. PL, phospholipid surface. (From Kumar V, Cotran RS, Robbins SL: Basic Pathology, 5th ed. Philadelphia, WB Saunders, 1994.)

Each step in a pathway results from a complex composed of an *enzyme* (activated coagulation factor), a *substrate* (proenzyme form of coagulation factor), and a *cofactor* (reaction accelerator), all held together by *calcium ions* on a *phospholipid complex*. Thus, clotting tends to remain localized to sites where such an assembly can occur (e.g., the surface of activated platelets or endothelium).

Besides catalyzing the final steps of the cascade, thrombin also exerts a wide variety of effects on the local vasculature and inflammatory cells; it even limits the extent of hemostasis (see later). Most of these effects are induced via *thrombin receptors*, seven-transmembrane spanner proteins. One end of the receptor is clipped by thrombin to yield a *tethered* peptide; this peptide binds to another site on the receptor and causes a conformational change that activates an associated G protein. This catalytic activity explains the impressive potency of even relatively small amounts of thrombin.

CONTROL MECHANISMS

Once activated, coagulation must be restricted to sites of vascular injury to prevent clotting of the entire vascular tree (see Fig. 5–1):

- Factor activation is restricted to sites of exposed phospholipids. Also, activated clotting factors are diluted by flow at sites distant from the original injury and are cleared by the liver and tissue macrophages.
- Antithrombins (e.g., *antithrombin III*), in the presence of heparin-like molecules on endothelium, inhibit thrombin and other serine proteases—factors IXa, Xa, XIa, and XIIa.
- In the presence of endothelial *thrombomodulin*, thrombin activates *proteins C and S*, which, in turn, inactivate factors Va and VIIIa.
- Thrombin induces endothelial release of t-PA, which converts inactive circulating *plasminogen* into active *plasmin*. Plasmin breaks down fibrin and interferes with its polymerization; the resulting *fibrin split products* also act as weak anticoagulants. Plasminogen can be converted to plasmin by a factor XII–dependent pathway. The functional activity of plasmin is restricted to sites of thrombosis because
  1. t-PA activates plasminogen most effectively when bound to fibrin meshwork.
  2. Free plasmin is rapidly neutralized by serum α_2-plasmin inhibitor.
  3. t-PA activity is blocked by *plasminogen activator inhibitor*.
- Endothelium modulates anticoagulation by releasing plasminogen activator inhibitors; these block fibrinolysis by inhibiting t-PA binding to fibrin. Plasminogen activator inhibitors are increased by thrombin as well as certain cytokines; they may cause the intravascular thrombosis accompanying severe inflammation.

Thrombosis (p. 124)

Thrombosis refers to inappropriate activation of blood clotting in uninjured vasculature or thrombotic occlusion of a vessel after relatively minor injury. Three primary influences on thrombus formation, so-called *Virchow's triad*, are as follows:

1. *Endothelial injury* is dominant and by itself can cause thrombosis, especially in the heart and arterial circulation (e.g., myocardial infarction, endocarditis, or ulcerated atherosclerotic plaque). Injury may occur from diverse causes, including hemodynamic stress (e.g., hypertension or turbulent flow over scarred valves), bacterial endotoxins, homocystinuria, hypercholesterolemia, radiation, or products absorbed from cigarette smoke. Thrombosis results from exposed subendothelial extracellular matrix and tissue factor, adherence of platelets, and depletion of prostaglandin I_2 and plasminogen activator inhibitors.
2. *Alterations occur in normal blood flow.* Normal blood flow is *laminar* (i.e., the cellular elements flow centrally in the vessel lumen, separated from endothelium by a clear zone of plasma). Stasis and turbulence (the latter forms eddy currents with local pockets of stasis):
   - ❏ Disrupt laminar flow and bring platelets into contact with the endothelium
   - ❏ Prevent dilution of activated clotting factors by fresh flowing blood

❑ Retard the inflow of clotting factor inhibitors and permit the build-up of thrombi
❑ Promote endothelial cell activation.

Stasis is important in causing thrombosis in the venous circulation, cardiac chambers, and arterial aneurysms; turbulence in the arterial circulation also directly causes endothelial injury and dysfunction. Hyperviscosity syndromes (e.g., *polycythemia*) or deformed erythrocytes (e.g., *sickle cell anemia*) result in small vessel stasis and also predispose to thrombosis.

3. *Hypercoagulability* contributes less frequently to thrombotic states but is an important component in certain conditions; it is loosely defined as any alteration of the coagulation pathways that predisposes to thrombosis (Table 5–2).

Of the heritable hypercoagulable states, factor V gene mutations are the most common; 2 to 15% of the white population (60% of patients with recurrent deep vein thrombosis) carry a mutation (called the *Leiden mutation*) that renders their factor V resistant to cleavage by activated protein C. Others with inherited lack of anticoagulants (e.g., antithrombin III, protein C, or protein S) also typically present with venous thrombosis and recurrent thromboembolism.

Acquired thrombotic diatheses have diverse causes. With oral contraceptive use or the hyperestrogenic state of pregnancy, hypercoagulability may result from increased hepatic synthesis of coagulation factors and reduced synthesis of antithrombin III. In disseminated cancers, release of procoagulant tumor products predisposes to thrombosis. In the *heparin-induced thrombocytopenia syndrome*, administration of unfractionated heparin induces circulating antibodies that cause platelet activation and endothelial cell injury. In the *antiphospholipid antibody syndrome*, patients have antibodies

Table 5–2.   HYPERCOAGULABLE STATES

Primary (Genetic)
Mutations in factor V
Antithrombin III deficiency
Protein C or S deficiency
Fibrinolysis defects
Homocysteinemia
Secondary (Acquired)
High risk for thrombosis
   Prolonged bed rest or immobilization
   Myocardial infarction
   Tissue damage (surgery, fracture, burns)
   Cancer
   Prosthetic cardiac valves
   Disseminated intravascular coagulation
   Heparin-induced thrombocytopenia
   Antiphospholipid antibody syndrome (lupus anticoagulant syndrome)
Lower risk for thrombosis
   Atrial fibrillation
   Cardiomyopathy
   Nephrotic syndrome
   Hyperestrogenic states
   Oral contraceptive use
   Sickle cell anemia
   Smoking

against anionic phospholipids, which presumably cause similar platelet activation; such patients may have a well-defined autoimmune disease, such as systemic lupus erythematosus (i.e., *lupus anticoagulant syndrome*), or may exhibit only the manifestations of a hypercoagulable state.

MORPHOLOGY OF THROMBI (p. 126)

Thrombi may form anywhere in the cardiovascular system. Aortic or cardiac thrombi are typically *nonocclusive (mural)* as a result of rapid and high-volume flow; smaller arterial thrombi may be *occlusive*. All these thrombi usually begin at sites of endothelial injury (e.g., atherosclerotic plaque) or turbulence (vessel bifurcation). Venous thrombi characteristically occur in sites of stasis and are *occlusive*.

At sites of origin, thrombi are generally firmly attached. Arterial thrombi tend to extend retrograde from the attachment point, whereas venous thrombi extend in the direction of blood flow. The propagating tail may not be well attached and may fragment to create an *embolus*.

Cardiac and arterial thrombi are gray-red and tend to have gross and microscopic laminations (*lines of Zahn*) produced by pale layers of platelets and fibrin alternating with darker red cell-rich layers. Major sites include the left ventricle overlying an infarct, ruptured atherosclerotic plaques, and aneurysmal sacs.

Venous thrombosis *(phlebothrombosis)* often creates a long red-blue cast of the vein lumen because it occurs in a relatively static environment, and the thrombus contains more enmeshed erythrocytes among sparse fibrin strands (*red* or *stasis thrombi*). Fibrin and attachment to the vessel wall distinguish stasis thrombi from postmortem clots. Phlebothrombosis most commonly affects the veins of the lower extremities ($> 90\%$ of cases).

Thrombi may also form on heart valves. In *infective endocarditis,* bacteria or fungi form large infected thrombotic masses (*vegetations*), causing underlying valve damage and systemic infection. Sterile vegetations *(nonbacterial thrombotic endocarditis)* can also develop on noninfected valves in patients with hypercoagulable states, particularly in those with disseminated cancer. Uncommonly, noninfective, *verrucous (Libman-Sacks) endocarditis* occurs in patients with systemic lupus erythematosus (owing to circulating immune complexes).

FATE OF THE THROMBUS

If a patient survives the immediate (generally ischemic or venous obstructive) effects of a thrombus, some combination of the following occurs:

- *Propagation,* causing complete vessel obstruction
- *Embolization* to other sites in the vasculature, particularly to the lungs with venous thrombi
- *Dissolution* by fibrinolytic activity
- *Organization and recanalization,* re-establishing vascular flow by ingrowth of endothelial cells, smooth muscle cells, and fibroblasts to create through-and-through capillary channels or by incorporating the thrombus as a subendothelial swelling of the vessel wall

Rarely, when bacterial seeding of a degrading thrombus occurs, a *mycotic aneurysm* may result.

CLINICAL SIGNIFICANCE (p. 129)

Thrombi are significant because

1. *They cause obstruction of arteries and veins.*
2. *They are possible sources of emboli.*

The particular relevance of each depends on the site of thrombosis. Thus, although venous thrombi may cause congestion and edema in distal vascular beds, a more dire consequence is that such thrombi (e.g., in deep leg veins) can result in pulmonary embolism and death. Conversely, although arterial thrombi can embolize, their role in local vascular obstruction (e.g., in causing myocardial or cerebral infarctions) is much more important.

Venous Thrombosis (Phlebothrombosis)

In most instances, venous thrombosis occurs in the superficial or deep leg veins.

- Superficial thrombi usually occur in varicose saphenous veins, where they cause local congestion and pain but rarely embolize. Local edema and impaired venous drainage can predispose to skin infections and to *varicose ulcers.*
- *Deep thrombi* in larger leg veins typically above the knee (e.g., popliteal, femoral, and iliac veins) more readily embolize. Although they may also cause pain and edema, the venous obstruction is usually offset by collateral flow. Thus, deep vein thromboses are entirely asymptomatic in *approximately 50% of affected patients* and are recognized only after embolization to the lungs.
- Deep venous thrombosis occurs in a variety of clinical settings:

  1. Advanced age, bed rest, or immobilization, which diminishes the milking action of muscles in the lower leg and slows venous return
  2. CHF
  3. Trauma, surgery, and burns resulting in reduced physical activity, injury to vessels, release of procoagulant substances from tissues, or reduced tPA
  4. The puerperal and postpartum states, which are associated with amniotic fluid embolization (see later) and hypercoagulability
  5. Tumor-associated procoagulant release, which causes the thromboses seen in disseminated cancers (*migratory thrombophlebitis* or *Trousseau syndrome*) and which may affect multiple sites simultaneously or sequentially

Arterial Thrombosis

Besides the obstructive consequences of arterial thrombi, cardiac and aortic mural thrombi can also embolize peripherally; the brain, kidneys, and spleen are prime targets. *Myocardial infarction* with dyskinesis and endocardial damage may result in mural thrombus. *Rheumatic valvular disease* can cause mitral valve stenosis, followed by left atrial dilation and thrombus formation within the atrium or auricular appendages; concurrent atrial fibrillation augments atrial blood stasis. *Atherosclerosis* is a major cause of arterial thrombi, related to abnormal vascular flow and loss of endothelial integrity.

Disseminated Intravascular Coagulation

Disseminated intravascular coagulation refers to widespread fibrin thrombi in the microcirculation, caused by a variety of disorders ranging from obstetric complications to advanced malignancy. Disseminated intravascular coagulation is not a primary disease but rather a complication of any diffuse activation of thrombin. The microthrombi can cause diffuse circulatory insufficiency, particularly in the brain, lungs, heart, and kidneys; in addition, there is a rapid concurrent consumption of platelets and coagulation factors (*consumption coagulopathy*) as well as activation of fibrinolysis, which can evolve into serious bleeding. Disseminated intravascular coagulation is discussed in greater detail along with the bleeding diatheses (p. 640).

EMBOLISM (p. 129)

Embolism refers to any intravascular solid, liquid, or gaseous mass carried by the blood to a site distant from its point of origin. Most (99%) arise from thrombi, hence the term *thromboembolism*; unless otherwise specified, embolism should be considered to be thrombotic in origin. Other forms include droplets of fat, gas bubbles, atherosclerotic debris (*atheroemboli*), tumor fragments, bone marrow, or foreign bodies such as bullets. Emboli lodge in vessels too small to permit further passage, resulting in partial or complete vascular occlusion and ischemic necrosis of distal tissue (*infarction*).

Pulmonary Thromboembolism (p. 130)

Pulmonary embolism has an incidence of 20 to 25 per 100,000 hospitalized patients, causing about 200,000 deaths per year in the United States. In more than 95%, pulmonary emboli originate from deep leg vein thrombi; depending on the size, a pulmonary embolus (PE) may occlude the main pulmonary artery, impact across the bifurcation (*saddle embolus*), or pass into smaller arterioles. Multiple emboli may occur, either sequentially or as a shower of small emboli from a single large mass; in general, *one PE puts a patient at risk for more*. Rarely, emboli pass through atrial or ventricular defects into the systemic circulation (*paradoxical embolism*).

- Most PEs (60 to 80%) are small and clinically silent. They eventually organize and get incorporated into the vessel wall or leave a delicate, bridging fibrous *web*. Embolic obstruction of small end-arteriolar pulmonary branches may cause infarction.
- Embolic obstruction of medium-sized arteries may result in pulmonary hemorrhage but usually does not cause pulmonary infarction because of collateral bronchial artery blood flow. In the setting of left-sided cardiac failure (with sluggish bronchial artery flow), infarcts may result.
- Sudden death, right heart failure (*cor pulmonale*), or cardiovascular collapse occurs when 60% or more of the pulmonary circulation is obstructed with emboli. Multiple emboli over time may cause pulmonary hypertension with right heart failure.

A more complete discussion of PEs is presented in the Lung Pathology chapter (p. 703).

Systemic Thromboembolism (p. 130)

Systemic thromboembolism refers to emboli in the arterial circulation. Some 80% arise from intracardiac mural thrombi; two thirds are secondary to myocardial infarcts, and 25% arise from within dilated left atria (e.g., owing to rheumatic valvular disease). The remainder of systemic emboli originate from aortic aneurysms, thrombi on ulcerated atherosclerotic plaques, or valvular vegetations and only rarely from paradoxical emboli. About 10% of systemic emboli are of unknown origin. Major sites for arteriolar embolization are the lower extremities (75%), brain (10%), viscera (10%), and upper extremities (5%). Consequences of systemic emboli depend on collateral vascular supplies, tissue vulnerability to ischemia, and vessel caliber; usually, arterial emboli cause distal infarction.

Fat Embolism (p. 130)

After thromboembolism, fat embolism is the most common form of embolism. Fat embolism occurs as a result of microscopic fat globules; it occurs after fractures of long bones or, rarely, with burns or soft tissue trauma. Fat embolism occurs in 90% of severe skeletal injuries, but fewer than 10% have any clinical findings. *Fat embolism syndrome*, fatal in up to 10% of cases, is heralded by sudden pulmonary insufficiency beginning 1 to 3 days after injury; 20 to 50% of patients have a diffuse petechial rash. Patients may have neurologic symptoms (irritability and restlessness), which can progress to delirium or coma. Thrombocytopenia and anemia may also occur.

Pathogenesis involves mechanical obstruction by microemboli of neutral fat, followed by local platelet and erythrocyte aggregation. Subsequent free fatty acid release causes toxic injury to endothelium; platelet activation and granulocyte recruitment (free radicals, proteases, and eicosanoids) contribute.

Diagnosis depends on identifying microvascular fat globules. Because lipids are dissolved out of tissue by routinely used solvents, documentation requires frozen sections and special fat stains. Associated edema and hemorrhage (and hyaline membranes in lungs) may also be seen microscopically.

Air Embolism (p. 131)

Air embolism refers to gas bubbles within the circulation obstructing vascular flow and causing ischemia. Air may enter the circulation during obstetric procedures or as a consequence of chest wall injury; generally more than 100 cc are required to have a clinical effect.

Decompression sickness is a special form of air embolism caused by sudden changes in atmospheric pressure; scuba and deep-sea divers and individuals in unpressurized aircraft in rapid ascent are at risk. Air breathed at high pressure (e.g., during a deep-sea dive) causes increasing amounts of gas (particularly nitrogen) to be dissolved in blood and tissues. Subsequent rapid ascent (depressurization) allows the dissolved gases to expand and bubble out of solution to form gas emboli.

Formation of gas bubbles in skeletal muscles and joints causes a painful condition called *the bends*. In lungs, edema, hemorrhage, and focal emphysema lead to respiratory distress, the so-called *chokes*. Gas emboli may also cause focal ischemia in a number of tissues, including brain and heart. Treatment consists of repressurizing the individual and forcing the gas bubbles back into solution, followed by subsequent slow decompression.

A more chronic form of decompression sickness is called *cais-

son disease; persistent gas emboli in the normally poorly vascularized portions of the skeleton (heads of the femurs, tibia, and humeri) lead to multiple foci of ischemic necrosis.

Amniotic Fluid Embolism (p. 131)

Amniotic fluid embolism is a serious (mortality rate > 80%) but uncommon (1 in 50,000 deliveries) complication of labor and the immediate postpartum period caused by amniotic fluid infusion into the maternal circulation. Classic findings include fetal squamous cells and mucin, lanugo hair, and vernix caseosa fat in the maternal pulmonary microcirculation. The syndrome is characterized by sudden severe dyspnea, cyanosis, and hypotensive shock, followed by seizures and coma. If the patient survives the initial crisis, pulmonary edema occurs; disseminated intravascular coagulation may ensue, owing to release of thrombogenic substances from amniotic fluid.

INFARCTION (p. 132)

Infarction refers to an area of ischemic necrosis usually caused by occlusion of the arterial supply (97% of cases). Almost all infarcts result from thrombotic or embolic events, although rarely there are other causes (e.g., vasospasm; extrinsic compression of a vessel by tumor, edema, or entrapment in a hernia sac; and twisting of vessels, such as testicular torsion or bowel volvulus); traumatic vessel rupture is a rare cause.

Occluded venous drainage (e.g., venous thrombosis) can cause infarction but more often induces congestion only; usually, bypass channels rapidly open, providing outflow. Infarcts resulting from venous thrombosis are more likely in organs with a single venous outflow, such as testis or ovary.

Factors That Influence Development of an Infarct (p. 133)

The effects of vascular occlusion can range from none to death of a tissue or even the individual. *The major determinants of outcome* are as follows:

- *Anatomic pattern of vascular supply* (i.e., availability of an alternative blood supply): Dual circulations (lung, liver) or anastomosing circulations (radial and ulnar arteries, circle of Willis, small intestine) protect against infarction. Obstruction of end-arterial vessels generally causes infarction (spleen, kidneys).
- *Rate of development of occlusion*: Slowly developing occlusions less often cause infarction by providing time to develop alternate perfusion pathways (e.g., collateral coronary circulation).
- *Vulnerability to hypoxia*: Neurons undergo irreversible damage after 3 to 4 minutes of ischemia; myocardial cells die only after 20 to 30 minutes. In contrast, fibroblasts within ischemic myocardium are viable even after many hours.
- *Oxygen content of blood*: Anemia, cyanosis, or CHF (with hypoxia) can cause infarction in an otherwise inconsequential blockage.

Morphology (p. 132)

Infarcts may be either *red (hemorrhagic)* or *white (pale, anemic)* and may be either *septic* or *bland.*

■ *Red infarcts* occur
   1. In venous occlusions (e.g., ovarian torsion)
   2. In loose tissues (such as lung)
   3. In tissues with dual circulations (e.g., lung and small intestine)
   4. In tissues previously congested because of sluggish venous outflow
   5. At a site of previous occlusion and necrosis when flow is re-established.
■ *White infarcts* occur in solid organs (such as heart, spleen, and kidney) with end-arterial circulations (i.e., few anastomoses).

All infarcts tend to be wedge-shaped; the occluded vessel marks the apex, and the organ periphery forms the base. Lateral margins may be irregular, reflecting the pattern of adjacent vascular supply. The dominant histologic characteristic of infarction is *ischemic coagulative necrosis*. An initial inflammatory response (lasting hours to days) is followed by a reparative response (lasting days to weeks) beginning in the preserved margins (p. 78). In stable or labile tissues, some parenchymal regeneration may occur where the underlying stromal architecture is spared; most infarcts are ultimately replaced by scar tissue. The brain is an exception; ischemic injury results in *liquefactive necrosis* (p. 17). Septic infarctions occur with embolization of infected heart valve vegetations or when microbes seed an area of necrosis; the infarct becomes an *abscess*, which only slowly organizes to scar.

SHOCK (p. 134)

Shock is systemic hypoperfusion resulting from reduction in either cardiac output or the effective circulating blood volume. This reduction results in *hypotension, followed by impaired tissue perfusion and cellular hypoxia.* Shock is the final common pathway for many lethal events, including severe hemorrhage, extensive trauma, large myocardial infarction, massive pulmonary embolism, and sepsis.

Shock is grouped into three major categories (Table 5–3). The basic mechanism underlying *cardiogenic* and *hypovolemic shock* is *low cardiac output. Septic shock* is caused by systemic microbial infection and has a more complicated pathogenesis (see below). Rarer causes of shock are *neurogenic*, with loss of vascular tone and peripheral pooling (anesthetic accident or spinal cord injury), and *anaphylactic*, with systemic vasodilation and increased vascular permeability (IgE-mediated hypersensitivity, p. 196).

Septic Shock (p. 134)

With a 25 to 75% mortality rate and 100,000 deaths annually in the United States, septic shock ranks first among the causes of death in intensive care units. The incidence is increasing (greater than twofold increase between 1979 and 1987) as a result of improved life support for high-risk patients who survive major crises only later to develop shock, increasing use of invasive

Table 5-3. THREE MAJOR TYPES OF SHOCK

Type of Shock	Clinical Examples	Principal Mechanisms
Cardiogenic	Myocardial infarction Ventricular rupture Arrhythmia Cardiac tamponade Pulmonary embolism	Failure of myocardial pump owing to intrinsic myocardial damage, extrinsic pressure, or obstruction to outflow
Hypovolemic	Hemorrhage Fluid loss, e.g., vomiting, diarrhea, burns, or trauma	Inadequate blood or plasma volume
Septic	Overwhelming microbial infections; endotoxic shock, gram-positive septicemia, or fungal sepsis; superantigens	Peripheral vasodilation and pooling of blood; endothelial activation and injury; leukocyte-induced damage; disseminated intravascular coagulation; activation of cytokine cascades

procedures, and more immunocompromised hosts vulnerable to infections.

Most cases of septic shock (70%) are caused by gram-negative bacilli expressing endotoxin *(endotoxic shock)*. Endotoxins are bacterial lipopolysaccharides (LPS) released when cell walls are degraded. LPS consists of a toxic fatty acid *(lipid A)* core and a complex polysaccharide coat. Analogous molecules in the walls of gram-positive bacteria and fungi can also elicit septic shock.

All of the effects of septic shock are reproduced by LPS alone. LPS binds (as a complex with a normal serum protein) to CD14 molecules on leukocytes (especially monocytes and macrophages), endothelial cells, and other cell types. Depending on dosage, the LPS conjugate activates vascular wall cells and leukocytes, induces cytokine mediators, or does both.

At *low doses*, LPS mainly activates complement and monocyte/macrophages, leading to enhanced bacterial eradication. Mononuclear phagocytes respond to LPS by producing tumor necrosis factor (TNF), which then induces interleukin-1 (IL-1) synthesis. TNF and IL-1 act on endothelial cells to produce further cytokines (e.g., IL-6 and IL-8) as well as induce adhesion molecules (p. 73). Thus, low-dose LPS results in a cytokine cascade, which augments *local* acute inflammation and improves microbe clearance.

With *moderate infections* and higher LPS levels, cytokine-induced secondary effectors (e.g., nitric oxide, p. 75 and platelet-activating factor, p. 72) become significant. Also, systemic effects of TNF and IL-1 are seen (e.g., fever and synthesis of acute-phase reactants). Higher-dose LPS also directly injures endothelial cells, triggering the coagulation cascade.

With *severe infection* (and high LPS levels), septic shock supervenes; high-dose cytokines and secondary mediators cause

- Systemic vasodilation (hypotension)
- Diminished myocardial contractility
- Widespread endothelial injury and activation, with systemic leukocyte adhesion and pulmonary alveolar capillary damage *(adult respiratory distress syndrome*, p. 700)
- Activation of the coagulation system, culminating in disseminated intravascular coagulation

The resulting hypoperfusion causes *multiorgan system failure* affecting the liver, kidneys, and central nervous system. Unless the underlying infection (and LPS overload) is brought under control, the patient usually dies. Certain bacterial proteins, called *superantigens*, are polyclonal T-lymphocyte activators; these induce systemic cytokine cascades (and clinical syndromes) similar to those occurring in septic shock (e.g., *toxic shock syndrome*).

Morphology (p. 136)

Cell and tissue changes occurring in shock of any form are essentially those of hypoxic injury and are nonspecific; particularly affected are the brain, heart, lungs, kidneys, adrenals, and gastrointestinal tract. With the exception of neuronal and myocyte loss, virtually all tissues may recover if the patient survives.

- The *brain* may show hypoxic encephalopathy (p. 1307).
- The *heart* shows areas of coagulation necrosis, with subendocardial hemorrhage, *contraction band necrosis*, or both kinds of necrosis (p. 554).
- The *kidneys* develop extensive tubular ischemic injury (*acute*

tubular necrosis, p. 969), causing oliguria, anuria, and electrolyte disturbances.

- The *lungs* are seldom affected in pure hypovolemic shock; however, diffuse alveolar damage (*shock lung*, p. 700) may occur in septic or traumatic shock.

Clinical Correlations (p. 137)

Shock of any cause evolves through three general phases:

1. Initial *nonprogressive* phase, in which reflex compensatory pathways (tachycardia, peripheral vasoconstriction, and renal conservation of fluid) are activated, and perfusion of vital organs (heart, brain) is maintained. Cutaneous vasoconstriction, for example, causes the pale, clammy skin of shock (although septic shock may initially cause warm, flushed skin as a result of vasodilation).

2. *Progressive stage*, characterized by tissue hypoperfusion and metabolic imbalances, including acidosis (owing to anaerobic glycolysis with lactic acid production as well as renal failure). Acidosis blunts the vasomotor response, dilating arterioles and causing blood to pool in the microcirculation. Peripheral pooling worsens the cardiac output and exacerbates endothelial anoxia, resulting in disseminated intravascular coagulation. Clinically the patient becomes confused, and urinary output declines.

3. *Irreversible stage*, after the body has incurred cellular and tissue injury so severe that even if the hemodynamic defects are corrected, survival is not possible. Widespread cell injury is reflected in lysosomal leakage. If ischemic bowel allows intestinal flora to enter the circulation, endotoxic shock may be superimposed.

The prognosis varies with the cause and duration of shock; treatment targets the underlying cause but is otherwise largely supportive. Most (80 to 90%) young, healthy patients with hypovolemic shock survive with appropriate management. Cardiogenic shock associated with extensive myocardial infarction and septic shock, however, have mortality rates of up to 75%.

Genetic Disorders

CLASSIFICATION

Genetic disorders can be classified as follows:

1. Mendelian disorders
2. Multifactorial disorders
3. Single-gene disorders with nonclassic inheritance
4. Chromosomal (cytogenetic) disorders

MENDELIAN DISORDERS (p. 143)

Mendelian disorders result from mutations in single genes of large effect.

DEFINITIONS

Penetrance   The percentage of individuals carrying an autosomal dominant gene and expressing the trait.

Variable expressivity   Variable expression of autosomal dominant trait in affected individuals.

Codominance   Full expression of both alleles of a given gene pair in a heterozygote.

Polymorphism   Multiple allelic forms of a single gene.

Pleiotropism   Multiple end effects of a single mutant gene.

Genetic heterogeneity   Production of a given trait by different mutations at multiple loci.

Autosomal Dominant Disorders (p. 144)

Some general features of autosomal dominant disorders are as follows:

■ Mutations affect structural (e.g., collagen) or regulatory (e.g., receptor) proteins. In some instances (e.g., collagen), the product of the mutant allele interferes with the function of the normal protein. Such mutant alleles, called *dominant negative*, can produce severe deficiency of protein, as in osteogenesis imperfecta (Chapter 28).
■ There is reduced penetrance and variable expressivity.
■ Onset of clinical features may be later than in autosomal recessive disorders.

Autosomal Recessive Disorders (p. 145)

Autosomal recessive disorders include most inborn errors of metabolism. In contrast to autosomal dominant disorders, the following features generally apply to most disorders in this category:

- Age of onset is frequently in early life.
- Clinical features tend to be more uniform.
- In many patients, enzyme proteins, rather than structural proteins, are affected.

Sex-Linked (X-Linked) Disorders (p. 146)

All sex-linked disorders are X-linked, and almost all are X-linked recessive. They are fully expressed in males because mutant genes on the X chromosome are not paired with alleles on the Y chromosome. In contrast, heterozygous females usually express the disease partially because the paired normal allele is randomly inactivated in some, but not all, cells (e.g., glucose-6-phosphate dehydrogenase [G6PD] deficiency). Fragile X syndrome is discussed later.

Biochemical and Molecular Basis of Mendelian Disorders (p. 146)

Virtually any type of protein may be affected in mendelian disorders. Some examples are provided in Table 6–1.

Disorders Associated with Defects in Structural Proteins (p. 148)

MARFAN SYNDROME (p. 148)

Marfan syndrome is a disorder of connective tissues affecting predominantly the skeletal, ocular, and cardiovascular systems.

Skeletal Changes

Skeletal changes are as follows:

- Tall stature with exceptionally long extremities
- Long, tapering fingers and toes (arachnodactyly)
- Laxity of joint ligaments, producing hyperextensibility
- Spinal deformities (e.g., kyphosis and scoliosis)

Ocular Changes

Ocular changes include:

- Bilateral dislocation of lenses (ectopia lentis)
- Increased axial length of the globe, giving rise to retinal detachments

Cardiovascular Lesions

Cardiovascular lesions include the following:

- Mitral valve prolapse is most common, although not life-threatening; affected valves are soft and billowy, producing a floppy valve associated with mitral regurgitation (discussed in more detail in Chapter 13).
- Cystic medionecrosis of the aorta is less common than mitral valve lesions but clinically more important. Histologically the

Table 6-1. BIOCHEMICAL AND MOLECULAR BASIS OF SOME MENDELIAN DISORDERS

Protein Type/Function	Example	Molecular Lesion	Disease
Enzyme	Phenylalanine hydroxylase	Splice site mutation: reduced amount	Phenylketonuria
	Hexosaminidase	Splice site mutation or frameshift mutation with stop codon: reduced amount	Tay-Sachs disease
Enzyme inhibitor	Adenosine deaminase	Point mutations; abnormal protein with reduced activity	Severe combined immunodeficiency
	α_1-Antitrypsin	Missense mutations; impair secretion from liver to serum	Emphysema and liver disease
Receptor	Low-density lipoprotein receptor	Deletions, point mutations: reduction of synthesis, transport to cell surface, or binding to low-density lipoprotein	Familial hypercholesterolemia
	Vitamin D receptor	Point mutations: failure of normal signaling	Vitamin D-resistant rickets
Transport			
Oxygen	Hemoglobin	Deletions: reduced amount	α-Thalassemia
		Defective mRNA processing; reduced amount	β-Thalassemia
		Point mutations: abnormal structure	Sickle cell anemia
Ions	Cystic fibrosis transmembrane conductance regulator	Deletions and other mutations	Cystic fibrosis
Structural			
Extracellular	Collagen	Deletions or point mutations cause reduced amount of normal collagen or normal amounts of mutant collagen	Osteogenesis imperfecta; Ehlers-Danlos syndromes
	Fibrillin	Missense mutations	Marfan syndrome
Cell membrane	Dystrophin	Deletion with reduced synthesis	Duchenne/Becker muscular dystrophy
	Spectrin, ankyrin, or protein 4.1	Heterogeneous	Hereditary spherocytosis
Hemostasis	Factor VIII	Deletions, insertions, nonsense mutations, and others; reduced synthesis or abnormal factor VIII	Hemophilia A
Growth regulation	Rb protein	Deletions	Hereditary retinoblastoma
	Neurofibromin		Neurofibromatosis type I

media undergoes softening with formation of cystlike spaces, giving rise to dilation of the aortic valve ring and valvular incompetence. More important, the cystic medionecrosis predisposes to an intimal tear through which the blood dissects into the media (a dissecting aneurysm); cleavage of the aortic wall may extend proximally or distally, often resulting in rupture of the aorta.

Death is usually caused by rupture of a dissecting aneurysm, followed in importance by cardiac failure.

Marfan syndrome results from mutations in the *fibrillin-1* gene. Fibrillin, a glycoprotein secreted by fibroblasts, is a component of microfibrils that provides a scaffolding for the deposition of elastin. Abnormal fibrillin disrupts assembly of microfibrils by a dominant negative effect. There is secondary weakness of the connective tissue, particularly in the aorta, mitral valve, and ciliary zonules. The fibrillin gene has been mapped to 15q21.1.

EHLERS-DANLOS SYNDROMES (p. 149)

Ehlers-Danlos syndromes (EDS) are a clinically and genetically heterogeneous group of disorders that result from some *defect in collagen*. They are divided into 12 variants on the basis of predominant clinical manifestations and pattern of inheritance. The following features are common to most variants:

- *Skin*: Skin is hyperextensible, extremely fragile, and vulnerable to trauma; surgical repair of wounds is markedly impaired owing to defective collagen.
- *Joints*: Joints are hypermobile and prone to dislocation.
- *Internal complications*: These affect several organs rich in collagen; manifestations include rupture of the colon and large arteries, ocular fragility with corneal rupture and retinal detachment, and diaphragmatic hernias.

The biochemical bases of abnormalities in collagen are extremely varied. Some of the better characterized defects are as follows:

- Reduced activity of lysyl hydroxylase, an enzyme essential for cross-linking of collagen fibers, is noted in type VI EDS, the most common autosomal recessive form. Collagens (types I and III) lack structural stability.
- Abnormalities of type III collagen, resulting from several distinct mutations in the structural gene, characterize type IV EDS. Because a structural rather than an enzyme protein is affected, the pattern of inheritance is autosomal dominant. Blood vessels and intestines, known to be rich in type III collagen, are prone to spontaneous rupture.
- Defective conversion of type I procollagen to collagen characterizes type VII EDS. It is caused by mutations affecting type I collagen genes. The mutant procollagen chains resist cleavage of *N*-terminal peptides, essential for the formation of normal collagen. Even if only one of the two alleles is mutant, their abnormal products interfere with the formation of normal collagen helices, and hence heterozygotes have severe disease.
- Defective copper metabolism is the basis of EDS type IX. Intracellular copper levels are high, but serum copper is low. Abnormality of copper metabolism secondarily reduces the activity of the enzyme lysyl oxidase, essential for cross-linking of collagen and elastin. It is inherited as an X-linked recessive trait.

Disorders Associated with Defects in Receptor Proteins

FAMILIAL HYPERCHOLESTEROLEMIA (p. 150)

Familial hypercholesterolemia results from a mutation in the gene encoding the receptor for low-density lipoprotein (LDL). At least 150 mutations that can be classified into five groups have been discovered.

1. *Class I* mutations impair transcription, resulting in failure of synthesis of receptor proteins.
2. *Class II* mutations prevent transport of the receptors from the endoplasmic reticulum to the Golgi complex.
3. *Class III* mutations are associated with production of a receptor protein that has reduced binding capacity.
4. *Class IV* mutations give rise to proteins that can bind LDL but cannot internalize the bound LDL.
5. *Class V* mutations give rise to LDL proteins that are expressed and internalized but are trapped in the endosomes and cannot be recycled.

Normal Cholesterol Transport and Metabolism

Figure 6–1 illustrates LDL metabolism. Only a few salient features are emphasized:

- LDL is the major transport form of cholesterol in plasma.
- Although many cells in the body possess high-affinity receptors that recognize apoprotein B-100 of the LDL molecule, about 70% of plasma LDL is cleared by the liver. The remaining 30% is transported into other cells, especially mononuclear phagocytes, by binding to distinct *scavenger* receptors for a chemically altered (e.g., acetylated) form of LDL.
- The transport of and metabolism of LDL into the liver can be resolved into several steps:
  1. Binding to surface receptors
  2. Internalization, followed by transport to and fusion with lysosomes
  3. Lysosomal processing, leading to release of free cholesterol into cytoplasm. Free cholesterol affects three processes:
     1. It suppresses cholesterol synthesis by inhibiting the enzyme hydroxymethylglutaryl coenzyme A reductase.
     2. It activates enzymes that favor esterification of cholesterol.
     3. It suppresses synthesis of LDL receptors, thereby preventing excessive transport of cholesterol into cells.

Clinical Features

Familial hyercholesterolemia is an extremely common disorder with a gene frequency of 1 in 500. Heterozygotes have the following features:

- Cells possess 50% of the normal number of high-affinity LDL receptors. Plasma LDL cholesterol level is two to three times higher than normal, resulting from both impaired clearance of plasma LDL and increased synthesis. The latter is secondary to decreased hepatic uptake of intermediate-density lipoprotein, the immediate precursor of plasma LDL.
- Hypercholesterolemia leads to premature atherosclerosis and accumulation of cholesterol in soft tissues and skin, producing xanthomas.

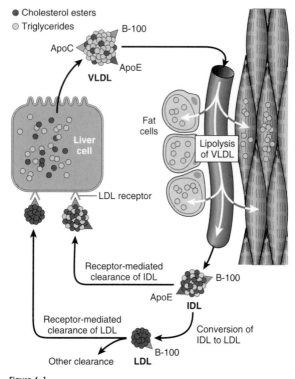

● Cholesterol esters
○ Triglycerides

Figure 6–1 ∎

Schematic illustration of low-density lipoprotein (LDL) metabolism and the role of the liver in its synthesis and clearance. Lipolysis of very-low-density lipoprotein (VLDL) by lipoprotein lipase in the capillaries releases triglycerides that are then stored in fat cells and used as a source of energy in skeletal muscles.

Homozygotes have much greater elevations of plasma LDL cholesterol and are at much greater risk of developing widespread atherosclerosis. Ischemic heart disease often develops before the age of 20. Xanthomas of the skin are also more prominent in homozygotes.

Disorders Associated with Defects in Enzymes (p. 153)

LYSOSOMAL STORAGE DISEASES
(pp. 153–160)

The synthesis, transport, and functions of lysosomal enzymes (p. 153 and Fig. 6–11 in *Robbins Pathologic Basis of Disease*) should be reviewed. *Lysosomal storage disorders result from an inherited lack of functional lysosomal enzymes or other proteins essential for their function.* In the absence of normal lysosomal processing, catabolism of complex substrates is impaired, leading to accumulation of partially degraded insoluble metabolites within lysosomes. The lysosomes, packed with undigested macromolecules, are enlarged and interfere with normal cell function.

Lysosomal storage diseases are classified on the basis of the biochemical nature of the accumulated metabolite (Table 6–2). Distribution of the stored material and resultant clinical features depend on

- The site where most of the material to be degraded is normally found
- The site where most of the degradation normally occurs

Because cells of the mononuclear phagocytic system are particularly rich in lysosomes and are responsible for degradation of several substrates, organs rich in phagocytic cells, such as liver and spleen, are often enlarged. Some of the more common disorders are described next.

TAY-SACHS DISEASE (GM$_2$-GANGLIOSIDOSIS: HEXOSAMINIDASE α-SUBUNIT DEFICIENCY)

Tay-Sachs disease results from mutations that affect the α-subunit of the hexosaminidase enzyme complex. The resultant deficiency of hexosaminidase A prevents degradation of GM$_2$-ganglioside. It is most common in Jews of Eastern European origin. The clinical features, which derive primarily from accumulation of GM$_2$-ganglioside in neurons of the central and autonomic nervous systems and retina, include

- Motor and mental deterioration commencing at about 6 months of age
- Blindness
- A cherry-red spot in the retina
- Death by 2 to 3 years of age

Morphologic Features

Morphologic features include

- Ballooning of neurons with cytoplasmic vacuoles that stain positive for lipids
- Whorled configurations in the cytoplasmic vacuoles, revealed by electron microscopy
- Progressive destruction of neurons with proliferation of microglia
- Accumulation of lipids in retinal ganglion cells, rendering them pale in color, thus accentuating the normal red color of the macular choroid (cherry-red spot)

Antenatal diagnosis and carrier detection are possible by DNA probe analysis and enzyme assays on cells obtained from amniocentesis.

NIEMANN-PICK DISEASE TYPES A AND B

Niemann-Pick disease types A and B are two related disorders that are associated with a deficiency of sphingomyelinase and consequent accumulation of sphingomyelin in mononuclear phagocytic and many other cell types. These syndromes must be distinguished from the so-called Niemann-Pick disease type C, which results from a defect in intracellular cholesterol esterification and transport. The molecular basis of type C is not known.

Table 6-2. LYSOSOMAL STORAGE DISEASES

Disease	Enzyme Deficiency	Major Accumulating Metabolites
Glycogenosis		
Type 2—Pompe disease	α-1,4-Glucosidase (lysosomal glucosidase)	Glycogen
Sphingolipidoses		
Tay-Sachs disease	Hexosaminidase-α subunit	G_{M2}-ganglioside
Sandhoff disease	Hexosaminidase-β subunit	G_{M2}-ganglioside, globoside
Sulfatidoses		
Gaucher disease	Glucocerebrosidase	Glucocerebroside
Niemann-Pick disease, types A and B	Sphingomyelinase	Sphingomyelin
Mucopolysaccharidoses		
MPS I (Hurler)	α-L-Iduronidase	Dermatan sulfate, heparan sulfate
MPS II (Hunter)	L-Iduronosulfate sulfatase	
Mucolipidoses (ML)		
I-cell disease (MLII) and pseudo-Hurler polydystrophy	Deficiency of phosphorylating enzymes essential for formation of mannose-6-phosphate recognition marker; acid hydrolases lacking recognition marker cannot be targeted to lysosomes but are secreted extracellularly	Mucopolysaccharide, glycolipid

Sphingomyelinase-deficient type A variant is the most common form and is associated with

- Diffuse neuronal involvement, leading eventually to cell death and shrinkage of the brain; there is a retinal cherry-red spot similar to that in Tay-Sachs disease.
- Massive accumulation of lipids in cells of the mononuclear phagocytic system, giving rise to massive splenomegaly, enlargement of liver and lymph nodes, and infiltration of bone marrow.
- Visceral involvement affecting the gastrointestinal tract and lungs.

Affected cells everywhere are enlarged and filled with numerous small vacuoles that impart foaminess to the cytoplasm. Clinical manifestations appear soon after birth and consist of hepatosplenomegaly, failure to thrive, and deterioration of psychomotor functions. Survival is limited to 1 or 2 years.

GAUCHER DISEASE

Gaucher disease refers to a cluster of autosomal recessive disorders in which mutations affecting the glucocerebrosidase locus reduce the levels of this enzyme. Consequently, cleavage of ceramide derived from cell membranes of senescent leukocytes and red cells as well as from turnover of gangliosides in the brains of neonates is impaired. Accumulation of glucocerebrosides occurs in the mononuclear phagocytic system and, in some forms, in the central nervous system. Two important variants of Gaucher disease can be distinguished:

1. *Type I*, the most common form, occurs in adults. This chronic, non-neuronopathic form is associated with storage of glucocerebrosides in the mononuclear phagocytic system; there is no brain involvement but massive splenomegaly; involvement of bone marrow produces small or large areas of bone erosions that can cause pathologic fractures; pancytopenia or thrombocytopenia results from hypersplenism; life span is not affected.

2. *Type II*, also known as the *acute neuronopathic form*, is associated with hepatosplenomegaly as well as central nervous system involvement; symptoms such as convulsions and mental deterioration dominate the clinical picture; death occurs at a young age.

These patterns, resulting from different allelic mutations in the structural gene for the enzyme, run within families. Prenatal diagnosis is possible by assay of enzymes in amniotic fluid cells and by DNA probe analysis. *Histologically*, affected cells (Gaucher cells) are distended with periodic acid–Schiff (PAS)–positive material that has a fibrillary appearance resembling crumpled tissue paper.

MUCOPOLYSACCHARIDOSES

The mucopolysaccharidoses (MPS) are a group of disorders resulting from inherited deficiencies of enzymes involved in the degradation of MPS. The mucopolysaccharides that accumulate in the cells include heparan sulfate, dermatan sulfate, keratan sulfate, and chondroitin sulfate. Histologically, affected cells are distended with clear cytoplasm (balloon cells) that contains PAS-positive material. Accumulated mucopolysaccharides are found in many cell types, including mononuclear phagocytic cells (giving rise to hepatosplenomegaly); fibroblasts throughout the body; endothelial cells and intimal smooth muscle cells (giving rise to narrowing of coronary arteries); and neurons.

Several clinical variants of MPS classified as MPS I through VII have been described, each resulting from the deficiency of one specific enzyme. Some better known examples are autosomal recessive Hurler disease (MPS I) and X-linked recessive Hunter disease (MPS II). In general, all forms are progressive disorders characterized by one or more of the following:

- Coarse facial features
- Hepatosplenomegaly
- Corneal clouding
- Lesions of cardiac valves
- Narrowing of coronary arteries
- Joint stiffness
- Mental retardation

GLYCOGEN STORAGE DISEASES
(pp. 160–162)

The glycogen storage diseases are a group of autosomal recessive disorders resulting from defects in the synthesis or catabolism of glycogen. On the basis of specific enzyme deficiencies and resultant clinical pictures, glycogen storage diseases have been divided into three major groups (Table 6–3):

1. *Hepatic forms*: The prototype is von Gierke disease (type I glycogenosis). This results from deficiency of the hepatic enzyme glucose-6-phosphatase, which is essential for conversion of glucose-6-phosphate to glucose. The major effects of this enzyme deficiency are
   1. Accumulation of glycogen because it cannot be broken down to free glucose
   2. Low blood glucose (hypoglycemia)
2. *Myopathic forms*: These result from deficiencies of enzymes that fuel glycolysis in striated muscles. McArdle disease (type V glycogenosis), the most important example, is caused by lack of muscle phosphorylase. Deficiency of this enzyme leads to
   1. Storage of glycogen in skeletal muscles
   2. Muscle weakness
   3. Muscle cramps after exercise
   4. Failure of exercise-induced rise in blood lactate.
3. *Miscellaneous forms*: There are several of these, the most important being type II glycogenosis, or Pompe disease, which results from deficiency of the lysosomal enzyme acid maltase (α-glucosidase). As in other lysosomal storage diseases, many organs are involved, but storage of glycogen is most prominent in the heart. Affected neonates have massive cardiomegaly, and death results from cardiac failure by 2 years of age.

ALKAPTONURIA

In alkaptonuria, the lack of homogentisic oxidase blocks the metabolism of phenylalanine and leads to accumulation of homogentisic acid. Excessive homogentisic acid is associated with the following:

- Excretion in urine, imparting to it a black color if allowed to stand.

Table 6-3. PRINCIPAL SUBGROUPS OF GLYCOGENOSES

Clinicopathologic Category	Specific Type	Enzyme Deficiency	Morphologic Changes	Clinical Features
Hepatic type	Hepatorenal—von Gierke disease (type I)	Glucose-6-phosphatase	Hepatomegaly—intracytoplasmic accumulations of glycogen and small amounts of lipid; intranuclear glycogen Renomegaly—intracytoplasmic accumulations of glycogen in cortical tubular epithelial cells	Failure to thrive, stunted growth, hepatomegaly, and renomegaly. Hypoglycemia owing to failure of glucose mobilization, often leading to convulsions. Hyperlipidemia and hyperuricemia resulting from deranged glucose metabolism; many patients develop gout and skin xanthomas. Bleeding tendency owing to platelet dysfunction. Mortality approximately 50%
Myopathic type	McArdle syndrome (type V)	Muscle phosphorylase	Skeletal muscle only—accumulations of glycogen predominantly in subsarcolemmal location	Painful cramps associated with strenuous exercise. Myoglobinuria occurs in 50% of cases. Onset in adulthood (>20 years). Muscular exercise fails to raise lactate level in venous blood. Compatible with normal longevity
Miscellaneous types	Generalized glycogenosis—Pompe disease (type II)	Lysosomal glucosidase (acid maltase)	Mild hepatomegaly—ballooning of lysosomes with glycogen creating lacy cytoplasmic pattern Cardiomegaly—glycogen within sarcoplasm as well as membrane-bound Skeletal muscle—similar to heart	Massive cardiomegaly, muscle hypotonia, and cardiorespiratory failure within 2 years. A milder adult form with only skeletal muscle involvement presenting with chronic myopathy

99

- Ochronosis—a blue-black pigmentation of the ears, nose, and cheeks resulting from binding of homogentisic acid to connective tissue and cartilage.
- Arthropathy associated with deposition in articular cartilage: The pigmented cartilage loses resilience and is readily eroded; the vertebral column, knee, shoulders, and hips are usually affected.

Disorders Associated with Defects in Proteins That Regulate Cell Growth (p. 162)

NEUROFIBROMATOSIS TYPES 1 AND 2
(p. 162)

Neurofibromatosis types 1 and 2 are two genetically distinct autosomal dominant disorders, both characterized by the presence of tumors of the nerves. Neurofibromatosis type 1 (also called von Recklinghausen disease) is characterized by three main features:

1. *Multiple neural tumors* involve nerve trunks in skin as well as internal organs. Three types of lesions are found: cutaneous, subcutaneous, and plexiform. The last-mentioned are subcutaneous tumors that contain numerous tortuous thickened nerves. They sometimes cause massive enlargement of a limb or other body parts. Histologically, neurofibromas reveal proliferation of neurites, Schwann cells, and fibroblasts, all embedded in loose myxoid stroma.

2. *Cutaneous pigmentations*, present in more than 90% of patients, take the form of light brown macules located over nerve trunks (*café au lait* spots).

3. *Lisch nodules* or pigmented iris hamartomas are present in almost all cases.

Several associated abnormalities are present; the important ones are as follows:

- There are skeletal lesions (bone cysts, scoliosis, and erosion of the bone surface) in 30 to 50% of patients.
- There is an increased risk of the development of other tumors, especially meningiomas, optic gliomas, and pheochromocytomas.
- There is a tendency toward reduced intelligence.

Loss by mutation of tumor suppressor genes underlies these conditions.

The NF-1 locus on chromosome 17 encodes neurofibromin, a protein that regulates the function of the p21 *ras* oncoprotein. NF-1 is a tumor-suppressor gene. The NF-2 locus on chromosome 22 also encodes a tumor-suppressor gene, of unknown function. These patients have the following features:

- Bilateral acoustic nerve tumors in all cases
- Gliomas, particularly ependymomas
- Café au lait spots
- Absence of Lisch nodules

Disorders with Multifactorial Inheritance
(p. 164)

Disorders with multifactorial inheritance result from the combined effects of two or more mutant genes combined with environmental factors and exhibit the following characteristics:

- The risk of expression is conditioned by the number of mutant genes inherited. Environmental influences significantly modify the risk of expression; hence the concordance rate in identical twins is 20 to 40%.

- The risk of recurrence of the disorder in first-degree relatives is 2 to 7%.
- The risk of recurrence in subsequent pregnancies increases with the birth of each affected child.

Multifactorial inheritance underlies many congenital malformations and common disorders, such as diabetes mellitus, gout, hypertension, and coronary heart disease.

CYTOGENETIC DISORDERS (p. 168)

Cytogenetic disorders may be due to

- Alterations in the number of chromosomes
- Alterations in the structure of chromosomes

Common Types of Numerical Disorders

Common types of numerical disorders are as follows:

- Monosomy, associated with one less normal chromosome (2n − 1)
- Trisomy, associated with one extra chromosome (2n + 1)
- Mosaicism, associated with one or more populations of cells, some with normal chromosomal complement, others with extra or missing chromosomes

Numerical disorders of chromosomes result from errors during cell division. Monosomy and trisomy usually result from nondisjunction of chromosomes during gametogenesis (the first meiotic division), whereas mosaics are produced when mitotic errors occur in the zygote. Monosomy or trisomy of autosomes usually results in early fetal death and spontaneous abortion, whereas similar imbalances in sex chromosomes are much better tolerated.

Structural Aberrations of Chromosomes

Structural aberrations of chromosomes include the following (Fig. 6–2):

- *Deletion*: Loss of a terminal or interstitial segment of a chromosome.
- *Translocation*: Involves transfer of a segment of one chromosome to another, as follows:
  - Balanced reciprocal, involving exchange of chromosomal material between two chromosomes with no net gain or loss of genetic material.
  - Robertsonian (centric) fusion, being reciprocal translocation between two acrocentric chromosomes involving the short arm of one and the long arm of the other; transfer of segments leads to formation of one abnormally large chromosome and one extremely small one. The latter is usually lost. This translocation predisposes to the formation of abnormal (unbalanced) gametes.
- *Isochromosome*: Formed when one arm (short or long) is lost and the remaining arm is duplicated, resulting in a chromosome of two short arms only or of two long arms. In live births, the most common isochromosome is designated i(Xq) with

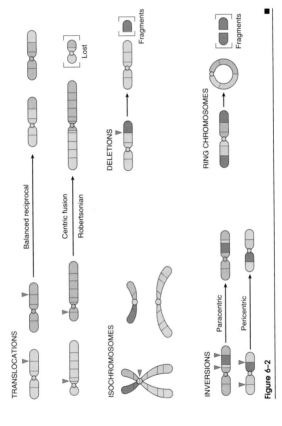

Figure 6–2 ■

Types of chromosomal rearrangements.

TRANSLOCATIONS

Balanced reciprocal

Centric fusion
Robertsonian

Lost

ISOCHROMOSOMES

INVERSIONS

Paracentric

Pericentric

DELETIONS

Fragments

RING CHROMOSOMES

Fragments

duplication of long arm and deletion of short arm of the X chromosome.
- *Inversion*: Rearrangement associated with two breaks in a chromosome, followed by inversion and reincorporation of the broken segment.
- *Ring chromosome*: Deletion affecting both ends, followed by fusion of the damaged ends.

Cytogenetic Disorders Involving Autosomes
(p. 170)

TRISOMY 21 (DOWN SYNDROME) (p. 170)

Down syndrome is the most common chromosomal disorder (1 in 800 births).

Karyotypic Features

Karyotypic features are as follows:

- About 95% have a complete extra chromosome 21 (47,XY,+21). The incidence of this form is strongly influenced by maternal age (1 in 1550 births in women younger than 20 years, increasing to 1 in 25 in women older than 45 years). In 95% of these cases, the extra chromosome is maternal in origin.
- A translocation variant, making up 4% of all cases, has extra chromosomal material derived from inheritance of a parental chromosome bearing a translocation of the long arm of chromosome 21 to chromosome 22 or 14 (e.g., 46,XX,der(14;21)(q10;q10),+21). Because the fertilized ovum already possesses two normal autosomes 21, the translocated chromosomal fragment provides the same triple-gene dosage as trisomy 21. Such cases are frequently (but not always) familial because the parent is a carrier of a robertsonian translocation. Such a rearrangement may also occur during gametogenesis.
- Mosaic variants make up about 1% of all cases; they have a mixture of cells with normal chromosome numbers and cells with an extra chromosome 21.

Clinical Features

Clinical features include the following:

- Flat facies with oblique palpebral fissures and epicanthic folds
- Severe mental retardation
- Congenital heart disease, especially septal defects, responsible for the majority of deaths in infancy and childhood
- Ten- to 20-fold increased risk of developing acute leukemia
- Serious infections resulting from abnormal immune responses
- Premature Alzheimer disease in those who survive after 35 years of age

OTHER TRISOMIES (p. 171)

Trisomy 18 (Edwards syndrome) and trisomy 13 (Patau syndrome) occur much less commonly than trisomy 21; affected infants have severe malformations and usually die within the first year of life.

CHROMOSOME 22Q11 DELETION SYNDROME (p. 173)

Karyotype

In chromosome 22Q11 deletion syndrome, a small deletion of band 11 on the long arm of chromosome 22 is best seen by fluorescence in situ hybridization.

Clinical Features

Clinical features are as follows:

- Congenital heart defects
- Abnormalities of palate
- Facial dysmorphism
- Developmental delay
- Variable T-cell deficiency
- Hypoparathyroidism

These clinical features are shared by the previously recognized DiGeorge syndrome (Chapter 7) and velocardiofacial syndrome. T-cell immunodeficiency and hypocalcemia are more prominent in some cases (DiGeorge syndrome), whereas facial dysmorphology and cardiac malformations are more prominent in others (velocardiofacial syndrome).

Cytogenetic Disorders Involving Sex Chromosomes (p. 173)

Imbalances of sex chromosomes are better tolerated than similar imbalances of autosomes, and hence sex chromosome disorders are more common than autosomal disorders. The milder nature of X-chromosome aberrations is, in part, related to the inactivation of one X chromosome, explained by the Lyon hypothesis:

- All but one X chromosome is genetically inactive.
- Random inactivation of either paternal or maternal X chromosome occurs early in embryogenesis and leads to the formation of a Barr body.
- Normal females are mosaics, having two cell populations, one with inactivated paternal X and the other with inactivated maternal X.

Because numerical aberrations of X chromosomes (extra or missing) are associated with somatic and gonadal abnormalities, the Lyon hypothesis has to be modified as follows:

- Both X chromosomes are required for normal gametogenesis; the inactivated X is selectively reactivated in germ cells during gamete formation.
- X inactivation spares certain regions of the chromosome necessary for normal growth and development.

KLINEFELTER SYNDROME (p. 174)

Klinefelter syndrome refers to male hypogonadism associated with two or more X chromosomes and at least one Y chromosome.

Karyotype

47,XXY is most common (80% of cases); others are mosaics (e.g., 46,XY/47,XXY).

Clinical Features

Clinical features include the following:

- Leading cause of male infertility
- Eunuchoid body habitus
- Minimal or no mental retardation
- Failure of male secondary sexual characteristics
- Gynecomastia; female distribution of hair
- Atrophic testis with hyperplasia of Leydig cells
- Plasma follicle-stimulating hormone and estrogen levels elevated; testosterone levels low

XYY SYNDROME (p. 174)

The clinical features of XYY syndrome are as follows:

- Affected individuals are usually tall; individuals are phenotypically normal.
- Some have behavioral difficulties (aggressive, antisocial, impulsive nature). This, however, is controversial.

TURNER SYNDROME (p. 174)

Turner syndrome refers to hypogonadism in phenotypic females resulting from complete or partial monosomy of X chromosome.

Karyotypes

Routine cytogenetics reveals the following:

- 45,X is most common (57% of cases).
- 46,X,i(Xq) (isochromosome of the long arm with deletion of the short arm) occurs.
- Mosaics occur (e.g., 45,X/46,XX).
- By using more sensitive techniques, mosaicism is revealed in up to 75% of cases. Some believe that most 45,X Turner syndrome patients are actually mosaics.

Clinical Features

Wide-ranging degrees of abnormalities occur, depending on karyotype; 45,X is most severely affected. Typical features include

- Lymphedema of neck, hands, and feet
- Webbing of neck
- Short stature
- Broad chest and widely spaced nipples
- Primary amenorrhea
- Failure of development of breasts
- Infantile external genitalia
- Ovaries severely atrophic and fibrous (streak ovaries)
- Congenital heart disease, particularly aortic coarctation

HERMAPHRODITISM AND PSEUDOHERMAPHRODITISM (p. 176)

True Hermaphrodites

True hermaphrodites are extremely rare. These individuals have both ovaries and testes, either combined as an ovotestis or with one gonad on each side. Fifty percent have 46,XX karyotype; of the remaining, approximately equal numbers have 46,XY and 45,X/46,XY karyotypes.

Pseudohermaphrodites

Pseudohermaphrodites have disparate gonadal and phenotypic sexual characteristics.

Female Pseudohermaphrodites. These have 46,XX karyotype. Ovaries and internal genitalia are normal, but external genitalia are ambiguous or virilized. The most common cause is inappropriate exposure to androgenic steroids during gestation. The condition may occur in congenital adrenal hyperplasia or in the presence of androgen-secreting maternal tumors.

Male Pseudohermaphrodites. Y chromosome is present, and therefore the gonads are exclusively testes, but external genitalia are either ambiguous or completely female. The condition results from defective virilization of the male embryo because of reduced androgen synthesis or resistance to action of androgens. The most common form is *complete testicular feminization* associated with mutation in the structural gene for androgen receptor located on Xq11-Xq12.

SINGLE-GENE DISORDERS WITH NONCLASSIC INHERITANCE (p. 176)

These are classified into four categories:

1. Triplet repeat mutations—fragile X syndrome
2. Mutations in mitochondrial genes—Leber hereditary optic neuropathy
3. Genomic imprinting—Prader-Willi and Angelman syndromes
4. Gonadal mosaicism

Triplet Repeat Mutations—Fragile X Syndrome (p. 177)

Several disorders, such as Huntington disease, myotonic dystrophy, and fragile X syndrome, are characterized by triplet repeat mutations. In these mutations, there is a long repeated sequence of three nucleotides, and most affected sequences share the nucleotides guanine (G) and cytosine (C).

Fragile X syndrome, the prototypic disorder in this category, is a common cause of familial mental retardation. It is characterized cytogenetically by a fragile site on Xq27.3, which is seen as a discontinuity of staining. At this site, there are multiple tandem repeats of the nucleotide sequence CGG in the 5′ untranslated region of the *FMR-1* gene. In normal individuals, the average number of repeats is 29, whereas affected individuals have 230 to 4000 repeats. In between are those with *premutations* characterized by 50 to 230 CGG repeats. In carrier females, the premutations undergo amplification during oogenesis, resulting in full mutations that are then passed on to their progeny. Because the mutations are carried on the X chromosome, this is an X-linked recessive disorder. Because premutations are silent, and they are amplified only during oogenesis in carrier females, however the transmission pattern differs from classic X-linked disorders. Thus, carrier males with premutations do not have any symptoms; approximately 50% of carrier females are affected. The molecular basis of fragile X syndrome is not clear. Presence of greater than 230 CGG repeats causes transcriptional suppression of the *FMR-1* gene.

Clinically, affected males have severe mental retardation, and 80% have an enlarged testis. Other physical features, such as an elongated face and large mandible, are inconsistent. The clinical features of fragile X syndrome worsen with each successive generation because of amplification of nucleotide repeats during oogenesis. This phenomenon is called *anticipation*.

In addition to fragile X syndrome, about 10 other disorders have been associated with a similar type of mutation. In all cases, neurodegenerative changes dominate the clinical picture.

Mutations in Mitochondrial Genes—Leber Hereditary Optic Neuropathy (p. 179)

Ova contain mitochondria, but spermatozoa contain few; hence the mitochondrial content of zygotes is derived almost entirely from the ovum. Thus, mitochondrial DNA is transmitted entirely by females, and diseases resulting from mutations in mitochondrial genes are *maternally inherited*. Affected females transmit the disease to all their offspring—male and female; however, daughters and not sons pass the disease further to their progeny. When a cell carrying normal and mutant mitochondrial DNA divides, the proportion of normal and mutant DNA in the daughter cells is random and quite variable. Hence, expression of disorders resulting from mutations in mitochondrial genes is quite variable. Genes contained in the mitochondria encode enzymes involved in oxidative phosphorylation, and hence diseases in this category predominantly affect organs heavily dependent on mitochondrial energy metabolism. These include the neuromuscular system, liver, heart, and kidney. As an example, Leber hereditary optic neuropathy causes blindness, neurologic dysfunction, and cardiac conduction defects.

Genomic Imprinting—Prader-Willi and Angelman Syndromes (p. 180)

Genomic imprinting is an epigenetic process that results in differential inactivation of either the maternal or the paternal alleles of certain genes. *Maternal imprinting* refers to transcriptional silencing of the maternal allele, whereas *paternal imprinting* refers to inactivation of the paternal allele. Two syndromes resulting from genomic imprinting are described.

Prader-Willi syndrome, characterized by mental retardation, short stature, hypotonia, obesity, and hypogonadism, results from the deletion of genes located at 15q12 in the paternally derived chromosome 15. In some cases, an entire chromosome 15 derived from the father is absent, replaced instead by two maternally derived chromosomes 15 (uniparental disomy). In the latter case, the patients do not exhibit any structural or numerical cytogenetic abnormality. In contrast with the Prader-Willi syndrome, patients with the phenotypically distinct *Angelman syndrome* are born with deletion of the same chromosomal region derived from their mothers, or uniparental disomy of paternal chromosome 15. These patients, in addition to mental retardation, have ataxia, seizures, and inappropriate laughter. The molecular mechanisms underlying these syndromes are not clear. It is believed that a gene or genes on maternal chromosome 15 is imprinted, and hence only the paternal allele is active. When there is a deletion affecting the paternal chromosome, no functional gene remains, and patients develop Prader-Willi syndrome. The converse is true in Angelman syndrome (Fig. 6–34, p. 180 in *Robbins Pathologic Basis of Disease*).

Gonadal Mosaicism (p. 181)

Gonadal mosaicism results from a mutation that selectively affects cells destined to form gonads during early embryogenesis. Because all somatic cells are normal, the affected individual is phenotypically normal. Because the germ cells are affected, however, one or more offspring of such an individual may manifest disease.

DIAGNOSIS OF GENETIC DISEASES
(p. 182)

Diagnosis of genetic diseases involves cytogenetic or molecular analyses.

Indications for Cytogenetic Analysis
(p. 182)

Indications for cytogenetic analysis are as follows:

1. Prenatal, performed on fetal cells obtained by amniocentesis or chorionic villus biopsy
    - ❏ Advanced maternal age (>34 years)
    - ❏ A parent with a structural chromosomal abnormality (e.g., robertsonian translocation)
    - ❏ Previous child with chromosomal abnormality
    - ❏ A parent who is carrier of an X-linked disease (to determine fetal sex)
2. Postnatal, performed on peripheral blood lymphocytes
    - ❏ Multiple congenital anomalies
    - ❏ Unexplained mental retardation
    - ❏ Suspected chromosomal abnormalities
    - ❏ Suspected fragile X syndrome
    - ❏ Infertility, to rule out sex chromosomal abnormality
    - ❏ Recurrent abortion (both parents must be evaluated to rule out carriers of balanced translocation)

Molecular Analyses (p. 182)

Two different approaches are applied to the diagnosis of genetic diseases by recombinant DNA technology:

1. *Direct gene diagnosis*, involving detection of the mutant gene
2. *Indirect gene diagnosis*, involving detection of linkage of the disease gene with a harmless *marker gene*

DIRECT GENE DIAGNOSIS (p. 182)

Direct gene diagnosis is based on the identification of a qualitative difference between DNA sequences in the normal and abnormal genes. Three methods are used:

1. One is based on the fact that some mutations alter or destroy certain restriction sites on normal DNA. For example, the normal

factor V gene has two restriction sites for the enzyme Mn11, one of which is lost if there is a mutation in the factor V gene. This results in the production of different-sized products when DNA from normal and affected individuals is amplified by polymerase chain reaction (PCR) then cut with Mnl1. The different products are visualized on gel electrophoresis.

2. Oligonucleotide probe analysis is used when the point mutation producing the abnormal gene does not alter any known restriction site. Two oligonucleotides 18 to 20 bases long are synthesized, having at their centers the single base by which the normal and mutant genes differ. Each oligonucleotide hybridizes strongly to the corresponding (normal) gene but weakly to the gene that does not share the exact sequence. Thus, after PCR amplification of target DNA, the normal and mutant genes can be distinguished on the basis of the *strength* of hybridization with the two oligonucleotide probes.

3. Mutations that affect the length of DNA (e.g., deletions or expansions) can also be detected by PCR analysis. For example, in the fragile X syndrome, amplifications of the DNA by primers that flank the region affected by trinucleotide repeats generate products of different sizes when DNA from normal carrier males and affected individuals is compared.

INDIRECT GENE DIAGNOSIS: GENE TRACKING (p. 184)

In many genetic diseases, the mutant gene and its normal counterpart have not yet been identified or sequenced, and thus direct gene diagnosis cannot be used. It is therefore necessary to employ *gene tracking*, which determines whether a given family member or fetus inherited the same relevant chromosomal region(s) as a previously affected family member. This technique requires that chromosomes carrying the normal and mutant genes in heterozygotes be distinguishable. To accomplish this, advantage is taken of naturally occurring variations in DNA sequences in the vicinity of (and linked to) the mutant gene. Such variations may result from differences in specific nucleotides (site polymorphisms) or differences in the number of nucleotide repeats (length polymorphisms). Site polymorphisms, also called *restriction fragment length polymorphisms*, result from DNA polymorphisms that give rise to fragments of different lengths in Southern blot analysis. In cystic fibrosis, for example, heterozygous parents and children have two bands derived from the normal and the affected chromosome. In contrast, an affected (homozygous) individual reveals a single band derived from two identical chromosomes carrying the mutant gene. Length polymorphisms result from differences between the number of repeats of short sequences of noncoding DNA. These can be detected by PCR analysis of the DNA because the product size depends on the number of nucleotide repeats.

Linkage analysis has proved useful in antenatal detection of several genetic disorders, such as cystic fibrosis, Huntington disease, polycystic kidney disease, fragile X syndrome, and Duchenne muscular dystrophy. It has certain limitations, however, as follows:

- For prenatal diagnosis, several affected and unaffected family members must be available for testing.
- Key family members (e.g., parents, siblings) must be heterozygous for the polymorphism (i.e., the normal chromosome and

that carrying the mutant gene must be distinguishable). Because length polymorphisms have multiple alleles, there are much greater chances of heterozygosity. These therefore are more useful than restriction site polymorphisms.

- Recombination between homologous chromosomes during gametogenesis may lead to loss of linkage between the DNA polymorphism and the mutant gene.

Disorders of Immunity

The immune system protects against exogenous (foreign) substances, microbial invasion, and possibly tumors, but occasionally immune responses also damage normal host tissues and react to *homologous antigens* (e.g., blood transfusions, transplanted tissues, fetal antigens in pregnancy) and sometimes *endogenous antigens*, the basis of autoimmune disorders. Pathology related to the immune system falls into three general categories:

1. *Hypersensitivity* (hyperactive) states (e.g., anaphylaxis)
2. *Autoimmunity* (e.g., systemic lupus erythematosus [SLE])
3. *Deficiency* states, congenital or acquired (e.g., acquired immunodeficiency syndrome [AIDS])

In addition, amyloidosis, in which immunoglobulin fragments are deposited in tissues, is also considered here.

MECHANISMS OF IMMUNE-MEDIATED INJURY (HYPERSENSITIVITY REACTIONS)

(p. 195)

Hypersensitivity reactions are subdivided on the basis of mechanisms of immune injury (Table 7–1).

Type I Hypersensitivity (Anaphylactic)

(p. 196)

Type I hypersensitivity is mediated by immunoglobulin E (IgE) antibodies formed in response to a particular antigen (allergen) and bound to mast cells and basophils. Synthesis of IgE antibody is highly dependent on the induction of CD4+ helper T cells of the T_H2 type. Interleukin-4 (IL-4) produced by T_H2 cells is essential for IgE synthesis, and IL-3, IL-5, and granulocyte macrophage–colony-stimulating factor (GM-CSF) promote production and survival of eosinophils. On re-exposure of sensitized individuals, allergen binds to and cross-links the IgE on mast cells and results in

■ Release *(degranulation)* of preformed vesicles containing *primary mediators*
■ De novo synthesis of *secondary mediators*

Degranulation may also be triggered by a variety of other physical and chemical stimuli, including

■ Complement fragments C3a and C5a *(anaphylatoxins)*
■ Certain drugs (codeine, morphine)
■ Mellitin (in bee venom)

Table 7-1. MECHANISMS OF IMMUNOLOGICALLY MEDIATED DISORDERS

Type	Prototype Disorder	Immune Mechanism
I. Anaphylactic type	Anaphylaxis, some forms of bronchial asthma	Formation of IgE (cytotropic) antibody → release of vasoactive amines and other mediators from basophils and mast cells
II. Cytotoxic type	Autoimmune hemolytic anemia, erythroblastosis fetalis, Goodpasture syndrome	Formation of IgG, IgM → binds to antigen on target cell surface → phagocytosis of target cell or lysis of target cell by C8,9 fraction of activated complement or antibody-dependent cellular cytotoxicity
III. Immune complex disease	Arthus reaction, serum sickness, systemic lupus erythematosus, certain forms of acute glomerulonephritis	Antigen-antibody complexes → activated complement → attracted neutrophils → release of lysosomal enzymes and other toxic moieties
IV. Cell-mediated (delayed) hypersensitivity	Tuberculosis, contact dermatitis, transplant rejection	Sensitized thymus-derived T lymphocytes → release of lymphokines and T cell–mediated cytotoxicity

- Sunlight
- Trauma
- Heat
- Cold

In many cases of type I hypersensitivity, two phases may be exhibited:

1. The initial (rapid) response, which becomes evident in 5 to 30 minutes after re-exposure, with resolution within 30 minutes

2. The second (delayed) phase, which sets in 2 to 8 hours later (without additional antigenic challenge), lasts for days, and is characterized by an intense infiltration by inflammatory cells and tissue damage.

Primary mast cell mediators typically induce the initial rapid response. These mediators include the following:

- *Biogenic amines* (e.g., histamine), which cause bronchial smooth muscle contraction, increased vascular permeability, and increased mucous gland secretions
- *Chemotactic mediators* (e.g., eosinophil chemotactic factors and neutrophil chemotactic factors)
- *Enzymes* contained in granule matrix (e.g., chymase, tryptase), which lead to generation of kinins and activated complement by acting on their precursor proteins
- *Proteoglycans* (e.g., heparin)

Secondary mediators include two classes:

1. Lipid mediators
2. Cytokines

The *lipid mediators* are as follows:

- *Leukotriene B_4* is highly chemotactic for neutrophils, monocytes, and eosinophils.
- *Leukotrienes C_4, D_4,* and *E_4* are 1000-fold more potent than histamine in increasing vascular permeability and causing bronchial smooth muscle contraction. These also cause marked mucous gland secretion.
- *Prostaglandin D_2* causes intense bronchospasm, vasodilation, and mucous secretion.
- *Platelet-activating factor* causes platelet aggregation, histamine release, bronchoconstriction, vasodilation, and increased vascular permeability. It also has proinflammatory effects, such as chemoattraction and degranulation of neutrophils.

The *cytokines*, which recruit and activate inflammatory cells, are thought to be produced by mast cells (tumor necrosis factor [TNF]-α, IL-1, IL-3, IL-4, IL-5, IL-6, GM-CSF, and chemokines). TNF-α is a powerful proinflammatory cytokine that recruits and activates many inflammatory cells. Additional cytokines are released by the recruited inflammatory cells. Eosinophils are particularly important in late-phase response. Their survival is favored by the T_H2 cell–derived and mast cell–derived cytokines (IL-3, IL-5, and GM-CSF). Epithelial cells activated by TNF-α secrete the chemokines eotaxin and RANTES, which are chemotactic for eosinophils. Eosinophils participate in tissue damage by producing major basic protein and eosinophil cationic protein.

SYSTEMIC ANAPHYLAXIS

Systemic anaphylaxis typically follows parenteral or oral administration of allergen, such as antisera, drugs, hormones, and enzymes. The severity reflects the level of sensitization, and even minuscule doses may induce shock in the appropriate host. Pruritus, urticaria, and erythema occur minutes after exposure, followed by bronchoconstriction and laryngeal edema, escalating into laryngeal obstruction, shock, and death within minutes to hours. Autopsy findings include pulmonary edema and hemorrhage (reflecting increased vascular permeability), lung hyperdistention, and right ventricular dilation (reflecting pulmonary vasoconstriction).

LOCAL ANAPHYLAXIS (ATOPIC ALLERGIES)

Atopy is a hereditary predisposition to develop local type I responses to inhaled or ingested allergens. It affects 10% of the population and includes urticaria, angioedema, rhinitis, and asthma (all described elsewhere). Candidate genes related to atopy have been mapped at 5q31, where many genes for T_H2-type cytokines are located.

Type II Hypersensitivity (Cytotoxic) (p. 199)

Type II hypersensitivity is mediated by antibodies against intrinsic antigens or extrinsic antigens adsorbed on the cell surface or on other tissue components. Subsequent injury may occur secondary to the following:

1. *Complement-dependent reactions*: These are either direct lysis via the C5–9 complement membrane attack complex (MAC) or by *opsonization* (enhanced phagocytosis) as a result of fixation of C3b fragments. Examples include the following:
   ❏ *Transfusion reactions*: Recipient antibodies against incompatible donor erythrocyte antigens.
   ❏ *Erythroblastosis fetalis*: Maternal IgG antibodies (capable of crossing the placenta) against fetal erythrocyte antigens.
   ❏ *Autoimmune thrombocytopenia, agranulocytosis*, or *hemolytic anemia*: Autoantibodies against one's own blood cells.
   ❏ *Certain drug reactions*: Antibodies against drugs that have complexed to erythrocyte or other protein antigens.
   ❏ *Goodpasture disease*: Antibodies against the common basement membrane component of kidneys and lungs.
2. *Antibody-dependent cell-mediated cytotoxicity (ADCC)*: Targets with low concentrations of bound antibody (IgG or IgE) are lysed (without phagocytosis) by nonsensitized cells with Fc receptors (e.g., monocytes, neutrophils, eosinophils, and natural killer [NK] cells). ADCC may be important for parasitic infections or tumors and may play a major role in graft rejection.
3. *Antibody-mediated cellular dysfunction*: Antiacetylcholine receptor antibodies impair neuromuscular transmission in myasthenia gravis; anti–thyroid-stimulating hormone receptor antibodies contribute to thyroid hyperfunction in Graves disease.

Type III Hypersensitivity (Immune Complex Mediated) (p. 201)

Type III hypersensitivity is mediated by antigen-antibody complexes—immune complexes—forming either in the circulation or at extravascular sites of antigen deposition; antigens may be exogenous (e.g., infectious agents) or endogenous. Subsequent injury derives from activation of various serum mediators, particularly complement.

SYSTEMIC IMMUNE COMPLEX DISEASE

In systemic immune complex disease, complexes form in the circulation and are systemically deposited.

Acute Serum Sickness

Acute serum sickness is the prototype caused by administration of large amounts of foreign serum (e.g., horse antithymocyte globulin). About 5 days after serum inoculation, newly synthesized antihorse serum antibodies complex with the foreign antigen to form circulating immune complexes. Small immune complexes (formed early in antigen excess) circulate for long periods and bind with low avidity to mononuclear phagocytes. Complexes deposit within a variety of capillary or arteriolar walls, causing vasculitis (see later). This deposition is promoted by increased vascular permeability secondary to activation of inflammatory cells via binding of immune complexes to Fc or C3b receptors. The activated inflammatory cells release vasoactive mediators, including cytokines. Affected tissues include renal glomeruli (causing glomerulonephritis), joints (arthritis), skin, heart, and serosal surfaces. With continued antibody production, large immune complexes eventually form (i.e., in antibody excess). These are cleared by phagocytes, ending the disease process.

Deposition of immune complexes activates the complement cascade with

- C3b release, enhancing opsonization
- C5a (chemotactic factor) release, with secondary neutrophil-mediated and monocyte-mediated injury
- C3a and C5a release, increasing vascular permeability and causing smooth muscle contraction
- Cytolysis mediated by the MAC
- A decrease in serum complement levels secondary to its consumption

Immune complexes also *aggregate platelets* (with subsequent degranulation) and *activate factor XII* (Hageman factor). The coagulation cascade and kinin systems are thus involved as well.

Morphology. Fibrinoid deposits within vessel walls with neutrophil infiltration and surrounding hemorrhage and edema—*acute necrotizing vasculitis (fibrinoid necrosis).* Superimposed thrombosis and downstream tissue necrosis may also be present. The immune complex and complement may be visualized by immunofluorescence as granular lumpy deposits or by electron microscopy as electron-dense deposits in the basement membranes. With time and clearance (catabolism) of the inciting antigen and immune complex, the lesions resolve.

Chronic Serum Sickness

Chronic serum sickness, resulting from recurrent or prolonged antigenemia (e.g., SLE), shows intimal thickening and vascular (or parenchymal or both) scarring.

LOCAL IMMUNE COMPLEX DISEASE (ARTHUS REACTION)

In local immune complex disease, localized tissue vasculitis and necrosis occur as a result of

- Local formation or deposition of immune complexes
- *Planting* of antigen within a particular tissue (e.g., the renal glomerulus) with subsequent in situ formation of immune complexes

This reaction may be produced experimentally by *intracutaneous* antigen injection in previously sensitized hosts carrying the appropriate circulating antibody. Antigen seeps into vascular walls where *large* immune complexes precipitate in situ (antibody excess). Complement and coagulation cascade activation and platelet aggregation lead to fibrinoid necrosis. Superimposed thrombosis may cause tissue necrosis.

Type IV Hypersensitivity (Cell Mediated)
(p. 204)

Type IV hypersensitivity is initiated by specifically sensitized T lymphocytes and includes delayed-type hypersensitivity and T cell–mediated cytotoxicity.

DELAYED-TYPE HYPERSENSITIVITY

Delayed-type hypersensitivity is the principal pattern of response to *Mycobacterium tuberculosis*, fungi, protozoa, and parasites as well as contact skin sensitivity. Delayed-type hypersensitivity also contributes to graft rejection. This hypersensitivity reaction is mediated by CD4+ (T_H1) cells that secrete specific cytokines after encounter with processed antigen in association with class II major histocompatibility complex (MHC). The induction of the T_H1 response is facilitated by IL-12, secreted by macrophages that have engulfed microbes or other antigen particles. T_H1 cells produce a variety of cytokines, such as interferon (IFN)-γ, IL-2, and TNF-α. These cytokines mediate injury primarily by recruiting and activating antigen-nonspecific monocytes and macrophages. The mechanisms of macrophage-mediated injury are discussed in Chapter 3. With persistent or nondegradable antigens, the initial nonspecific infiltrate of T cells and macrophages is replaced by a collection of macrophages that transform into epithelioid cells, thus forming a focal granuloma.

T CELL–MEDIATED CYTOTOXICITY

Generation of CD8+ cytotoxic T lymphocytes (CTL) is the principal pattern of response to many viral infections and to tumor cells. CTL also contribute to graft rejection. CTL recognize processed antigen in association with class I MHC. CTL-induced injury is mediated by the perforin-granzyme pathway and Fas-Fas L pathway.

TISSUE TRANSPLANTATION (p. 207)

To understand transplant rejection, a brief review of histocompatibility antigens is given.

Histocompatibility Antigens (p. 207)

The most important histocompatibility antigens are grouped in the MHC (also known as *human leukocyte antigen* or *HLA cluster*) on chromosome 6; they are highly polymorphic (i.e., with several alternative genes [alleles] for each locus). This complexity is a formidable barrier to transplantation.

CLASS I ANTIGENS

Present on virtually all nucleated cells and platelets, class I antigens are polymorphic heavy chain glycoproteins (coded on three closely linked loci: HLA-A, HLA-B, and HLA-C) and a nonpolymorphic β_2-microglobulin (coded by a gene on chromosome 15); they elicit antibodies in nonidentical individuals and are typed by conventional serologic techniques.

- These antigens typically bind only those processed antigens that are initially synthesized *endogenously* (e.g., viral products in a virally infected cell). The peptides derived from the processing of antigens bind to the *peptide-binding groove*, which faces outward from the cell membrane and is composed of the α_1 and α_2 domains of the class I heavy chain.
- MHC-I antigens *present* processed antigens to *CD8+ cytotoxic T cells* (with the appropriate receptor specificity), resulting in T-cell activation.
- Because T-cell receptors recognize only *antigen-MHC complexes*, CD8+ T cells bind and kill only infected cells that bear self–class I antigens; this is called *MHC restriction*.

CLASS II ANTIGENS

Class II antigens are characteristically confined to *antigen-presenting cells*, including dendritic cells, macrophages, B cells, and activated T cells.

- MHC-II antigens are coded in the HLA-D region with three serologically defined subloci (DP, DQ, and DR). Each class II molecule is a heterodimer of noncovalently associated α and β chains.
- MHC-II antigens typically bind and present *exogenous* (then internalized and processed) antigens to CD4+ T cells. *CD4+ helper T lymphocytes* also exhibit MHC restriction, recognizing processed antigen only in the context of self–class II MHC.

CLASS III PROTEINS

Some components of the complement system (C2, C4, Bf), and some cytokines (TNF-α and TNF-β) are encoded within the MHC cluster. Although linked to class I and II antigens, these are not histocompatibility antigens.

Transplant Rejection (p. 206)

Renal transplant rejection is described in some detail, followed by a brief comment on bone marrow transplantation. With minor variations, however, the same concepts are true for other tissues and organs (e.g., liver and heart).

CD8+ and CD4+ T cells react to processed MHC antigens in grafts. Consequences include direct CTL-mediated cytolysis as well as microvascular injury, tissue ischemia, and macrophage-mediated destruction. *Antibody-mediated responses* may also be important in some circumstances. They involve initial endothelial cell injury and subsequent vasculitis. This pattern of rejection, in general, responds poorly to immunosuppressive drugs.

HYPERACUTE REJECTION (p. 207)

When the recipient has been previously sensitized to antigens in graft (e.g., by blood transfusion, previous pregnancy, infections with HLA cross-reactive microorganisms), there is an immediate *hyperacute rejection* (minutes to 1 to 2 days) in which preformed circulating antibody fixes to antigens in the graft vascular bed and induces complement-mediated and ADCC-mediated injury.

The gross image is reflected in a cyanotic, mottled, flaccid organ. Microscopically the lesions resemble an Arthus reaction (described earlier). Immunoglobulin and complement are deposited in the vessel walls with endothelial injury, fibrin-platelet microthrombi, neutrophil infiltrates, and arteriolar fibrinoid necrosis followed by distal parenchymal infarction.

ACUTE REJECTION (p. 209)

Acute rejection typically occurs within a few days of transplantation or after cessation of immunosuppressive therapy. Both cellular and humoral mechanisms contribute to variable degrees.

Acute cellular rejection is characterized by an interstitial mononuclear cell infiltrate (macrophages, plasma cells, and both CD4+ and CD8+ T cells). CD8+ CTL damage tubular epithelial cells and vascular endothelial cells. CD4+ T cells inflict damage by inducing a delayed hypersensitivity reaction. Cellular rejection typically responds promptly to immunosuppressive drugs.

Acute rejection vasculitis is mediated by antidonor antibodies. It typically occurs in the first few months after transplantation. It causes necrotizing vasculitis and consequent thrombosis. A subacute vasculitis may also occur; it causes thickening of intima by proliferating fibroblasts and by accumulation of foamy macrophages. The resultant narrowing of blood vessels can cause infarction.

CHRONIC REJECTION (p. 210)

Chronic rejection occurs over months to years and is characterized by progressive organ dysfunction (i.e., rising serum creatinine). *Morphologically* the arteries show dense intimal fibrosis, probably the end stage of recurrent episodes of acute rejection leading to parenchymal ischemic injury. Frequently, there is a mononuclear interstitial infiltrate with numerous plasma cells and eosinophils.

BONE MARROW TRANSPLANTATION (p. 210)

Bone marrow transplantation presents special problems. Bone marrow transplantation is used for hematologic malignancies (e.g., leukemia), aplastic anemia, or immunodeficiency states. The recipient receives lethal levels of irradiation (or chemotherapy or both) to eradicate malignant cells, create a satisfactory graft bed, and minimize host rejection of the grafted marrow. Recipient NK cells or radiation-resistant T cells, however, may mediate significant transplant rejection.

The unique problem with marrow transplantation is *graft-versus-host disease (GVHD)*, in which donor immunocompetent cells or precursors are introduced into MHC-nonidentical, now immunocompromised recipients. The host cells are recognized by the transplanted cells as being foreign. CD8+ and CD4+ T cell–mediated injury ensues. Liver, skin, and gastrointestinal mucosa are most typically affected. There is also profound immunosuppression and reactivation of cytomegalovirus infection, particularly in the lung. Chronic GVHD produces skin changes similar to those seen in systemic sclerosis.

GVHD and complications (e.g., infections) are often lethal. Aside from close MHC matching, selective T-cell depletion from donor marrow is attempted to reduce the severity of GVHD. T cell–depleted marrow engrafts poorly, however, and in leukemic patients the relapse rate of leukemia is increased when T cell–depleted marrow is transplanted. Donor T cells in the marrow seem to exert a graft-versus-leukemia effect.

AUTOIMMUNE DISEASES (p. 211)

Autoimmune diseases result from some breakdown in *self-tolerance*, which is the lack of responsiveness to one's own antigens. Tolerance may be central or peripheral:

- *Central tolerance*: Many self-antigens are expressed in the thymus and presented by thymic antigen-presenting cells in association with MHC molecules. Immature T-cell clones with T-cell receptors that have high affinity for self-antigens are deleted in the thymus during development. A similar negative selection also occurs during B-cell development. Clonal deletion is not perfect, however, and normal B cells can be found with surface immunoglobulin against self-antigens (e.g., DNA, myelin, collagen, and thyroglobulin).
- *Peripheral tolerance*: Autoreactive cells that escape the thymus may be deleted or inactivated in the periphery. This may occur by three mechanisms:
  1. Clonal deletion by activation-induced death: Those self-antigens that are abundant in the peripheral tissue may cause persistent activation of self-reactive T cells, leading to expression of Fas-L on these cells. Such cells undergo apoptosis by engaging Fas coexpressed on these cells.
  2. Clonal anergy: Irreversible functional inactivation of T cells may occur when they recognize self-antigen in the absence of costimulatory signals from normal parenchymal cells.
  3. Peripheral suppression by T cells: CD4+ T cells of the T_H2 type may inhibit the functions of autoreactive T_H1-type cells by secreting cytokines such as IL-10 and transforming growth factor (TGF)-β.

Tolerance may be maintained if either helper T cells or B cells (or both) are rendered inactive. Because helper T cells control both cellular and humoral immunity, tolerance of T-helper cells is considered critical for prevention of autoimmune diseases. Autoimmune reactions may result from failure of peripheral tolerance:

- *Breakdown of T-cell anergy*: T-cell anergy may be broken if the antigen-presenting cells in the tissues are induced to express costimulator molecules, such as B7-1, thus providing the two signals (antigen plus costimulation) required for an immune response. Such induction may occur if infection of the tissue results in localized inflammation and release of cytokines and mediators that influence expression of costimulatory molecules.

■ *Failure of activation-induced cell death*: Defects in the Fas-Fas L pathway or other molecules involved in activation-induced death may prevent apoptosis of autoreactive T cells.

■ *Failure of T cell–mediated suppression*: Loss of suppressor T cells may prevent regulation of autoreactive T cells.

■ *Molecular mimicry*: Some infectious agents share epitopes with self-antigens, and hence antibodies against such epitopes may damage normal tissues.

■ *Polyclonal lymphocyte activation*: If anergic self-reactive clones are stimulated by antigen-independent mechanisms, autoimmunity may occur. A nonantigen-specific, polyclonal B-cell activator is bacterial endotoxin (lipopolysaccharide). Some microbial products, called superantigens, can activate multiple clones of CD4+ T cells by binding to class II MHC molecules and certain Vβ T-cell receptor chains. Among the polyclonally stimulated T and B cells, some may be autoreactive.

■ *Release of sequestered antigens*: Some antigens, such as lens crystallin and sperm that are sequestered from the developing immune system, do not induce self-tolerance. When released by trauma they can induce autoimmunity.

■ *Exposure of cryptic self and epitope spreading*: The molecular structure of certain self-antigens prevents exposure of some self-epitopes to developing T cells, and hence T cells are not tolerized to such *cryptic* epitopes. If such epitopes become recognizable in postnatal life as a result of molecular alteration in self-antigens, T cells reactive to such epitopes can cause autoimmunity. This phenomenon, called *epitope spreading*, is believed to be important in the pathogenesis of chronic autoimmune diseases.

HLA linkage (especially to the DR antigens) and familial clustering in some autoimmune diseases suggest a genetic component. Exogenous infection with bacteria, mycoplasmas, or especially viruses may also trigger autoimmunity, suggesting an exogenous component as well.

Autoimmunity may be tissue specific (e.g., autoimmune thyroiditis) or systemic (e.g., SLE). The following are systemic diseases (the single tissue diseases are discussed in their own chapters).

Systemic Lupus Erythematosus (p. 216)

SLE is the prototypical systemic autoimmune disorder, characterized by numerous autoantibodies, especially *antinuclear antibodies (ANAs)*. Incidence approaches 1 in 2500 in some general populations; the female-male ratio is 9:1.

ANAs are commonly detected by indirect immunofluorescence. The patterns of immunofluorescence (e.g., homogeneous, peripheral, speckled, nucleolar), although nonspecific, suggest the type of circulating antibody. ANAs occur in other autoimmune disorders, however, and in up to 10% of normal individuals (Table 7–2), but *anti–double-stranded (native) DNA and anti-Smith antigen antibodies strongly suggest SLE.*

ANAs cannot penetrate intact cells. Nuclei of damaged cells react with ANA, lose their chromatin patterns, and become homogeneous *lupus erythematosus (LE) bodies* (hematoxylin bodies).

Table 7-2. ANTINUCLEAR ANTIBODIES IN VARIOUS AUTOIMMUNE DISEASES

Nature of Antigen	Antibody System	Disease, % Positive					
		Systemic Lupus Erythematosus	Drug-Induced Lupus Erythematosus	Systemic Sclerosis—Diffuse	Limited Scleroderma—CREST	Sjögren Syndrome	Inflammatory Myopathies
Many nuclear antigens (DNA, RNA, proteins)	Generic ANA (indirect IF)	>95	>95	70-90	70-90	50-80	40-60
Native DNA	Anti-double-stranded DNA	40-60	<5	<5	<5	<5	<5
Histones	Antihistone	50-70	>95	<5	<5	<5	<5
Ribonucleoprotein (Smith antigen)	Anti-Sm	20-30	<5	<5	<5	<5	<5
Ribonucleoprotein (U1RNP)	Nuclear RNP	30-40	<5	<15	<10	<5	<5
Ribonucleoprotein Ribonucleoprotein	SS-A(Ro) SS-B(La)	30-50 10-15	<5 <5	<5 <5	<5 <5	70-95 60-90	<10 <5
DNA topoisomerase I	Scl-70	<5	<5	28-70	10-18	<5	<5
Centromeric proteins	Anticentromere	<5	<5	22-36	90	<5	<5
Histidyl-tRNA synthetase	Jo-1	<5	<5	<5	<5	<5	25

Boxed entries indicate high correlation.
ANA, antinuclear antibodies; RNP, ribonucleoprotein.

Phagocytosis of LE bodies by neutrophils or macrophages in vitro forms *LE cells* in up to 70% of patients with SLE.

In addition to ANAs, patients with SLE produce many other autoantibodies, some directed against blood elements (red cells, platelets, leukocytes). In addition, up to 40 to 50% of patients have antibodies to certain proteins complexed to phospholipids. Some bind to cardiolipin antigen, giving rise to false-positive Venereal Disease Research Laboratory (VDRL) tests. Others interfere with (prolong) in vitro tests for clotting. These so-called *lupus anticoagulants* actually exert a *pro*coagulant effect in vivo, causing recurrent vascular thromboses, miscarriages, and cerebral ischemia. Their mechanism of action in vivo is unknown.

ETIOLOGY AND PATHOGENESIS

Monozygotic twin concordance (24%) and familial and HLA clustering suggest a *genetic predisposition*. In addition, *exogenous factors*, such as drug exposure (see later), ultraviolet irradiation, and estrogens, are also involved. Although the cause is unknown, the pathogenesis is thought to involve some basic defect in the maintenance of self-tolerance with activation of B cells. This may occur secondary to some combination of

- Heritable defects in the regulation of B-cell proliferation
- Helper T-cell hyperactivity

It is thought that the primary defect is in CD4+ helper T cells that drive self-antigen–specific B cells to produce autoantibodies. Tissue damage occurs by formation of immune complexes (type III hypersensitivity) or by antibody-mediated injury to blood cells (type II hypersensitivity).

MORPHOLOGY

Typical in all tissues is an acute necrotizing vasculitis with fibrinoid deposits, involving small arteries and arterioles. Immunoglobulin, DNA, and C3 may be found within vessel walls. Skin and muscle are most commonly involved. A perivascular lymphocytic infiltrate is frequently present. In chronic cases, vessels show a fibrous thickening and luminal narrowing.

Kidney

The kidney is involved in virtually all cases of SLE. There are five patterns of *lupus nephritis*:

1. *Class I:* Normal by light, electron, and fluorescence microscopy; rare.
2. *Class II:* Mesangial lupus glomerulonephritis (GN); present in about 20% of patients. Associated with minimal hematuria or proteinuria. Slight increase in mesangial matrix and cells with granular mesangial immunoglobulins and complement deposits.
3. *Class III:* Focal proliferative GN; 20% of patients. Associated with recurrent hematuria, moderate proteinuria, and occasional mild renal insufficiency. Focal and segmental glomerular swelling with endothelial and mesangial proliferation, neutrophil infiltration, and sometimes fibrinoid deposits and capillary thrombi.
4. *Class IV:* Diffuse proliferative GN; 40 to 50% of patients, many of whom are overtly symptomatic, with microscopic to gross hematuria, proteinuria (sometimes nephrotic range), hypertension,

and diminished glomerular filtration rate. Most glomeruli show endothelial, mesangial, and occasionally epithelial proliferation. Immune complex deposits are typically *subendothelial* and when extensive form *wire loops*. Frequently, there are also tubular changes with granular immune complex deposits in basement membranes and interstitial changes. Most severe form of lupus nephritis, carrying the worst prognosis.

5. *Class V:* Membranous GN; 15% of patients. Induces severe proteinuria or nephrotic syndrome. Diffusely thickened capillary walls similar to idiopathic membranous GN and characterized by *subepithelial* immune complex deposits.

Skin

Classically, malar erythema, including bridge of nose *(butterfly rash)*, occurs. Also, variable cutaneous lesions ranging from erythema to bullae occur elsewhere. Sunlight exacerbates the lesions. Microscopically, there is basal layer degeneration with dermalepidermal junction immunoglobulin and complement deposits. The dermis shows variable fibrosis, perivascular mononuclear cell infiltrates, and vascular fibrinoid change.

Joints

Typically a nonspecific, nonerosive synovitis occurs. There is minimal joint deformity in contrast to rheumatoid arthritis.

Central Nervous System

Neuropsychiatric manifestations are probably secondary to endothelial injury and occlusion (antiphospholipid antibodies) or impaired neuronal function as a result of antibodies to a synaptic membrane antigen.

Serositis

Serositis is initially fibrinous with focal vasculitis, fibrinoid necrosis, and edema, progressing to adhesions, possibly obliterating serosal cavities (i.e., the pericardial sac).

Heart

Characteristic *nonbacterial verrucous (Libman-Sacks) endocarditis* occurs much less frequently with the use of steroids. Typically, numerous small, warty vegetations (0.5 to 4 mm) occur on the inflow or outflow surfaces (or both) of the mitral and tricuspid valves. Subtle or overt valvular abnormalities readily detected by echocardiography are common. They affect mitral and aortic valves and may cause stenosis or regurgitation.

An increasing number of younger patients, especially those treated with corticosteroids, have clinical evidence of coronary artery disease. The pathogenesis of the coronary atherosclerosis is not clear.

Spleen

Moderate splenomegaly occurs with capsular thickening and follicular hyperplasia. Marked perivascular fibrosis around penicilliary arteries is characteristic, producing an *onion-skin* appearance. Immunoglobulin, C3, and DNA are found within these vessels.

Lungs

Pleuritis occurs with pleural effusions, interstitial pneumonitis, and diffuse fibrosing alveolitis, all probably related to immune complex deposition.

CLINICAL COURSE

SLE presents insidiously as a systemic, chronic, recurrent, febrile illness with symptoms referable to virtually any tissue but especially joints, skin, kidneys, and serosal membranes. Autoantibodies to hematologic components may induce thrombocytopenia, leukopenia, and anemia. The clinical manifestations are protean (Table 7–3). The course of the disease is highly variable; rarely, it is fulminant with death in weeks to months.

- Sometimes the disease may cause minimal symptoms (hematuria, rash) and remit even without treatment.
- More often, the disease is characterized by recurrent flares and remissions over many years and is held in check by immunosuppressive regimens.
- Ten-year survival is approximately 80%; death is most commonly caused by renal failure or intercurrent infections.

DISCOID LUPUS ERYTHEMATOSUS

Discoid lupus erythematosus is a disease limited to cutaneous lesions that grossly and microscopically mimic SLE. Only 35% of patients have a positive ANA. As in SLE, there is deposition of immunoglobulin and C3 at the dermal-epidermal junction. After many years, 5 to 10% of affected individuals develop systemic manifestations.

Table 7–3. MANIFESTATIONS OF SYSTEMIC LUPUS ERYTHEMATOSUS

Clinical Manifestation	Prevalence in Patients (%)
Hematologic	100
Arthritis	90
Skin	85
Fever	83
Fatigue	81
Weight loss	63
Renal	50
Pleurisy	46
Myalgia	33
Pericarditis	25
Gastrointestinal	21
Raynaud phenomenon	20
Central nervous system	20
Ocular	15
Peripheral neuropathy	14
Pneumonitis	11
Parotid gland enlargement	8
Liver disease	2

From Condemi JJ: The autoimmune diseases. JAMA *258*:2920–2929, 1987. Copyright 1987, American Medical Association.

DRUG-INDUCED LUPUS ERYTHEMATOSUS

Drugs such as hydralazine, procainamide, isoniazid, and D-penicillamine frequently induce a positive ANA and less often a lupus erythematosus–like syndrome. With the latter, although there is multiorgan involvement, renal and central nervous system disease is uncommon. Anti–double-stranded DNA antibodies are rare, but antihistone antibodies are common. There is linkage with HLA-DR4. Drug-related lupus erythematosus usually remits after cessation of the offending agent.

Sjögren Syndrome (p. 225)

Sjögren syndrome is characterized by dry eyes *(keratoconjunctivitis sicca)* and dry mouth *(xerostomia)*, resulting from immune-mediated lacrimal and salivary gland destruction. Forty per cent of cases occur in isolation (the primary form or *sicca syndrome*), and the remaining 60% occur in association with other autoimmune diseases, such as rheumatoid arthritis (most common), SLE, or scleroderma.

- Ninety per cent of patients are women between 35 and 45 years of age.
- Most patients have rheumatoid factor in the absence of rheumatoid arthritis and ANAs especially against ribonucleoproteins SS-A and SS-B (see Table 7–2).
- Injury is probably a consequence of both cellular and humoral mechanisms. Injury is most likely initiated by activation of CD4+ T cells reacting to an unknown self-antigen. There is some association with human T-cell lymphotropic virus (HTLV)-1 infection, and patients with human immunodeficiency virus (HIV)-1 infection can develop similar lesions.

Morphologically the lacrimal and salivary glands (other exocrine glands may also be involved) initially show a periductal lymphocytic infiltrate (predominantly CD4+ T cells with some B cells) with ductal epithelial hyperplasia and luminal obstruction. This is followed by acinar atrophy, fibrosis, and eventual fatty replacement. Secondary changes include

- Corneal inflammation, erosion, and ulceration
- Atrophy of oral mucosa with inflammatory fissuring and ulceration
- Difficulty in swallowing solid foods
- Nasal drying and crusting with ulceration and, rarely, septal perforation
- Laryngitis, bronchitis, or pneumonitis resulting from respiratory involvement

To distinguish lacrimal and salivary gland enlargements by themselves (called *Mikulicz syndrome*) caused by Sjögren syndrome from other causes (sarcoidosis, leukemia, lymphoma), lip biopsy (to examine minor salivary glands) is helpful.

Some cases of Sjögren syndrome have extraglandular involvement, as follows:

- Commonly a tubulointerstitial nephritis occurs with tubular atrophy causing renal tubular acidosis with excess urate and phosphate excretion. Glomerular involvement is rare.
- Adenopathy may occur with pleomorphic lymph node infiltrates. There is a 40-fold increased risk of developing a B-cell lymphoma in involved glands.

Systemic Sclerosis (Scleroderma) (p. 227)

Systemic sclerosis involves excessive systemic fibrosis, most commonly in the skin (where it may be confined for years) but also eventually in the gastrointestinal tract, kidneys, heart, muscles, and lung in most patients. The female-male ratio is 3:1, with peak incidence in the 50- to 60-year age group. The disease initially presents with symmetric edema and thickening skin of hands and fingers or with Raynaud phenomenon (paroxysmal pallor or cyanosis of tips of fingers or toes). This initial presentation is followed by

- Articular symptoms that may mimic rheumatoid arthritis
- Dysphagia from esophageal fibrosis (up to 50% of patients)
- GI involvement leading to malabsorption or intestinal pain or obstruction
- Pulmonary fibrosis, which may cause respiratory or right-sided heart dysfunction
- Direct cardiac involvement, which may induce arrhythmias or heart failure
- Development of malignant hypertension, which may result in fatal renal failure.

Systemic sclerosis is subclassified into the following:

- *Diffuse scleroderma*: Widespread cutaneous and early visceral involvement with rapid progression. Associated more or less with specific ANA (see Table 7–2).
- Localized scleroderma *(CREST syndrome)*: Acronym for calcinosis, *R*aynaud phenomenon, *e*sophageal dysmotility, *s*clerodactyly, and *t*elangiectasia. Minimal cutaneous involvement (typically fingers and face) with late visceral involvement and a relatively benign course. Associated with anticentromere antibodies.

PATHOGENESIS

Although the genesis is unknown (and may be multifactorial), the final common pathway of systemic sclerosis involves fibroblast activation and endothelial injury. Possibilities include the following:

- Activation of CD4+ T cells by an unidentified antigen with production of cytokines (TNF-α, IL-1, IL-4, platelet-derived growth factor, or TGF-β) which promotes collagen synthesis
- Recurrent endothelial injury (owing to toxic mediators released by activated T cells or environmental triggers) causing platelet aggregation and subsequent release of activating factors that alter vascular permeability and stimulate fibroblasts

In addition, a host of autoantibodies, reflecting deranged humoral immunity, is also present. Of importance are

1. Antibodies to DNA topoisomerase I (anti-Scl 70), which is highly specific for diffuse scleroderma
2. Anticentromere antibody, characteristic of the CREST syndrome

There is no evidence that these antibodies cause injury.

MORPHOLOGY

Skin

Grossly, there is diffuse sclerosis with atrophy. Initially, affected areas are edematous with a doughy consistency. Eventually, fibrotic fingers become tapered and clawlike with diminished mobility, and the face becomes a drawn mask.

- Focal obliteration of the vascular supply causes ulceration. Occasionally, fingertips undergo autoamputation.
- Microscopically, there are perivascular lymphocytic infiltrates with early capillary and arteriolar injury and partial occlusion; edema and collagen fiber degeneration are followed by progressive dermal fibrosis and vascular hyaline thickening.

Gastrointestinal Tract

Progressive atrophy and collagenization of muscularis occurs, mostly in the esophagus; the lower two thirds may develop rubber-hose inflexibility.

- Throughout the alimentary tract, mucosa may be thinned and ulcerated with mural collagenization.
- Vascular changes are as described for skin.

Musculoskeletal System

Typically an inflammatory synovitis progressing to fibrosis is present; joint destruction is uncommon.

- Muscle involvement begins proximally with edema and mono-nuclear-perivascular infiltrates, progressing to interstitial fibrosis with myofiber degeneration.
- Vessels show basement membrane thickening.

Kidneys

The kidneys are affected in two thirds of patients with systemic sclerosis.

- *Renal failure accounts for 50% of deaths in systemic sclerosis.*
- The most prominent changes are in vessel walls (especially interlobular arteries) with intimal proliferation and deposition of mucinous or collagenous material.
- Hypertension is present in 30% of cases, 10% of which have a malignant course. Hypertension further accentuates the vascular changes, often resulting in fibrinoid necrosis with thrombosis and necrosis.

Lungs

Variable fibrosis of small pulmonary vessels with diffuse interstitial and alveolar fibrosis progresses in some cases to honeycombing.

Heart

Perivascular infiltrates with interstitial fibrosis occasionally evolve into a restrictive cardiomyopathy. There may also be conduction system involvement with resultant arrhythmias.

Nervous System

The central nervous system may have arterial lesions similar to those in the kidney with distal ischemic changes. Peripheral neuropathy may occur owing to perineural vascular sclerosis.

Inflammatory Myopathies (p. 229)

Inflammatory myopathies are an uncommon group of immunologically mediated inflammatory disorders that injure skeletal muscles. Included are *dermatomyositis*, *polymyositis*, and *inclusion body myositis*.

- *Dermatomyositis*: Dermatomyositis is characterized by involvement of skin and skeletal muscles, and affects children as well as adults.
  - Classic skin rash is seen as lilac or heliotrope discoloration of upper eyelids with periorbital edema. Scaling red eruptions (Grotton lesions) are often present on knuckles, elbows, and knees.
  - Muscle weakness is gradual and bilaterally symmetric and typically affects proximal muscles first.
  - Women have a slightly higher risk of developing visceral cancers—lung, ovary, stomach.
  - Dermatomyositis is most likely caused by antibody-mediated injury to the microvasculature in the perimysial connective tissue. The resultant perifascicular atrophy of myofibers is characteristic.
- *Polymyositis*: Muscle involvement resembles dermatomyositis, but skin involvement and association with cancers are lacking. Polymyositis is caused by damage to muscle fibers by CD8+ cytotoxic T cells, which can be seen to invade and surround muscle fibers. Both necrotic and regenerating fibers are present.
- *Inclusion body myositis*: In contrast to the two other forms, the muscle involvement in inclusion body myositis is asymmetric and involves distal muscles (extensors of foot and flexors of fingers) first. Histologically characterized by the presence of vacuoles in affected myocytes, which are rimmed by basophilic granules.

The diagnosis of these disorders is based on clinical features, electromyography, increase in serum creatinine kinase, and biopsy.

Mixed Connective Tissue Disease (p. 231)

It is controversial whether mixed connective tissue disease represents a heterogeneous subgroup of other autoimmune disorders or is a separate clinical entity. It is characterized by the following:

- Features suggestive of SLE, polymyositis, and systemic sclerosis (e.g., Raynaud phenomenon, esophageal dysmotility, myositis, leukopenia-anemia, fever, lymphadenopathy, and hypergammaglobulinemia)
- High ANA titers to ribonucleoproteins (and in contrast to SLE *no* antibodies to native DNA or Smith antigens)
- Infrequency of renal disease
- Excellent response to steroids

Polyarteritis Nodosa and Other Vasculitides (p. 231)

Polyarteritis nodosa and other vasculitides comprise a group of noninfectious necrotizing vasculitides detailed in Chapter 12.

IMMUNOLOGIC DEFICIENCY SYNDROMES (p. 231)

Immunologic deficiency syndromes may be subdivided into primary and secondary forms:

- *Primary immunodeficiency disorders* are usually hereditary, typically manifesting between 6 months and 2 years of life as maternal antibody protection is lost.
- *Secondary immunodeficiencies* result from altered immune function because of infections, malnutrition, aging, immunosuppression, irradiation, chemotherapy, or autoimmunity.

X-Linked Agammaglobulinemia of Bruton
(p. 232)

X-linked agammaglobulinemia of Bruton is one of the most common primary immunodeficiency syndromes. This X-linked disorder presents as *recurrent bacterial infections* (e.g., *Staphylococcus, Haemophilus influenzae, Streptococcus pneumoniae*) beginning after 6 months of age. There is virtually no serum immunoglobulin, but cell-mediated immune function is normal; consequently, most viral and fungal infections are handled appropriately. Exceptions include enterovirus, echovirus (causing a fatal encephalitis), and vaccine-associated poliovirus (causing paralysis) because these viruses are neutralized by antibodies in the bloodstream. *Giardia lamblia*, an intestinal parasite that is normally resisted by secreted IgA, can also cause persistent infections.

- The basic defect is lack of *mature* B cells because of mutations in Bruton tyrosine-kinase gene expressed in early B cells. Pre-B cells are present in normal numbers in marrow, but lymph nodes and spleen lack germinal centers, and plasma cells are absent from all tissues.
- T-cell numbers and function are entirely normal.
- For unknown reasons, these patients have an increased frequency (up to 20%) of autoimmune connective tissue diseases, including a rheumatoid-like arthritis that responds to gammaglobulin therapy.

Common Variable Immunodeficiency
(p. 233)

Common variable immunodeficiency comprises a heterogeneous group of disorders, congenital or acquired, sporadic or familial. *The common feature is hypogammaglobulinemia, generally affecting all immunoglobulin classes but occasionally only IgG.*

The pathogenesis of antibody deficiency is not clear and may differ among patients. There may be intrinsic B-cell defects or, more commonly, defective B-cell maturation as a result of defects in T cells. Some patients show linkage with the complement genes within HLA complex, as do certain patients with selective IgA deficiency, suggesting some genetically determined defect in B-cell differentiation. Clinical features resemble X-linked agammaglobulinemia (i.e., recurrent sinopulmonary infections, serious enterovirus infections, and persistent *G. lamblia* infections). In contrast to X-linked agammaglobulinemia, symptoms start in childhood or adolescence. These patients are also prone to autoimmune diseases and lymphoid malignancies.

Isolated IgA Deficiency (p. 234)

Isolated IgA deficiency is a common immunodeficiency (1 in 600 people) with *virtual absence of serum and secretory IgA and occasionally of IgG$_2$ and IgG$_4$ subclasses.* This immunodeficiency may be familial or acquired after toxoplasmosis, measles, or other viral infection.

- Although usually asymptomatic, patients may have recurrent sinopulmonary and gastrointestinal infections and are prone to respiratory tract allergies and autoimmune diseases (SLE, rheumatoid arthritis).
- The basic defect is failure of maturation of IgA-positive B cells. Immature forms are present in normal numbers.
- Forty per cent of patients have antibodies to IgA. Transfusion of IgA-containing blood products may induce anaphylaxis.

Hyper-IgM Syndrome

Hyper-IgM syndrome is characterized by the production of IgM but failure to produce IgG, IgA, and IgE antibodies. This syndrome results from failure of T cells to cause B cells to switch to the formation of immunoglobulins other than IgM. Such isotype switching depends on interaction of CD40L on T cells with CD40 on B cells. In 70% of patients, there is mutation of CD40L gene encoded on X chromosome; hence the disease is X-linked. In others, precise mutation is not yet identified.

Clinically, lack of IgG leads to recurrent bacterial infections; in addition, because T-cell/macrophage interactions also involve CD40–CD40L, there is also susceptibility to *Pneumocystis carinii* pneumonia.

DiGeorge Syndrome (Thymic Hypoplasia)
(p. 235)

DiGeorge syndrome is a multiorgan congenital disorder resulting from failure of development of the third and fourth pharyngeal pouches before the eighth week of gestation. Characteristics are as follows:

- *Thymic hypoplasia or aplasia*: T-cell deficiency with lack of cell-mediated responses (especially to fungi and viruses); B cells and immunoglobulin levels are usually normal.
- *Parathyroid hypoplasia*: Abnormal calcium regulation with hypocalcemic tetany.
- *Congenital defects of heart and great vessels.*
- *Dysmorphic facies.*

DiGeorge syndrome results from the deletion of some unidentified genes on 22q11; this chromosomal abnormality is seen in 90% of cases. Patients may be treated with fetal thymus or thymic epithelium transplants. If children survive into their fifth year, T-cell function tends to normalize even with thymic aplasia.

Severe Combined Immunodeficiency Disease (p. 235)

Severe combined immunodeficiency disease (SCID) refers to a heterogeneous group of autosomal or X-linked recessive disorders *characterized by lymphopenia and defects in T-cell and B-cell function*, particularly in the former. Pathogenetic mechanisms fall into two general categories:

1. In 50 to 60% of cases, SCID is an X-linked disorder resulting from a mutation in the common γ chain (γc) subunit of several cytokine receptors. Because of the defective receptor subunit, lymphoid progenitors fail to be stimulated by IL-2, IL-4, IL-7, IL-9, IL-11, and IL-15, and consequently there is a severe defect in T-cell development and a lesser defect in B-cell development.

2. The remaining cases of SCID are inherited as autosomal recessives, and in this group the most common cause is deficiency of the enzyme adenosine deaminase. This deficiency leads to an accumulation of metabolites, such as deoxy–adenosine triphosphate (ATP), that are toxic to lymphocytes.

Because T-cell defects lead to secondary B-cell defects, patients with SCID have impairment of cellular and humoral immunity, manifested as recurrent bacterial, viral, and fungal infections. Their lymphoid tissue (thymus, lymph nodes) is hypoplastic. Bone marrow transplantation is the only treatment at present.

Immunodeficiency with Thrombocytopenia and Eczema (Wiskott-Aldrich Syndrome)
(p. 236)

Wiskott-Aldrich syndrome is an *X-linked recessive disease characterized by thrombocytopenia, eczema, and recurrent infections* with a predilection for the development of lymphomas.

- The thymus is morphologically normal, but there is peripheral T-cell depletion in lymphoid tissues with an associated defect in cellular immunity.
- Antibody responses are variable but are characteristically poor to polysaccharide antigens.
- The pathogenesis is unknown; bone marrow transplantation has occasionally been curative.

GENETIC DEFICIENCIES OF THE COMPLEMENT SYSTEM (p. 236)

Genetic deficiencies of the complement system have been described for virtually all complement components and for two inhibitors. A deficiency of C2 is the most common, but it is not associated with serious infections, presumably because the alternative complement pathway is unaffected. Deficiency of C3 impairs both complement pathways and hence leads to increased susceptibility to bacterial infections. Inherited deficiencies of C1q, C2, and C4 impair clearance of immune complexes and hence increase the risk of immune complex–mediated diseases (e.g., SLE). An absence of C1 esterase inhibitor is associated with *hereditary angioedema* as a result of uncontrolled generation of vasoactive kinins. Defects in later-acting components (C5–C8) result in recurrent neisserial infections.

Acquired Immunodeficiency Syndrome
(p. 236)

AIDS is an infectious secondary form of immunodeficiency caused by HIV-1. It is characterized by profound suppression of T cell–mediated immunity, opportunistic infections, secondary neoplasms, and neurologic disease.

EPIDEMIOLOGY AND MODES OF TRANSMISSION

Transmission of HIV occurs through

1. Sexual contact
2. Parenteral inoculation
3. Passage from infected mothers to fetuses or newborns.

In the United States, there are five major risk groups:

1. *Homosexual/bisexual men*: Approximately 57% of reported cases of AIDS (in homosexual men the virus enters via lymphocytes in semen through traumatized rectal mucosa).
2. *Intravenous drug users* (without a history of homosexual contact): Approximately 25% of all patients. Caused by sharing of contaminated needles and paraphernalia.
3. *Hemophiliacs*: Especially those receiving large amounts of pooled factor VIII concentrate before 1985; 0.8% of cases.
4. *Blood/component recipients (excluding hemophiliacs)*: 1.2% of all patients. Transmission by this route has been virtually eliminated in the United States.
5. *Other high-risk groups*: Ten per cent of patients acquire disease through heterosexual contacts with members of other high-risk groups.

In approximately 6% of cases, no risk factors can be identified. Ninety per cent of children with AIDS have an HIV-infected mother and suffer transplacental or perinatal transmission. Ten per cent of pediatric AIDS patients are those who received blood or blood products before 1985.

Some other aspects of transmission are as follows:

- The risk of seroconversion after an accidental needle-stick with infected blood is approximately 0.3%.
- HIV is *not* transmitted by casual (nonsexual) contact.
- Outside the United States and Europe, male-to-female transmission (most through vaginal intercourse) is the most common mode of spread.
- Increased heterosexual transmission is beginning to outpace other modes in the United States.
- Although HIV has been found in vaginal and cervical secretions, monocytes, and endothelium, female-to-male transmission is not common in the United States.
- All forms of sexual transmission are facilitated by coexistence of sexually transmitted diseases with genital ulcerations.

BIOLOGY OF HIV-1

HIV-1 is a human type C retrovirus in the same family as the animal lentivirus family. It is also closely related to HIV-2, which causes a similar disease, primarily in West Africa.

- HIV is a *nontransforming cytopathic retrovirus* inducing immunodeficiency by destruction of target T cells.
- The HIV-1 lipid envelope, derived from the infected host membrane during budding, is studded with two viral glycoproteins, gp120 and gp41, the former important in binding to host CD4 molecules to initiate viral infection.

- The virus core contains major capsid protein p24, nucleocapsid protein, genomic RNA, and three viral enzymes: protease, integrase, and reverse transcriptase. Antiviral therapy is directed against reverse transcriptase and protease.
- It has several genes not present in the other retroviruses. These include *tat, vpu, vif, nef,* and *rev.* Many, such as *tat* and *rev,* regulate HIV transcription and hence may be targeted for therapy.

HIV INFECTION OF LYMPHOCYTES AND MONOCYTES

Central to the pathogenesis of AIDS is depletion of CD4+ helper T cells. The CD4 antigen (also present at lower levels on monocytes and macrophages) is the high-affinity receptor for the gp120 protein on HIV-1. In addition to CD4, the gp120 must also bind to coreceptors on its target cells. The major coreceptors are CCRS and CXCR4, which also serve as receptors for chemokines. Some individuals who have mutations in the genes that encode CCR5 are resistant to HIV infection.

- After binding, the virus is internalized; the genome undergoes reverse transcription; the proviral DNA is then integrated into the host genome.
- *Transcription/translation and viral propagation may subsequently occur only with T-cell activation (e.g., antigenic stimulation). In the absence of T-cell activation, the infection enters a latent phase.*
- Early in the course of the disease, HIV colonizes the lymphoid organs; this is followed by T-cell depletion. The mechanism by which T cells are lost is not certain. According to one view, approximately 1 to 2 billion T cells are lysed every day by viral infection in the lymphoid tissues, but early in the disease this loss is largely replenished by regeneration, and hence T-cell loss appears to be deceptively small. According to other views, T-cell destruction by viral infection is not sufficient to explain the T-cell loss, and additional mechanisms must exist including reduced T-cell production and apoptosis of uninfected T cells.
- Infected monocytes and macrophages refractory to HIV cytopathic effects act
  1. As reservoirs for HIV (perhaps transferring virus to T cells during antigen presentation).
  2. As vehicles for viral transport, especially to the central nervous system.
- In addition to macrophages, the follicular dendritic cells in the germinal center of lymph nodes are also important reservoirs of HIV. The viral particles coated with anti-HIV antibodies are found attached to the Fc receptor for immunoglobulin on the surface of follicular dendritic cells. These HIV virions continually infect T cells as they come in close contact with the follicular dendritic cells during passage through lymph nodes.
- The consequences of CD4+ cell depletion on immune function are listed in Table 7–4.
- In addition to T-cell depletion, there are also qualitative defects in T-cell function, with a selective loss of T-cell memory early in the course of disease.
- There is paradoxic B-cell activation, but nonetheless patients with AIDS are unable to mount appreciable antibody responses to new antigens, probably owing to CD4+ T-cell depletion, intrinsic B-cell defects, or both.

Table 7-4. MAJOR ABNORMALITIES OF IMMUNE
FUNCTION IN AIDS

Lymphopenia
Predominantly due to selective loss of the CD4+ helper-inducer T-cell
  subset; inversion of CD4–CD8 ratio
Decreased T-Cell Function in Vivo
Preferential loss of memory T cells
Susceptibility to opportunistic infections
Susceptibility to neoplasms
Decreased delayed-type hypersensitivity
Altered T-Cell Function in Vitro
Decreased proliferative response to mitogens, alloantigens, and soluble
  antigens
Decreased specific cytotoxicity
Decreased helper function for pokeweed mitogen-induced B-cell
  immunoglobulin production
Decreased IL-2 and IFN-γ production
Polyclonal B-Cell Activation
Hypergammaglobulinemia and circulating immune complexes
Inability to mount de novo antibody response to a new antigen
Refractoriness to the normal signals for B-cell activation in vitro
Altered Monocyte or Macrophage Functions
Decreased chemotaxis and phagocytosis
Decreased HLA class II antigen expression
Diminished capacity to present antigen to T cells
Increased spontaneous secretion of IL-1, TNF-α, IL-6

IL, interleukin; IFN, interferon; TNF, tumor necrosis factor.

CENTRAL NERVOUS SYSTEM INVOLVEMENT BY HIV

The central nervous system is a major target in HIV infection. This occurs predominantly, if not exclusively, via monocytes. Infected monocytes circulate to the brain and are somehow activated either to release toxic cytokines directly or to recruit other neuron-damaging inflammatory cells.

NATURAL HISTORY OF HIV INFECTION

On the basis of interactions of HIV with the host immune system, HIV infection can be divided into three phases (Fig. 7–1).

1. *Early, acute phase*: Characterized by transient viremia, widespread seeding of lymphoid tissue, a temporary fall in CD4+ T cells, followed by seroconversion and control of viral replication by generation of CD8+ antiviral T cells. Clinically a self-limited acute illness with sore throat, nonspecific myalgias, and aseptic meningitis may develop. Clinical recovery and near-normal CD4+ T-cell counts occur within 6 to 12 weeks. The viral load at the end of the acute phase reflects the balance between HIV production and host defenses. This viral set-point is an important predictor of the rate of progression of HIV disease. Those with high viral loads at the end of the acute phase progress to AIDS more rapidly.

2. *Middle, chronic phase*: Characterized by clinical latency with continued vigorous viral replication mainly in the lymphoid tissue but gradual decline of CD4+ counts owing to brisk regeneration of the T cells. Patients may develop persistent generalized lymph

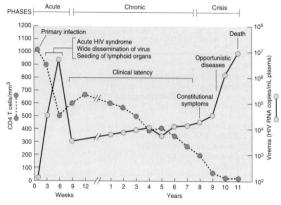

Figure 7-1   ∎

Typical course of human immunodeficiency virus (HIV) infection. During the early period after primary infection, there is widespread dissemination of virus and a sharp decrease in the number of CD4 + T cells in peripheral blood. An immune response to HIV ensues, with a decrease in viremia followed by a prolonged period of clinical latency. During this period, viral replication continues. The CD4 + T-cell count gradually decreases during the following years, until it reaches a critical level below which there is a substantial risk of opportunistic diseases. (Redrawn from Fauci AS, Lane HC: Human immunodeficiency virus disease: AIDS and related conditions. In Fauci AS, et al (eds): Harrison's Principles of Internal Medicine, 14th ed. New York, McGraw-Hill, 1997, p 1791.)

node enlargement, with no constitutional symptoms. This phase may last for years. Toward the end of this phase, fever, rash, fatigue, and viremia appear. The chronic phase may last from 7 to 10 years.

3. *Final, crisis phase*: Characterized by rapid decline in host defenses manifested by low CD4+ counts, weight loss, diarrhea, opportunistic infections, and secondary neoplasms. This phase is usually recognized as full-blown AIDS. Centers for Disease Control guidelines consider anyone with HIV infection and CD4+ T-cell count less than 200 cells/μl as having AIDS, even if all clinical features are not present.

In each of the three phases of HIV infection, viral replication continues, and hence HIV infection lacks a phase of true microbiologic latency.

The clinical features of full-blown AIDS include the following:

- A variety of opportunistic infections occur (Table 7–5). *Pneumocystis carinii* pneumonia occurs in 50% of patients; other pathogens are *Candida*, cytomegalovirus, typical and atypical mycobacteria, *Cryptococcus neoformans, Toxoplasma gondii, Cryptosporidium*, herpes simplex virus, papovaviruses, and *Histoplasma capsulatum*.
- A wide spectrum of pyogenic bacterial infections (reflecting altered humoral immunity) occurs.
- A variety of malignant neoplasms occur (see Table 7–5). Aggressive *Kaposi sarcoma* (KS) is the most common; it is more common in homosexuals than in other risk groups.
- KS lesions are composed of spindle cells that form vascular channels. These lesions are monoclonal neoplasms that are

Table 7-5. AIDS-DEFINING OPPORTUNISTIC
INFECTIONS AND NEOPLASMS FOUND
IN PATIENTS WITH HIV INFECTION

Infections

Protozoal and helminthic infections
  Cryptosporidiosis or isosporidiosis (enteritis)
  Pneumocytosis (pneumonia or disseminated infection)
  Toxoplasmosis (pneumonia or CNS infection)

Fungal infections
  Candidiasis (esophageal, tracheal, or pulmonary)
  Cryptococcosis (CNS infection)
  Coccidioidomycosis (disseminated)
  Histoplasmosis (disseminated)

Bacterial infections
  Mycobacteriosis (*atypical*, e.g., *M. avium-intracellulare*, disseminated or
    extrapulmonary; *M. tuberculosis*, pulmonary or extrapulmonary)
  Nocardiosis (pneumonia, meningitis, disseminated)
  Salmonella infections, disseminated

Viral infections
  Cytomegalovirus (pulmonary, intestinal, retinitis, or CNS infections)
  Herpes simplex virus (localized or disseminated)
  Varicella-zoster virus (localized or disseminated)
  Progressive multifocal leukoencephalopathy

Neoplasms

  Kaposi sarcoma
  Non-Hodgkin lymphomas (Burkitt, immunoblastic)
  Primary lymphoma of the brain
  Invasive cancer of uterine cervix

CNS, central nervous system.

strongly associated with human herpesvirus-8 (HHV-8), also called *KS herpesvirus*. It is thought that proliferation of the spindle cells in KS is driven by cytokines derived from HHV-8-infected mesenchymal cells, HIV-infected T cells, and HHV-8-infected B cells. KS also occurs in non-HIV–infected individuals (Chapter 12).

■ Aggressive B-cell non-Hodgkin lymphomas, especially at extra-nodal sites, frequently involving the brain, occur at rates 120-fold higher than in the general population. In addition, an uncommon body cavity lymphoma that involves pleural, peritoneal, and pericardial spaces is also found. Epstein-Barr virus is important in the pathogenesis of AIDS-associated lymphomas. Fifty percent of systemic lymphomas and 100% of central nervous system lymphomas carry the Epstein-Barr virus genome. Body cavity lymphomas are associated with HHV-8 infection. Patients with AIDS also have increased incidence of squamous cell carcinoma of the uterine cervix most likely caused by greater susceptibility to HIV infection.

■ Clinical neurologic involvement occurs in 40 to 60% of patients, manifesting as
  1. Acute aseptic meningitis
  2. A vacuolar myelopathy
  3. A peripheral neuropathy
  4. Most commonly, a progressive encephalopathy designated AIDS-dementia complex.

■ With AIDS, the 5-year mortality rate is 85%, and with longer intervals the rate approaches 100%.

MORPHOLOGY

With the exception of the central nervous system, the tissue changes in AIDS are neither specific nor diagnostic. Basically the pathologic features are those of the various opportunistic infections and the specific neoplasms. These infections and those in the central nervous system and in AIDS-associated nephropathy are discussed elsewhere in the chapters devoted to each particular organ. Following is a description of lymph node pathology.

Lymph Nodes

Adenopathy in early HIV infection reflects the initial polyclonal B-cell proliferation and hypergammaglobulinemia, showing nonspecific, predominantly follicular hyperplasia with mantle zone attenuation and intense medullary plasmacytosis. HIV particles can be demonstrated in germinal centers by in situ hybridization, localized mainly on the surface of follicular dendritic cells.

- With progression to full-blown AIDS, the lymphoid follicles become involuted *(burned out)*, with general lymphocyte depletion and disruption of the organized follicular dendritic cell network.
- Inflammatory responses to infections may be sparse or atypical, and infectious organisms may not be apparent without special stains.
- Similar lymphoid depletion occurs in the spleen and thymus.
- Patients frequently develop diffuse high-grade malignant B-cell lymphomas (the second most common malignancy, after KS), perhaps because of prolonged B-cell proliferation in the face of deteriorating regulatory controls.

AMYLOIDOSIS (p. 251)

Amyloid is a heterogeneous group of pathogenetic fibrillar proteins that accumulate within tissues and organs, either because of excess synthesis or because of resistance to catabolism. *All these proteins share the ability to aggregate into an insoluble, cross-beta–pleated sheet tertiary conformation; are all deposited extracellularly in a variety of tissues* and in a large array of clinical settings. As the material accumulates, it produces pressure atrophy of adjacent parenchyma. Depending on tissue distribution and degree of involvement, amyloid may be asymptomatic and found only as an unsuspected anatomic change or may be life-threatening.

Ultrastructure (p. 251)

By electron microscopy, amyloid is composed predominantly (90%) of nonbranching fibrils of indeterminate length and a diameter of 7.5 to 10 nm. These fibrils are associated with a minor (10%) *P component*, consisting of stacks of pentagonal, doughnut-shaped structures with homology to C-reactive protein.

Chemical Nature (p. 252)

There are three major and several minor chemically distinct classes of amyloid fibrils (Table 7–6):

Table 7-6. CLASSIFICATION OF AMYLOIDOSIS

Clinicopathologic Category	Associated Diseases	Major Fibril Protein	Chemically Related Precursor Protein
Systemic (Generalized) Amyloidosis			
Immunocyte dyscrasias with amyloidosis (primary amyloidosis)	Multiple myeloma and other monoclonal B-cell proliferations	AL	Immunoglobulin light chains, chiefly λ type
Reactive systemic amyloidosis (secondary amyloidosis)	Chronic inflammatory conditions	AA	SAA
Hemodialysis-associated amyloidosis	Chronic renal failure	$A\beta_2M$	β_2-Microglobulin
Hereditary amyloidosis			
Familial Mediterranean fever	—	AA	SAA
Familial amyloidotic neuropathies (several types)	—	ATTR	Transthyretin*
Systemic senile amyloidosis	—	ATTR	Transthyretin*
Localized Amyloidosis			
Senile cerebral	Alzheimer disease	$A\beta_2$	APP
Endocrine, e.g., medullary carcinoma of thyroid	—	ACal	Calcitonin

*Transthyretin is also known as prealbumin. The transthyretins deposited as amyloid are mutant forms of normal transthyretin.
AL, amyloid light chain; AA, amyloid associated (protein); SAA, serum amyloid associated (protein).

1. *AL (amyloid light-chain protein)*: Immunoglobulin light chains (or amino-terminal fragments thereof) derived from plasma cells; lambda much more often than kappa. *Frequently associated with B-cell dyscrasias (e.g., multiple myeloma).*

2. *AA (amyloid-associated protein)*: A nonimmunoglobulin protein derived from a 12,000-dalton serum precursor called *SAA* (serum amyloid–associated) protein synthesized in liver and elevated in inflammatory states.

3. *β_2-amyloid protein* ($A\beta_2$): A peptide found in Alzheimer disease that forms the core of cerebral plaques and deposits within cerebral vessel walls. It derives from a transmembrane glycoprotein precursor (APP).

Some less common forms of amyloid in particular clinical settings include

- *Transthyretin (TTR)*: A normal serum protein that binds and transports thyroxine and retinol. A mutant form is deposited as amyloid in a group of hereditary diseases called *familial amyloid polyneuropathy.*

- *β_2-microglobulin*: The smaller nonpolymorphic peptide component of class I MHC molecules and a normal serum protein; deposited in amyloidosis complicating long-term hemodialysis.

Clinical Forms of Amyloidosis (p. 252)

Amyloidosis is subdivided into *systemic* (generalized) and *localized* (tissue-specific) forms and is further classified on the basis of predisposing conditions (see Table 7–6).

SYSTEMIC AMYLOIDOSIS

Systemic amyloidosis is associated with the following conditions:

1. *B-cell dyscrasias (also called primary amyloidosis)*: The most common form in the United States. Composed of AL-type amyloid.
  - AL-type systemic amyloidosis occurs in 5 to 15% of patients with multiple myeloma.
  - Tumorous plasma cells synthesize abnormal quantities of a single immunoglobulin (*M spike* on serum protein electrophoresis) or immunoglobulin light chain (*Bence Jones* protein). By virtue of their smaller size, Bence Jones proteins are frequently excreted in the urine.
  - The vast majority of cases of AL-type systemic amyloidosis are *not* associated with *overt* B-cell neoplasms. Nevertheless, they have monoclonal immunoglobulins, light chains, or both.
  - Typically (but not always), this type involves the heart, gastrointestinal tract, peripheral nerves, skin, and tongue more than other organs.

2. *Secondary or reactive amyloidosis*: Marked by AA-type amyloid.
  - *Secondary amyloidosis is associated with chronic inflammatory states (infectious and noninfectious) producing protracted cell breakdown* (e.g., rheumatoid arthritis, scleroderma, dermatomyositis, bronchiectasis, chronic osteomyelitis).
  - Typically, kidneys, liver, spleen, lymph nodes, adrenals, and thyroid are involved.

3. *Hemodialysis related*: Affects up to 70% of patients on chronic hemodialysis. Due to deposition (in joints, synovium, and tendon sheaths) of β2-microglobulin not filtered by normal dialysis membranes.

4. *Hereditary forms*: Include many rare entities, often confined to specific geographic locations.

- Most common and best characterized is *familial Mediterranean fever*, a recurrent, febrile illness typically in Sephardic Jews, Armenians, and Arabs, characterized by bouts of serosal inflammation. The systemic amyloid is of AA type, suggesting that chronic inflammation plays a pivotal role.
- *Familial amyloidotic polyneuropathies* have autosomal dominant transmission and show deposition of variant transthyretins principally in peripheral and autonomic nerves.

LOCALIZED AMYLOIDOSIS

Localized amyloidosis is confined to amyloid in a single organ or tissue. The following conditions are associated:

1. *Nodular (tumor-forming) deposits*: Often AL protein with associated plasma cell infiltrates. Occur most frequently in lung, larynx, skin, bladder, tongue, and periorbitally. May represent localized forms of B-cell dyscrasias.

2. *Endocrine amyloid*: Deposition in a variety of tumors associated with catabolism of polypeptide hormones or prohormones (e.g., thyroid medullary carcinoma [procalcitonin]).

AMYLOIDOSIS OF AGING

Amyloidosis of aging occurs typically in the eighth and ninth decades and is most commonly due to deposition of transthyretin. Although amyloid distribution is systemic, the dominant involvement is of the heart, and it presents with cardiomyopathy or arrhythmias. In addition to the sporadic senile systemic amyloidosis, there is another form, affecting predominantly the heart, in which mutant transthyretin is deposited. This condition is more common in blacks.

Morphology

Macroscopically, affected tissues are stained blue-violet with iodine and dilute sulfuric acid. Microscopically with routine stains, amyloid is amorphous, acellular, hyaline, and eosinophilic. With special stains (e.g., Congo red), it is salmon-red, and characteristic yellow-green birefringence may be seen by means of polarized light.

KIDNEYS

Kidneys are classically enlarged, pale gray, waxy, and firm. In advanced disease, chronic vascular occlusion (owing to amyloid deposits) may result in a shrunken, contracted organ. Amyloid deposits in the following places:

- *Glomeruli*, initially mesangial and subendothelial: With continued accumulation, there is hyalinization of glomeruli.
- *Peritubular regions* begin in the tubular basement membrane and gradually extend into the interstitium.

■ *Blood vessels*: Hyaline thickening of arterial and arteriolar walls with narrowing lumen eventually causes ischemia with tubular atrophy and interstitial fibrosis.

SPLEEN

The spleen may be enlarged (up to 800 gm). Amyloid deposits begin between cells. With time, one of two patterns emerges:

1. *Sago spleen*: Deposits are limited to the splenic follicles, giving rise to *tapioca-like* granules on gross inspection.
2. *Lardaceous spleen*: Amyloid largely spares the follicles and is deposited in the pulp. Fusion of deposits forms large geographic areas.

LIVER

Amyloid induces hepatomegaly with a pale, waxy gray, firm appearance. Microscopically, amyloid first deposits in the space of Disse, gradually encroaching on parenchyma and sinusoids to produce pressure atrophy with massive hepatic replacement.

HEART

Distinctive (although not always present) are minute, typically atrial, pink-to-gray subendocardial droplets representing focal amyloid accumulations. Vascular and subepicardial deposits may also occur. Microscopically, there are interstitial and perimyocyte deposits, progressively leading to pressure atrophy.

Clinical Features

Diagnosis is made on the basis of biopsy and characteristic Congo red stain. Favored biopsy sites are the kidney (when renal manifestations are present) and the rectum or gingiva (in systemic disease).

■ Abdominal fat pad aspirates may also yield diagnostic tissue.
■ In amyloidosis suspected of being associated with B-cell dyscrasias, serum and urine electrophoresis and bone marrow biopsy (for plasmacytosis) are indicated.
■ In systemic amyloidosis, the prognosis is poor. Median survival after diagnosis in the setting of B-cell dyscrasias is about 24 months. Reactive amyloidosis may have a slightly better outlook, depending on the ability to control the underlying condition.

Neoplasia

A tumor is an abnormal mass of tissue, the growth of which is virtually autonomous and exceeds that of normal tissues. In contrast to non-neoplastic proliferations (Chapter 2), the growth of tumors persists after cessation of the stimuli that initiated the change. Tumors are classified into two broad categories: benign and malignant.

NOMENCLATURE (p. 261)

All tumors have two basic components:

1. The *transformed* neoplastic cells
2. The supporting stroma composed of nontransformed elements, such as connective tissues and blood vessels

Classification of neoplasms is based on the characteristics of their parenchyma.

Benign Tumors (p. 261)

In general, the names of benign tumors end with the suffix *oma*. For example, benign mesenchymal tumors include lipoma, fibroma, angioma, osteoma, and leiomyoma. The nomenclature of benign epithelial tumors is somewhat complex and is based on both histogenesis and architecture. Some examples follow:

■ *Adenomas*: Benign epithelial tumors arising in glands or forming glandular patterns.
■ *Cystadenomas*: Adenomas producing large cystic masses, seen typically in the ovary.
■ *Papillomas*: Epithelial tumors forming microscopic or macroscopic finger-like projections.
■ *Polyp*: A tumor projecting from the mucosa into the lumen of a hollow viscus (e.g., stomach or colon).

Malignant Tumors (p. 261)

Malignant tumors are often called *cancers* and are broadly divided into two categories:

1. *Carcinomas*, arising from epithelial cells
2. *Sarcomas*, arising from mesenchymal tissues

The nomenclature of specific types of carcinomas or sarcomas is based on their appearance and presumed histogenetic origin. Thus, malignant epithelial tumors with glandular growth patterns are referred to as *adenocarcinomas*, whereas sarcomas arising from or resembling smooth muscle cells are called *leiomyosarcomas*.

Some tumors appear to have more than one parenchymal cell type. Two important members of this category are as follows:

1. *Mixed tumors*, derived from one germ cell layer that differentiates into more than one parenchymal cell type. For example, mixed salivary gland tumor contains epithelial cells as well as myxoid stroma and cartilage-like tissue. All elements arise from altered differentiation of ductal epithelial cells.
2. *Teratomas*, made up of a variety of parenchymal cell types representative of more than one germ cell layer, usually all three. They arise from totipotential cells that retain the ability to form endodermal (e.g., gut epithelium), ectodermal (e.g., skin), and mesenchymal (e.g., fat) tissues. Such tumors are found principally in the testis and ovary.

A summary of tumor nomenclature is given in Table 8–1. Two non-neoplastic lesions simulating tumors bear names that are deceptively similar to tumors:

1. *Choristomas*: Ectopic, sometimes nodular, rests of nontransformed tissues (e.g., pancreatic cells under the small bowel mucosa).
2. *Hamartomas*: Malformations that present as a mass of disorganized tissue indigenous to the particular site (i.e., a hamartomatous nodule in the lung may contain islands of cartilage, bronchi, and blood vessels).

CHARACTERISTICS OF BENIGN AND MALIGNANT NEOPLASMS (p. 264)

The distinction between benign and malignant tumors is based on appearance (morphology) and ultimately on behavior (clinical course), using four criteria:

1. Differentiation and anaplasia
2. Rate of growth
3. Local invasion
4. Metastases

Differentiation and Anaplasia (p. 264)

Differentiation is the extent to which tumor cells resemble comparable normal cells. Cells within most benign tumors closely mimic corresponding normal cells. Thus, thyroid adenomas are composed of normal-looking thyroid acini, and the cells in lipomas look like those in normal adipose tissue. Although malignant neoplasms are in general less well differentiated than their benign counterparts, they nevertheless display patterns ranging from well differentiated to very poorly differentiated. Lack of differentiation, also called *anaplasia*, is a hallmark of malignant cells. The following cytologic features characterize anaplastic, or poorly differentiated, tumors:

- *Nuclear and cellular pleomorphism*: Wide variation in the shape and size of cells and nuclei.
- *Hyperchromatism*: Darkly stained nuclei that frequently contain prominent nucleoli.
- *Nuclear-cytoplasmic ratio*: Approaches 1:1 instead of 1:4 or 1:6, reflecting enlargement of nuclei.
- *Abundant mitoses*: Reflect proliferative activity. Mitotic figures may be abnormal (e.g., tripolar spindles).

- *Tumor giant cells*: Contain a single large polyploid nucleus or multiple nuclei; sometimes seen.

Poorly differentiated, anaplastic tumors also demonstrate a total disarray of tissue architecture. For example, in an anaplastic tumor of the uterine cervix, the normal orientation of squamous epithelial cells with respect to each other is lost. Well-differentiated tumors, whether benign or malignant, tend to retain the functional characteristics of their normal counterparts. There may be attributes such as production of hormones in tumors of endocrine origin or keratin in squamous epithelial tumors.

Dysplasia refers to disorderly but non-neoplastic growth. It is characterized by pleomorphism, hyperchromatism, and loss of normal orientation. Dysplastic changes are usually encountered in epithelia, especially in the uterine cervix. When dysplastic changes are marked and *involve the entire thickness of the epithelium*, the lesion is considered a preinvasive neoplasm and is referred to as *carcinoma in situ*. This is a forerunner, in many cases, of invasive carcinoma. Mild degrees of dysplasia, however, common in the uterine cervix, do not always lead to cancer and are often reversible when the inciting cause (e.g., chronic irritation) is removed.

Rate of Growth (p. 267)

Most malignant tumors grow more rapidly than benign tumors. Some cancers grow slowly for years, however, and then enter a phase of rapid growth; others expand rapidly from the outset. Growth of cancers arising from hormone-sensitive tissues, such as the uterus, may be affected by the variations in hormone levels associated with pregnancy and menopause. Rapidly growing malignant tumors often contain central areas of ischemic necrosis because the tumor blood supply fails to keep pace with the oxygen needs of the expanding mass of cells.

Local Invasion (p. 267)

Local invasion is characterized as follows:

- Most benign tumors grow as cohesive expansile masses that develop a rim of condensed connective tissue, or *capsule*, at the periphery.
- They do not penetrate the capsule or the surrounding normal tissues.
- The plane of cleavage between the capsule and the surrounding tissues facilitates surgical enucleation.
- Malignant neoplasms are invasive, infiltrating and destroying normal tissues surrounding them.
- A well-defined capsule and plane of cleavage are lacking, making enucleation difficult or impossible.
- Surgical treatment of such tumors requires removal of a considerable margin of healthy and apparently uninvolved tissue.

Metastasis (p. 268)

The process of metastasis involves invasion of the lymphatics, blood vessels, and body cavities by the tumor, followed by transport and growth of secondary tumor cell masses that are discontinuous with the primary tumor. *This is the single most important feature distinguishing benign from malignant tumors.* With the notable exception of tumors in the brain and basal cell carcinomas

Table 8-1. NOMENCLATURE OF TUMORS

Tissue of Origin	Benign	Malignant
Composed of One Parenchymal Cell Type		
Tumors of mesenchymal origin		
Connective tissue and derivatives	Fibroma	Fibrosarcoma
	Lipoma	Liposarcoma
	Chondroma	Chondrosarcoma
	Osteoma	Osteogenic sarcoma
Endothelial and related tissues		
Blood vessels	Hemangioma	Angiosarcoma
Lymph vessels	Lymphangioma	Lymphangiosarcoma
Synovium		Synovioma (synoviosarcoma)
Mesothelium		Mesothelioma
Brain coverings	Meningioma	Invasive meningioma
Blood cells and related cells		
Hematopoietic cells		Leukemias
Lymphoid tissue		Malignant lymphomas
Muscle		
Smooth muscle	Leiomyoma	Leiomyosarcoma
Striated muscle	Rhabdomyoma	Rhabdomyosarcoma

Tissue of Origin	Benign	Malignant
Epithelial tumors		
Stratified squamous		
Basal cells of skin or adnexa	Squamous cell papilloma	Squamous cell or epidermoid carcinoma Basal cell carcinoma
Epithelial lining		
Glands or ducts	Adenoma Papilloma Cystadenoma	Adenocarcinoma Papillary carcinoma Cystadenocarcinoma
Respiratory passages		Bronchogenic carcinoma Bronchial adenoma (carcinoid)
Neuroectoderm	Nevus	Malignant melanoma
Renal epithelium	Renal tubular adenoma	Renal cell carcinoma (hypernephroma)
Urinary tract epithelium (transitional)	Transitional cell papilloma	Transitional cell carcinoma
Placental epithelium (trophoblast)	Hydatidiform mole	Choriocarcinoma
Testicular epithelium (germ cells)		Seminoma
More Than One Neoplastic Cell Type—Mixed Tumors—Usually Derived from One Germ Layer		
Salivary glands	Pleomorphic adenoma (mixed tumor of salivary gland origin)	Malignant mixed tumor of salivary gland origin
Breast	Fibroadenoma	Malignant cystosarcoma phyllodes
Renal anlage		Wilms tumor
More Than One Neoplastic Cell Type Derived from More Than One Germ Layer—Teratogenous		
Totipotential cells in gonads or in embryonic rests	Mature teratoma, dermoid cyst	Immature teratoma

of the skin, almost all malignant tumors have the capacity to metastasize.

Distant spread of tumors occurs by three routes:

1. *Spread into body cavities*: This occurs by seeding of surfaces in peritoneal, pleural, pericardial, and subarachnoid spaces. Carcinoma of the ovary, for example, spreads transperitoneally to the surface of the liver or other abdominal viscera.

2. *Invasion of lymphatics*: This is followed by transport of tumor cells to regional nodes and, ultimately, other parts of the body and is common in the initial spread of carcinomas. Thus, carcinomas of the breast spread to either axillary or internal mammary lymph nodes, depending on the location (and therefore lymphatic drainage) of the tumor. Lymph nodes that are the sites of metastases are frequently enlarged. Such enlargement usually results from the growth of tumor cells in nodes but in some cases may result primarily from a reactive hyperplasia of the lymph nodes in response to the tumor antigens.

3. *Hematogenous spread*: This is typical of all sarcomas but also is the favored route for certain carcinomas, such as those originating in the kidney. Because of their thinner walls, veins are more frequently invaded than arteries. Lung and liver are common sites of hematogenous metastases because they receive the systemic and venous outflow. Other major sites of hematogenous spread include brain and bones.

EPIDEMIOLOGY (p. 271)

A variety of factors predispose an individual or a population to the development of cancer.

Geographic and Environmental Factors
(p. 273)

In the United States, cancer is responsible for approximately 23% of all deaths annually. Cancers of the lung, colon, and prostate are the leading causes of cancer death in men. In women, lung, breast, and colon cancers are the most common forms.

Environmental factors significantly influence the occurrence of specific forms of cancer in different parts of the world. In Japan, for example, the death rate from cancer of the stomach is about seven times that in the United States. Conversely, carcinoma of the colon is much less common as a cause of death in Japan. In Japanese immigrants to the United States, the death rates for stomach and colon cancer are intermediate between those of natives of Japan and the United States, pointing to environmental and cultural influences. Other examples of environmental factors in carcinogenesis are

- Increased risk of certain cancers with exposure to asbestos, vinyl chloride, and 2-naphthylamine
- Association of carcinomas of the oropharynx, larynx, and lung with cigarette smoking

Age (p. 273)

Cancer is most common in those older than 55 years of age. Certain cancers are particularly common in children younger than 15 years of age:

- Tumors of the hematopoietic system (leukemias and lymphomas)

- Neuroblastomas
- Wilms tumors
- Retinoblastomas
- Sarcomas of bone and skeletal muscle

Heredity (p. 275)

Heredity plays a role in the development of cancer even in the presence of clearly defined environmental factors. Hereditary forms of cancers can be divided into three categories:

1. *Inherited cancer syndromes* are characterized by inheritance of single mutant genes that greatly increase the risk of developing a certain type of tumor. The predisposition to the tumor is thus an autosomal dominant trait, as exemplified by familial retinoblastoma and familial adenomatous polyposis. These syndromes are associated with inheritance of a single mutant allele of the *cancer-suppressor genes*. In each of these syndromes, only specific sites or tissues are affected, and usually there is an associated *marker phenotype* (e.g., the presence of multiple benign tumors in familial polyposis of colon and benign endocrine gland tumors in multiple endocrine neoplasia).

2. *Familial cancers* are characterized by familial clustering of specific forms of cancer, but the transmission pattern is not clear in an individual case. Familial forms of common cancers (e.g., breast, colon, brain, and ovary) are recorded. In contrast to inherited cancer syndromes, there is no marker phenotype (e.g., familial colon cancers do not arise in preexisting polyps).

3. *Autosomal recessive syndromes of defective DNA repair* are characterized by chromosome or DNA instability that greatly increases the predisposition to environmental carcinogens.

Acquired Preneoplastic Disorders (p. 276)

Certain clinical conditions are associated with an increased risk of developing cancers:

- Cirrhosis of the liver—hepatocellular carcinoma
- Atrophic gastritis of pernicious anemia—stomach cancer
- Chronic ulcerative colitis—carcinoma of the colon
- Leukoplakia of the oral and genital mucosa—squamous cell cancers

Certain benign tumors are also associated with the subsequent development of cancer. Although the development of cancers in benign tumors is uncommon, there are a few exceptions (e.g., villous adenomas of the colon often develop into cancer). Most malignant tumors, however, arise de novo.

MOLECULAR BASIS OF CANCER

(p. 276)

A simplified scheme of the molecular pathogenesis of cancer is provided in Figure 8–1 and recapitulated here:

- Cancer is a genetic disease. The genetic injury may be acquired in somatic cells by environmental agents or inherited in the germ line. Tumors develop as clonal progeny of a single genetically damaged progenitor cell. The monoclonality of tumors can be verified by study of X-linked markers (e.g., glucose-6-

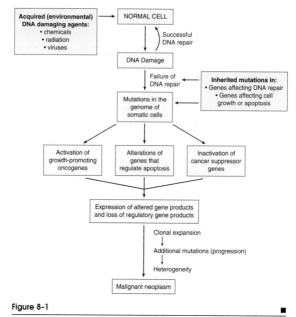

Figure 8-1   ∎

Flow chart depicting a simplified scheme of the molecular basis of cancer.

phosphate dehydrogenase isoenzymes or X-linked restriction fragment length polymorphisms).
- Four classes of genes are the targets of genetic damage:
  1. Growth-promoting protooncogenes
  2. Growth-inhibiting tumor-suppressor genes
  3. Genes that regulate apoptosis
  4. Genes that regulate DNA repair
- Carcinogenesis is a multistep process. The attributes of malignancy (e.g., invasiveness, excessive growth, escape from the immune system) are acquired in a stepwise fashion—a process called *tumor progression*. At the genetic level, progression results from accumulation of successive mutations.

Oncogenes and Cancer (p. 277)

Oncogenes and *protooncogenes* are defined as follows:

- *Oncogenes* are genes whose products are associated with neoplastic transformation.
- *Protooncogenes* are normal cellular genes that affect growth and differentiation. They can be converted into oncogenes by
  1. Transduction into retroviruses (v-*onc*)
  2. Changes in situ that affect their expression, function, or both, thereby converting them into c-*onc*

Most human tumors are not caused by v-*oncs*. The presence of c-*onc* is detected by transfection of tumor-derived DNA into the NIH/3T3 mouse fibroblast cell line. If the tumor DNA contains transforming sequences (c-*onc*), the transfected fibroblasts acquire the growth characteristics of neoplastic cells: loss of contact inhibition, growth in soft agar, and tumor formation in immunosuppressed mice. DNA transfection has revealed the presence of c-*oncs* in many human tumors.

Protein Products of Oncogenes (p. 279)

To understand the transforming activity of oncogenes, it is essential to consider their functions in normal cell growth. Stimulation of normal cell proliferation is often triggered by growth factors that bind to cell membrane receptors. The signal received on the cell membrane is transduced to the cytoplasm and ultimately to the nucleus by the generation of second messengers such as Ca^{2+}. These signals activate nuclear regulatory factors that initiate DNA transcription, and the cells then go into cycle.

The products of protooncogenes are grouped in the following list and in Table 8–2 on the basis of their role in signal transduction.

- *Growth factors*: Some protooncogenes (e.g., c-*sis*) code for growth factors, such as platelet-derived growth factor. Many tumors that produce growth factors are also responsive to the growth-promoting effects of the secreted growth factors and hence subject to autocrine stimulation.
- *Growth factor receptors*: Several oncogenes encode growth factor receptors. Both structural alterations (mutations) and overexpression of the receptor genes have been found in association with malignant transformation. Mutations in several tyrosine-kinase types of growth factor receptors lead to their constitutive activation without binding to their ligands. As an example, mutations and rearrangements of the *ret* gene are detected in MEN2A, MEN2B, and papillary carcinoma of the thyroid. Overexpression commonly involves members of the epidermal growth factor receptor family (e.g., c-*erb* B1 is overexpressed in the majority of squamous cell carcinomas of lung; c-*erb* B2 [also called c-*neu*] is amplified in adenocarcinomas of the breast, ovary, lung, stomach, and so on). In breast cancers that have amplified c-*erb* B2, the prognosis is poor, presumably because their cells are sensitive to smaller quantities of growth factors.
- *Signal-transducing proteins*: These proteins are biochemically heterogeneous and grouped into two major categories:
  1. *Guanosine triphosphate (GTP)–binding proteins*: To this family belongs the *ras* family of proteins and G proteins. Approximately 10% to 20% of all human tumors carry mutant *ras* proteins. Normal *ras* proteins flip back and forth between an activated (GTP-bound) signal-transmitting form and an inactive (guanosine diphosphate [GDP]–bound) quiescent form. The conversion of active *ras* to inactive *ras* is mediated by its intrinsic GTPase activity, which is augmented by a family of GTPase-activating proteins (GAPs). Mutant *ras* proteins bind GAPs, but their GTPase activity fails to be augmented, and hence they are trapped in the signal-transmitting GTP-bound form.
  2. *Non–receptor-associated tyrosine kinases*: An example in this category is the c-*abl* gene, which in its normal form exerts a regulated tyrosine-kinase activity. In chronic myeloid leukemia, translocation of c-*abl* and its fusion to the *bcr* gene produce a hybrid gene with potent, unregulated tyrosine-kinase activity.
- *Nuclear transcription proteins*: The products of *myc, jun, fos,*

Table 8-2. SELECTED ONCOGENES, THEIR MODE OF ACTIVATION, AND ASSOCIATED HUMAN TUMORS

Category	Protooncogene	Mechanism	Associated Human Tumor
Growth Factors			
PDGF-β chain	*sis*	Overexpression	Astrocytoma
			Osteosarcoma
Fibroblast growth factors	*hist*-1	Overexpression	Stomach cancer
	int-2	Amplification	Bladder cancer
			Breast cancer
			Melanoma
Growth Factor Receptors			
EGF-receptor family	*erb*-B1	Overexpression	Squamous cell carcinomas of lung
	erb-B2	Amplification	Breast, ovarian, lung, and stomach cancers
	erb-B3	Overexpression	Breast cancers
CSF-1 receptor	*fms*	Point mutation	Leukemia
	*ret**	Point mutation	Multiple endocrine neoplasia 2A and B. Familial medullary thyroid carcinoma
		Rearrangement	Sporadic papillary carcinomas of thyroid

Proteins Involved in Signal Transduction			
GTP-binding	*ras*	Point mutations	A variety of human cancers, including lung, colon, pancreas; many leukemias
Nonreceptor tyrosine kinase	*abl*	Translocation	Chronic myeloid leukemia
			Acute lymphoblastic leukemia
Nuclear Regulatory Proteins			
Transcriptional activators	*myc*	Translocation	Burkitt lymphoma
	N-*myc*	Amplification	Neuroblastoma
			Small cell carcinoma of lung
	L-*myc*	Amplification	Small cell carcinoma of lung
Cell Cycle Regulators			
Cyclins	cyclin D	Translocation	Mantle cell lymphoma
		Amplification	Breast, liver, esophageal cancers
Cyclin-dependent kinase	CDK4	Amplification	Glioblastoma, melanoma, sarcoma
		Point mutation	

PDGF-platelet-derived growth factor; EGF, epidermal growth factor; CSF, colony-stimulating factor; GTP, guanosine triphosphate.
*ret protooncogene is a receptor for glial cell line–derived neurotrophic factor.

and *myb* oncogenes are nuclear proteins. They are expressed in a highly regulated fashion during proliferation of normal cells, and they are believed to regulate transcription of growth-related genes. Their oncogenic versions are associated with persistent expression. Dysregulation of *myc* expression occurs in Burkitt's lymphoma, neuroblastomas, and small cell cancer of the lung.

- *Cyclins and cyclin-dependent kinases (CDKs).* These regulate the progression of cells through the cell cycle. Inactive CDKs are expressed constitutively during the cell cycle; they are activated by cyclins that are synthesized during specific phases of the cell cycle. D-type cyclins facilitate the transition from G_1 to S phase by activating CDK4 and CDK6. These two CDKs phosphorylate the retinoblastoma protein (pRb). Phosphorylated pRb releases E2F transcription factors, which then allow synthesis of S-phase genes. The activity of CDKs is inhibited by CDK inhibitors, and hence the latter inhibit cell division. Overexpression of cyclin D and CDK4 is common in many types of cancer.

Activation of Oncogenes (p. 284)

Protooncogenes may be converted to oncogenes by one of three mechanisms:

1. Point mutations
2. Chromosomal rearrangements
3. Gene amplification

POINT MUTATIONS

The *ras* protooncogenes are activated by point mutations. Approximately 15% of all human tumors carry mutated H-*ras* or K-*ras* oncogenes. One possible mechanism of these mutations is exposure to cancer-causing chemicals.

CHROMOSOMAL REARRANGEMENTS

Chromosomal rearrangements are believed to activate protooncogenes by one of two mechanisms:

1. Placement of the genes next to strong promoter/enhancer elements of immunoglobulin or T-cell receptor loci in lymphoid cells. In Burkitt lymphoma, the t(8;14) translocation places the c-*myc*-containing segment of chromosome 8 in close proximity to the actively expressed immunoglobulin heavy chain gene on chromosome 14.
2. Fusion of the gene with new genetic sequences. In chronic myelogenous leukemia, the t(9;22) translocation relocates the c-*abl* gene from chromosome 9 to the *bcr* locus on chromosome 22. The c-*abl-bcr* hybrid gene codes for a chimeric protein that exhibits tyrosine kinase activity. EWS, another transcription factor on 22q12, is frequently translocated in many sarcomas, including Ewing sarcoma.

GENE AMPLIFICATION

Reduplication of protooncogenes can lead to increased expression or activity. Examples include

- N-*myc* amplification (3 to 300 copies) in neuroblastomas; there seems to be a strong correlation among N-*myc* amplification, advanced stage, and poor prognosis.

- Amplification of the c-*erb* B2 gene in 30 to 40% of breast cancers; there is a correlation between c-*erb* B2 amplification and prognosis.

Cancer-Suppressor Genes (p. 286)

Cancer may arise not only by activation of growth-promoting oncogenes, but also by inactivation of genes that normally suppress cell proliferation (cancer-suppressor genes, or antioncogenes). The *Rb* gene located on chromosome 13q14 is the prototypic cancer-suppressor gene. It is relevant to the pathogenesis of the childhood tumor, retinoblastoma. Forty per cent of retinoblastomas are familial; the rest are sporadic. To account for the familial and sporadic occurrence, the *two-hit* hypothesis has been proposed:

- Both normal alleles of the *Rb* locus must be inactivated (two hits) for the development of retinoblastoma.
- In familial cases, children inherit one defective copy of the *Rb* gene in the germ line; the other copy is normal. Retinoblastoma develops when the normal *Rb* gene is lost in the retinoblasts as a result of somatic mutation.
- In sporadic cases, both normal *Rb* alleles are lost by somatic mutation in one of the retinoblasts.
- Cancer develops when the cells become homozygous for the mutant cancer-suppressor genes. Because heterozygous cells are normal, these genes are also called *recessive cancer genes*.
- The *Rb* locus may be involved in the pathogenesis of several cancers because patients with familial retinoblastoma are at greatly increased risk of developing osteosarcomas and soft tissue sarcomas.

PROTEIN PRODUCTS OF TUMOR-SUPPRESSOR GENES

Protein products of tumor-suppressor genes are as follows:

- *Rb gene*: The *Rb* gene product regulates the advancement of cells from the G_1 to S phase of the cell cycle. In its hypophosphorylated state, it prevents cells from entering the S phase by binding to and inactivating the E2F transcription factors. When the cell is stimulated by growth factors, the cyclins D and E are up-regulated, and they activate CDKs (CDK4 and CDK6); these, in turn, cause phosphorylation of pRb and release of E2F transcription factors. Thus, transcription of genes essential for the S phase is triggered. With mutations in the *Rb* gene, the regulation of E2F transcription factors is lost, and cells continue to cycle in the absence of a growth stimulus. Several other mechanisms that regulate the cell cycle do so via the *Rb* protein. These include the following:
  1. Transforming growth factor-β (TGF-β) is a growth-inhibiting cytokine that up-regulates inhibitors of CDKs and thus prevents pRb phosphorylation.
  2. The tumor-suppressor gene *p53* also exerts its growth-inhibiting effect by up-regulating synthesis of p21, a CDK inhibitor.
  3. Several oncogenic DNA viruses (e.g., human papillomavirus [HPV]) cause functional deletion of pRb by binding to pRb and displacing the E2F transcription factors.

- *p53*: The *p53* tumor-suppressor gene, located on 17p13.1, is mutated in greater than 50% of all human cancers. Those who inherit a mutant copy of the *p53* gene *(Li-Fraumeni syndrome)* are at a high risk of developing a malignant tumor by inactivation of the second normal allele in somatic cells. Patients with the Li-Fraumeni syndrome develop many different types of tumors, including leukemias, sarcomas, breast cancer, and brain tumors. The function of the normal *p53* gene is to prevent the propagation of genetically damaged cells. When the DNA is damaged by ultraviolet (UV) light, chemicals, or irradiation, the normal *p53* gene is up-regulated, and it initiates transcription of several genes that cause cell cycle arrest and DNA repair. The cell cycle arrest in the G_1 phase is mediated by *p53*-dependent transcription of the CDK inhibitor *p21*. If during the pause in cell cycle the DNA can be repaired, the cell is allowed to continue to S phase; however, if DNA damage cannot be repaired, *p53* induces apoptosis by increasing transcription of the proapoptic gene *bax*. With homozygous loss of *p53*, DNA damage goes unrepaired, and cells carrying mutant genes continue to divide and eventually give rise to cancer. Similar to the *Rb* gene, *p53* can also be functionally inactivated by products of DNA oncogenic viruses.
- *BRCA-1 and BRCA-2*: About 5 to 10% of breast cancers are familial, and mutations in *BRCA-1* or *BRCA-2* can account for 80% of such cases. Individuals who inherit defective copies of *BRCA-1* are also at an increased risk of developing ovarian cancers, and those with germ line mutations of *BRCA-2* have an increased risk of cancers of the ovary and male breast cancer and possibly others. The function of these genes is not fully understood; their products are located in the nucleus and are believed to play a role in DNA repair.
- *APC gene*: Those born with one mutant allele of this gene develop hundreds of adenomatous polyps in the colon, of which one or more develop into colonic cancers. *APC* mutations with homozygous loss are also found in 70 to 80% of sporadic colon cancers. Normal APC protein binds to and degrades another molecule, called β-catenin, in the cytoplasm. In the absence of the APC protein, β-catenin levels go up, and it translocates to the nucleus and up-regulates cellular proliferation. Thus, *APC* is a negative regulator of β-catenin.
- *NF-1 gene*: This tumor-suppressor gene regulates signal transduction by the *ras* pathway. Homozygous loss of *NF-1* impairs the conversion of active (GTP-bound) *ras* to inactive (GDP-bound) *ras*, and thus cells are continuously stimulated to divide. As with *APC*, germ line inheritance of one mutant allele of *NF-1* predisposes to the development of numerous benign neurofibromas; some of these tumors progress to malignancy.
- *Cell surface receptors*: TGF-β up-regulates growth inhibitory genes, including CDK inhibitors, by binding to TGF-β receptors. In many colon cancers, TGF-β receptors are mutated, preventing the growth-restraining effects of TGF-β. E-cadherin, on the surface of many epithelial cells, acts as a glue to keep cells together. Loss of these glycoproteins in many cancers facilitates disaggregation of neoplastic cells and local or distant invasion.
- *WT-1*: This *tumor-suppressor gene* is of unknown function. Mutational inactivation of WT-1, either in the germ line or in the somatic cells, is associated with the development of Wilms tumors.

The locations and functions of tumor-suppressor genes are summarized in Table 8–3.

Genes That Regulate Apoptosis (p. 294)

The prototypic gene in this group, *bcl-2*, prevents programmed cell death, or apoptosis. Overexpression of *bcl-2* presumably extends cell survival, and if the cells are genetically damaged, they continue to suffer additional mutations in oncogenes and cancer-suppressor genes. The most dramatic example of *bcl-2* overexpression is seen in B-cell lymphomas of the follicular type. Here a t(14;18) translocation juxtaposes *bcl-2* with transcriptionally active immunoglobulin heavy chain locus, resulting in overexpression of *bcl-2*. Some other genes of the bcl-2 family (e.g., *bax*) favor apoptosis. *bcl-2* and related genes seem to control apoptosis by regulating the exit of cytochrome *c* from the mitochondrion. Cytochrome *c* activates the proteolytic enzyme caspase 9 (Chapter 1). Genes unrelated to the bcl-2 family can also regulate apoptosis. *p53* was already mentioned. In addition, if c-*myc*-driven cells do not have sufficient growth factors in their environs, they undergo apoptosis, which can be prevented by *bcl-2* overexpression.

Genes That Regulate DNA Repair (p. 295)

The DNA repair genes do not contribute directly to cell growth or proliferation. They act indirectly by correcting errors in DNA that occur spontaneously during cell division or those that follow exposure to mutagenic chemicals or irradiation. Patients with *hereditary nonpolyposis colon cancer* are born with one defective copy of one of several DNA repair genes. They develop carcinomas of the cecum or proximal colon without a preneoplastic stage of an adenomatous polyps. The affected genes, including *hMSH2* and *hMLH1*, are involved in DNA mismatch repair. When errors involving DNA mismatch accumulate in protooncogenes and tumor-suppressor genes, the carcinomas develop.

Patients with *xeroderma pigmentosum* develop skin cancers as a result of the mutagenic effects of UV light. These patients have mutations in the nucleotide excision repair genes required for correcting UV light–induced pyrimidine dimer formation. Other syndromes of defective DNA repair and cancer susceptibility include Bloom syndrome, Fanconi anemia, and ataxia telangiectasia.

Molecular Basis of Multistep Carcinogenesis (p. 296)

No single genetic alteration is sufficient to induce cancers in vivo. Multiple controls exerted by all three categories of genes—oncogenes, tumor-suppressor genes, and apoptosis-regulating genes—must be lost for the emergence of cancer cells. This situation is best exemplified by the adenoma-carcinoma sequence in the colon. In this sequence, the evolution of benign adenomas to carcinomas is marked by increasing and additive effects of mutations, affecting *ras*, *APC*, *p53*, and other unidentified genes on 18q. The accumulation of mutations, resulting perhaps from genetic instability of cancer cells, may be promoted by loss of *p53*, DNA repair genes, or both. Genes that regulate cellular proliferation in a more or less tissue-specific manner, such as *APC*, *NF-1*, and *Rb*, are called *gatekeeper* genes, whereas those that regulate genomic stability (DNA repair genes) are called *caretaker*

Table 8-3. SELECTED TUMOR-SUPPRESSOR GENES INVOLVED IN HUMAN NEOPLASMS

Subcellular Location	Gene	Function	Tumors Associated with Somatic Mutations	Tumors Associated with Inherited Mutations
Cell surface	TGF-β receptor	Growth inhibition	Carcinomas of colon	Unknown
	E-cadherin	Cell adhesion	Carcinomas of stomach, breast	Familial gastric cancer
Under plasma membrane	APC	Inhibition of signal transduction	Carcinomas of stomach, colon, pancreas; melanoma	Familial adenomatosis polyposis coli; colon cancer
	NF-1	Inhibition of *ras* signal transduction	Schwannomas	Neurofibromatosis type I and sarcomas
Cytoskeleton	NF-2	Unknown	Schwannomas and meningiomas	Neurofibromatosis type II; acoustic schwannomas and meningiomas
Nucleus	Rb	Regulation of cell cycle	Retinoblastoma; osteosarcoma; carcinomas of breast, colon, lung	Retinoblastomas, osteosarcoma
	p53	Regulation of cell cycle and apoptosis in response to DNA damage	Most human cancers	Li-Fraumeni syndrome; multiple carcinomas and sarcomas
	WT-1	Nuclear transcription	Wilms tumor	Wilms tumor
	p16	Regulation of cell cycle by inhibiting cyclin-dependent kinases	Pancreatic, esophageal cancers	Malignant melanoma
	BRCA-1	DNA repair	Rare breast carcinomas	Carcinomas of female breast and ovary
	BRCA-2	DNA repair	Rare breast carcinomas	Carcinomas of male and female breast

genes. These latter genes regulate the likelihood of mutations in the gatekeeper genes.

KARYOTYPIC CHANGES IN TUMOR CELLS (p. 298)

Many human neoplasms are associated with nonrandom chromosomal abnormalities, suggesting that certain cytogenetic abnormalities may be important and possibly primary events in neoplastic transformation. They are also of diagnostic and prognostic significance in some cases. Three types of nonrandom chromosomal abnormalities have been described:

- Translocations
- Deletions
- Amplifications

These abnormalities were described earlier and are discussed again in specific chapters.

BIOLOGY OF TUMOR GROWTH (p. 298)

Kinetics of Tumor Cell Growth (p. 299)

Three variables influence tumor cell growth:

1. *Doubling time of tumor cells*: The cell cycle of transformed cells has the same five phases (G_0, G_1, S, G_2, and M) noted in normal cells. The total cell cycle time for many tumors is equal to or longer than that of corresponding normal cells. Hence, progressive and rapid tumor growth cannot always be ascribed to a shortening of tumor cell cycle time.

2. *Growth fraction (GF)*: This refers to the proportion of cells within the tumor population that are in the replicative pool (i.e., out of G_0). Most cells within clinically detectable tumors are not in the proliferative pool. Even in some rapidly growing tumors, the GF is approximately 20%. Cells leave the replicative pool by being shed, by differentiating, and by reverting to G_0. Thus, progressive tumor growth cannot be ascribed to an inordinately high GF.

3. *Cell production and loss*: Tumor cell accumulation resulting in progressive growth of tumors can best be explained by an imbalance between cell production and cell loss. In some tumors (especially those with a high GF), the imbalance is large, resulting in more rapid growth than in those in which cell production exceeds cell loss by only a small margin.

Knowledge of tumor cell kinetics has the following clinical implications:

- The rate of tumor growth depends on the GF and the degree of imbalance between tumor cell production and loss. High GF, as in certain lymphomas, is associated with rapid growth.
- *Susceptibility of tumors to chemotherapy*: Because most antineoplastic agents act on dividing cells, tumors with higher GFs are the most susceptible to anticancer agents. They are also the most rapidly growing if left untreated.
- *Latent period of tumors*: If all descendants of an originally transformed cell remained in the replicative pool, most tumors would become clinically detectable within a few months after

the initiation of tumor cell growth. Because most tumor cells leave the replicative pool, however, the accumulation of tumor cells is a relatively slow process. This, in turn, results in a latent period of several months to years before a tumor becomes clinically detectable.

Tumor Angiogenesis
(p. 301)

Because tumor cells, similar to normal cells, need oxygen to survive, vascularization of tumors by host-derived blood vessels has a profound influence on tumor growth. In rapidly growing tumors, the rate of growth sometimes exceeds the pace of vascularization, causing areas of ischemic necrosis. Vascularization of tumors is effected by the release of tumor-associated angiogenic factors derived from tumor cells or inflammatory cells (e.g., macrophages) that enter the tumors. The two most important tumor angiogenic factors are vascular endothelial growth factor (VEGF) and basic fibroblast growth factor (bFGF). In addition to angiogenic factors, tumor cells or host cells also produce antiangiogenic factors. These include angiostatin, endostatin, and vasculostatin. Tumor growth is controlled by the balance between angiogenic and antiangiogenic factors. The latter is under study therapeutically to retard tumor growth.

Tumor Progression and Heterogeneity
(p. 302)

Tumor progression refers to the phenomenon whereby tumors become progressively more aggressive and acquire greater malignant potential. Progression is related to the sequential appearance within the tumor of cells that differ with respect to invasiveness, rate of growth, ability to form metastases, ability to evade immunosurveillance, and several other attributes. Thus, a clinically detectable tumor, although monoclonal, is usually made up of phenotypically and genetically heterogeneous cells. The heterogeneity is believed to result from genetic instability of tumor cells, which are subject to a high rate of random mutations, possibly because of loss of *p53*, DNA repair genes, or both. Tumor cell heterogeneity and progression begin well before clinical detection of tumors (latent period) and continue thereafter.

Mechanisms of Invasion and Metastasis
(p. 302)

The sequential steps involved in invasion and metastasis are depicted in Figure 8–2. This sequence may be interrupted at any stage by host factors. Experimental studies in animals indicate that cells within a primary tumor are heterogeneous with respect to metastatic abilities. Only certain subclones can complete all the steps outlined in Figure 8–2 and are able to form secondary tumors at distant sites.

INVASION OF EXTRACELLULAR MATRIX
(p. 302)

Tumor cells must attach to, degrade, and penetrate the extracellular matrix at several steps of the metastatic cascade. Invasion

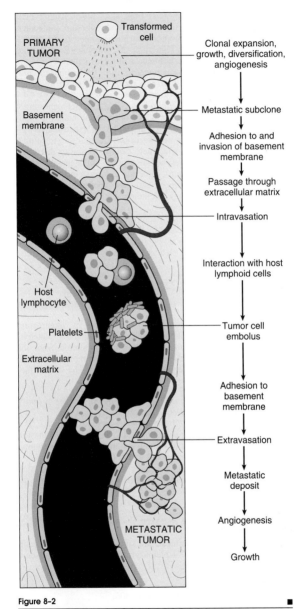

Figure 8-2 ∎

The metastatic cascade. The sequential steps involved in the hematogenous spread of a tumor are illustrated.

of extracellular matrix can be resolved into the following four steps:

1. *Detachment of tumor cells from each other*: Tumor cells remain attached to each other by several adhesion molecules, including a family of glycoproteins called *cadherins*. In several carcinomas, there is down-regulation of epithelial (E) cadherins, presumably reducing the cohesiveness of tumor cells.

2. *Attachment to matrix components*: Tumor cells bind to laminin and fibronectin via cell surface receptors. Receptor-mediated binding is an important step in invasion.

3. *Degradation of extracellular matrix*: After attachment, tumor cells secrete proteolytic enzymes that degrade the matrix components and create passageways for migration. In experimental systems, the ability of tumor cell variants to degrade extracellular matrix can be correlated with their metastatic ability. Enzymes that are important in this respect are type IV collagenases (cleave basement membrane collagen), cathepsin D (a cysteine proteinase), and urokinase-type plasminogen activator. These enzymes act on a large variety of substrates, including laminin, fibronectin, and protein cores of proteoglycans.

4. *Migration of tumor cells*: Factors that favor tumor cell migration in the passageways created by the degradation of extracellular matrix are poorly understood. Implicated in this process are autocrine motility factors and cleavage products of the extracellular matrix.

VASCULAR DISSEMINATION AND HOMING OF TUMOR CELLS (p. 305)

In the circulation, tumor cells form emboli by aggregation and by adhering to circulating leukocytes, particularly platelets. Aggregated tumor cells are afforded some protection from the antitumor host effector cells. The site where tumor cell emboli lodge and produce secondary growths is influenced by several factors:

- *Vascular and lymphatic drainage from the site of the primary tumor, as discussed earlier.*
- *Interaction of tumor cells with organ-specific receptors.* For example, certain tumor cells have high levels of an adhesion molecule, CD44, that binds to high endothelial venules in lymph nodes, thereby facilitating nodal metastases.
- *The microenvironment of the organ or site (e.g., a tissue rich in protease inhibitors might be resistant to penetration by tumor cells).*

CARCINOGENIC AGENTS (p. 305)

Radiation and many chemicals are known to be carcinogenic in animals and humans, and suspicion grows stronger that the same is true for viruses.

Chemical Carcinogenesis (p. 306)

Neoplastic transformation brought about by chemicals is a dynamic multistep process. It can be broadly divided into two stages:

1. *Initiation* refers to the induction of certain irreversible changes (mutations) in the genome of cells. Initiated cells are not

transformed cells; they do not have growth autonomy or unique phenotypic characteristics. In contrast to normal cells, however, they give rise to tumors when appropriately stimulated by promoting agents.

2. *Promotion* refers to the process of tumor induction in previously initiated cells by chemicals referred to as *promoters*. The effect of promoters is relatively short-lived and reversible; they do not affect DNA and are nontumorigenic by themselves.

MECHANISMS OF INITIATION (p. 306)

The vast majority of chemicals are referred to as *procarcinogens* because they require metabolic activation in vivo to produce ultimate carcinogens. Only a few alkylating and acylating agents are direct-acting carcinogens. The activation of procarcinogens in most cases depends on microsomal cytochrome P-450 oxygenases. Individuals who inherit highly inducible forms of these enzymes incur a higher risk of smoking-related lung cancers. Several factors, such as age, sex, and hormones, also modulate the activity of microsomal enzymes and hence the potency of procarcinogens.

Molecular Targets of Chemical Carcinogens (p. 307)

All direct-acting and ultimate carcinogens are highly reactive electrophilic compounds that can react with nucleophilic sites in the cell. DNA is the primary and most important target of chemical carcinogens; thus, chemical carcinogens are mutagens that induce mutations in protooncogenes, cancer-suppressor genes, and, possibly, genes that regulate apoptosis. As an example, the *ras* oncogene is frequently mutated in chemically induced tumors in rodents. Because specific sequences are targeted by different chemicals, an analysis of the mutations found in human tumors may allow linkage to specific carcinogens. Carcinogen-induced changes in DNA, however, do not necessarily lead to the initiation of carcinogenesis because the damage to DNA can be repaired by cellular enzymes. If the ability to repair DNA is impaired, as in xeroderma pigmentosum, the risk of cancer development significantly increases. Because chemical carcinogens are mutagenic, a simple in vitro test for carcinogenicity is the *Ames test*, using the ability of potential carcinogens to induce mutations in selected strains of the bacterium *Salmonella typhimurium*.

PROMOTION OF CARCINOGENESIS (p. 308)

As discussed earlier, the expression of the initial mutagenic event in most instances requires subsequent exposure to promoters, which can include various hormones, drugs, phenols, and phorbol esters. Phorbol esters are the most widely used promoters in experimental systems; they are not mutagenic and seem to exert their effects by epigenetic mechanisms.

Tetradecanoyl phorbol acetate (TPA), a commonly used promoter, is a powerful activator of protein kinase C, an enzyme that is a key element in the signal transduction pathways. Activation of protein kinase C leads to a series of phosphorylation reactions that ultimately affect cell proliferation and differentiation. Thus, promoters appear to be involved in the clonal expansion and aberrant differentiation of initiated cells.

Carcinogenic Chemicals (p. 308)

Carcinogenic chemicals include the following:

- *Alkylating agents*: These include direct-acting agents, such as cyclophosphamide and busulfan, used in the treatment of cancer as well as immunosuppressants. Patients receiving such therapy are at increased risk of developing another cancer.
- *Aromatic hydrocarbons*: These are present in cigarette smoke and may therefore be relevant to the pathogenesis of lung cancer.
- *Azo dyes*: β-naphthylamine, an aniline dye used in the rubber industries, was in the past responsible for bladder cancers in exposed workers.
- *Naturally occurring carcinogens*: Aflatoxin B_1, produced by the fungus *Aspergillus flavus*, is a potent hepatocarcinogen in animals and is believed to be a factor in the high incidence of liver cancer in Africa. The fungus grows on moldy grains and peanuts, and the toxin is ingested with contaminated foods.
- *Nitrosamines and amides*: These can be synthesized in the gastrointestinal tract from ingested nitrites or derived from digested proteins and may contribute to the induction of gastric cancer.
- *Miscellaneous agents*: Asbestos, vinyl chloride, and metals such as nickel are carcinogenic. They predispose exposed individuals to the development of cancer. Hormones such as estrogens may play a role in the causation of endometrial cancer.

Radiation Carcinogenesis (p. 309)

Radiant energy in the form of UV rays and ionizing radiations can cause cancer.

ULTRAVIOLET RAYS

Natural UV radiation, especially UVB, derived from the sun can cause skin cancer. At greatest risk are fair-skinned people who live in locales that receive a great deal of sunlight. Thus, carcinomas and melanomas of exposed skin are particularly common in Australia and New Zealand. Two mechanisms may be involved in induction of cancer by UV rays:

1. Damage to DNA by the formation of pyrimidine dimers
2. Immunosuppression, demonstrated only in animal models

IONIZING RADIATION

Electromagnetic and particulate radiations are carcinogenic. Evidence for the carcinogenicity of ionizing radiation comes from several sources:

- Miners of radioactive ores have an increased risk of lung cancer.
- The incidence of certain forms of leukemia is greatly increased in survivors of atomic bombs in Japan.
- Therapeutic radiation to the neck in children has been associated with the later development of thyroid cancer.

In humans, there is a hierarchy of cellular vulnerability to radiation-induced neoplasms:

- Most common are myeloid leukemias, followed by thyroid cancer in children.

- Cancers of the breast and lung are less commonly radiation induced.
- Skin, bone, and gut are the least susceptible to radiation carcinogenesis.

The ability of ionizing radiations to cause cancer lies in their ability to induce mutations. Such mutations may result from a direct effect of the radiant energy or an indirect effect mediated by the generation of free radicals from water or oxygen. Particulate radiations (such as α particles and neutrons) are more carcinogenic than electromagnetic radiation (x-rays, gamma rays).

Viral and Microbial Carcinogenesis (p. 311)

A variety of DNA and RNA viruses are known to cause cancer in animals, and some are implicated in human cancer.

DNA VIRUSES (p. 311)

Many cause tumors in animals. Three have associations with human tumors:

1. HPV
2. Epstein-Barr virus (EBV)
3. Hepatitis B virus (HBV)

Human Papillomavirus

Approximately 70 genetically distinct types of HPV have been identified. Some types (e.g., 1, 2, 4, and 7) definitely cause benign squamous papillomas (warts) in humans. Evidence supporting the role of HPV in human cancers is as follows:

- Squamous cell cancers of the uterine cervix contain HPV types 16 or 18 in greater than 90% of cases. These viruses are also contained in presumed precursors (e.g., carcinoma in situ) of the invasive cancer.
- Genital warts with low malignant potential are caused by distinct HPV types (*low-risk* types, e.g., HPV-6 and HPV-11).
- Molecular analysis of HPV-associated cervical carcinomas reveals clonal integration of the viral genomes in the host cell DNA. During integration, the viral DNA is interrupted in a manner that leads to overexpression of the E6 and E7 viral proteins. These proteins have the potential to transform cells by binding to and inhibiting the functions of *Rb* and *p53* tumor-suppressor gene products.

Epstein-Barr Virus

EBV is a member of the herpesvirus family and is associated with four human cancers:

1. Burkitt lymphoma
2. Nasopharyngeal cancer
3. B-cell lymphomas in immunosuppressed patients, especially those with acquired immunodeficiency syndrome (AIDS)
4. Some forms of Hodgkin disease

Burkitt Lymphoma. Burkitt lymphoma is a tumor of B lymphocytes that is consistently associated with a t(8;14) translocation. In certain parts of Africa, Burkitt lymphoma is endemic, and virtually all of these patients' tumor cells carry the EBV genome. It is unlikely, however, that EBV alone can cause Burkitt lymphoma. In normal individuals, EBV-driven B-cell proliferation is self-limited and controlled. In patients with subtle or overt immune dysregulation, EBV causes sustained B-cell proliferation because EBV genes dysregulate growth-controlling pathways of B cells. Such B cells acquire additional mutations and sometimes the translocation t(8;14) and eventually become autonomous. The role of normal immune responses in control of EBV-induced B-cell proliferation is illustrated by the occurrence of B-cell lymphomas in patients with AIDS and recipients of immunosuppressive drugs. These patients have polyclonal B-cell proliferations that transform into monoclonal lymphomas. In transplant recipients, withdrawal of immunosuppressive drugs can cause regression of such EBV-induced proliferations.

Nasopharyngeal Cancer. Nasopharyngeal cancer is endemic in southern China and some other locales, and the EBV genome is found in all such tumors. As in Burkitt lymphoma, EBV probably acts in concert with other factors.

Hepatitis B Virus

There is a close association between HBV infection and liver cancer in many parts of the world. In Taiwan, the risk of developing hepatic cancer is increased 200-fold in those infected with HBV. Cofactors other than HBV are also believed to play roles in the genesis of liver cancer. The mechanism by which HBV causes cancer is probably multifactorial:

- By causing hepatocellular injury and resulting regenerative hyperplasia, the pool of mitotically active cells subject to mutational damage by environmental agents such as aflatoxins is increased.
- HBV encodes a regulatory element called *HBx*, which seems to cause transcriptional activation of several protooncogenes.
- HBx protein also binds to *p53* and may thus inactivate it.

Hepatitis C virus, like HBV, is associated with liver cancer. This is believed to be due to the ability of HCV to cause liver injury and subsequent regeneration as discussed.

RNA ONCOGENIC VIRUSES (p. 314)

Only one human retrovirus, human T-cell lymphotropic virus type 1 (HTLV-1), has been firmly implicated in carcinogenesis:

- This virus has a strong tropism for CD4+ T cells and is believed to cause a leukemia/lymphoma of these lymphocytes.
- HTLV-1-associated leukemia/lymphoma is endemic in parts of Japan and the Caribbean basin. It is sporadic elsewhere, including the United States.
- HTLV-1 proviral DNA is detected in DNA of leukemic T cells. The integration shows a clonal pattern.
- The mechanism of HTLV-1-induced transformation is not clear; HTLV-1 does not contain a v-*onc*, and it is not found integrated near a protooncogene.
- The HTLV-1 genome contains a unique segment referred to as the *tax* region. The proteins encoded by the *tax* gene activate the transcription of the T-cell growth factor IL-2 and its receptor IL-2R, thus setting up an autocrine loop. The resulting polyclonal expansion of T cells is at increased risk of developing additional mutations to give rise eventually to a monoclonal T-cell tumor.

Helicobacter pylori (p. 315)

Helicobacter pylori has been linked to peptic ulcer, gastric lymphoma, and carcinoma. Its role in peptic ulcers is described in Chapter 18. Chronic infection with *H. pylori* is thought to induce *H. pylori*–reactive T cells that cause proliferation of polyclonal B-cell populations via cytokine secretion. These T cell–dependent B cells eventually become monoclonal and T independent by accumulating mutations. The resultant tumor is called *marginal zone lymphoma* or, sometimes, *MALTOMA*. Before becoming T cell independent, such B-cell proliferations respond to antibiotic treatment.

HOST DEFENSE AGAINST TUMORS (p. 315)
Tumor Antigens (p. 315)

Tumor antigens can be classified into two groups: tumor-specific antigens, present only on tumor cells, and tumor-associated antigens, present on tumor cells and also on some normal cells.

Tumor-specific antigens are readily demonstrated in chemically induced tumors in rodents and some human tumors. Tumor-specific antigens are composed of tumor-derived peptides that are presented on the cell surface by major histocompatibility complex class I molecules and recognized by CD8 + T cells. There are several mechanisms by which tumor antigens recognized by autologous CD8 + cells are formed:

- *Tumor-specific shared antigens*: These antigens are expressed on many tumor cells but not on any normal tissues. They represent peptides derived from genes whose products are present only in the testis, where they cannot be expressed on the cell surface because of lack of human leukocyte antigen (HLA) antigens. Such tumor antigens include MAGE-1, expressed in a subset of melanomas, and cancers of lung, breast, liver, stomach, and ovaries. MAGE antigens can be recognized by autologous cytotoxic T cells and could be used for immunotherapy.
- *Differentiation antigens*: Certain antigens are expressed selectively in some normal cells and in cancer derived from such tissues. For example, a peptide derived from the enzyme tyrosinase is expressed in normal melanocytes as well as melanomas.
- *Antigens resulting from mutations*: These are derived from mutated protooncogenes and cancer-suppressor genes. Hence, they are truly tumor specific. Examples include antigenic peptides derived from mutant forms of *p53*, K-*ras*, and *bcr-c-abl*.
- *Overexpressed antigens*: Some molecules overexpressed in tumor cells (e.g., the c-erbB2 receptor in breast cancer) can give rise to peptides recognized by CD8 + T cells.
- *Viral antigens*: These are derived from proteins encoded by oncogenic viruses such as HPV-16.

Tumor-associated antigens include oncofetal antigens (e.g., carcinoembryonic antigen [CEA]) and lineage-specific antigens (e.g., CD10 on B cells). They do not evoke immune responses but are useful for tumor diagnosis.

Immunosurveillance (p. 318)

A putative immunosurveillance against tumors has been hypothesized. Evidence for its existence consists of

- Increased frequency of cancers in patients with congenital or acquired (drug-induced, AIDS) immunodeficiency

- Increased susceptibility to EBV infections and EBV-associated lymphoma in boys with X-linked immunodeficiency

Tumors may escape immunosurveillance by

- Selective outgrowth of antigen-negative variants
- Loss or reduced expression of histocompatibility antigens, thus becoming less susceptible to cytotoxic T-cell lysis
- Tumor-induced immunosuppression
- Failure of sensitization because tumor cells do not express costimulatory molecules such as B7-1
- Apoptosis of cytotoxic T cells because tumor cells express Fas; the FasL-expressing T cells undergo death when engaged by tumor-associated Fas.

An argument against immunosurveillance is as follows: Tumors that develop in immunodeficient patients are mainly lymphomas, which could be the consequence of an abnormal immune system rather than failure of immunosurveillance.

CLINICAL FEATURES OF TUMORS (p. 319)
Local and Hormonal Effects (p. 319)

Local and hormonal effects of tumors are as follows:

- *Related to location*: Intracranial tumors (e.g., pituitary adenoma) can expand and destroy the remaining pituitary gland, giving rise to an endocrine disorder; tumors of the gastrointestinal tract may cause obstruction of the bowel or may ulcerate and cause bleeding.
- *Hormone production*: Tumors of endocrine glands may elaborate hormones; this is more common in benign than in malignant tumors.

Cancer Cachexia (p. 319)

Loss of body fat, wasting, and profound weakness are referred to as *cancer cachexia*. The basis of cachexia is multifactorial:

- Loss of appetite
- Poorly understood metabolic changes that lead to reduced synthesis and storage of fat and increased mobilization of fatty acids from adipocytes
- Production of cachectin (tumor necrosis factor-α) by activated macrophages and other humoral factors, such as protein mobilizing factors, which can mimic some of the metabolic effects of tumors and hence may be involved

Paraneoplastic Syndromes (p. 320)

Paraneoplastic syndromes refers to symptoms not directly related to the spread of the tumor or elaboration of hormones indigenous to the tissue from which the tumor arose. Paraneoplastic syndromes may be the earliest clinical manifestations of a neoplasm and may mimic distant spread. The most common syndromes are the following:

- *Endocrinopathies*: Some nonendocrine cancers produce hormones or hormone-like factors (ectopic hormone production); for example, certain cancers of the lung (small cell type) produce *Cushing syndrome* by elaborating adrenocorticotropic hormone or related peptides.

- *Hypercalcemia*: Hypercalcemia may occur owing to resorption of bone resulting from the elaboration of parathyroid hormone (PTH)–like peptides (PTH-related protein) or, in some cases, of TGF-α by certain tumors (e.g., squamous cell cancer of the lung, T-cell leukemias/lymphomas). Cancer-associated hypercalcemia also results from osteolysis induced by bony metastases; this, however, is not to be considered a paraneoplastic syndrome.
- *Acanthosis nigricans*: The acquired (nongenetic) form of this verrucous pigmented lesion of the skin is frequently associated with visceral malignancy.
- *Clubbing of fingers and hypertrophic osteoarthropathy*: These conditions are associated with lung cancers and other thoracic lesions.
- *Thrombotic diatheses*: Thrombotic diatheses resulting from production of thromboplastic substance by tumor cells may manifest as disseminated intravascular coagulation or as vegetations on heart valves (nonbacterial thrombotic endocarditis).

GRADING AND STAGING OF TUMORS

(p. 321)

The grade and stage of malignant neoplasms provide a semiquantitative estimate of the clinical gravity of a tumor:

- *Grading* is based on the degree of differentiation and the number of mitoses within the tumor. Cancers are classified as grades I to IV with increasing anaplasia. In general, higher-grade tumors are more aggressive than lower-grade tumors. Grading is imperfect because
  1. Different parts of the same tumor may display different degrees of differentiation.
  2. The grade of tumor may change as the tumor grows.
- *Staging* is based on the anatomic extent of the tumor. Relevant to staging are the size of the primary tumor and the extent of local and distant spread. Two methods of staging are in current use: the TNM (*t*umor, *n*ode, *m*etastases) and the AJC (*A*merican *J*oint *C*ommittee) systems. Both systems assign to higher stages those tumors that are larger, locally invasive, and metastatic.

Both histologic grading and clinical staging are valuable for prognostication and for planning therapy, although staging has proved to be of greater clinical value.

LABORATORY DIAGNOSIS OF CANCER

(p. 322)

Histologic and Cytologic Methods (p. 322)

Histologic examination is the most important method of diagnosis. Proper histologic diagnosis is greatly aided by

- Availability of all relevant clinical data
- Adequate preservation and sampling of the specimen
- In some cases, examination of the frozen specimen to detect cell surface receptors

In addition to the usual fixed and paraffin-embedded sections, quick-frozen sections are employed to obtain a rapid diagnosis while the patient is still under anesthesia.

FINE-NEEDLE ASPIRATION

Fine-needle aspiration involves aspiration of cells and fluids from tumors or masses that occur in readily palpable sites (e.g., breast, thyroid, lymph nodes). The aspirated cells are smeared, stained, and examined.

CYTOLOGIC (PAPANICOLAOU) SMEARS

Cytologic or Papanicolaou smears involve examination of cancer cells that are readily shed. Exfoliative cytology is used most commonly in the diagnosis of dysplasia, carcinoma in situ, and invasive cancer of the uterine cervix and tumors of the stomach, bronchus, and urinary bladder.

Interpretation is based chiefly on changes in the appearance of individual cells. In the hands of experts, false-positive results are uncommon, but false-negative results do occur because of sampling errors. When possible, cytologic diagnosis must be confirmed by biopsy before therapeutic intervention.

IMMUNOCYTOCHEMISTRY

Immunocytochemistry involves detection of cell products or surface markers by monoclonal antibodies. The binding of antibodies can be revealed by fluorescent labels or chemical reactions that result in the generation of a colored product. This technique is useful in the following settings:

- Diagnosis of undifferentiated tumors by the detection of tissue-specific intermediate filaments
- Categorization of leukemias and lymphomas by using monoclonal antibodies specific for various lymphohematopoietic cells
- Determination of the site of origin of metastases by using reagents that identify specific cell types (e.g., prostate specific antigen for prostate cancer)
- Detection of molecules that have prognostic or therapeutic significance (e.g., immunochemical detection of hormone receptors and products of protooncogenes, such as c-erbB2, on breast cancers)

DNA PROBE ANALYSIS

DNA probe analysis involves polymerase chain reaction or FISH analysis. This technique is currently used most extensively in the diagnosis of lymphoid neoplasms because such tumors are associated with clonal rearrangements of T-cell and B-cell antigen receptor genes. Detection of oncogenes such as N-*myc* is also valuable in assessing the prognosis of certain tumors. Diagnosis of chronic myeloid leukemia can be made by detection of the *bcr-c-abl* fusion gene product, even in the absence of the Ph1 chromosome. Specific translocations detected by polymerase chain reaction can distinguish between similar-appearing tumors (e.g., small round blue cell tumors in children). Hereditary predisposition to certain tumors (e.g., breast cancer and endocrine neoplasms) can be detected by mutational analysis of *BRCA-1*, *BRCA-2*, and *RET* genes.

FLOW CYTOMETRY

Measurement of the DNA content of tumor cells by flow cytometry is useful because with several tumors there is a relationship between abnormal DNA content and prognosis. Flow cytometric detection of cell surface antigens is of value in the diagnosis of leukemias and lymphomas.

TUMOR MARKERS

Tumor markers are tumor-derived or tumor-associated molecules that can be detected in blood or other body fluids. They are not primary methods of diagnosis but rather adjuncts to the diagnosis. They may also be of value in determining the response to therapy. Examples of tumor markers follow:

- *CEA*, normally produced by fetal gut, liver, and pancreas, may be elaborated by cancers of the colon, pancreas, stomach, and breast. Less consistently, the levels are elevated in non-neoplastic conditions (e.g., alcoholic cirrhosis, hepatitis, and ulcerative colitis). This antigen is of value in estimating tumor burden in colorectal cancer and in detecting recurrences after surgery.
- α-*fetoprotein* is normally produced by fetal yolk sac and liver. Markedly elevated levels are noted in cancers of the liver and testicular germ cells. Non-neoplastic conditions, such as cirrhosis and hepatitis, are also associated with less marked elevations of α-fetoprotein. Measurements of α-fetoprotein levels are useful in indicating the presence of liver or testicular cancer and in assessing recurrence and response to therapy.

Infectious Diseases

In the United States, serious infections affect persons immunosuppressed by acquired immunodeficiency syndrome (AIDS), chronic disease, or anticancer drugs. Infectious diseases kill more than 10 million persons each year in developing countries, where mostly children die from respiratory and diarrheal infections caused by common viruses and bacteria. Koch's postulates link a specific microorganism to a specific disease.

Helicobacter gastritis, hepatitis B virus (HBV) and hepatitis C virus (HCV) hepatitis, rotavirus diarrhea, and legionnaires' pneumonia are all more recently discovered infectious diseases, in which the pathogen was difficult to culture. Other infections may genuinely be new to humans (e.g., human immunodeficiency virus [HIV], which causes AIDS, and *Borrelia burgdorferi*, which causes Lyme disease) or may be secondary to severe immunosuppression caused by AIDS (e.g., cytomegalovirus [CMV], human herpesvirus type 8, *Mycobacterium avium-intracellulare*, *Pneumocystis carinii*, and *Cryptosporidium parvum*).

To understand the mechanisms of infectious disease, one must consider

1. Virulence properties of the organism
2. The host response to the infectious agent

CATEGORIES OF INFECTIOUS AGENTS
(p. 332)

Prions

- Are composed only of a modified host protein (PrP^{Sc}).
- Are not viruses because they lack RNA or DNA.
- Cause spongiform encephalopathies (kuru and Creutzfeldt-Jakob disease).
- Are associated with neurodegenerative diseases, including fatal familial insomnia.

Viruses

- Are obligate intracellular organisms.
- Contain DNA or RNA within a cylindrical or spherical protein coat or capsid, which may be surrounded by a lipid bilayer (envelope).
- Cause acute illness (e.g., colds, influenza epidemics), lifelong

latency and long-term reactivation (e.g., herpesviruses), or chronic disease (e.g., HBV, HIV).

Bacteriophages and Plasmids

Bacteriophages and plasmids are mobile genetic elements that encode bacterial virulence factors (e.g., adhesins, toxins, or antibiotic resistance).

Bacteria

- Lack nuclei but have rigid cell walls containing two phospholipid bilayers (gram-negative species) or a single bilayer (gram-positive species).
- Are major causes of severe infectious disease.
- Grow extracellularly (e.g., *Pneumococcus*) or intracellularly (e.g., *Mycobacterium tuberculosis*).

Normal persons carry 10^{12} bacteria on the skin, including *Staphylococcus epidermidis* and *Propionibacterium acnes*, and 10^{14} bacteria in the gastrointestinal tract, 99.9% of which are anaerobic.

Chlamydiae, Rickettsiae, and Mycoplasmas

Chlamydiae, rickettsiae, and mycoplasmas are similar to bacteria but lack certain structures (a cell wall in mycoplasmas) or metabolic capabilities (adenosine triphosphate [ATP] synthesis in chlamydiae). Other characteristics are as follows:

- Chlamydiae cause genitourinary infections, conjunctivitis, and respiratory infections of newborns.
- Rickettsiae are transmitted by insect vectors, including lice (epidemic typhus), ticks (Rocky Mountain spotted fever [RMSF], Q fever), and mites (scrub typhus) and cause a hemorrhagic vasculitis, pneumonia, hepatitis (Q fever), or encephalitis (RMSF).
- Mycoplasmas bind to the surface of epithelial cells and cause atypical pneumonia or nongonococcal urethritis.

Fungi

Fungi have thick, chitin-containing cell walls and grow in humans as budding yeast cells and slender tubes (hyphae). Other characteristics are as follows:

- In otherwise healthy persons, fungi produce
  1. Superficial infections (e.g., *athlete's foot* caused by tinea)
  2. Abscesses (e.g., sporotrichosis)
  3. Granulomas (e.g., *Coccidioides, Histoplasma*, and *Blastomyces*)
- In immunocompromised hosts, opportunistic fungi (e.g., *Candida, Aspergillus*, and *Mucor*) cause systemic infections characterized by tissue necrosis, hemorrhage, and vascular occlusion.
- In AIDS patients, the opportunistic fungus-like organism *P. carinii* causes a lethal pneumonia.

Protozoa

Protozoa are single cells with a nucleus, a pliable plasma membrane, and complex cytoplasmic organelles. Other characteristics are as follows:

- *Trichomonas vaginalis* is transmitted sexually.
- Intestinal protozoa (e.g., *Entamoeba histolytica* and *Giardia lamblia*) are infective when swallowed.
- Blood-borne protozoa (e.g., *Plasmodium* species and *Leishmania* species) are transmitted by blood-sucking insects.

Helminths

- Are highly differentiated multicellular organisms with complex life cycles.
- Cause disease in proportion to the number of infecting organisms.

Roundworms (nematodes) infect the intestines (e.g., *Ascaris*, hookworms, and *Strongyloides*) or tissues (e.g., filariae and *Trichinella*). *Flatworms* (cestodes) are segmented tapeworms in the intestines or form tissue cysts (e.g., cysticerci and hydatids). The most important *fluke* (trematode) is the blood-dwelling schistosome.

Ectoparasites

- Are arthropods (e.g., lice, ticks, bedbugs, fleas) that attach to and live on the skin.
- May be vectors for other pathogens (e.g., Lyme disease spirochetes transmitted by ticks).

HOST BARRIERS TO INFECTION (p. 338)

Host barriers to infection include intact skin and mucosal surfaces and secretory products (e.g., lysozyme in tears and acid in stomach).

- Commensal skin bacteria cause infections when they enter through cuts or burns.
- Respiratory, gastrointestinal, and urogenital infections are caused by virulent organisms penetrating intact mucosal barriers.

HOW MICROORGANISMS CAUSE DISEASE (p. 340)

Infectious agents damage tissues directly by entering cells, releasing toxins, or damaging blood vessels. Microbes induce host cellular responses that cause additional tissue damage, including suppuration, scarring, and hypersensitivity reactions.

Viral Injury to Host Tissues (p. 340)

- Viruses enter host cells by
  1. Binding to host cell surface proteins (e.g., HIV to CD4 and CCR5 on helper lymphocytes)

2. Translocation into the cytosol from the plasma membrane or endosomal membranes
3. Replication via virus-specific enzymes

- Viral infection can be abortive, latent (e.g., varicella-zoster virus [VZV]), or persistent (e.g., HBV).
- Viruses kill host cells by
  - Inhibiting host cell DNA, RNA, or protein synthesis (e.g., poliovirus)
  - Damaging the plasma membrane (e.g., HIV)
  - Lysing cells (e.g., rhinoviruses and influenza viruses)
  - Inducing a host immune response to virus-infected cells (e.g., HBV).

Bacterial Injury to Host Tissues (p. 341)

- Bacterial injury depends on the ability to deliver toxins (e.g., *Vibrio cholerae*) or to adhere to host cells and enter them (e.g., *Listeria monocytogenes*).
- Bacterial adhesins include filamentous pili (e.g., *Escherichia coli* and *Neisseria gonorrhoeae*) that determine to which host cells the microbes will attach (bacterial tropism).
- Most bacterial virulence factors are also found in avirulent organisms.
- Some virulence genes are organized into pathogenicity islands, which are located on chromosomes or plasmids and encode type III secretory apparatus as well as adherence proteins and toxins.
- Bacterial endotoxin is a lipopolysaccharide that induces fever via host lymphokines, including tumor necrosis factor (TNF) and interleukin-1 (IL-1).
- Bacterial exotoxins are composed of a binding part and a catalytic part, which adenosine diphosphate (ADP) ribosylates and inactivates host proteins (e.g., diphtheria or cholera toxins) or degrades host proteins (e.g., botulinum toxin).
- Bacteria may reproduce within the phagolysosomes (e.g., *Mycobacterium* and *Legionella*) or cytosol (e.g., *Shigella* and *Listeria*).

Immune Evasion by Microbes (p. 344)

Microbes avoid the host immune response by

- Remaining inaccessible within the lumen of the small intestine (e.g., toxin-producing *Clostridium difficile*) or rapidly entering host cells (e.g., malaria sporozoites into the liver).
- Producing a capsule that covers antigens and prevents phagocytosis (e.g., *Streptococcus pneumoniae*).
- Changing their surface antigens (e.g., rhinoviruses, *N. gonorrhoeae*, and African trypanosomes).
- Infecting lymphocytes (e.g., HIV and Epstein-Barr virus [EBV]) and damaging the host immune system.

SPECIAL TECHNIQUES FOR DIAGNOSING INFECTIOUS AGENTS (p. 344)

Some infectious agents can be directly observed in hematoxylin and eosin–stained sections (e.g., the inclusion bodies formed by CMV and herpesvirus; bacterial clumps, which usually stain blue; *Candida* and *Mucor*, among the fungi; most protozoans; and all helminths). Many infectious agents, however, are best visualized

Table 9-1. SPECIAL TECHNIQUES FOR
DIAGNOSING INFECTIOUS AGENTS

Gram stain	Most bacteria
Acid-fast stain	Mycobacteria, *Nocardia* (modified)
Silver stains	Fungi, *Legionella, Pneumocystis*
Periodic acid–Schiff	Fungi, amebae
Mucicarmine	Cryptococci
Giemsa	Campylobacteria, *Leishmania,* malaria
Antibody probes	Viruses, rickettsiae
Culture	All classes
DNA probes	Viruses, bacteria, protozoa

after special stains that identify organisms based on particular
characteristics of their cell walls or coat (Table 9–1). In addition,
cultures of lesional tissues are performed to speciate organisms
and determine drug sensitivity.

SPECTRUM OF INFLAMMATORY
RESPONSES TO INFECTION (p. 345)

In contrast to the vast molecular diversity of microorganisms,
the tissue responses to these agents are limited to five microscopic patterns.

Suppurative Inflammation (Neutrophils)

- Suppurative inflammation is caused by *pyogenic* bacteria,
  mostly extracellular gram-positive cocci and gram-negative
  rods.
- Suppurative inflammation is secondary to increased vascular
  permeability and leukotaxis of neutrophils attracted by bacterial
  peptides, which contain *N*-formyl methionine residues.
- The sizes of exudative lesions vary from tiny microabscesses
  formed during sepsis to diffuse involvement of the meninges
  (e.g., *Haemophilus influenzae*) or entire lobes of the lung (e.g.,
  S. pneumoniae).

Mononuclear Inflammation

- Mononuclear inflammation is induced by
  - Viruses
  - Intracellular bacteria
  - Spirochetes
  - Intracellular parasites
  - Helminths
- Mononuclear inflammation includes mostly lymphocytes (e.g.,
  chancres of primary syphilis) or macrophages (e.g., granulomas
  of mycobacteria), depending on the characteristics of the organ-
  ism and the host.

Cytopathic-Cytoproliferative Inflammation

- Cytopathic-cytoproliferative inflammation is characterized by
  virus-mediated damage to individual host cells in the absence
  of host inflammatory response.

- Cytopathic-cytoproliferative inflammation may show
  - Inclusion bodies (e.g., CMV)
  - Polykaryons (e.g., measles viruses)
  - Blisters (e.g., herpesviruses)
  - Warty changes (e.g., papillomaviruses)

Necrotizing Inflammation

- Necrotizing inflammation is caused by uncontrolled viral infection (e.g., fulminant HBV infection), secreted bacterial toxins (e.g., those of *Clostridium perfringens*), or contact-mediated cytolysis of host cells by protozoa (e.g., *Entamoeba histolytica*).
- Necrotizing inflammation results in severe tissue necrosis in the absence of inflammatory infiltrates.

Chronic Inflammation and Scarring

- Chronic inflammation and scarring are caused by certain acute infections (e.g., gonococcal salpingitis) or chronic infections (e.g., schistosomiasis).
- Chronic inflammation and scarring may be severe despite a paucity of organisms present (e.g., *M. tuberculosis*).

Pattern of Inflammation

- Pattern of inflammation may be mixed because of multiple simultaneous infections (e.g., AIDS pneumonitis with CMV, *Pneumocystis*, and *Mycobacterium*).
- Pattern of inflammation may vary based on host response (e.g., mostly lymphocytes in tuberculoid leprosy and mostly macrophages in lepromatous leprosy).
- Pattern should be consistent with the organisms cultured or identified by microscopy.

RESPIRATORY INFECTIONS (p. 347)

Viral respiratory disorders are the most frequent and least preventable of all infectious diseases and range in severity from the discomforting but self-limited common cold to life-threatening pneumonias.

Rhinoviruses (Common Cold) (p. 347)

- Rhinoviruses are unencapsulated, icosahedral viruses that contain single-stranded RNA.
- Rhinoviruses bind to intercellular adhesion molecule (ICAM-1) on epithelial cells of the upper respiratory tract and induce mucus secretion via bradykinin release.
- Rhinoviruses induce serotype-specific immunoglobulin G (IgG) and IgA antibodies, which prevent reinfection with the same rhinovirus but not with 100 other serotypes.

Influenza Viruses (p. 348)

- Influenza viruses have eight single-stranded RNAs, each bound by a nucleoprotein that determines the type of influenza virus (A, B, or C).

- Influenza viruses have envelopes containing a hemagglutinin and neuraminidase, which project outward and determine the subtype of the virus (H1 to H3; N1 or N2).
- Nasal channels, sinuses, eustachian tubes, tonsils, and bronchioles are affected.
- Infection produces mucosal hyperemia and swelling with a predominantly lymphomonocytic and plasmacytic infiltration of the submucosa accompanied by overproduction of mucus secretions.
- Clearance of the primary influenza virus infection occurs when cytotoxic T cells kill virus-infected cells.
- Host antibodies to the hemagglutinin and neuraminidase prevent future infection with that influenza virus.
- A single subtype of influenza virus A is present throughout the world at a given time.
- Epidemics of influenza occur through mutations of the hemagglutinin and neuraminidase (antigenic drift) that allow the virus to escape most, although not necessarily all, host antibodies.
- The pandemic of influenza in 1918 that killed 20 million people was caused by a swine influenza virus.
- A major complication of viral damage to bronchial epithelium is bacterial superinfection (e.g., *Pneumococcus*, *Staphylococcus*, and *Haemophilus*).

Haemophilus influenzae (p. 348)

- *H. influenzae* is a pleomorphic gram-negative organism, which is a major cause of life-threatening epiglottitis, laryngotracheobronchitis, and meningitis in young children.
  - A polyribose capsule determines serotype and prevents opsonization by complement and phagocytosis by host cells.
  - Children are vaccinated against the capsular polysaccharide b.
  - Lesions feature dense, fibrin-rich exudates of polymorphonuclear cells.

Tuberculosis (p. 349)

- Tuberculosis is caused by the aerobic, non–spore-forming, nonmotile bacillus *M. tuberculosis*, which has a waxy coat that stains red with acid-fast stains.
- Tuberculosis is the most important infectious disease, killing about 3 million persons each year, mostly in developing countries.
- Urban AIDS patients in the United States frequently have florid infections with *M. tuberculosis*, which may be multidrug resistant, or with *M. avium* and *M. intracellulare*, which are opportunistic pathogens.
- In *primary tuberculosis*, inhaled mycobacteria briefly proliferate in macrophages but are controlled in 95% of cases by T cell–mediated immune response, which is demonstrable by a positive purified protein derivative (PPD) test.
  - Mycobacteria may block vacuolar acidification by nonactivated macrophages.
  - CD4 + helper T cells secrete TNF-γ, which activates macrophages to kill intracellular mycobacteria via reactive nitrogen intermediates and also to form *epithelioid cell granulomas.*
  - CD8 + suppresser T cells kill macrophages that are infected with mycobacteria, resulting in the formation of *caseating (cheeselike) granulomas* (delayed-type hypersensitivity reactions).

- The residual lesion is a calcified scar in the lung parenchyma and in the hilar lymph node *(Ghon complex).*
- In *secondary tuberculosis,* mycobacteria associated with granulomas may remain confined to the lung or may spread hematogenously throughout the lungs, kidneys, meninges, marrow, and in series of organs.
  - Granulomas, which fail to control the mycobacteria, are the major cause of tissue damage in tuberculosis.
  - Cavities formed by caseating granulomas may rupture into blood vessels, causing further hematogenous spread of mycobacteria, or into airways, releasing infectious bacteria into aerosols.
  - In AIDS, disseminated granulomas containing abundant *M. tuberculosis, M. avium,* and *M. intracellulare* organisms are poorly formed and are also frequent in lymph nodes and bowel.

Histoplasma capsulatum and Coccidioides immitis (p. 352)

- *H. capsulatum* and *C. immitis* are dimorphic fungi, which are endemic along the Ohio and Mississippi Rivers *(Histoplasma)* and in the western United States *(Coccidioides).*
- *H. capsulatum* and *C. immitis* cause granulomatous disease, which may resemble primary and secondary tuberculosis in normal hosts and disseminated tuberculosis in AIDS patients.
- *Histoplasma,* which stain black with silver methenamine, bind to complement receptors on macrophages and reproduce within the phagolysosomes.
- In endemic areas, 80% of persons have delayed-type sensitivity (response to PPD-like challenge) to *Coccidioides,* which blocks fusion of the macrophage phagosome with the lysosome.

GASTROINTESTINAL INFECTIONS (p. 353)

An overview of gastrointestinal infections is presented in Table 9–2.

- Normal host defenses include
  - Gastric acid
  - Duodenal bile and lytic enzymes
  - Mucous layer
  - Secreted IgA
- Nonenveloped viruses (hepatitis A virus, rotavirus, and Norwalk viruses) resist stomach acid.
- Enterobacteria cause illness by releasing toxins, invading epithelium, or causing bacteremia.

Viral Enteritis (p. 354)

- Viral enteritis is caused by single-stranded RNA (Norwalk virus), double-stranded RNA (rotavirus), and double-stranded DNA viruses (enteric adenoviruses).
- Diarrhea results from malabsorption of sodium and water by blunted or destroyed villous epithelial cells.

Table 9-2. MAJOR INFECTIOUS CAUSES OF DIARRHEA

Organism	Comment
Viruses	
Rotaviruses	Principally in children under age 6. Sporadic—from contaminated water, may become epidemic; also direct fecal-oral transmission
Enteric adenoviruses	Common in infants and children, mostly sporadic
Norwalk virus	Young and old, mainly epidemic; fecal-oral
Bacteria	
Enterotoxigenic *E. coli*	Major cause of traveler's diarrhea, food- and water-borne, previously unencountered strains
Campylobacter jejuni	Major global cause, any age, mainly children, transmission by contaminated water and food
Yersinia enterocolitica	Similar to above
Shigella	Major global offender, children and adults, fecal-oral direct transmission and contaminated water and food, endemic and epidemic
Enteropathogenic *E. coli*	Children and nursery outbreaks
Salmonella spp.	Large number serotypes with range of clinical syndromes, children and adults, food- and water-borne, human and animal reservoirs
Clostridium difficile	Antibiotic-associated, hospital-acquired, mainly in predisposed adults
Vibrio cholerae	Major cause of pandemic and epidemic diarrhea
Parasites	
Giardia lamblia	Carrier state common, major cause of traveler's diarrhea, contaminated drinking water, high infection rate in Russia, northwestern United States, other locales; may become epidemic
Entamoeba histolytica	Large reservoir of asymptomatic carriers in developed countries and endemic in developing areas, fecal-oral, sexual transmission particularly among homosexuals, and from contaminated water and food

Bacterial Enteritis (p. 355)

SHIGELLA SPECIES AND O-TYPE ENTEROTOXIC *E. COLI* (p. 355)

- *Shigella* species and O-type enterotoxic *E. coli* cause dysentery (diarrhea with blood and mucus in the stool) as well as hemolytic-uremic syndrome.
- Shiga toxin, similar to *E. coli* verotoxins, binds to host cell glycolipids and blocks protein synthesis.
- *Shigella* reproduce within the cytosol of intestinal epithelial cells and destroy them, producing numerous ulcers, featuring a fibrin-rich and neutrophil-rich exudate.

CAMPYLOBACTER JEJUNI (p. 355)

- *C. jejuni* is a comma-shaped bacterium that
  1. Secretes toxins and causes diarrhea
  2. Invades the colonic epithelium and causes dysentery
  3. Reproduces in mesenteric lymph nodes and causes enteric fever
- *C. jejuni* is a major contaminant of poultry along with *Salmonella.*
- Infection is dependent on intact host signal-transduction pathways for invasion.
- A related bacterium, *Helicobacter pylori*, causes chronic gastritis and gastric ulcers.

YERSINIA SPECIES (p. 356)

- *Y. enterocolitis* and *Y. pseudotuberculosis* are facultative intracellular bacteria, which cause ileitis and lymphadenitis.
- A pathogenicity island encodes bacterial proteins, which disrupt normal host signaling.

SALMONELLA SPECIES (p. 356)

- *S. enteritidis*–contaminated chicken and beef are important causes of food poisoning.
- *S. typhi*, which is spread from person-to-person via the fecal-oral route, causes systemic typhoid fever.
- Greater than 20 *Salmonella* virulence genes are induced by low oxygen tension in the colon and acidity within the macrophage lysosome.
- *S. typhi* multiplies within macrophages of intestinal Peyer patches (causing ulceration of the overlying mucosa), spleen, liver, and bone marrow.
- Chronic carriers of *S. typhi* (e.g., *typhoid Mary*) have asymptomatic gallbladder colonization.

VIBRIO CHOLERAE (p. 357)

- *V. cholerae* is a noninvasive, toxin-producing bacterium that causes pandemics (long-lasting epidemics) of severe watery diarrhea, originating in India and Bangladesh.
- Serotype O139 (Bengal strain) has replaced serotype O1—either classic or El Tor—as predominant *Vibrio* in South Asia.
- *V. cholerae* virulence factors include flagellar proteins important for motility and attachment and a toxin, similar in structure to the heat-labile toxin of *E. coli* that causes traveler's diarrhea.

- Cholera toxin binds to GM_1 ganglioside on epithelial cells and ADP-ribosylates host G-proteins, which activate adenyl cyclase, increase levels of intracellular cyclic adenosine monophosphate (cAMP), and cause massive secretion of chloride, sodium, and water.

Parasitic Intestinal Infections (p. 358)

ENTAMOEBA HISTOLYTICA (p. 358)

- *E. histolytica* causes dysentery when organisms attach via an adherence lectin to the colonic epithelium, lyse colonic epithelial cells by means of a channel-forming protein, and invade the bowel wall.
- *E. histolytica* causes disease, whereas *E. dispar* does not.
- Flask-shaped colonic ulcers contain few inflammatory cells, extensive liquefactive necrosis, and amebae, which resemble macrophages with a small single nucleus and frequently contain engulfed red blood cells.

GIARDIA LAMBLIA (p. 359)

- *G. lamblia* is the most prevalent pathogenic gut protozoan worldwide.
- *G. lamblia* causes acute or chronic diarrhea when binucleate parasites adhere to the duodenal epithelium via sucker-discs.
- The parasites show antigenic variation of their major surface protein, which may allow them to escape host IgA.
- Infection causes

  - Clubbing of villi
  - A decreased villus-crypt ratio
  - A mixed inflammatory infiltrate of the lamina propria

- Infection produces diarrhea by blocking absorption.

SKIN INFECTIONS AND SEXUALLY TRANSMITTED DISEASES (p. 359)

Most sexually transmitted diseases are transmitted through the skin and present initially as skin lesions. Skin pathogens enter through moist skin, cuts, or insect bites.

Herpesviruses (p. 359)

- Herpesviruses are large, double-stranded DNA viruses surrounded by an envelope, which are neurotropic and cause cold sores (herpes simplex virus type 1), genital sores (herpes simplex virus type 2), corneal blindness, and encephalitis (rarely).
- Human herpesvirus-8 causes Kaposi's sarcoma.
- In primary infections, herpes simplex virus type 1 and herpes simplex virus type 2 replicate and cause vesicular lesions in the epidermis of the skin and mucous membranes.
- In secondary infections, herpesviruses, which have remained latent in the neurons, spread from the regional ganglia to the skin or to mucous membranes.
- Herpesvirus lesions show large, pink-to-purple (Cowdry type A), virion-containing intranuclear inclusions, which push darkly stained host cell chromatin to the edges of the nucleus.
- Herpesviruses also produce multinucleated syncytia, which are

diagnostic in smears of fluid from intraepithelial blisters (Tzanck preparations).
- In herpes stromal keratitis, which is treated with steroids, infiltrates of mononuclear cells surround keratinocytes and endothelial cells and may lead to neovascularization, scarring, opacification of the cornea, and blindness.

Chlamydia trachomatis (p. 361)

- *C. trachomatis* is an obligate intracellular pathogen of columnar epithelial cells that causes nongonococcal urethritis, lymphogranuloma venereum, and trachoma.
- In some males, *C. trachomatis* infection causes Reiter syndrome, which is a triad of conjunctivitis, polyarthritis, and genital infection.
- Infants born to mothers with *C. trachomatis* cervicitis may develop self-limited inclusion conjunctivitis or neonatal pneumonia.
- Chlamydiae exist in two forms:
  1. Elementary bodies, which never divide but are infectious
  2. Reticulate bodies, which multiply within vacuoles of host cells but are not infectious
- In lymphogranuloma venereum, inguinal, pelvic, and rectal lymph nodes are enlarged and contain a mixture of suppurative and granulomatous inflammation.
- In inclusion conjunctivitis, conjunctivae are hyperemic, are edematous, and show a monocytic infiltrate.

Neisseria gonorrhoeae (p. 362)

- *N. gonorrhoeae* is an encapsulated, gram-negative diplococcus that causes urethritis (*clap*), pharyngitis, or proctitis, depending on sexual practices.
- *N. gonorrhoeae* may cause urethral strictures and chronic infections of the epididymis, prostate, and seminal vesicles.
- *N. gonorrhoeae* may infect the fallopian tubes (salpingitis), resulting in tubo-ovarian abscesses and scars, sterility, and ectopic pregnancy.
- *N. gonorrhoeae* binds to host epithelial cells via pili, which show antigenic variation based on intragenomic recombination and on recombination after incorporation of exogenous DNA from lysed gonococci.
- Perinatal ophthalmic infection was a major cause of blindness before prophylactic administration of silver nitrate to neonates became routine.
- Internalization is based on a second set of adhesins called the *opacity outer membrane proteins* or *P.II*, which also show antigenic variation.
- Gonococcal lesions show exudative and purulent reactions, followed by granulation tissue, plasma cell infiltrates, and scarring as chronicity increases.

Treponema pallidum (Syphilis) (p. 362)

- *T. pallidum* is a microaerophilic spirochete with an axial periplasmic flagella wound around a slender, helical protoplasm, all of which is covered by an outer membrane.
- *Primary syphilis*, which occurs approximately 3 weeks after contact with an infected individual, features a single firm, non-

tender, raised, red lesion (*chancre*) located at the site of treponemal invasion on the penis, cervix, vaginal wall, or anus.

- *Secondary syphilis*, which occurs 2 to 10 weeks after the primary chancre, is characterized by a diffuse rash, particularly of the palms and soles, that may be accompanied by white oral lesions, fever, lymphadenopathy, headache, arthritis, and (rarely) immune complex nephritis.
- *Tertiary syphilis*, which occurs years after the primary lesion, is characterized by
  1. Active inflammatory lesions of the aorta, heart, and central nervous system
  2. Quiescent lesions (gummas) involving the liver, bones, and skin
- *Congenital syphilis*
  1. Causes late abortion, stillbirth, or death soon after delivery
  2. May persist in latent form to become apparent only during childhood

Whatever the stage of the disease and location of the lesions, the histologic hallmarks of syphilis are obliterative endarteritis and plasma cell infiltrates. The endarteritis is secondary to the binding of spirochetes to endothelial cells, mediated by host fibronectin molecules bound to the surface of the spirochetes. Syphilitic gummas are white-gray and rubbery, occur singly or multiply, and vary in size from microscopic defects resembling tubercles to large, tumor-like masses.

Sequelae of congenital syphilis include

1. An extensive cutaneous rash containing many spirochetes
2. Osteochondritis with collapse of the bridge of the nose
3. Periostitis with bowing of the tibia
4. Keratitis
5. Hutchinson teeth (peg-shaped incisors)
6. Eighth nerve deafness

Trichomonas vaginalis (p. 364)

- *T. vaginalis* is a noninvasive anaerobic, flagellated protozoan parasite, which frequently causes vaginal itching and a profuse watery discharge containing the parasites.
- The vaginal mucosa and superficial submucosa are infiltrated by lymphocytes, plasma cells, and polymorphonuclear leukocytes.

GRAM-POSITIVE BACTERIAL INFECTIONS
(p. 365)

Staphylococcus aureus (p. 365)

- *S. aureus* is a gram-positive coccus that forms grapelike clusters and causes
  - Skin lesions (boils, carbuncles, impetigo, and scalded skin)
  - Pharyngitis
  - Pneumonia
  - Endocarditis
  - Food poisoning
  - Toxic shock syndrome
- *S. aureus* is a major cause of infection of persons with severe burns and surgical wounds and second only to *E. coli* as a cause of hospital-acquired infections.

- Virulence factors, which are controlled by an autoinducing peptide, include
  - Surface proteins involved in adherence to host cells
  - Enzymes that degrade host proteins
  - Toxins that lyse host cells and cause scalded skin syndrome (exotoxins), cause food poisoning (enterotoxins), and produce shock (endotoxin and toxic shock syndrome toxin, which is a superantigen).
- Whether the lesion is located in the skin, lungs, bones, or heart valves, *S. aureus* causes pyogenic inflammation, which is remarkable for its local destructiveness.

Streptococcus Species (p. 367)

- Streptococci are gram-positive cocci that grow in pairs or chains, which are typed according to their surface antigens.
- *S. pneumoniae* is the major cause of community-acquired pneumonia and causes adult bacterial meningitis.
- *S. pyogenes* produces
  - Pharyngitis
  - Scarlet fever
  - Erysipelas (swelling skin rash)
  - Impetigo
  - Rheumatic fever
  - Glomerulonephritis
- *S. agalactiae* causes neonatal sepsis and urinary tract infections.
- *Enterococcus faecalis* and *S. viridans* cause endocarditis.
- *S. mutans* causes dental caries.
- Streptococcal virulence factors include
  1. Rodlike surface M-proteins and a polysaccharide capsule that prevent bacteria from being phagocytosed
  2. A pneumolysin that lyses host cells and wastes host complement
  3. Exotoxins that produce the rash in scarlet fever
  4. Proteases that degrade chemotactic peptides and immunoglobulins
  5. Lactic acid that demineralizes tooth enamel
- Streptococcal lesions are remarkable for their diffuse spreading neutrophilic infiltrates with minimal destruction of host tissues.

Clostridium Species (p. 368)

- Clostridia are gram-positive, box-shaped bacilli that grow under anaerobic conditions and produce spores frequently present in the soil.
- *C. perfringens* and *C. septicum*, which invade traumatic and surgical wounds and cause gas gangrene, also contaminate illegal abortions and cause uterine myonecrosis.
- *C. tetani*, which proliferates in puncture wounds and in the umbilical stump of newborn infants in developing countries, releases a potent neurotoxin, called *tetanospasmin*, that causes convulsive contractions of skeletal muscles (lockjaw). Tetanus toxoid (formalin-fixed neurotoxin) is part of the diphtheria, pertussis, and tetanus (DPT) immunization.
- *C. botulinum* grows in inadequately sterilized canned foods and releases a potent neurotoxin that causes a severe paralysis of respiratory and skeletal muscles (botulism).
- *C. difficile* overgrows other intestinal flora in antibiotic-treated patients, releases multiple toxins, and causes a pseudomembranous colitis.

- Clostridial toxins
  1. Block acetylcholine release (*C. botulinum* and *C. tetani* neurotoxins)
  2. Degrade host membranes (*C. perfringens* α-toxin)
  3. Glucosylate rho proteins (*C. difficile* toxins)
  4. ADP-ribosylate G proteins (*C. botulinum* exoenzyme C3).
- Clostridial cellulitis and gas gangrene are remarkable for a foul odor; marked edema or exudate with thin, discolored fluid; and wide, deep tissue destruction.
- Microscopically the extent of tissue necrosis is disproportionate to the number of neutrophils and clostridia present.

INFECTIONS OF CHILDHOOD AND ADOLESCENCE (p. 370)

With the exception of EBV, the cause of infectious mononucleosis, all of the infectious agents described here are now preventable by vaccination. Still, these viruses and bacteria cause not infrequent miniepidemics in the United States and are responsible for considerable morbidity and mortality in the developing world.

Measles Virus (Rubeola) (p. 370)

- Measles virus is a paramyxovirus that causes 1.5 million deaths per year among children in the developing world, who by reasons of poor nutrition are 10 to 1000 times more likely to die of measles pneumonia than Western children.
- Most children develop T cell–mediated immunity to measles virus that controls the viral infection and produces the measles rash, which is a hypersensitivity reaction to viral antigens in the skin.
- Subacute sclerosing panencephalitis and measles inclusion-body encephalitis (in immunocompromised individuals) are rare late complications of measles, caused by hypermutated, *defective* viruses.
- Ulcerated mucosal lesions in the oral cavity near the opening of Stensen ducts (pathognomonic Koplik spots) show necrosis, neutrophils, and neovascularization.
- The lymphoid organs typically have marked follicular hyperplasia, large germinal centers, and randomly distributed multinucleate giant cells, called *Warthin-Finkeldey cells*, which have eosinophilic nuclear and cytoplasmic inclusion bodies and are pathognomonic of measles.

Mumps Virus (p. 370)

- Mumps virus is an RNA virus of the paramyxovirus family that includes
  1. Measles virus
  2. Respiratory syncytial virus (the major cause of lower respiratory infections in infants)
  3. Parainfluenza virus (the cause of croup)
- Mumps virus causes a transient inflammation and enlargement of the parotid glands and, less often, of the testes, pancreas, and central nervous system.
- Mumps lesions show interstitial edema and diffuse infiltrates of histiocytes, lymphocytes, and plasma cells.

Epstein-Barr Virus (Infectious Mononucleosis) (p. 371)

- EBV is a γ-group herpesvirus that causes a benign, self-limited lymphoproliferative disease that is characterized by
  - Fever
  - Generalized lymphadenopathy
  - Splenomegaly
  - Sore throat
  - The appearance in the blood of atypical activated T lymphocytes
- EBV enters the epithelial cell cytoplasm by directly fusing with the plasma membrane.
- EBV enters the B-cell cytoplasm by fusing with endosomal membranes.
- Two EBV proteins, EBNA2 and LMP-1, are associated with B-cell immortalization, which may occur in latently infected lymphocytes.
- In *mononucleosis*, the total white cell count increases to as many as 18,000, 95% of which are atypical T lymphocytes with an abundant, finely granular, basophilic cytoplasm, containing small fenestrations.
- The lymph nodes in the posterior cervical, axillary, and groin regions have the following characteristics:
  1. Are enlarged
  2. Show increased number of T cells in their paracortical zones
  3. Contain large binucleate cells, Reed-Sternberg–like cells
- With impaired immunity, mononucleosis may become chronic and transform into B-cell lymphoma.
- In *Burkitt lymphoma* associated with EBV, there is a characteristic 8:14 translocation, in which the c-*myc* oncogene is placed into the immunoglobulin heavy chain expression region.

Poliovirus (p. 373)

- Poliovirus is a spherical, unencapsulated RNA virus, which is a member of the enterovirus family. Other members cause
  - Childhood diarrhea
  - Rashes (coxsackievirus A)
  - Conjunctivitis (enterovirus 70)
  - Viral meningitis (coxsackievirus and echovirus)
  - Myopericarditis (coxsackievirus B)
  - Jaundice (hepatitis A virus)
- Poliovirus is the target of a vaccination campaign to eliminate the virus worldwide.
- There are three major strains of poliovirus, each of which is included in the Salk formalin-fixed (killed) vaccine and the Sabin oral, attenuated (live) vaccine.
- In 1 of 100 infected persons, poliovirus invades the central nervous system and replicates in motor neurons of the spinal cord (spinal poliomyelitis resulting in muscular paralysis) or brain stem (bulbar poliomyelitis possibly resulting in respiratory paralysis).

Varicella-Zoster Virus (Chickenpox and Shingles) (p. 373)

- VZV is an α-herpesvirus, which infects mucous membranes, skin, and neurons.

188

- VZV is transmitted in epidemic fashion by aerosols, disseminates hematogenously, and causes widespread vesicular skin lesions (chickenpox).
- VZV infects satellite cells around neurons in the dorsal root ganglia and may recur many years after the primary infection in the form of shingles.
- One reason why VZV recurs less frequently than herpes simplex virus is that the genes involved in reactivation in herpes simplex virus are missing in VZV.
- The chickenpox rash occurs approximately 2 weeks after respiratory infection and travels in multiple waves centrifugally from the torso to the head and extremities.
- Each lesion progresses rapidly from a macule to a vesicle, which resembles "a dew drop on a rose petal."
- Histologically, chickenpox vesicles contain intranuclear inclusions of the epithelial cells, and the blisters are identical to those of herpes simplex virus type 1 (p. 360).

Whooping Cough (p. 374)

- Whooping cough is caused by the gram-negative coccobacillus *Bordetella pertussis* in persons not given the DPT vaccine.
- Virulence factors include a filamentous hemagglutinin, pertussis toxin that ADP-ribosylates the same G proteins as cholera toxin, and a hemolysin important in early colonization.
- Laryngotracheobronchitis may include mucosal erosion, hyperemia, and copious mucopurulent exudates.
- Mucosal and peribronchial lymph follicles are hypercellular and enlarged, and there is a striking peripheral lymphocytosis.

Diphtheria (p. 375)

- Diphtheria is caused by the gram-positive rod *Corynebacterium diphtheriae* and is prevented by immunization with a formalin-fixed toxoid in the DPT vaccine.
- Phage-encoded diphtheria toxin, similar to *Pseudomonas* exoenzyme A, ADP-ribosylates and inactivates the ribosomal protein elongation factor-2.
- Tracheal colonization may lead to
  - Mucosal erosion
  - Formation of a suffocating pharyngeal fibrinosuppurative exudate (pseudomembrane)
  - Toxin-mediated damage to the heart, nerves, liver, or kidneys

OPPORTUNISTIC AND AIDS-ASSOCIATED INFECTIONS (p. 375)

Opportunistic pathogens are those that cause no or mild infections in immunocompetent individuals but may cause devastating disease in infants or in individuals with genetic or acquired immunodeficiencies.

Cytomegalovirus (p. 376)

- CMV is a β-group herpesvirus, which causes esophagitis, colitis, hepatitis, pneumonitis, renal tubulitis, chorioretinitis, and meningoencephalitis in neonates and in persons immunosuppressed secondary to transplant chemotherapy or AIDS.

- CMV is spread
  - By intrauterine or perinatal transmission at childbirth
  - In mother's milk
  - In respiratory droplets
  - In semen and vaginal fluid
  - In blood transfusions
  - By transplantation of virus-infected grafts from a donor with latent infection
- Affected infants manifest the following:
  - Hemolytic form of anemia
  - Jaundice
  - Thrombocytopenia
  - Purpura
  - Hepatosplenomegaly (owing to extramedullary hematopoiesis)
  - Pneumonitis
  - Deafness
  - Chorioretinitis
  - Extensive brain damage
- CMV chorioretinitis is a frequent cause of blindness in AIDS patients.
- Disseminated CMV in the immunoincompetent individual causes focal necrosis with minimal inflammation in virtually any organ.
- Endothelial and epithelial cells infected with CMV are markedly enlarged, with large purple intranuclear inclusions surrounded by a clear halo and smaller basophilic cytoplasmic inclusions.

Pseudomonas aeruginosa (p. 376)

- *P. aeruginosa* is an opportunistic gram-negative bacterium that is a frequent and deadly pathogen of persons with cystic fibrosis, severe burns, or neutropenia.
- Most cystic fibrosis patients die of pulmonary failure secondary to chronic infection with *P. aeruginosa.*
- *P. aeruginosa* also causes
  - Corneal keratitis in wearers of contact lenses
  - Endocarditis and osteomyelitis in intravenous drug abusers
  - External otitis (swimmer's ear) in normal individuals
  - Malignant external otitis in diabetics
- Distinctive virulence factors of *Pseudomonas* include
  1. Formation of mucoid colonies that are resistant to antilipopolysaccharide antibodies, complement, and phagocytes
  2. Exotoxins A and exoenzyme S that ADP-ribosylate elongation factor 2 and p21^{ras}
  3. Iron-containing compounds that are extremely toxic to endothelial cells and so may cause the vascular lesions characteristic of this bacterium
- *Pseudomonas* pneumonia in the neutropenic host shows necrotizing inflammation with a striking alternation of whitish necrotic and dark red hemorrhagic areas.
- Microscopically, masses of organisms cloud the host tissue with a bluish haze, concentrating in the walls of blood vessels, where host cells undergo coagulation necrosis and nuclei fade away.
- In cystic fibrosis, *Pseudomonas* causes mucous plugging, bronchiectasis, and chronic pulmonary fibrosis.

Legionella pneumophila (Legionnaires' Disease) (p. 377)

- *L. pneumophila* is a gram-negative bacterium identified only by special stains or culture methods.
- *L. pneumophila* causes miniepidemics of severe pneumonia in susceptible individuals exposed to aerosols from cooling systems of buildings.
- *L. pneumophila* is a facultative intracellular parasite of macrophages, in which bacteria fail to induce a respiratory burst and block phagosome fusion with the lysosome.
- *L. pneumophila* produces a multifocal pneumonia of fibrinopurulent type that is initially nodular but may become confluent or lobar.
- A high ratio of mononuclear phagocytes to neutrophils is characteristic, with many destroyed phagocytes at the center of the lesions (leukocytoclasis), surrounded by intact macrophages.

Listeria monocytogenes (p. 378)

- *L. monocytogenes* is a gram-positive, motile facultative intracellular bacterium, which causes severe food-borne infections.
- *L. monocytogenes* causes severe disease in pregnant women, their neonates, and persons immunosuppresed subsequent to organ transplantation or AIDS.
- *L. monocytogenes* has on its surface leucine-rich internalins, which bind to E-cadherin on host epithelial cells and induce phagocytosis of the bacterium.
- *L. monocytogenes* escapes from the phagosome via lysteriolysin O and multiplies in the cytosol.
- *L. monocytogenes* uses ActA proteins on its surface to polymerize host actin and move the bacterium to cell surface filopodia.
- Meningitis caused by *L. monocytogenes* is similar to that caused by other pyogenic bacteria (e.g., *Haemophilus* or *Neisseria*) with numerous neutrophils. The finding of gram-positive, mostly intracellular bacillary rods in the cerebrospinal fluid is virtually diagnostic.

Candidiasis *(Candida albicans, Candida tropicalis)* (p. 378)

- *C. albicans* and *C. tropicalis* are part of the normal flora of the skin, mouth, and gastrointestinal tract but cause disseminated visceral infections in neutropenic patients.
- *C. albicans* and *C. tropicalis* grow best on warm, moist surfaces and so frequently cause vaginitis (particularly during pregnancy), diaper rash, and oral thrush.
- Chronic mucocutaneous candidiasis occurs in the following:
  1. Persons with AIDS
  2. Individuals with inherited or iatrogenic defects in T cell–mediated immunity
  3. Persons with polyendocrine deficiencies (e.g., hypoparathyroidism, hypoadrenalism, and hypothyroidism)
- Virulence factors include surface molecules that bind host cells, a proteinase that degrades host tissues, and released adenosine that blocks neutrophil oxygen radical production.
- The transition from yeast to hyphal form may be another virulence factor.
- *Candida* infections of the oral cavity (thrush) and vagina pro-

duce superficial curdy white patches or large, almost fluffy membranes that are easily detached, revealing a reddened, irritated mucosa.
- Microscopically, lesions contain yeast, hyphae, and pseudohyphae; acute and chronic inflammation; and (sometimes) granulomas.
- Severe, invasive candidiasis in neutropenic persons causes microabscesses in which fungi in the centers of the lesions are surrounded by areas of necrosis.

Cryptococcus neoformans (p. 379)

- *C. neoformans* is a yeast acquired by inhalation that causes meningoencephalitis in AIDS patients and in persons with leukemia, lymphoma, systemic lupus, Hodgkin disease, sarcoidosis, or organ transplants.
- High-dose corticosteroids are a major risk factor for *Cryptococcus* infection.
- *C. neoformans* virulence is associated with its capsular polysaccharide, which is stained bright red with mucicarmine in tissues or negatively stained with India ink in cerebrospinal fluid.
- In normal persons, *C. neoformans* may form a solitary pulmonary granuloma similar to the coin lesions caused by *Histoplasma*.
- In immunosuppressed patients, *Cryptococcus* forms small cysts within the gray matter (soap bubble lesions) as well as a diffuse meningitis with a chronic granulomatous reaction.

Aspergillus fumigatus (p. 380)

- *A. fumigatus* is a ubiquitous mold that causes allergies (brewer's lung) and colonization in otherwise healthy persons and a severe sinusitis and pneumonia in neutropenic persons.
- *Aspergillus* species growing on the surface of peanuts secrete the carcinogen aflatoxin, which may be a major cause of liver cancer in Africa.
- Allergic bronchopulmonary aspergillosis is a hypersensitivity reaction, often in association with asthma.
- Preexisting lesions in the lungs caused by tuberculosis, bronchiectasis, old infarcts, or abscesses may develop brownish colonies of *Aspergillus* (aspergillomas) without invasion of the tissues.
- In debilitated hosts, *Aspergillus* with septate filaments branching at acute angles causes a necrotizing pneumonia with sharply delineated, rounded gray foci with hemorrhagic borders, often referred to as *target lesions*.

Mucormycosis (p. 380)

- Mucormycosis is an opportunistic infection of neutropenic persons and ketoacidotic diabetics, caused by *bread mold fungi*, including *Mucor*, *Absidia*, *Rhizopus*, and *Cunninghamella*.
- The three primary sites of *Mucor* invasion, depending on whether the spores (widespread in dust and air) are inhaled or ingested, are
  1. The nasal sinuses
  2. The lungs
  3. The gastrointestinal tract

- In diabetics, the fungus may spread from nasal sinuses to the orbit and the brain.
- In the lungs, gut, or meninges, phycomycetes, which are non-septate with right-angle branches, cause local tissue necrosis and invade arterial walls.

Pneumocystis carinii (Pneumocystis Pneumonia) (p. 381)

- *P. carinii* is often the first opportunistic infection in HIV-1-infected persons and was the leading cause of death in AIDS until prophylactic antibiotic therapy reduced its frequency and severity.
- *P. carinii* is likely a fungus, based on the following characteristics:

  1. Properties of its cell wall
  2. The paucity of its intracellular organelles
  3. Phylogenetic analysis of its small-subunit ribosomal RNA sequence

- *P. carinii* causes a diffuse and dense pneumonia, in which the alveolar spaces are filled by a foamy, proteinaceous edema fluid, containing 4- to 6-mm-long organisms that stain with silver or Giemsa.
- Frequently, there is concurrent respiratory infection by opportunistic bacteria, fungi, or CMV.

Cryptosporidium parvum and *Cyclospora cayetanensis* (p. 382)

- *C. parvum* is a protozoan parasite, which causes a transient watery diarrhea in normal persons and a chronic and debilitating diarrhea in AIDS patients.
- *C. parvum* oocytes are not killed by chlorine but instead must be removed by filtration through sand, so that epidemics of cryptosporidiosis occur when municipal water filtration systems break down.
- Acid-fast cryptosporidia enter the cytosol of intestinal epithelial cells and cause mixed inflammation of the lamina propria.
- Guatemalan raspberries contaminated with *Cyclospora cayetanensis*, another coccidian parasite, caused diarrhea in 20 states in 1996.

Toxoplasma gondii (Toxoplasmosis) (p. 382)

- *T. gondii* is an obligate intracellular protozoan, which causes a mild lymphadenopathy in normal persons yet produces severe opportunistic infections in the following:
  - Fetuses
  - AIDS patients
  - Persons receiving bone marrow and organ transplants
- *T. gondii* infects persons who ingest oocysts within cat feces or incompletely cooked lamb or pork.
- *T. gondii* penetrates any type of host cell, a unique property of this parasite.
- *T. gondii* travels through the placenta into the fetus and destroys the developing heart, brain, and lung tissues.
- In AIDS patients, *Toxoplasma* frequently cause space-occupying lesions in the central nervous system.

TROPICAL, ZOONOTIC, AND VECTOR-BORNE INFECTIONS (p. 383)

Most of the infectious agents discussed here are common in the tropics and are vector-borne. Other tropical infectious agents are associated with poor living conditions (e.g., *M. leprae*, tapeworm, trichinella, and schistosomes). Arthropod-borne infections of temperate climates include Rocky Mountain Spotted Fever (RMSF), ehrlichiosis, Lyme disease, and babesiosis.

Dengue Fever (Denguevirus) (p. 383)

- Dengue fever is caused by an arthropod-borne virus (Arbovirus), which also includes those viruses that cause Eastern encephalitis and yellow fever.
- Dengue fever is considered an emerging infectious disease because its incidence is increasing in Central America and Mexico, with failure to control its mosquito vector.
- In persons previously exposed to Denguevirus, antiviral antibodies may enhance the uptake of virus into host cells and cause disseminated intravascular coagulation, shock, and death (hemorrhagic dengue).

Rickettsiae (p. 383)

- Rickettsiae are obligate intracellular bacteria that cause epidemic typhus (*R. prowazekii*), scrub typhus (*R. tsutsugamushi*), and spotted fevers (*R. rickettsii* and others) (Table 9–3).
- *Epidemic typhus*, which is transmitted from person to person via body lice, is particularly associated with wars and human suffering, when persons are forced to live in close contact without changing clothes.
- *Scrub typhus*, transmitted by chiggers, was a major problem for U.S. soldiers in the Pacific in World War II and in Vietnam.
- *RMSF* infections, accidentally transmitted to humans by rodent and dog ticks, is actually most frequent in the Southeastern and Southwestern United States.
- *Q fever*, which is caused by the related organism *Coxiella burnetii* that produces pneumonia and fever, is transmitted by aerosols.
- Ehrlichia, which are tick-borne, infect neutrophils or macrophages.
- Rickettsiae predominantly infect host endothelial and vascular smooth muscle cells, causing a widespread vasculitis with perivascular mixed infiltrates, which may be complicated by thrombi and hemorrhages.
- In *typhus fever*, lesions vary from a skin rash to gangrene of the tips of fingers, nose, ear lobes, penis, and vulva.
- In *RMSF*, an eschar at the site of the tick bite is followed by a hemorrhagic rash that extends over the entire body. Other tissues frequently involved include brain, skeletal muscle, lungs, kidneys, testes, and heart.

Trachoma (Chlamydia trachomatis) (p. 385)

- *C. trachomatis* causes a chronic, suppurative eye disease and is a leading global cause of blindness.
- Closely related *C. pneumoniae* and *C. psittaci* cause mild and severe pneumonias.

Table 9-3. RICKETTSIAL DISEASES AND PATHOGENS

Disease	Geography	Agent	Transmission	Distinctive Features
Typhus Group (No Eschar)				
Epidemic typhus	Worldwide (war, famine)	*R. prowazekii*	Louse feces	Endothelial infection; centrifugal type rash
Brill-Zinsser disease	That of epidemic typhus	*R. prowazekii*	Late reactivation	Those of epidemic typhus, but generally milder
Flying squirrel typhus	Southeastern United States	*R. prowazekii*	Fleas, lice of flying squirrel	Similar to epidemic typhus, but mortality is lower
Murine typhus	Worldwide (rat-related)	*R. typhi (mooseri)*	Rat flea feces	Similar to epidemic typhus, but mortality is lower
Spotted Fever Group				
Rocky Mountain spotted fever	North and South America	*R. rickettsii*	Tick bite	Endothelia and vascular smooth muscle infected; rash is centripetal; eschar rarely seen
Boutonneuse fever	Mediterranean, India	*R. conorii*	Tick bite	Prominent eschar, *tache noire*
North Asian and Queensland tick typhus	Russia, China, Australia	*R. sibirica* *R. australia*	Tick bite	Both diseases are typical spotted fevers commonly with eschar
Rickettsial pox	United States, Russia, Korea, Africa	*R. akari*	Mite bite	Prominent eschar; papulovesicular rash (milder than RMSF)
Scrub Typhus				
	East Asia, Pacific	*R. tsutsugamushi*	Chigger bite	Frequent eschar and lymphadenopathy
Q Fever	Worldwide	*Coxiella burnetii*	Droplet inhalation	No eschar or rash; fever, pneumonia, ring granuloma
Ehrlichiosis	Not yet fully known	*Ehrlichia sennetsu, E. canis*	Tick bite	Fever, lymphadenopathy, no eschar or rash

In progressive trachoma, there is a suppurative stage resembling inclusion conjunctivitis, followed by deeper tissue involvement with lymphoplasmacytic infiltrates. When the conjunctiva ulcerates, penetration of the cornea leads to pannus formation, fibroblast overgrowth, scarring, and eventual blindness.

In *C. psittaci* pneumonia (also known as *ornithosis*), alveolar septa show edema and mononuclear infiltrates. Alveolar spaces are filled with mononuclear cells and seroproteinaceous fluid.

Leprosy *(Mycobacterium leprae)* (p. 385)

■ Leprosy is a slowly progressive infection caused by *M. leprae*, which results in unsightly or disabling deformities and peripheral neural sensory deficits.

■ Although *M. leprae* is for the most part contained within the skin and nerves, leprosy is believed to be transmitted from person to person via aerosols from lesions in the upper respiratory tract.

■ *M. leprae* is an acid-fast obligate intracellular organism; it has not been grown in culture but can be grown in the nine-banded armadillo.

■ Leprosy is a bipolar disease, determined by the host cellular immune response:

1. Patients with *tuberculoid leprosy* and a normal immune response form granulomas similar to those seen in tuberculosis that contain epithelioid macrophages, giant cells, and few surviving mycobacteria. The 48-hour lepromin skin test is strongly positive, and damage to the nervous system comes from granulomas in the nerve sheaths.

2. Patients with *lepromatous leprosy* lack T cell–mediated immunity (are anergic to lepromin) and have diffuse nodular lesions containing macrophages stuffed with enormous numbers of mycobacteria, as is seen in disseminated *M. avium* or *M. intracellulare* of AIDS patients. Nodular lesions coalesce to yield a distinctive leonine facies, whereas peripheral nerves are symmetrically invaded with mycobacteria, with minimal inflammation but with loss of sensation.

■ Because leprosy pursues an extremely slow course, spanning decades, most patients die with leprosy rather than of it.

Plague *(Yersinia pestis)* (p. 387)

■ Also called the *Black Death*, plague is caused by *Y. pestis*, a gram-negative facultative intracellular bacterium that is transmitted by flea bites or by aerosols.

■ *Y. pestis* caused three great pandemics that killed an estimated 100 million persons in Egypt and Byzantium in the 6th century; one quarter of Europe's population in the 14th and 15th centuries; and tens of millions in India, Burma, and China at the beginning of the 20th century.

■ *Y. pestis* secretes a protease that activates plasminogen and cleaves complement and is essential for spread of the bacterium from the local site of inoculation into the bloodstream.

■ *Y. pestis* causes lymph node enlargement (bubos), pneumonia, or sepsis, all with
• Dramatic proliferation of the organisms
• Necrosis of tissues and blood vessels
• Neutrophilic infiltrates adjacent to necrotic areas

Relapsing Fever (*Borrelia* Species) (p. 388)

- Relapsing fever is caused by helical *Borrelia* spirochetes, which are transmitted from person to person by body lice (*B. recurrentis*) or from animals to humans by soft ticks (*Borrelia* species, each named for the tick species transmitting them).
- The relapsing fever is caused by successive waves of spirochetes in the blood, each of which contains a single variant surface protein, which is eventually recognized by host antibodies (antigenic variation).
- Antibiotic treatment of *Borrelia* may cause a massive release of endotoxin, resulting in rigors, fall in blood pressure, and leukopenia (the Jarisch-Herxheimer reaction).
- Microscopically the spleen shows focal areas of necrosis with numerous neutrophils and borreliae.

Lyme Disease (*Borrelia burgdorferi*) (p. 388)

- Lyme disease is named for the Connecticut town where in the mid-1970s there was an epidemic of arthritis associated with skin erythema, caused by the spirochete *B. burgdorferi*.
- Lyme disease is transmitted from rodents to humans by tiny, hard deer ticks and is the major arthropod-borne disease presently in the United States.
- Similar to syphilis, Lyme disease has three stages:
  1. An expanding area of redness appears with an indurated or necrotic center at the site of the tick bite (called *erythema chronicum migrans*).
  2. Early hematogenous spread of spirochetes results in secondary annular skin lesions (erythema migrans), lymphadenopathy, migratory joint and muscle pain, cardiac arrhythmias, and meningitis, often with cranial nerve involvement.
  3. Two or 3 years after the initial bite, a chronic arthritis ensues, sometimes with severe damage to large joints and an encephalitis that varies from mild to debilitating. The host immune response, which is out of proportion to the scant number of organisms detectable, may be caused by antibodies to spirochete heat-shock proteins that cross-react with host tissues.
- Skin lesions caused by *B. burgdorferi* contain lymphocytes and plasma cells with local edema.
- In early Lyme arthritis, the synovium resembles that of early rheumatoid arthritis, with villous hypertrophy, lining cell hyperplasia, and abundant lymphocytes and plasma cells in the subsynovium.
- A distinctive feature of Lyme disease is an arteritis with onion skin–like lesions.

Malaria (*Plasmodium* Species) (p. 389)

- In its severest form, malaria is caused by the protozoan parasite *P. falciparum*, which kills 1 to 1.5 million persons per year and so is the major parasitic cause of death.
- *P. vivax* and *P. malariae*, which are also transmitted by Anopheles mosquitoes, cause mild anemia and may cause splenic rupture and nephrotic syndrome.
- *P. falciparum* parasites infect liver cells and then red blood cells, cause severe anemia when red blood cells lyse, and produce cerebral infarcts when infected red blood cells bind to endothelial cells in the central nervous system.

- Genetic resistance to malaria is associated with the ability of HLA-B53 liver cells to present malaria antigens to cytotoxic T cells and the increased rate of splenic clearance of infected red blood cells by individuals with the sickle trait.
- *P. falciparum var* proteins form knobs on infected red blood cells, which show antigenic variation and bind red blood cells to endothelia.
- *P. falciparum* infection initially causes congestion and enlargement of the spleen, whereas in chronic malaria infection, the spleen becomes increasingly fibrotic and brittle.
- Pigmented phagocytic cells may be found dispersed throughout the bone marrow, lymph nodes, subcutaneous tissues, and lungs.
- In malignant cerebral malaria caused by *P. falciparum*, brain vessels are plugged with parasitized red cells, causing ring hemorrhages.

Babesia microti (p. 391)

- *B. microti* is a malaria-like protozoan that is transmitted by the same deer ticks that carry Lyme disease.
- *B. microti* parasitizes red blood cells and causes a mild fever and hemolytic anemia, which is often subclinical except in debilitated or splenectomized individuals, who develop severe or fatal parasitemias.
- In blood smears, *B. microti* resembles *P. falciparum* ring stages, although *B. microti* lacks hemozoin pigment and may form tetrads, which are diagnostic.

Leishmaniasis (*Leishmania* Species) (p. 391)

- Leishmaniasis is a chronic inflammatory disease of
  - The skin (*L. major* and *L. aethiopica* in the Old World and *L. mexicana* and *L. brasiliensis* in the New World)
  - Mucous membranes (*L. brasiliensis*)
  - Viscera (*L. donovani* in the Old World and *L. chagasi* in the New World)
- Leishmaniasis is caused by obligate intracellular, kinetoplastid protozoan parasites, which are transmitted through the bite of infected sandflies.
- *Leishmania* are able to resist acid and proteases in lysosomes of host macrophages.
- Host T cell–mediated responses determine the course of infection.
- In *simple cutaneous leishmaniasis*, an itchy, indurated papule changes into a shallow, slowly expanding ulcer with irregular borders and heals by involution within 6 months without treatment. Microscopically the lesion is granulomatous, usually with foreign body giant cells and few parasites.
- In *diffuse cutaneous leishmaniasis* (rare), the entire body is covered by bizarre nodular lesions, which resemble keloids and contain vast aggregates of foamy macrophages stuffed with *Leishmania*. The patients are anergic to leishmanin and other skin antigens.
- In *mucocutaneous leishmaniasis*, sometimes disfiguring lesions, which contain numerous parasite-containing histiocytes, lymphocytes, and plasma cells, develop at the mucocutaneous junctions of the larynx, nasal septum, anus, or vulva.
- In *visceral leishmaniasis*, parasites invade macrophages throughout the reticuloendothelial system and cause severe sys-

temic disease marked by hepatosplenomegaly, lymphadenopathy, pancytopenia, fever, and weight loss. Often, there is hyperpigmentation of the skin in the extremities, which is why the disease is called *kala-azar (black fever)* in Hindi.

African Trypanosomiasis *(Trypanosoma rhodesiense, Trypanosoma gambiense)*
(p. 393)

- African Trypanosomiasis is caused by kinetoplastid parasites that proliferate as extracellular forms in the blood and cause sustained or intermittent fevers, lymphadenopathy, splenomegaly, progressive brain dysfunction (sleeping sickness), cachexia, and death.
- *T. rhodesiense* infection is often acute and virulent; its tsetse fly vector prefers the savannah plains of East Africa.
- *T. gambiense* infection tends to be chronic and occurs most frequently in the West African bush.
- African trypanosomes are covered by a single, abundant, glycolipid-anchored protein called the *variable surface glycoprotein*, which varies in response to host antibodies.
- Human high-density lipoprotein kills *T. brucei*, which devastate cattle and sheep in East Africa.
- A large, red, rubbery chancre forms at the site of the insect bite, where numerous parasites are surrounded by a dense, largely mononuclear, inflammatory infiltrate.
- With chronicity, the lymph nodes and spleen enlarge as a result of hyperplasia and infiltration by lymphocytes, plasma cells, and macrophages, which are filled with killed parasites.
- In the central nervous system, there is a leptomeningitis extending into the perivascular Virchow-Robin spaces and eventually a demyelinating panencephalitis.

Chagas Disease *(Trypanosoma cruzi)*
(p. 393)

- Caused by a kinetoplastid, intracellular protozoan parasite, *T. cruzi*, Chagas disease is the most frequent cause of heart failure in Brazil and neighboring Latin American countries.
- Chagas disease is transmitted from person to person via *kissing bugs* (triatomids), which hide in the cracks of rickety houses.
- *T. cruzi* resist complement by means of a surface protein homologous to the human complement regulatory protein, decay accelerating factor.
- A protein called *penetrin* on the surface of *T. cruzi* binds the extracellular matrix proteins heparin, heparin sulfate, and collagen and mediates invasion of the parasites into host cells, where parasites escape from the phagolysosome into the cytosol.
- In *acute Chagas disease*, which is mild in most individuals, focal myocardial cell necrosis is accompanied by interstitial inflammatory infiltrates.
- In *chronic Chagas disease*, which occurs in 20% of infected patients 5 to 15 years after initial infection, the heart is typically dilated and contains mural thrombi. There is interstitial and perivascular mononuclear inflammatory infiltrate, which is heaviest in the right bundle branch and causes cardiac arrhythmias. Many patients also have dilation of the esophagus or colon owing to invasion of the myenteric ganglia.

Trichinella spiralis (Trichinosis) (p. 394)

- *T. spiralis* is a nematode parasite that is acquired by ingestion of improperly cooked meat from pigs that have eaten *T. spiralis*-infected rats or pork.
- In the human gut, *T. spiralis* parasites develop into adults that mate and release larvae, which penetrate into the tissues.
- Larvae disseminate hematogenously and penetrate muscle cells, causing
  - Fever, myalgias, and marked eosinophilia (frequently)
  - Periorbital edema, dyspnea (with invasion of the diaphragm), encephalitis (with invasion of the central nervous system), and cardiac failure (rarely).
- *T. spiralis* larvae, approximately 1 mm long and coiled, encyst in striated skeletal muscles (nurse cells), which are surrounded by new blood vessels, lymphoplasmacytic infiltrates, or both.

Hookworm (p. 394)

- Hookworms infect nearly 1 billion persons and cause anemia by consuming 0.2 ml blood per worm per day (*Ancylostoma duodenale*) or 0.02 ml (*Necator americanus*).
- Anemia is aggravated by increased worm burden and by iron deficiency and malnutrition.
- Hookworm virulence factors include secreted anticoagulants, antioxidants, anticholinesterase, and hyaluronidase.

Cysticercosis *(Taenia solium)* and Hydatid Disease (*Echinococcus* Species) (p. 395)

CYSTICERCOSIS

- *T. solium* is a cestode parasite that produces mild abdominal symptoms, caused by a solitary tapeworm in the gut lumen (hence its name) or convulsions, intracranial hypertension, and mental disturbances (cysticercosis caused by 1 to 100 *T. solium* cysts in brain tissues).
- Adult tapeworms result from ingestion of undercooked pork that contains *T. solium* cysticerci.
- *T. solium* tapeworms, which may be many inches long and resemble the beef tapeworm *T. saginatum* (which does not cause cerebral infections), attach to the stomach wall via hooklike scolices and release thousands of eggs in the feces each day.
- Ingested eggs cause cerebral cysticercosis when larvae hatch, penetrate the gut wall, disseminate hematogenously, and encyst in the central nervous system.
- Cerebral *T. solium* cysts rarely exceed 1 cm and have a cyst wall that induces little host inflammatory response.

HYDATID DISEASE

- Hydatid disease is caused by ingestion of tapeworm eggs in dog feces, which hatch in the duodenum and invade into the liver, lungs, or bones.
- Unilocular cysts caused by *E. granulosus*, which also infects sheep, is most common.
- Multilocular cysts caused by *E. multilocularis*, which also infects rodents, or *E. vogeli*, which infects pacas, is less common.
- The cysts begin at microscopic levels and progressively increase

in size, so that in 5 years they may be greater than 10 cm in diameter.

Schistosomiasis (p. 396)

- Schistosomiasis is transmitted by fresh water snails and is the most important helminth disease, infecting approximately 200 million persons and killing approximately 250,000 annually.
- Most of the mortality comes from hepatic granulomas and fibrosis, caused by *Schistosoma mansoni* in Latin America, Africa, and the Middle East and *S. japonicum* and *S. mekongi* in East Asia.
- In Africa, *S. haematobium* causes hematuria and granulomatous disease of the bladder, resulting in chronic obstructive uropathy.
- Female schistosomes produce hundreds of eggs per day, around which granulomas are formed composed of macrophages, lymphocytes, neutrophils, and eosinophils.
- *Schistosoma mansoni* eggs cause liver pathology in three ways:
  1. Substances released from schistosome eggs are directly hepatotoxic.
  2. Carbohydrate antigens in eggs induce macrophage accumulation and granuloma formation, mediated by TNF and TH2 helper cells.
  3. Eggs release factors that stimulate lymphocytes to secrete a fibrogenic lymphokine that stimulates fibroblast proliferation and portal fibrosis.
- In some 10% of heavily infected persons, schistosomes induce an exuberant periportal fibrosis, called *pipe-stem* fibrosis, or Symmer fibrosis.
- In portal triads, vein lumens are obliterated, causing presinusoidal portal hypertension and severe congestive splenomegaly, esophageal varices, and ascites.
- In *S. haematobium* infection, granulomas may cause blood in the urine, stenoses of the ureters, and an increased rate of squamous carcinoma of the bladder.

Elephantiasis *(Wuchereria bancrofti, Brugia malayi)* (p. 397)

- Lymphatic filariasis is transmitted by mosquitoes and is caused by two closely related nematodes, *Wuchereria bancrofti* and *Brugia malayi.*
- Filariasis causes a spectrum of diseases including
  1. Asymptomatic microfilaremia
  2. Chronic lymphadenitis with swelling of the dependent limb or scrotum (elephantiasis)
  3. Tropical pulmonary eosinophilia
- In microfilaremic individuals who appear healthy, there is a hypoimmune response to circulating parasites.
- In chronic lymphatic filariasis, there is no filaremia but instead a persistent lymphedema of the scrotum, penis, vulva, leg, or arm.
- Hyperkeratotic and fibrotic elephantoid skin overlies dilated lymphatics that contain adult filarial worms surrounded by eosinophils, hemorrhage, and fibrin or granulomas.
- In tropical pulmonary eosinophilia, there is an IgE-mediated hypersensitivity to microfilariae in which dead microfilariae are surrounded by stellate, hyaline eosinophilic precipitates embed-

ded in small epithelioid granulomas (Meyers-Kouvenaar bodies).

River Blindness *(Onchocerca volvulus)*
(p. 398)

- River blindness is a major cause of blindness in equatorial Africa, caused by *O. volvulus*, a filarial nematode transmitted by blackflies.
- River blindness is being dramatically reduced in West Africa by the aggressive distribution of the antihelminth drug ivermectin.
- Adult parasites mate in the dermis, where they are surrounded by a mixed infiltrate of host cells that produces a characteristic subcutaneous nodule (onchocercomata).
- The major pathology, which includes blindness and chronic pruritic dermatitis, is caused by large numbers of microfilariae, released by females, that accumulate in the skin and in the eye chambers.
- *Leopard* skin shows foci of epidermal atrophy and elastic fiber breakdown alternating with areas of hyperkeratosis, hyperpigmentation with pigment incontinence, dermal atrophy, and fibrosis.
- Degenerating microfilaria and a surrounding eosinophilic infiltrate cause blindness by means of a sclerosing keratitis, which may opacify the cornea and cause choroid and retinal atrophy.

Environmental and Nutritional Pathology

HUMANS AND THE ENVIRONMENT (p. 403)

Environmental and occupational health encompasses the diagnosis, treatment, and prevention of injuries and illnesses resulting from exposure to exogenous chemical or physical agents. Such exposure may occur in the workplace or as a result of personal habits, such as drug or alcohol abuse or cigarette smoking. These destructive habits may involuntarily expose fetuses and children to these adverse influences. There is also substantial concern about the potential chronic effects of exposure to low levels of contaminants in air, water, and food.

Recognition of Occupational and Environmental Diseases (p. 404)

The magnitude of adverse health effects caused by occupational and environmental diseases is enormous. Accidents, illness, and premature deaths caused by occupational exposures affect 120 million workers in the United States. The annual number of fatal workplace injuries is about 10,000. The incidence of nonfatal injuries is highest among construction workers followed by workers in agriculture, forestry, fishing, and manufacturing. In addition to injuries, occupational exposures contribute to a wide range of common causes of death (Table 10–1).

The risk of environmental exposure to chemicals is also substantial. Estimates suggest that more than 60,000 chemicals are currently used in the United States; about 1500 are pesticides and 5500 are food additives that affect water and food supplies. Some of these chemicals produce cancer in rodents. Industrial chemicals and metals are common at hazardous waste sites. It is estimated that 4 million people live within 1 mile of 785 heavily contaminated sites that are slated for clean-up *(Superfund sites)*. Physicians in these locales should be familiar with the evidence (or lack of it) relating these potential hazards to the causation of disease.

Mechanisms of Toxicity (p. 404)

Toxicology is the scientific discipline that studies the detection, effects, and mechanisms of action of poisons and toxic chemicals. Toxicity is a relative phenomenon that depends on the dose and

Table 10–1. ESTIMATED OCCUPATIONAL DISEASE
MORTALITY IN THE UNITED STATES
IN 1992

Cause of Death	No. of Deaths	Percentage Attributed to Occupation
Cancer	517,090	6–10
Cardiovascular and cerebrovascular disease	101,846	5–10
Chronic respiratory disease	91,541	10
Pneumoconioses	1136	100
Nervous system disease	26,936	1–3
Renal disease	22,957	1–3

From Leigh JP, et al: Occupational injury and illness in the United States: Estimates
of cost, morbidity, and mortality. Arch Intern Med 157:1557, 1997.

the inherent chemical properties of a chemical. Dose-response
curves are usually produced in laboratory animals exposed to
various amounts of a test substance. From these curves, several
key points about chemical toxicity can be obtained:

- *Threshold dose* is the amount of chemical producing a measurable response.
- *No observed effect level* is a dose lower than the threshold dose.
- *Ceiling effect* is a plateau that is reached at which the response is not increased.

From this information, it is possible to establish the *daily (or
annual) threshold limit* for the permissible level for occupational
exposures.

Several important toxicologic principles have been established
(Fig. 10–1):

- Exogenous chemicals are absorbed after ingestion, inhalation, or skin contact, then distributed to various organs.
- Chemicals are metabolized to products that may be more or less toxic than the parent chemical. These products then interact with a target molecule resulting in a toxic effect.
- The site of toxicity is where metabolism or excretion of toxic metabolites occurs.
- The dose administered (external dose) may not be the same as the biologic effective dose delivered to the target organ and target macromolecule.

The basic principles of xenobiotic metabolism include the following (Fig. 10–2):

- Most xenobiotics are *lipophilic*, which facilitates transport in the bloodstream and penetration of membranes.
- Lipophilic toxicants are metabolized to hydrophilic metabolites by two steps:
  1. In *phase I reactions*, a polar functional group is added to the parent compound.
  2. In *phase II reactions*, conjugation products are produced with endogenous substances that are more soluble and more readily excreted.
- *There are genetic variations in the level of activity of these xenobiotic-metabolizing enzymes*, such as the cytochrome P-

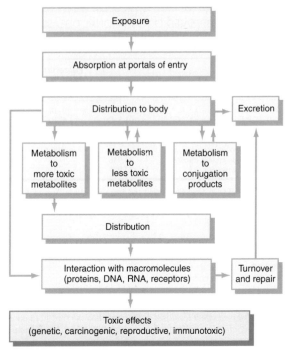

Figure 10-1 ∎

Absorption and distribution of toxicants. (From Hodgson E, Levi PE: Absorption and distribution of toxicants. In Hodgson E, Levi PE [eds]): A Textbook of Modern Toxicology. Stamford, CT, Appleton & Lange, 1997, p 52.)

450–dependent monooxygenase system (P-450). These enzymes detoxify endogenous products as well as activate xenobiotics to reactive intermediates and carcinogens. People who have inherited alleles of the P-450 gene that confer higher activity are at increased risk of developing lung cancer.

- Multiple pathways may be involved in metabolism of a chemical toxicant. Predominance of one pathway over another may account for differences in toxicity and carcinogenicity.
- Endogenous factors, such as nutritional and hormonal status, alter enzyme activities involved in xenobiotic metabolism.
- Exogenous factors, such as drugs or ethanol, can increase or inhibit activities of xenobiotic metabolizing enzymes.
- Repair pathways may modify the interaction between the active metabolite and the target molecule.

Phase I reactions are mediated by the following:

- A *cytochrome P-450–dependent monooxygenase system* located in the smooth endoplasmic reticulum. It is composed of a complex containing a heme protein (P-450), NADPH-P-450 reductase, and phosphatidylcholine. The activity of this system is greatest in the liver. Different P-450 isozymes have specific tissue distributions and show preferential activity toward differ-

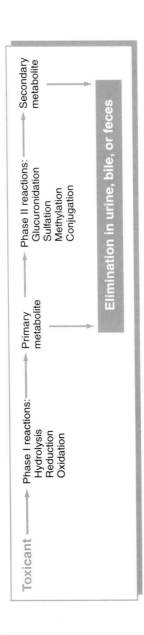

Figure 10–2

Biotransformation of lipophilic toxicants to hydrophilic metabolites. (Adapted from Hodgson E: Metabolism of toxicants. In Hodgson E, Levi PE [eds]: A Textbook of Modern Toxicology, Stamford, CT, Appleton & Lange, 1997, p. 57.)

ent substrates. Notable among the broad range of substrates metabolized by this system is benzo[a]pyrene, which is converted to a secondary metabolite that binds covalently to DNA and causes lung and skin tumors. Benzo[a]pyrene is one of several chemical carcinogens present in cigarette smoke.

- A *flavin-containing monooxygenase system* also located in the smooth endoplasmic reticulum in the liver. It oxidizes nicotine in cigarette smoke as well as other amines.
- *Peroxidase-dependent co-oxidation*, conjugated by prostaglandin H synthase, which is found in the smooth endoplasmic reticulum in seminal vesicles, kidneys, and the urinary bladder. It metabolizes 2-naphthylamine, a chemical found in dyes associated with bladder cancer.

All of these oxidative reactions generate oxygen free radicals as byproducts. Reduced glutathione is a major defense mechanism against oxygen free radicals and toxic metabolites of xenobiotics. The products of phase I reactions are often conjugated with endogenous substrates to yield water-soluble end products that can be excreted from the body.

Phase II reactions include the following:

- *Glucuronidation*: An alternative pathway for metabolism of naphthylamine is oxidation by cytochrome P-450 followed by glucuronidation in the liver. The secondary glucuronide is excreted in the urine, where it can form a carcinogen. This sequence of reactions leads to the increased incidence of cancer of the urinary bladder in workers exposed to synthetic dyes.
- *Biomethylation*: Occupational exposure to inorganic mercury ($HgCl_2$) occurs during the manufacture of germicides, fungicides, electronics, and plastics. Inorganic mercury causes necrosis of the proximal convoluted tubule. Mercury can be methylated by aquatic microorganisms that are subsequently ingested by herbivorous fish, which, in turn, are consumed by carnivorous fish, which may be eaten by humans. This is an example of *bioaccumulation* of a toxic chemical in the environment. Industrial discharge of mercury into a bay in Minamato, Japan, resulted in bioaccumulation of this toxicant a millionfold in fish. Individuals who ingested these fish developed paralysis and subsequently died. Methyl mercury is readily absorbed from the gastrointestinal tract. Dimethyl mercury is even more toxic; it can be absorbed via the skin or inhaled and can lead to severe neurotoxicity.
- *Glutathione conjugation*: A common pathway for detoxification of primary metabolites is conjugation to reduced glutathione. These water-soluble metabolites are readily excreted in the bile and urine.

COMMON ENVIRONMENTAL AND OCCUPATIONAL EXPOSURES (p. 408)

Personal Exposures (p. 408)

TOBACCO USE

Use of tobacco products, including cigarettes, cigars, pipes, and snuff, is associated with more mortality and morbidity than any other personal, environmental, or occupational exposure.

- Tobacco use is estimated to contribute to 390,000 deaths per year in the United States and is associated with 10 million cases of chronic diseases.

- Smoking is a major risk factor for lung cancer and can interact with other environmental and occupational exposures in an additive or synergistic fashion.
- Cigarette smoke consists of a particulate phase and a gas phase. There are more than 4000 constituents, including 43 known carcinogens, in tobacco smoke. These include
  - *Chemical carcinogens* and *carcinogenic metals* (e.g., arsenic, nickel, cadmium)
  - *Promoters* (e.g., acetaldehyde)
  - *Irritants* (e.g., nitrogen dioxide)
  - *Cilia toxins* (e.g., hydrogen cyanide)
  - *Carbon monoxide*, which binds to hemoglobin with high affinity and decreases the delivery of oxygen to the peripheral tissues
- Cigarette smoke contains nicotine, an alkaloid that readily crosses the blood-brain barrier and stimulates nicotine receptors in the brain. It is responsible for tobacco addiction.
- The inhaled agents in cigarette smoke may act directly on the mucous membranes, may be swallowed in saliva, or may be absorbed into the bloodstream from the alveolar capillary bed. They may act on distant target organs and cause a variety of systemic diseases, including *lung cancer, ischemic heart disease*, and *chronic obstructive pulmonary disease*. Cigarette smoking is a multiplicative risk factor for the development of coronary artery disease and atherosclerosis. Cessation of smoking reduces but does not eliminate the risk of lung cancer as well as coronary artery disease.
- The fetus is especially vulnerable to the consequences of maternal smoking: As few as 10 cigarettes per day can cause fetal hypoxia, resulting in low birth weight, prematurity, increased incidence of spontaneous abortion, and complications at the time of delivery.
- Cigarette smoking may facilitate transport of other hazardous agents to the lungs and exacerbate bronchitis, asthma, and pneumoconiosis associated with particulates such as silica or coal dust.
- Tobacco use also increases the prevalence of peptic ulcers, impairs their healing, and increases the likelihood of recurrences.
- There are risks associated with exposure to sidestream smoke (*second-hand* smoke), also called *passive smoking* or *environmental tobacco smoke*. Reports from the National Research Council and the Surgeon General concluded that passive smoking increases the risk of lung cancer, ischemic heart disease, and acute myocardial infarction. Maternal smoking increases the risk of sudden infant death syndrome, and young children in households with smokers suffer from an increased incidence of respiratory and ear infections and exacerbations of asthma.

"It's time we made smoking history," a slogan of the public health agencies in the United States, has a great deal of merit.

ALCOHOL (ETHANOL) ABUSE

Ethanol is the most widely used and abused agent throughout the world.

- There are 15 to 20 million alcoholics in the United States, and approximately 100,000 deaths in the United States are attributed to alcohol abuse per year.

- A blood alcohol concentration of 100 mg/dl is the legal definition for drunk driving in many states. The effects of drinking depend on the amount of ethanol consumed per unit of body weight and the time period in which the ethanol is ingested. Approximately 12 oz (340 ml) of beer, 4 oz (115 ml) of nonfortified wine and 1.5 oz (43 ml) of an 86 proof beverage each contain approximately 10 g of ethanol.
- Chronic alcohol use results in psychological and physical dependence. The biologic basis for ethanol addiction is unknown, although genetic factors may be involved.
- Ethanol is metabolized by alcohol dehydrogenase in the gastric mucosa and liver and by cytochrome P-450 and catalase in the liver, yielding acetaldehyde, which, in turn, is converted to acetic acid by aldehyde dehydrogenase. There are genetic polymorphisms in aldehyde dehydrogenase that slow ethanol metabolism, encountered in about 50% of Chinese, Vietnamese, and Japanese people.

The metabolism of ethanol is directly responsible for most of its toxic and chronic effects (Table 10–2).

- *Liver*: Ethanol can causes *fatty change*, *acute alcoholic hepatitis*, and *cirrhosis* (Chapter 19). Fatty change is an acute but reversible accumulation of fat in hepatocytes. In chronic alcoholism, it can cause massive enlargement of the liver. Alcoholic hepatitis can produce fever, liver tenderness, and jaundice because of a direct toxic effect of ethanol. With chronic ethanol use, 10 to 15% of alcoholics develop irreversible liver damage or alcoholic cirrhosis. This condition is characterized by a hard, shrunken liver with formation of micronodules of regenerating hepatocytes surrounded by dense bands of collagen.
- *Nervous system*: The acute depressive effects and addiction pro-

Table 10–2. MECHANISMS OF DISEASE CAUSED BY ETHANOL ABUSE

Organ System	Lesion	Mechanism
Liver	Fatty change	Toxicity
	Acute hepatitis	
	Alcoholic cirrhosis	
Nervous system	Wernicke syndrome	Thiamine deficiency
	Korsakoff syndrome	Toxicity and thiamine deficiency
	Cerebellar degeneration	Nutritional deficiency
	Peripheral neuropathy	Thiamine deficiency
Cardiovascular system	Cardiomyopathy	Toxicity
	Hypertension	Vasopressor
Gastrointestinal tract	Gastritis	Toxicity
	Pancreatitis	Toxicity
Skeletal muscle	Rhabdomyolysis	Toxicity
Reproductive system	Testicular atrophy	?
	Spontaneous abortion	?
Fetal alcohol syndrome	Growth retardation	Toxicity
	Mental retardation	
	Birth defects	

From Rubin E: Alcohol abuse. In Craighead JE [ed]: Pathology of Environmental and Occupational Disease. St. Louis, Mosby–Year Book, p. 249; and Lewis DD, Woods SE: Fetal alcohol syndrome. Am Fam Physician 50:1025, 1994.

duced by ethanol are believed to be related to changes in membrane fluidity and altered signal transduction. Chronic thiamine deficiency, common in chronic alcoholics, contributes to degeneration of nerve cells, reactive gliosis, and atrophy of the cerebellum and peripheral nerves. It produces the ataxia, disturbed cognition, ophthalmoplegia, and nystagmus characteristic of *Wernicke syndrome*. Some alcoholics with poor nutrition develop severe memory loss characteristic of *Korsakoff syndrome*.

- *Cardiovascular system*: Chronic ethanol abuse can cause a cardiomyopathy resulting in dilation of the heart.
- *Gastrointestinal tract*: Acute gastritis is a direct toxic effect of ethanol use.
- *Skeletal muscle*: Direct ethanol toxicity can also injure skeletal muscles leading to muscle weakness and pain.
- *Reproductive system*: Ethanol abuse leads to testicular atrophy in men and decreased fertility in both men and women.
- *Fetal alcohol syndrome*: A devastating consequence of as little as one maternal drink per day is the fetal alcohol syndrome. First recognized in 1968, this syndrome is characterized by growth and developmental defects, including microcephaly; facial dysmorphology; and malformations of the brain, cardiovascular system, and genitourinary system. Fetal alcohol syndrome is the most common type of preventable mental retardation in the United States, affecting 1200 children per year.
- *Ethanol and cancer*: Use of alcoholic beverages is associated with increased incidence of cancer of the oral cavity, pharynx, esophagus, liver, and possibly breast. Although ethanol is not a direct-acting carcinogen, one of its metabolites, acetaldehyde, may act as a tumor promoter. Additionally, ethanol may induce the P-450 enzyme complex and enhance metabolic activation of other carcinogens.

Methanol and ethylene glycol may be ingested accidentally or as inexpensive substitutes for ethanol. They are metabolized by alcohol dehydrogenase more slowly than ethanol, resulting in initial symptoms of intoxication, followed by possible blindness and kidney toxicity.

DRUG ABUSE

Drug abuse, addiction, and overdose are serious public health problems. Commonly abused drugs can be classified as central nervous system depressants, stimulants, narcotics, or hallucinogens.

- *Central nervous system depressants*: Ethanol is the most widely abused central nervous system depressant. Barbiturates are circulated illegally and are known as *downers*. Both types of drugs induce sedation and decrease anxiety. Tolerance develops rapidly, causing drug users to increase the dose.
- *Central nervous system stimulants*: *Cocaine* abuse is a serious public health problem. Cocaine produces a rapid *high* of short duration characterized by euphoria and increased energy. It inhibits the reuptake of neurotransmitters dopamine and norepinephrine in the central and peripheral nervous systems, resulting in excess catecholamine stimulation. Acute cocaine overdose produces seizures, cardiac arrhythmias, and respiratory arrest. Chronic abuse causes insomnia, increased anxiety, paranoia, and hallucinations. Chronic use of cocaine is associated with hypertension, strokes, and sudden death. *Amphetamines* are also potent central nervous system stimulants. Overdose causes

sweating, tremors, restlessness, and confusion that may progress to delirium, convulsions, coma, and death.

■ *Narcotics*: These drugs are prescribed to relieve pain, but they also cause sedation and altered mood. Intravenous heroin abuse induces suppression of anxiety, sedation, mood changes, nausea, and respiratory depression. Chronic abuse induces tolerance as well as psychological dependence. Overdose can cause convulsions, cardiorespiratory arrest, and death. Intravenous drug users are susceptible to *infections* of the skin and subcutaneous tissue; heart valves, particularly the tricuspid valve; liver; and lungs. Most cases are caused by staphylococci. Viral hepatitis and acquired immunodeficiency syndrome (AIDS) are common among drug addicts and are acquired by sharing contaminated needles.

■ *Hallucinogens*: Both natural and chemical substances have hallucinogenic properties. Among the natural hallucinogens are the alkaloid mescaline, which can be isolated from the peyote cactus, and marijuana, isolated from the hemp plant *Cannabis sativa*. The active ingredient in marijuana is tetrahydrocannabinol, which produces a state of relaxation and heightened sensation. Notable among the chemical hallucinogens are phencyclidine (PCP), which causes inebriation, disorientation, and numbness, and lysergic acid diethylamide (LSD), which is absorbed rapidly and causes psychic effects and visual illusions.

Therapeutic Drugs (p. 414)

Adverse drug reactions occur frequently and refer to untoward effects of drugs that are given in conventional therapeutic settings (Table 10–3). Several widely used drugs are discussed in more detail.

EXOGENOUS ESTROGENS AND ORAL CONTRACEPTIVES

Estrogens and oral contraceptives are discussed separately because

1. Estrogens for postmenopausal syndrome may be given alone and are usually natural estrogens.
2. Oral contraceptives contain synthetic estrogens, which are always given with progesterone.

Exogenous Estrogens

Estrogen therapy is currently used widely in postmenopausal women to prevent or slow the progression of osteoporosis (Chapter 28). Exogenous estrogen therapy is associated with the following adverse effects:

■ *Endometrial carcinoma*: Unopposed estrogen therapy increases the risk of endometrial cancer 3-fold to 6-fold after 5 years and more than 10-fold after 10 years, compared with the risk of untreated women. This risk is substantially reduced when progestins are added to the therapeutic regimen.
■ *Breast carcinoma*: Although controversial, the bulk of evidence suggests that the increased risk of breast carcinoma is small, if any, and is not influenced by the addition of progestins (Chapter 25).
■ *Thromboembolism*: Estrogen therapy does not increase the risk of thromboembolism.
■ *Cardiovascular disease*: Myocardial infarction and stroke are among the leading causes of death in postmenopausal women.

Table 10-3. SOME COMMON ADVERSE DRUG REACTIONS AND THEIR AGENTS

Reaction	Major Offenders
Blood dyscrasias (feature of almost half of all drug-related deaths)	
Granulocytopenia, aplastic anemia, pancytopenia	Antineoplastic agents, immunosuppressives, and chloramphenicol
Hemolytic anemia, thrombocytopenia	Penicillin, methyldopa, quinidine
Cutaneous	
Urticaria, macules, papules, vesicles, petechiae, exfoliative dermatitis, fixed drug eruptions	Antineoplastic agents, sulfonamides, hydantoins, many others
Cardiac	
Arrhythmias	Theophylline, hydantoins
Cardiomyopathy	Doxorubicin, daunorubicin
Renal	
Glomerulonephritis	Penicillamine
Acute tubular necrosis	Aminoglycoside antibiotics, cyclosporine, amphotericin B
Tubulointerstitial disease with papillary necrosis	Phenacetin, salicylates
Pulmonary	
Asthma	Salicylates
Acute pneumonitis	Nitrofurantoin
Interstitial fibrosis	Busulfan, nitrofurantoin, bleomycin
Hepatic	
Fatty change	Tetracycline
Diffuse hepatocellular damage	Halothane, isoniazid, acetaminophen
Cholestasis	Chlorpromazine, estrogens, contraceptive agents
Systemic	
Anaphylaxis	Penicillin
Lupus erythematosus syndrome (drug-induced lupus)	Hydralazine, procainamide
Central nervous system	
Tinnitus and dizziness	Salicylates
Acute dystonic reactions and parkinsonian syndrome	Phenothiazine antipsychotics
Respiratory depression	Sedatives

Estrogens elevate the level of high-density lipoproteins (HDL) and reduce the level of low-density lipoproteins (LDL). This lipid profile is protective against the development of atherosclerosis. Epidemiologic studies have shown a 40 to 50% decrease in the risk of ischemic heart disease in women who received postmenopausal estrogen therapy. The addition of sequential progestins, which tend to counter the estrogen effect on the lipid profile, does not alter the benefit of estrogen therapy.

Oral Contraceptives

Oral contraceptives usually contain a synthetic estradiol and variable amounts of a progestin (combined oral contraceptives). Currently prescribed oral contraceptives contain smaller amounts of estrogens and are associated with fewer side effects.

■ *Breast carcinoma*: There may be a slight increase in breast cancer risk when combined oral contraceptives are used by younger women, particularly nulliparous women less than 25 years old. A multiplicative effect may be caused by cigarette smoking.

- *Endometrial cancer*: There is no increased risk of endometrial cancer, and these drugs probably exert a protective effect.
- *Cervical cancer*: Although there may be some increased risk of cervical cancer, it could be correlated with life style rather than the drugs.
- *Ovarian cancer*: Oral contraceptives protect against ovarian cancer.
- *Thromboembolism*: Earlier formulations with high estrogen levels were clearly associated with an increased risk of thromboembolism because of increased hepatic synthesis of coagulation factors. Second-generation drugs with lower estrogen levels suggest that the overall risk is much less. Third-generation contraceptives, which combine low-dose estrogens with synthetic progestins, confer a higher risk of venous thrombosis.
- *Hypertension*: The new formulations cause a slight increase in blood pressure.
- *Cardiovascular disease*: There is some uncertainty regarding the risk of atherosclerosis and myocardial infarction. Evidence suggests that nonsmoking, healthy women younger than 45 years of age who use the newer low-estrogen formulations do not incur an increased risk of ischemic heart disease.
- *Hepatic adenoma*: There is a well-defined association between the use of oral contraceptives and this benign tumor.

The various pros and cons of oral contraceptives must be balanced against the risk of an unwanted pregnancy.

ACETAMINOPHEN

Acetaminophen is a commonly used nonprescription analgesic and antipyretic. When taken in large doses, it causes hepatic necrosis and liver failure.

ASPIRIN (ACETYLSALICYLIC ACID)

Aspirin overdoses occur from accidental ingestion by young children and in suicide attempts by adults. The initial consequences of an overdose are respiratory alkalosis, followed by metabolic acidosis that can prove fatal before anatomic changes occur. *Chronic aspirin toxicity (salicylism)* may develop in persons who take 3 gm or more daily, for long periods of time, for chronic inflammatory conditions. Aspirin toxicity is manifested by headache, dizziness, ringing in the ears (tinnitus), difficulty in hearing, mental confusion, drowsiness, nausea, vomiting, and diarrhea. More serious is the development of acute erosive gastritis. Proprietary analgesic mixtures containing aspirin and phenacetin when taken for years have been associated with potentially fatal renal papillary necrosis *(analgesic nephropathy)*.

Outdoor Air Pollution (p. 416)

Air pollution is a serious problem in the United States and in most other industrial countries. Epidemiologic research as well as clinical and toxicologic studies provides evidence for adverse health effects of air pollutants. The major sources of air pollution are from

- Combustion of fossil fuels in motor vehicles and industry
- Photochemical reactions
- Power plant emissions

The lungs are the major target of common outdoor air pollution. Especially vulnerable are children and people with chronic lung and heart disease. Some of the major air pollutants and their adverse health effects are as follows (Table 10–4):

- *Ozone*: Ozone is a major component of smog. Exposure to as little as 0.08 ppm produces cough, chest discomfort, and inflammation in the lungs. Ozone is highly reactive and oxidizes polyunsaturated lipids to hydrogen peroxide and lipid aldehydes, which act as irritants and induce the release of inflammatory mediators.
- *Nitrogen dioxide*: Nitrogen dioxide is less reactive than ozone. It dissolves in water in the airways to form acids that damage the airway lining.
- *Sulfur dioxide*: Sulfur dioxide is absorbed in the airways where it releases products that cause local irritation.
- *Acid aerosols*: Combustion products of fossil fuels are released into the atmosphere, where the sulfur and nitrogen dioxide are oxidized to sulfuric acid and nitric acid. These products are dissolved in water droplets or absorbed onto particulates and become irritants to the airway epithelium.
- *Particulates*: The deposition and clearance of inhaled particulates depend on their size and shape (Chapter 16). Although it is unclear which characteristics of the heterogeneous ambient particles contribute to their adverse health effects, it is suspected that these effects may be related to free radical generation at the surface of fine particles.

The growing numbers and activities of humans have resulted in serious air pollution. A layer of *ozone in the upper atmosphere* is critically important for human survival because it prevents the sun's ultraviolet (UV) light from penetrating the environment. A large number of chemicals used by humans destroy ozone. The major offenders are chlorofluorocarbons (CFCs) used as aerosols and refrigerants, and nitrogen dioxide, produced by internal combustion engines. The consequences of the depletion of the ozone layer include an increased incidence of skin cancers in humans and damaging effects on other life forms. A closely related problem is global warming. The accumulation of carbon dioxide and other gases in the atmosphere traps the earth's infrared radiation while permitting free penetrance of visible light and warming solar radiation. The net effect is the accumulation of heat at the earth's surface or the *greenhouse* phenomenon. The interrelated problems of ozone loss and global warming are paradigms of environmental problems that constitute clear and present threats.

Indoor Air Pollution (p. 418)

Levels of indoor air pollutants have increased during the last 20 years because of increased insulation and decreased ventilation in homes. The major categories of these pollutants and their health effects are cited in Table 10–5.

- *Carbon monoxide* is an odorless, colorless gas that is a byproduct of combustion produced by burning gasoline, oil, coal, wood, and natural gas. Carbon monoxide levels in ambient air should not exceed 9 ppm. Poisoning is manifested as headaches, dizziness, loss of motor control, and coma.
- *Nitrogen dioxide* is produced by gas stoves and kerosene heaters and impairs lung defenses.
- *Wood smoke* is a complex mixture of particulates and other

Table 10–4. HEALTH EFFECTS OF OUTDOOR AIR POLLUTANTS

Pollutant	Populations at Risk	Effects
Ozone	Healthy adults and children	Decreased lung function
		Increased airway reactivity
		Lung inflammation
	Athletes, outdoor workers	Decreased exercise capacity
	Asthmatics	Increased hospitalizations
Nitrogen dioxide	Healthy adults	Increased airway reactivity
	Asthmatics	Decreased lung function
	Children	Increased respiratory infection
Sulfur dioxide	Healthy adults	Increased respiratory symptoms
	Patients with chronic lung disease	Increased mortality
		Increased hospitalization
	Asthmatics	Decreased lung function
Acid aerosols	Healthy adults	Altered mucociliary clearance
	Children	Increased respiratory infections
	Asthmatics	Decreased lung function
		Increased hospitalizations
Particulates	Children	Increased respiratory infections
		Decreased lung function
	Patients with chronic lung or heart disease	Excess mortality
	Asthmatics	Increased attacks

From Bascom R, et al: Health effects of outdoor air pollution. Am J Respir Crit Care Med 153:3, 1996.

Table 10-5. HEALTH EFFECTS OF INDOOR AIR POLLUTANTS

Pollutant	Populations at Risk	Effects
Carbon monoxide	Adults and children	Acute poisoning
Nitrogen dioxide	Children	Increased respiratory infections
Wood smoke	Children	Increased respiratory infections
Formaldehyde	Adults and children	Eye and nose irritation
Radon	Adults and children	Lung cancer
Asbestos fibers	Maintenance and abatement workers	Lung cancer; mesothelioma
Man-made mineral fibers	Maintenance and construction workers	Skin and airway irritation
Bioaerosols	Adults and children	Allergic rhinitis, asthma

From Bascom R, et al: Health effects of outdoor air pollution. Am J Respir Crit Care Med 153:3, 477, 1996.

toxic components that can increase the incidence of respiratory infections, especially in children.

- *Formaldehyde* is a soluble, volatile chemical used in the manufacture of many consumer products that can cause acute irritation of the eyes and upper respiratory tract.
- *Radon* is a radioactive gas that is a decay product of uranium widely distributed in the soil. Radon gas emanating from the earth is prevalent in some mines and homes and may be a cause of lung cancer.
- *Asbestos fibers* were used in homes and public buildings before the 1970s, and low levels of fibers have been found in indoor air. Workers who repair or remove asbestos-containing materials are at risk for lung cancer and mesothelioma if they do not use respirators.
- *Manufactured mineral fibers*, such as fiberglass, have been used as an asbestos substitute for home insulation and can cause skin and lung irritation.
- *Bioaerosols*, such as aerosolization of bacteria responsible for *Legionella* pneumonia, has been associated with contaminated heating and cooling systems in public buildings (Chapter 9).

Industrial Exposures (p. 419)

Occupational exposures contribute to diseases that can affect almost all organ systems and result in acute toxicity, hypersensitivity reactions, chronic toxicity, and cancer (Table 10–6).

- *Volatile organic compounds* are used in industry and in homes. High levels of exposure cause headaches, dizziness, and liver or kidney toxicity. These agents include *aliphatic hydrocarbons*, such as chloroform and carbon tetrachloride, which are widely used industrial solvents and cleaning agents. All of these compounds are readily absorbed through the lungs, skin, and gastrointestinal tract. In addition to acute central nervous system depression, they can cause liver and kidney toxicity. *Petroleum products*, such as gasoline and kerosene, are quite volatile and are a common cause of poisoning in children. When accidentally swallowed by children, they produce a violent pneumonitis. Inhalation of these products causes dizziness, incoordination, and central nervous system depression. *Aromatic hydrocarbons*, such as benzene and toluene, are widely used solvents that are hazardous when inhaled. For example, benzene causes bone marrow toxicity, aplastic anemia, and acute leukemia.
- *Polycyclic aromatic hydrocarbons* (three or more fused benzene rings) are produced by combustion of fossil fuels and by iron and steel foundries. Benzo[a]pyrene is the prototype of this class of compounds, which is metabolized to reactive intermediates capable of binding DNA. Occupational exposure is associated with an increased risk of lung and bladder cancers. Cigarette smoking is another important source of benzo[a]pyrene.
- *Plastics*, *rubber*, and *polymers*: Occupational exposure to vinyl chloride monomers used to produce polyvinyl chloride resins is associated with angiosarcoma of the liver.
- *Metals*: Occupational exposure to metals in mining and manufacturing is associated with acute and chronic toxicity as well as carcinogenicity. These associations are summarized in Table 10–7. Although exposure to cobalt, cadmium, chromium, and nickel may present significant occupational hazards, exposure

Table 10-6. HUMAN DISEASES ASSOCIATED WITH OCCUPATIONAL EXPOSURES

Organ	Effect	Toxicant
Cardiovascular system	Heart disease	Carbon monoxide, lead, solvents, cobalt, cadmium
Pulmonary system	Lung cancer	Radon, asbestos, silica, bis-chloromethyl ether, nickel, arsenic, chromium, mustard gas
	Chronic obstructive lung disease	Grain dust, coal dust, cadmium
	Hypersensitivity	Beryllium, isocyanates
	Irritation	Ammonia, sulfur oxides, formaldehyde
	Fibrosis	Silica, asbestos, cobalt
Nervous system	Nasal cancer	Isopropyl alcohol, wood dust
	Peripheral neuropathies	Solvents, acrylamide, methyl chloride, mercury, lead, arsenic, DDT
	Ataxic gait	Chlordane, toluene, acrylamide, mercury
	Central nervous system depression	Alcohols, ketones, aldehydes, solvents
	Cataracts	Ultraviolet radiation
Renal system	Toxicity	Mercury, lead, glycol ethers, solvents
	Bladder cancer	Naphthylamines, 4-aminobiphenyl, benzidine, rubber products
Reproductive system	Male infertility	Lead, phthalate plasticizers
	Female infertility	Cadmium, lead
	Teratogenesis	Mercury, PCBs
Reticuloendothelial system	Leukemia	Benzene, radon, uranium
Skin	Folliculitis and acneiform dermatosis	PCBs, dioxins, herbicides
	Cancer	Ultraviolet radiation
Gastrointestinal tract	Liver angiosarcoma	Vinyl chloride

DDT, dichlorodiphenyltrichloroethane; PCBs, polychlorinated biphenyls. Adapted from Leigh JP, et al: Occupational injury and illness in the United States. Estimates of costs, morbidity, and mortality. Arch Intern Med 157:1557, 1997; Mitchell FL: Hazardous waste. In Rom WN (ed): Environmental and Occupational Medicine, 2nd ed. Boston, Little, Brown, 1992, p. 1275; and Levi PE: Classes of toxic chemicals. In Hodgson E, Levi PE (eds): A Textbook of Modern Toxicology. Stamford, CT, Appleton & Lange, 1997, p. 229.

Table 10-7. TOXIC AND CARCINOGENIC METALS

Metal	Disease	Occupation
Lead	Renal toxicity Anemia, colic Peripheral neuropathy Insomnia, fatigue Cognitive deficits Cerebral edema in children	Battery and ammunition workers, foundry workers, spray painting, radiator repair
Mercury	Renal toxicity Muscle tremors, dementia Cerebral palsy Mental retardation	Chlorine-alkali industry
Arsenic	Cancer of skin, lung, liver	Miners, smelters, oil refinery workers, farm workers
Beryllium	Acute lung irritant Chronic lung hypersensitivity ? Lung cancer	Beryllium refining, aerospace manufacturing, ceramics
Cobalt + tungsten carbide	Lung fibrosis Asthma	Toolmakers, grinders, diamond polishers
Cadmium	Renal toxicity ? Prostate cancer	Battery workers, smelters, welders, soldering
Chromium	Cancer of lung and nasal cavity	Pigment workers, smelters, smelters, steel workers
Nickel	Cancer of lung and nasal sinuses	Smelters, steel workers, electroplating

Adapted from Levi PE: Classes of toxic chemicals. In Hodgson E, Levi PE (eds): A Textbook of Modern Toxicology. Stamford, CT, Appleton & Lange, 1997, p. 229; and Sprince NL: Hard metal disease. In Rom WN (eds): Environmental and Occupational Medicine, 2nd ed. Boston, Little, Brown, 1992, p. 791.

to lead continues to be a serious public health problem and is discussed in detail.

Lead

Lead is used in the production of batteries and ammunition as well as in foundries. In some parts of the world, tetraethyl lead is used as a gasoline additive. Environmental sources of lead are urban air because of the use of leaded gasoline, soil contaminated with exterior lead paint, the water supply because of lead plumbing, and house dust in homes with interior lead paint. Although inhalation is the most important route of occupational exposure, ingested lead from contaminated food and beverages can be absorbed in the gastrointestinal tract. Absorbed lead accumulates in the bones and developing teeth in children.

Lead toxicity is due to

- High affinity for sulfhydryl groups, which inhibits enzyme function, such as those involved in the incorporation of iron into the heme molecule (hence patients develop hypochromic anemia)
- Competition with calcium ions for storage in bone
- Inhibition of membrane-associated enzymes leading to impaired red blood cell survival (hemolysis) and renal damage
- Impaired metabolism of 1,25-dihydroxyvitamin D

Lead contributes to multiple chronic health effects (Fig. 10–3):

- Injury to the central and peripheral nervous systems causes headache, dizziness, and memory deficits in the adult; encephalopathy with acute cerebral edema and mental deterioration occurs in children.
- Blood changes include a characteristic punctate basophilic stippling of erythrocytes, microcytic hypochromic anemia, and hemolysis.
- Gastrointestinal changes include abdominal pain and anorexia.

Infants and children are particularly vulnerable to lead toxicity. Ten percent of preschool children in urban areas may have significant blood lead levels (>15 µg/dl). Even at low levels, intellectual impairment, behavioral abnormalities, and learning deficits have been described.

Agricultural Hazards (p. 422)

Agricultural productivity has been increased with the use of fertilizers and pesticides. Pesticide residues can be found on foods and contaminate soil and water supplies. Agricultural pesticides are divided into five categories, depending on the target:

1. Insecticides
2. Herbicides
3. Fungicides
4. Rodenticides
5. Fumigants

All pesticides are toxic to some plant or rodent species, and at higher doses, they can also be toxic to farm animals, pets, and humans (Table 10–8). The acute toxicity of pesticides has been established, but the chronic toxicity of these chemicals is less certain. Selected examples of the adverse heath effects of the most common pesticides are outlined:

- *Organochlorine* insecticides such as *DDT* (dichlorodiphenyl-trichloroethane) and *dioxins*, such as TCDD (2,3,7,8-tetrachlo-

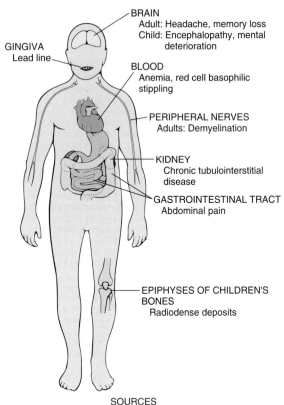

Figure 10–3 ■

Consequences of lead exposure.

rodibenzo-p-dioxin), have low acute toxicity for humans; however, they *bioaccumulate and persist* in the environment and in fat tissue. DDT may cause reproductive dysfunction and cancer in humans, although this is controversial. During the Vietnam War, the defoliant agent orange was contaminated with TCDD. In animal studies, TCDD is highly toxic, immunosuppressive, teratogenic, and carcinogenic.

■ *Organophosphate* insecticides, such as malathion, are irreversible inhibitors of cholinesterases resulting in abnormal transmission at peripheral and central nerve endings. These chemicals are absorbed through the skin, gastrointestinal tract, and lungs and can cause neurotoxicity and delayed neuropathy.

Table 10–8. HEALTH EFFECTS OF AGRICULTURAL PESTICIDES

Category	Example	Effect
Insecticides	Organochlorines DDT Chlordane Lindane Methoxychlor	Neurotoxicity, hepatotoxicity
	Organophosphates Parathion Diazinon Malathion	Neurotoxicity; delayed neuropathy
	Carbamates Aldicarb Carbaryl	Neurotoxicity (reversible)
	Botanical agents Nicotine Pyrethrins Rotenone	Paresthesia, lung irritant, allergic dermatitis
Herbicides	Arsenic compounds	Hyperpigmentation, gangrene, anemia, sensory neuropathy, cancer
	Dinitrophenols	Hyperthermia, sweating
	Chlorophenoxy herbicides	
	2,4-D and 2,4,5-T	? Lymphoma, sarcoma
	TCCD	Fetotoxicity, immunotoxicity, cancer
	Paraquat	Acute lung injury
	Atrazine	? Cancer
	Alachlor	? Cancer
Fungicides	Captan Maneb Benomyl	? Reproductive toxicity
Rodenticides	Fluoroacetate	Cardiac and respiratory failure
	Warfarin	Hemorrhage
	Strychnine	Respiratory failure
Fumigants	Carbon disulfide	Cardiac toxicity
	Ethylene dibromide	Neurotoxicity
	Phosphine	Lung edema, brain damage
	Chloropicrin	Eye irritation, lung edema, arrhythmias

DDT, dichlorodiphenyltrichloroethane. Adapted from Hodgson E: Introduction to toxicology. In Hodgson E, Levi PE (eds): A Textbook of Modern Toxicology. Stamford, CT, Appleton & Lange, 1997, p. 1; and Levi PE: Classes of toxic chemicals. In Hodgson E, Levi PE (eds): A Textbook of Modern Toxicology. Stamford, CT, Appleton & Lange, 1997, p. 229.

Natural Toxins (p. 424)

Potent toxins and carcinogens are present in the natural environment. These include mycotoxins, such as ergot alkaloids, and phytotoxins, such as cycasin, which may contaminate food. Animal toxins include venoms produced by snakes and bees as well as the toxins produced by dinoflagellates. Animal toxins can be ingested by consuming fish, snails, or mollusks that have eaten dinoflagellates containing ciguatoxin or saxitoxin. Aflatoxin B_1 is produced by fungi that contaminate stored peanuts, corn, and other grains. It is a potent carcinogen, particularly for the liver, and contributes to the high incidence of liver cancer in Africa and the Far East. The mushroom *Amanita phalloides* may cause hepatic necrosis or even death.

Radiation Injury (p. 424)

Radiation is energy distributed across the electromagnetic spectrum as waves (long wavelengths, low frequency) or particles (short wavelengths, high frequency). Approximately 80% of radiation is derived from natural sources, including cosmic radiation, UV light, and natural radioisotopes, especially radon gas. The remaining 20% is derived from man-made sources, such as medical and dental diagnostic and therapeutic procedures, consumer products, and occupational exposures.

Electromagnetic radiation characterized by long wavelengths and low frequencies (e.g., radio waves and microwaves) produces vibration and rotation of atoms in biologic molecules and is described as *nonionizing radiation*. Radiation energy of short wavelengths and high frequency can ionize biologic target molecules and eject electrons. X-rays, gamma rays, and cosmic rays are forms of *ionizing radiation*. *Particulate radiation* is classified by the type of particles emitted (e.g., alpha or beta particles). The energy of these particles is measured in million electron volts (MeV). The decay of radioisotopes is expressed by the *curie*—3.7 $\times$ 10^{10} disintegrations per second (Ci)—or the *becquerel*—1 disintegration per second (Bq). The rate of decay of radioisotopes is usually expressed as the *half-life* and ranges from a few seconds to centuries.

IONIZING RADIATION

The dose of ionizing radiation is measured in several units:

- *Roentgen*: Unit of charge produced by x-rays or gamma rays that ionize a specific volume of air.
- *Rad*: The dose of radiation that produces absorption of 100 ergs of energy per gram of tissue.
- *Gray* (Gy): The dose of radiation that produces absorption of 1 joule of energy per kilogram of tissue. 1 Gy corresponds to 100 rad.
- *Rem*: The dose of radiation that causes a biologic effect equivalent to 1 rad of x-rays or gamma rays.

These measurements do not directly quantify energy absorbed per unit of tissue and therefore do not predict the biologic effects of radiation. These effects depend on several factors, in addition to the physical properties of the radioactive material and the dose:

- Dose rate is important; a single dose can cause greater injury than divided or fractionated doses that allow time for cellular repair.
- Because DNA is the most important subcellular target of ionizing radiation, rapidly dividing cells (e.g., hematopoietic cells, gastrointestinal epithelium) are more radiosensitive than quiescent cells (e.g., bone, muscle).
- A single dose of external radiation administered to the whole body is more lethal than regional doses with shielding.
- Different cell types differ in the extent of their adaptive and reparative responses to radiation.
- Cells in the G_2 and mitotic phases of the cell cycle are most sensitive to ionizing radiation.
- Ionizing radiation can penetrate tissue and ionize atoms or molecules within cells with secondary generation of ions and free radicals, such as oxygen-derived radicals from the radiolytic cleavage of water (Chapter 1). Free radical scavengers and antioxidants protect against radiation injury.

Cellular Mechanisms of Radiation Injury

The acute effects of ionizing radiation range from overt necrosis at high doses (>10 Gy), killing of proliferating cells at intermediate doses (1 to 2 Gy), and no histopathologic effect at doses less than 0.5 Gy. If cells undergo extensive DNA damage or if they are unable to repair this damage, they may undergo apoptosis. Surviving cells may show delayed effects of radiation injury: mutations, chromosomal aberrations, and genetic instability. These genetically damaged cells may become malignant and cause cancers.

- *Acute effects*: Ionizing radiation produces a variety of lesions in cellular DNA, including DNA-protein cross-links and DNA strand breaks. DNA damage stimulates expression of several genes involved in DNA repair. The tumor-suppressor gene *p53* is activated after DNA damage and increases expression of several downstream effector genes, which, in turn, induce cell cycle arrest and, in some cases, apoptosis.
- *Chronic effects*: Chronic effects are caused by a combination of atrophy of parenchymal cells, ischemia as a result of vascular damage, and fibrosis resulting in scarring.
- *Carcinogenesis*: Occupational or accidental exposure to ionizing radiation produces an increased incidence of skin, thyroid, and lung cancers as well as leukemia and osteogenic sarcomas. A notable example is the increased incidence of thyroid cancer seen in children exposed to radiation from atomic bombs or from the nuclear power plant accident at Chernobyl. The mechanism responsible for the delayed carcinogenic effect of ionizing radiation may be due to *latent genetic instability*, in which mutations persist and accumulate.

Clinical Manifestations of Exposure to Ionizing Radiation

Acute, whole-body exposure can be described as the *acute radiation syndrome* or *radiation sickness*. Depending on the dose, four syndromes are produced:

1. Subclinical
2. Hematopoietic
3. Gastrointestinal
4. Central nervous system

These syndromes are summarized in Table 10–9.

Radiation Therapy

External radiation is delivered to malignant neoplasms at fractionated doses, with shielding of normal tissues. Patients may experience transient fatigue, vomiting, and anorexia.

Growth and Developmental Abnormalities

Developing fetuses and young children are highly sensitive to growth and developmental abnormalities induced by ionizing radiation. Four susceptible phases can be defined:

1. Preimplantation embryo: Irradiation of the mother before implantation can be lethal to the embryo.
2. Organogenesis: Critical stages of organogenesis are from implantation to 9 weeks of gestation.
3. Fetal period: From 6 weeks of gestation until birth, functional

Table 10-9. CLINICAL FEATURES OF ACUTE RADIATION SYNDROMES

Category	Whole-Body Dose (rem)	Symptoms	Prognosis
Subclinical	<200	Mild nausea and vomiting; lymphocytes <1500/mm³	100% survival
Hematopoietic	200–600	Intermittent nausea and vomiting; petechiae, hemorrhage; maximum neutrophil and platelet depression in 3 weeks; lymphocytes <1000/mm³	Infections May require bone marrow transplant
Gastrointestinal	600–1000	Nausea, vomiting, diarrhea; hemorrhage and infection in 1–3 weeks; severe neutrophil and platelet depression; lymphocytes <500/mm³	Shock and death in 10–14 days
Central nervous system	>1000	Intractable nausea and vomiting; confusion, somnolence, convulsions, coma in 15 minutes–3 hours; lymphocytes absent	Death in 14–36 hours

abnormalities of the central nervous system and reproductive systems may be produced by maternal irradiation.

4. Postnatal period: Infants and young children exposed to radiation may cease bone growth and maturation. Development of the central nervous system, eyes, and teeth may also be perturbed.

Heritable mutations and chromosomal abnormalities leading to the induction of cancer may follow exposure to ionizing radiation.

Delayed Radiation Injury

Months and years after irradiation, delayed complications may occur. The most vulnerable sites of delayed radiation injury are the following:

■ *Blood vessels*: Blood vessels in the field of irradiation show subintimal fibrosis, fibrosis of the muscle wall, degeneration of the internal elastic lamina, and severe narrowing of the lumen.
■ *Skin*: Atrophy of the epidermis, dermal fibrosis, and dilation and weakening of the subcutaneous vessels comprise changes that are called *radiation dermatitis*.
■ *Heart*: Radiotherapy to the chest for malignant disease may damage the heart and pericardium.
■ *Lungs*: Radiation causes acute injury as well as delayed radiation pneumonitis as a result of intra-alveolar and interstitial fibrosis.
■ *Kidneys and urinary bladder*: Delayed renal peritubular fibrosis, vascular damage, and hyalinization of glomeruli develop gradually, leading to hypertension and atrophy. The bladder is sensitive to radiation injury, with acute necrosis of the epithelium followed by submucosal fibrosis, contracture, bleeding, and ulceration.
■ *Gastrointestinal tract*: Esophagitis, gastritis, enteritis, colitis, and proctitis can result from local irradiation.
■ *Eyes and central nervous system*: Radiation gives rise to cataracts. The brain may show focal necrosis and demyelination of white matter. Irradiation of the spinal cord can damage small blood vessels, leading to necrosis, demyelination, and paraplegia, called *transverse myelitis*.

ULTRAVIOLET INJURY

UV radiation is divided into UVA, UVB, and UVC; 3 to 5% of the total solar radiation that penetrates to the earth's surface is UV radiation. Ozone in the atmosphere is an important protection against UV radiation: Ozone completely absorbs all UVC and partially absorbs UVB. Ozone depletion by atmospheric pollutants is predicted to contribute to an increase in UVB and possibly UVC at the earth's surface, triggering a 2 to 4% increase in the incidence of skin cancers. The effects of UV radiation are summarized in Table 10–10.

■ The acute effects of UVA and UVB are short-lived and reversible and include erythema, pigmentation, and injury to Langerhans cells and keratinocytes in the epidermis. Erythema, edema, and acute inflammation are mediated by release of histamine from mast cells in the dermis.
■ Tanning induced by UVA and UVB is due to a delayed increase in the number of melanocytes, elongation and extension of dendritic processes, and transfer of melanin to keratinocytes.

Table 10-10. ACUTE AND DELAYED EFFECTS OF ULTRAVIOLET RADIATION

Radiation	Wavelength (nm)	Acute Effects	Delayed Effects
UVA	320–400	Erythema 8–48 hours	Tanning
		Depletion of Langerhans cells	? Skin cancer
		Pigment darkening	
		Dermal inflammation	
UVB	290–320	Erythema 3–24 hours	Tanning
		Apoptosis of keratinocytes	Solar elastosis
		Depletion of Langerhans cells	Premature aging
			Actinic keratosis
			Skin cancer
UVC	200–290		? Skin cancer

- Repeated exposures to UV radiation produce changes in the skin characteristic of premature aging:
  - Wrinkling
  - Solar elastosis
  - Irregularities in pigmentation
- Skin damage induced by UVB may be mediated by reactive oxygen species and damage to endogenous chromophores, such as melanin. UV radiation also damages DNA and generates pyrimidine dimers, such as those found in malignant skin lesions. A series of molecular changes (collectively referred to as the *UV response pathway*) leads to a protective cellular response consisting of DNA repair, cell cycle arrest, or apoptosis. The importance of DNA repair as a defense mechanism against skin cancer is illustrated by increased sensitivity of patients with *xeroderma pigmentosum*, who lack repair enzymes, to UV-induced skin cancers.

ELECTROMAGNETIC FIELDS

Nonionizing electromagnetic fields range between less than 1 cycle/sec (Hertz) for DC power lines up to 100 GHz for long-distance microwaves and radar. There was public concern that residential exposure to ambient 50- to 60-Hz magnetic fields might be a health threat and contribute to an increased incidence of leukemia in children. This concern has been allayed by an epidemiologic study that failed to establish such a relationship.

Physical Environment (p. 431)

Human injury, death, and disability are major public health problems in modern industrialized societies. Injuries caused by the physical environment, resulting from human activities as well as external forces, can be divided into four categories:

1. Mechanical force
2. Heat and cold
3. Electrical injuries
4. High altitudes

MECHANICAL FORCE

Mechanical force may inflict soft tissue injuries, bone injuries, and head injuries. Soft tissue injuries can be superficial, involving mainly the skin, or deep, associated with visceral damage. The skin injuries can be further described as follows:

- *Abrasion*: This type of skin injury represents a scrape, in which the superficial epidermis is torn off by friction or force. Regeneration without scarring usually occurs promptly unless infection complicates the process.
- *Laceration versus incision*: A laceration is an irregular tear in the skin produced by overstretching. It may be linear or stellate, depending on the tearing force. In contrast, an incision is made by a sharp cutting object, such as a knife (scalpel) or a piece of glass. The incision, in contrast to the laceration, can usually be neatly approximated by sutures, leaving little or no scar. Deep tissues and organs may sustain lacerations from an external blow with or without apparent superficial injury.
- *Contusion*: A contusion is an injury caused by a blunt force that injures small blood vessels and causes interstitial bleeding usually without disruption of the continuity of the tissue.

GUNSHOT WOUNDS

Gunshot wounds are part of forensic pathology, a subspecialty dealing with trauma and the associated medicolegal issues. The character of a gunshot wound at entry and exit and the extent of injury depend on the type of gun used (handgun or rifle) and on a large number of variables, including the caliber of the bullet, the type of ammunition, the distance of the firearm from the body, the locus of the injury, the trajectory of the missile (at right angles to the skin or oblique), and the gyroscopic stability of the bullet (the presence or absence of wobbling or tumbling). With handguns held at close range (within a foot of the skin surface), there is a gray-black discoloration about the wound of entrance (fouling) produced by the heat, smoke, and burned powder deposits exiting with the bullet from the muzzle. When firearms are held more than a foot away but within 3 feet, there may be only stippling without fouling. At greater distances, neither is present. Cutaneous exit wounds are generally more irregular than wounds of entrance because in passing through the tissues the bullet almost inevitably develops a wobbling trajectory.

THERMAL INJURIES

Cutaneous burns are responsible for about 4500 deaths annually in the United States, a large proportion involving children and the elderly. The clinical significance of a burn depends on many factors:

- Depth of the burn
- Percentage of body surface involved
- Possible presence of internal injuries from inhalation of hot gases and fumes
- Promptness and efficacy of the postburn therapy, in particular, fluid and electrolyte management, prevention of shock, and prevention or control of wound infection

Any burn exceeding 50% of the total body surface, whether superficial or deep, is grave and potentially fatal. In *partial-*

thickness burns, characterized by blistering, the dermis and its skin appendages are spared, and complete regeneration is possible. By contrast, a *full-thickness burn* implies total destruction of the entire epidermis, extending into the dermis and sometimes even more deeply; regeneration of the epidermis is possible only from the margins or spared deeper appendages. The *systemic consequences* of a burn are far more important than the local injury. In large burns, neurogenic shock may appear almost immediately. Neurogenic shock may be followed by hypovolemic shock, owing to the copious loss of exudate from the burn surface. Secondary burn *infection* is an important complication in all burn patients who have lost epidermis. With excess heat loss from the burn wound, a *hypermetabolic state* develops that, together with the loss of plasma proteins, may induce serious fluid, electrolyte, and nutritional imbalances. Collectively, burn patients present a set of complex clinical problems that require specialized care.

Hyperthermia

Prolonged exposure to elevated ambient temperatures can result in the following conditions:

- *Heat cramps* occur from loss of electrolytes through sweating.
- *Heat exhaustion* is the most common heat syndrome. It results from a failure of the cardiovascular system to compensate for hypovolemia, secondary to water depletion. Its onset is sudden with prostration and collapse.
- *Heat stroke* is associated with high ambient temperatures and high humidity. Thermoregulatory mechanisms fail, sweating ceases, and core body temperature rises to high (e.g., 106°F) levels. This situation results from a marked generalized peripheral vasodilation with peripheral pooling of blood and a decreased effective circulating blood volume. Necrosis of muscles and myocardium may occur associated with systemic effects, such as arrhythmias and disseminated intravascular coagulation. Heat stroke typically occurs in individuals undergoing intense physical training and in people with cardiovascular disease.

Hypothermia

Prolonged exposure to low ambient temperature leads to hypothermia. At about 90°F, loss of consciousness occurs, followed by bradycardia and atrial fibrillation at lower core temperatures. Freezing of cells and tissues causes injury by direct effects of the crystallization of intracellular and extracellular water and by indirect effects exerted by circulatory changes. Slowly falling temperatures may induce vasoconstriction and increased permeability, leading to edematous changes (e.g., *trench foot*). Sudden falls in temperature that are persistent may cause ischemic injuries.

ELECTRICAL INJURIES

The passage of an electric current through the body may be without effect; may cause sudden death by disruption of neural regulatory impulses, producing cardiac arrest; or may cause thermal injury to organs interposed in the pathway of the current. Many variables are involved in electrical injuries, but the most important are the resistance of the tissues to the conductance of the electric current and the intensity of the current. The resistance of the tissues of the body to the flow of electricity varies inversely to their water content. Dry skin is particularly resistant, but when skin is wet or immersed in water its resistance is greatly decreased. The greater the resistance of tissues, the greater the heat generated. Thus, an electric current may cause a surface burn of dry skin but may cause death by disruption of regulatory pathways when it is transmitted through wet skin. The thermal effects of the passage of the electric current also depend on its intensity. High-intensity current, such as lightning, may course along the skin producing linear arborizing burns known as *lightning marks* or be conducted around the victim *(flashover)*.

INJURIES RELATED TO CHANGES IN ATMOSPHERIC PRESSURE

Depending on the direction of change (increase or decrease), its rate of development, and the magnitude of change, four syndromes can be produced in relation to changes in atmospheric pressure:

1. *High-altitude illness* is encountered in mountain climbers in the rarefied atmosphere encountered at altitudes above 4000 m. The lowered oxygen tension produces progressive mental obtundation and may be accompanied by increased capillary permeability with cerebral and pulmonary edema.

2. *Blast injury* implies a violent increase in pressure either in the atmosphere (air blast) or in water (immersion blast).

3. *Air or gas embolism* may occur as a complication of scuba diving, mechanical positive-pressure ventilatory support, and hyperbaric oxygen therapy and rarely as a manifestation of decompression disease. The abnormal increase in intra-alveolar air pressure leads to entrance of air into the interstitium and small blood vessels. Pulmonary, mediastinal, and subcutaneous emphysema may result. In some instances, the coalescence of numerous small air emboli that gain access to the arterial circulation may lead acutely to strokelike syndromes or a myocardial ischemic episode.

4. *Decompression (caisson) disease* is encountered in deep-sea divers who spend long periods of time in caissons or tunnels, under increased atmospheric pressure. The injury is encountered with too-rapid decompression. As the underwater depth and consequent atmospheric pressure increase, larger and larger amounts of oxygen and accompanying gases (nitrogen) dissolve in the blood and tissue fluids. Once too-rapid ascent begins, the dissolved gases come out of solution and form minute bubbles in the bloodstream and tissues. Coalescence of these bubbles produces even larger masses capable of becoming significant emboli in the bloodstream. Periarticular bubbles produce the *bends*. Bubbles formed within the lung or gaseous emboli give rise to respiratory difficulties, with severe substernal pain referred to as the *chokes*. Days after the dive, *caisson disease of bone* may appear. It takes the form of foci of aseptic necrosis typically of femoral and humeral heads, attributed to embolic occlusion of the vascular supply.

FOOD AND NUTRITION (p. 436)

Food Safety: Additives and Contaminants
(p. 436)

Food contains numerous natural constituents and additives that may threaten human health. A wide range of chemicals are natural constituents of foods, including carcinogens and natural pesticides. Food may also be contaminated by natural toxicants or microorganisms, such as hepatitis A virus or *Salmonella enteritidis, Escherichia coli,* or *Cryptosporidium.*

Additional chemicals are added to foods either directly (chemical sweeteners, preservatives, food colors) or indirectly (agricultural pesticides, residues of drugs or hormones given to animals, industrial contaminants). Low levels of metals, chlorinated hydrocarbons, and polychlorinated biphenyls are present in the food supply.

Nutritional Deficiencies (p. 436)

In developing countries, undernutrition or protein-energy malnutrition (PEM) continues to be common. It continues to occur even in affluent societies in low economic pockets. In industrialized societies, the most common diseases (atherosclerosis, cancer, diabetes, and hypertension) have all been linked to some form of dietary impropriety.

An adequate diet should provide

- Energy, in the form of carbohydrates, fats, and proteins
- Essential (and nonessential) amino acids and fatty acids
- Vitamins and minerals

In *primary malnutrition*, one or all of these components are missing from the diet. By contrast, in *secondary* or *conditional malnutrition*, the supply of nutrients is adequate, but malnutrition results from nutrient malabsorption, impaired nutrient use or storage, excess nutrient losses, or increased need for nutrients. Undernutrition in affluent societies is associated with the following:

- *Ignorance and poverty*: The homeless, elderly, and children of the poor demonstrate the effects of undernutrition.
- *Chronic alcoholism*: Alcoholics can have vitamin deficiencies as well as PEM.
- *Acute and chronic illnesses*: In some illnesses, the basal metabolic rate becomes elevated (e.g., burns).
- *Self-imposed dietary restriction*: Eating disorders such as anorexia nervosa and bulimia nervosa affect a large population concerned about body image.

PROTEIN-ENERGY MALNUTRITION

Severe PEM is common in developing countries, where up to 25% of children may be affected. PEM refers to a range of clinical syndromes characterized by a dietary intake of protein and calories inadequate to meet the body's needs. The diagnosis of PEM is usually made by comparing the body weight for a given height with a standard table, although evaluation of fat stores, muscle mass, and serum proteins can also be helpful. The most common victims of PEM worldwide are children. A child whose weight falls to less than 80% of normal is considered to be malnourished. When the level falls to 60% of normal weight for sex and age, the child is considered to have *marasmus*, which has the following features (Table 10–11):

- Growth retardation and loss of muscle mass occur.
- Subcutaneous fat is mobilized.
- Extremities are emaciated, and the head appears too large for the body.
- Serum albumin levels are near-normal.
- Immune deficiency results in concurrent infections.

Table 10-11. COMPARISON OF SEVERE MARASMUS-LIKE AND KWASHIORKOR-LIKE SECONDARY PROTEIN-ENERGY MALNUTRITION

Syndrome	Clinical Setting	Time Course	Clinical Features	Laboratory Findings	Prognosis
Marasmus-like protein-energy malnutrition	Chronic illness (e.g., chronic lung disease, cancer)	Months	History of weight loss Muscle wasting Absent subcutaneous fat	Normal or mildly reduced serum proteins	Variable; depends on underlying disease
Kwashiorkor-like protein-energy malnutrition	Acute, catabolic illness (e.g., severe trauma, burns, sepsis)	Weeks	Normal fat and muscle Edema Easily pluckable hair	Serum albumin <2.8 gm/dl	Poor

Modified from Bennett JC, Plum F (eds): Cecil Textbook of Medicine, 20th ed. Philadelphia, WB Saunders, 1996, p 1156.

The other form of severe malnutrition is *kwashiorkor*, which occurs when protein deprivation is relatively greater than the reduction in total calories. It has the following features (Table 10–11):

- Kwashiorkor is most commonly seen in impoverished African and Southeast Asian children.
- *Kwashiorkor is a more severe form of malnutrition than marasmus.* There are two protein compartments in the body: the *visceral protein compartment*, consisting of the protein stores in the visceral organs, such as the liver, and the *somatic protein compartment*, represented by skeletal muscles. These two compartments are regulated differently. The visceral compartment is depleted more severely in kwashiorkor, whereas the somatic compartment is affected more severely in marasmus. The marked loss of the visceral protein compartment in kwashiorkor results in hypoalbuminemia, giving rise to a generalized or dependent edema.
- Skin lesions give a *flaky paint* appearance.
- Hair changes include loss of normal color and texture.
- Fatty liver results from decreased synthesis of carrier proteins.
- Immune defects and secondary infections occur.

Secondary PEM occurs in chronically ill or hospitalized patients. Both marasmus-like and kwashiorkor-like syndromes (with intermediate forms) may develop. Secondary PEM is common in advanced cancer and AIDS patients. The malnutrition in these settings is sometimes called *cachexia*.

Morphology

The major anatomic features of PEM include

- Growth failure
- Peripheral edema
- Loss of body fat and atrophy of muscle
- Enlarged and fatty liver in kwashiorkor but not in marasmus
- Hypoplastic bone marrow in both kwashiorkor and marasmus because of decreased numbers of red cell precursors

ANOREXIA NERVOSA AND BULIMIA

Anorexia nervosa is self-induced starvation, resulting in marked loss of weight; bulimia is a condition in which the patient binges on food and then induces vomiting. These eating disorders occur primarily in previously healthy young women who have developed an obsession with a thin body image. The clinical findings are similar to those in severe PEM.

Vitamin Deficiencies (p. 439)

Thirteen vitamins are necessary for health; four—A, D, E, and K—are fat soluble, and the remainder are water soluble. A summary of all of the essential vitamins along with their functions and deficiency syndromes is presented in Table 10–12.

VITAMIN A

Vitamin A is a group of related chemicals that have a hormone-like function. *Retinol* is the transport and also the storage form of vitamin A. Carotenoids, found in yellow and leafy green vegeta-

Table 10-12 VIATMINS: MAJOR FUNCTIONS AND DEFICIENCY SYNDROMES

Vitamin	Functions	Deficiency Syndromes
Fat-Soluble		
Vitamin A	A component of visual pigment Maintenance of specialized epithelia Maintenance of resistance to infection	Night blindness, xerophthalmia, blindness Squamous metaplasia Vulnerability to infection, particularly measles
Vitamin D	Facilitates intestinal absorption of calcium and phosphorus and mineralization of bone	Rickets in children Osteomalacia in adults
Vitamin E	Major antioxidant; scavenges free radicals	Spinocerebellar degeneration
Vitamin K	Cofactor in hepatic carboxylation of procoagulants—factors II (prothrombin), VII, IX, and X; and protein C and protein S	Bleeding diathesis
Water-Soluble		
Vitamin B_1 (thiamine)	As pyrophosphate, is coenzyme in decarboxylation reactions	Dry and wet beriberi, Wernicke syndrome ?Korsakoff syndrome
Vitamin B_2 (riboflavin)	Converted to coenzymes flavin mononucleotide and flavin adenine dinucleotide, cofactors for many enzymes in intermediary metabolism	Ariboflavinosis, cheilosis, stomatitis, glossitis, dermatitis, corneal vascularization
Niacin	Incorporated into nicotinamide adenine dinucleotide (NAD) and NAD phosphate involved in a variety of redox reactions	Pellagra—three Ds: dementia, dermatitis, diarrhea
Vitamin B_6 (pyridoxine)	Derivatives serve as coenzymes in many intermediary reactions	Cheilosis, glossitis, dermatitis, peripheral neuropathy
Vitamin B_{12}	Requisite for normal folate metabolism and DNA synthesis Maintenance of myelinization of spinal cord tracts	Combined system disease (megaloblastic pernicious anemia and degeneration of posterolateral spinal cord tracts)
Vitamin C	Serves in many oxidation-reduction (redox) reactions and hydroxylation of collagen	Scurvy
Folate	Essential for transfer and use of 1-carbon units in DNA synthesis	Megaloblastic anemia, neural tube defects
Pantothenic acid	Incorporated in coenzyme A	No nonexperimental syndrome recognized
Biotin	Cofactor in carboxylation reactions	No clearly defined clinical syndrome

bles, can be metabolized to active vitamin A. About 90% of the body's vitamin A reserve is found in the perisinusoidal stellate (Ito) cells in the liver.

Functions

Functions of vitamin A include

- Maintaining normal vision in reduced light
- Potentiating the differentiation of mucus-secreting epithelial cells
- Enhancing immunity to infections, particularly in children
- Acting as photoprotective and antioxidant agents

Deficiency State

Vitamin A deficiency results in the following conditions:

- Impaired vision occurs, particularly night blindness.
- *Xerophthalmia* (dry eye) refers to a collection of ocular changes, including dryness of the conjunctivae (xerosis), formation of small opaque spots (Bitot spots) or ulcers on the corneal surface, and eventual destruction of the cornea (keratomalacia).
- Production of keratinizing metaplasia of epithelial surfaces results in infections of the respiratory tract because of squamous epithelial metaplasia of the airways and renal and urinary bladder stones because of desquamation of keratinized epithelium.
- Immune deficiency occurs.

Vitamin A Toxicity

Both short-term and long-term excess of vitamin A produce clinical consequences, an issue of some concern because of the availability of large doses at health food stores. Acute toxic manifestations include headache, vomiting, stupor, and papilledema. Chronic toxicity is associated with weight loss, nausea, and vomiting; dryness of the lips; and bone and joint pain.

VITAMIN D

The major function of vitamin D is the maintenance of normal plasma levels of calcium and phosphorus. It is required for the prevention of rickets in growing children whose epiphyses have not already closed and osteomalacia in adults as well as prevention of hypocalcemic tetany.

The metabolism of vitamin D can be outlined as follows (Fig. 10–4A):

- Absorption of vitamin D in the gut or synthesis from precursors in the skin
- Binding to a plasma α_1-globulin and transport to liver
- Conversion to 25-hydroxyvitamin D (25(OH)D) by 25-hydroxylase in the liver
- Conversion of 25(OH)D to 1,25(OH)$_2$D by α_1-hydroxylase in the kidney

Biologically, 1,25(OH)$_2$D is the most active form. The production of 1,25(OH)$_2$D by the kidney is regulated by three mechanisms:

1. In a feedback loop, increased levels of 1,25(OH)$_2$D down-regulate synthesis of this metabolite by inhibiting the action of α_1-hydroxylase.
2. Hypocalcemia stimulates secretion of parathyroid hormone

NORMAL VITAMIN D METABOLISM

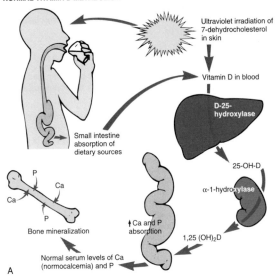

A

VITAMIN D DEFICIENCY

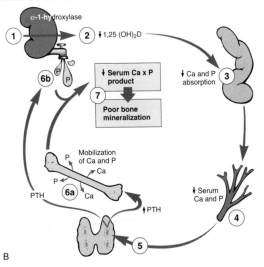

B

Figure 10-4 ∎

A, Schema of normal vitamin D metabolism. *B,* Vitamin D deficiency. There is inadequate substrate for the renal hydroxylase (1), yielding a deficiency of 1,25(OH)₂D (2), and deficient absorption of calcium and phosphorus from the gut (3), with consequent depressed serum levels of both (4). The hypocalcemia activates the parathyroid glands (5), causing mobilization of calcium and phosphorus from bone (6a). Simultaneously the parathyroid hormone (PTH) induces wasting of phosphate in the urine (6b) and calcium retention. Consequently the serum levels of calcium are normal or nearly normal, but the phosphate is low; hence mineralization is impaired (7).

(PTH), which, in turn, augments the conversion of 25(OH)D to 1,25(OH)$_2$D by activating α_1-hydroxylase.

3. Hypophosphatemia directly activates α_1-hydroxylase and thus increases formation of 1,25(OH)$_2$D.

Functions

1,25(OH)$_2$D can be thought of as a steroid hormone that binds to a widely expressed receptor. Vitamin D has the following functions:

- Stimulates intestinal absorption of calcium and phosphorus
- Collaborates with PTH in the mobilization of calcium from bone
- Stimulates PTH-dependent reabsorption of calcium in the distal renal tubules

Vitamin D deficiency causes *rickets* in growing children and *osteomalacia* in adults. Both forms of skeletal disease result from altered vitamin D absorption or metabolism or, less commonly, from disorders that affect the function of vitamin D or disturb calcium or phosphorus homeostasis (Fig. 10–4B). An inadequacy of vitamin D causes a deficiency of 1,25(OH)$_2$D and deficient absorption of calcium and phosphorus from the gut with consequent depressed serum levels of both. The hypocalcemia activates the parathyroid glands, causing mobilization of calcium and phosphorus from bone. PTH induces wasting of phosphate in the urine and calcium retention. Consequently, serum levels of calcium are nearly normal, but the phosphate level is low, impairing bone mineralization.

Morphology

The basic alteration in both rickets and osteomalacia is an excess of unmineralized matrix. In children, inadequate provisional calcification of epiphyseal cartilage deranges endochondral bone growth, resulting in

- Overgrowth of epiphyseal cartilage
- Persistence of distorted masses of cartilage
- Deposition of osteoid matrix on inadequately mineralized cartilaginous remnants
- Disruption of the orderly replacement of cartilage by osteoid matrix
- Deformation of the skeleton as a result of disordered endochondral bone growth

The skeletal changes depend on the severity of the rachitic process and its duration:

- Frontal bossing and a squared appearance to the head occurs in infants.
- Deformation of the chest resulting from overgrowth of cartilage at the costochondral junction produces the *rachitic rosary*. The sternum protrudes anteriorly causing a *pigeon breast* deformity.
- In ambulating children, deformities affect the long bones, spine, and pelvis causing bowing of the legs and lumbar lordosis.
- In adults, the lack of vitamin D produces an excess of osteoid, which weakens the bone and makes it susceptible to fracture. Persistent failure of mineralization in adults leads to loss of skeletal mass, or *osteopenia*, which can be difficult to differentiate from osteoporosis.

VITAMIN E

Vitamin E comprises a group of eight closely related fat-soluble compounds; α-tocopherol is the most active and widely available. Vitamin E is abundant in most foods. The absorption of the tocopherols, similar to other fat-soluble vitamins, requires normal biliary and pancreatic function. After absorption, vitamin E is transported in the blood by chylomicrons, which equilibrate with LDLs. It accumulates throughout the body, mostly in fat depots. Vitamin E serves as a *scavenger of free radicals* formed in redox reactions throughout the body. Vitamin E may inhibit atheroma formation in atherosclerosis by reducing the oxidation of LDL. In the context of cancer, the antioxidant effect may reduce mutagenesis.

Hypovitaminosis E resulting from a deficient diet is uncommon and occurs in association with malabsorption syndromes, infants of low birth weight, developmental defects in the gastrointestinal tract, or lipoprotein disorders. The central nervous system is particularly vulnerable to vitamin E deficiency where axons in the posterior columns of the spinal cord degenerate, with loss of nerve cells in the dorsal root ganglia and degenerative changes in the spinocerebellar tracts. The neurologic manifestations of vitamin E deficiency are absent tendon reflexes, ataxia, dysarthria, and loss of position sense and pain sensation.

VITAMIN K

Vitamin K is a required cofactor for a liver enzyme to carboxylate specific glutamate residues found in a variety of proteins, including

- Clotting factors VII, IX, and X and prothrombin, in which carboxylation facilitates calcium binding and interactions involved in the generation of thrombin (Chapter 5)
- Anticoagulant proteins C and S
- Osteocalcin, a protein made by osteoblasts, in which vitamin K appears to favor calcification

Vitamin K is converted from its reduced form to an oxidized state during interactions with its substrate proteins but then is rapidly recycled by the healthy liver to its original form. Additionally the endogenous intestinal bacterial flora synthesizes the vitamin. Despite both of these sources of the vitamin, there is a definite need for a small amount of the exogenous vitamin. Deficiency occurs in the following settings:

- Fat malabsorption syndromes
- After destruction of the vitamin K–synthesizing flora by antibiotics
- In the neonatal period, because liver reserves are small, the bacterial flora has not developed, and the level of vitamin K in breast milk is small
- In diffuse liver disease

The major consequence of vitamin K deficiency in adults is the development of a *bleeding diathesis*, characterized by hematomas, hematuria, melena, ecchymoses, and bleeding from the gums.

THIAMINE

Thiamine is widely available in the diet, although refined foods, such as polished rice and white flour, contain little. Thiamine is absorbed from the gut and phosphorylated to produce the functionally active form of the vitamin, which is then used as an enzyme cofactor or in the maintenance of neural membranes and nerve conductance.

In underdeveloped countries, where a large part of the scant diet consists of polished rice, as occurs in many areas in Southeast Asia, thiamine deficiency sometimes develops. In developed countries, *thiamine deficiency affects one fourth of chronic alcoholics admitted to general hospitals.* Because a subclinical deficiency state may be converted to an overt deficiency when refeeding chronically malnourished persons, such as alcoholics, adequate amounts of thiamine must be administered concurrently. The three major targets of thiamine deficiency are the peripheral nerves, the heart, and the brain, so persistent thiamine deficiency gives rise to three distinctive syndromes, which typically appear in sequence.

1. A *polyneuropathy (dry beriberi)* is symmetric and takes the form of a nonspecific peripheral neuropathy with myelin degeneration of axons involving motor, sensory, and reflex arcs, leading to footdrop, wristdrop, and sensory changes.

2. A *cardiovascular syndrome (wet beriberi)* is associated with peripheral vasodilation, high-output cardiac failure. and a flabby four-chambered dilated heart.

3. *Wernicke-Korsakoff syndrome* (Chapter 30) is seen in protracted severe deficiency states, typically in chronic alcoholics. Wernicke encephalopathy is marked by ophthalmoplegia, nystagmus, ataxia of gait and stance, and derangement of mental function, typically confusion. Korsakoff psychosis consists of impairment of remote recall, confabulation, and inability to acquire new information. Lesions in the central nervous system take the form of hemorrhages into the mammillary bodies.

RIBOFLAVIN

Riboflavin is a critical component of the flavin-containing nucleotides, which participate in a range of oxidation-reduction reactions. Riboflavin is found in many different meat and dairy products and in vegetables.

Riboflavin deficiency (ariboflavinosis) still occurs as a primary deficiency state among persons in economically deprived and developing countries. In developed nations, it is found in alcoholics and in individuals with debilitating diseases, such as cancer. It is associated with

- Cheilosis, or fissures at the angles of the mouth, which tend to become infected
- Glossitis, in which the tongue becomes atrophic and magenta in color
- Ocular changes, in which an inflammatory reaction in the cornea can cause opacities and sometimes ulcerations
- Dermatitis, greasy and scaling skin involving the nasolabial folds, which may extend into a butterfly distribution to involve the cheeks

NIACIN

Niacin is the generic designation for nicotinic acid, an essential component of two cofactors nicotinamide adenine dinucleotide (NAD) and nicotinamide adenine dinucleotide phosphate (NADP). NAD functions as a coenzyme for multiple dehydrogenases involved in the metabolism of fat, carbohydrate, and amino acids. NADP participates in similar reactions, notably in the hexose-monophosphate shunt of glucose metabolism.

Niacin can be derived from the dietary grains or may be synthesized endogenously from tryptophan. Thus, *pellagra* may result from either a niacin or a tryptophan deficiency.

Pellagra is identified by the *three Ds*: dermatitis, diarrhea, and dementia.

- *Dermatitis* is bilaterally symmetric and is found on exposed areas of the body and consists of sharply demarcated scaling and desquamation.
- *Diarrhea* is caused by atrophy of the gastrointestinal epithelium.
- *Dementia* results from neuron degeneration in the brain, accompanied by similar changes in the spinal cord.

PYRIDOXINE (VITAMIN B$_6$)

Vitamin B$_6$ comprises a group of naturally occurring substances, generically referred to as pyridoxine, that participate as cofactors for enzymes involved in the metabolism of lipids and amino acids. Vitamin B$_6$ is present in most foods; however, food processing may destroy pyridoxine and in the past was responsible for severe deficiency in infants fed dried milk preparations. Secondary hypovitaminosis B$_6$ is produced by a variety of drugs that act as pyridoxine antagonists, including isoniazid (used to treat tuberculosis). Clinical findings in vitamin B$_6$-deficient patients may be related to those of concomitant riboflavin and niacin deficiency, including cheilosis, glossitis, dermatitis, and peripheral neuropathy.

VITAMIN C (ASCORBIC ACID)

A deficiency of vitamin C leads to the development of *scurvy*, characterized by bone disease in children and hemorrhages and healing defects in both children and adults. Scurvy in a growing child is more dramatic than in an adult. Vitamin C is present in most foods and is abundant in fruits and vegetables, so that all but the most restricted diets provide adequate amounts. Ascorbic acid activates prolyl and lysyl hydroxylases, providing for *hydroxylation of procollagen*. Inadequately hydroxylated precursors cannot be appropriately cross-linked, and so collagen lacks tensile strength. Additionally, lack of vitamin C leads to suppression of the rate of synthesis of collagen peptides. The defects in collagen synthesis affect the integrity of blood vessels and account for the predisposition to hemorrhages in scurvy. Vitamin C can scavenge free radicals directly and can act indirectly by regenerating the antioxidant form of vitamin E. The synergistic antioxidant properties of both of these vitamins may retard atherosclerosis by reducing the oxidation of LDL.

Morphology

- *Hemorrhages* often appear in the skin and in the gingival mucosa and cause subperiosteal hematomas and bleeding into joint spaces after minimal trauma.
- *Skeletal changes* occur because of inadequate formation of osteoid matrix. There is no defect in mineralization.
- *Gingival* swelling and secondary bacterial periodontal infections occur.

- *Skin lesions* are characterized by a perifollicular, hyperkeratotic, papular rash.
- *Wound healing* is impaired.

FOLATE

Folates are essential cofactors in the transfer and use of single-carbon units in DNA synthesis. They are found in whole-wheat flour, beans, nuts, and leafy green vegetables. Folate is heat labile and depleted in cooked and processed foods. In the United States, 15 to 20% of adults have low serum folate. In developing countries with diets based on corn, folate deficiency is even more common. Some drugs (e.g., anticonvulsants), personal habits (e.g., ethanol use), and chronic diseases (malabsorption syndromes) interfere with folate absorption and metabolism and are associated with folate deficiency. Folate deficiency is associated with megaloblastic anemia and neural tube defects in the developing fetus. Combined folate and vitamin B_{12} deficiency has been postulated to contribute to the development of colon cancer.

MINERAL DEFICIENCIES

A number of minerals are essential for health. Of the trace elements found in the body, *only five—iron, zinc, copper, selenium, and iodine—have been associated with well-characterized deficiency states* (Table 10–13). Three influences are particularly relevant to mineral deficiencies:

1. Inadequate supplementation in preparations used for total parenteral nutrition
2. Interference with absorption by dietary constituents
3. Inborn errors of metabolism leading to abnormalities of absorption

Zinc deficiency is characterized by a distinctive rash most often around the eyes, nose, mouth, and distal parts called *acrodermatitis enteropathica*; growth retardation in children; and diminished reproductive capacity. *Selenium*, similar to vitamin E, protects against oxidative damage of membrane lipids. The deficiency of this element is known in China as *Keshan disease*, which presents as a congestive cardiomyopathy, mainly in children and young women. Comments on the role of these and other trace elements in health and disease are presented in Table 10–13.

Obesity (p. 452)

Obesity is a massive problem in the United States, where 25% of the population older than age 20 is clinically obese. Fat accumulation is measured in several ways:

- Some expression of weight in relation to height (e.g., body mass index; the body mass index is closely correlated with body fat)
- Skinfold measurements
- Various body circumferences, particularly the ratio of the waist-hip circumference.

A 20% excess in body weight imparts a health risk. The adverse health effects of obesity are related not only to the total body weight, but also to the distribution of stored fat. Central or visceral

Table 10-13. FUNCTIONS OF TRACE METALS AND DEFICIENCY SYNDROMES

Nutrient	Functions	Deficiency Syndromes
Iron	Essential component of hemoglobin as well as a number of iron-containing metalloenzymes	Hypochromic microcytic anemia
Zinc	Component of enzymes, principally oxidases	Acrodermatitis enteropathica, growth retardation, infertility
Iodine	Component of thyroid hormone	Goiter and hypothyroidism
Selenium	Component of glutathione peroxidase	Myopathy, rarely cardiomyopathy
Copper	Component of cytochrome peroxidase oxidase, dopamine β-hydroxylase, tyrosinase, lysyl oxidase, and unknown enzyme involved in cross-linking keratin	Muscle weakness, neurologic defects, hypopigmentation, abnormal collagen cross-linking
Manganese	Component of metalloenzymes, including oxidoreductases, hydrolases, and lipases	No well-defined deficiency syndrome
Fluoride	Mechanism unknown	Dental caries

241

fat is associated with a much greater health risk than is excess accumulation of fat in subcutaneous tissue.

Obesity is a disorder of *energy balance*. When food-derived energy chronically exceeds energy expenditure, the excess calories are stored as triglycerides in adipose tissue. The balance between intake and expenditure is controlled by neural and hormonal mechanisms (Fig. 10–5). Adipocytes communicate with the hypothalamic centers that control appetite and energy expenditure by secreting a polypeptide hormone called *leptin*. Leptin acts as an antiobesity factor by binding to and activating leptin receptors in the hypothalamus. These receptors suppress appetite and increase energy expenditure, physical activity, and production of heat. Leptin decreases secretion of the appetite stimulant neurotransmitter neuropeptide Y. In addition, through neuronal pathways, activation of leptin receptors in the hypothalamus increases the release of norepinephrine from sympathetic nerve terminals that innervate adipose tissue. Norepinephrine binds to the β_3-adrenergic receptors on fat cells and leads to increased metabolism of fatty acids and dissipation of the energy as heat.

Dysfunction of the leptin system likely plays a role in human obesity. The majority of obese patients have a high level of plasma leptin, indicating that there is some form of leptin resistance. Such resistance is most likely at the level of transport of leptin into the central nervous system or in abnormalities in hypothalamic pathways that are normally regulated by leptin. It is unlikely that mutational inactivation of the leptin gene or its downstream targets

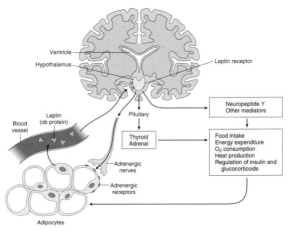

Figure 10–5 ■

The hormonal and neural circuits that regulate body weight. Adipocytes secrete a hormone called *leptin* in response to increased fat stores and hormones such as insulin and glucocorticoids. Leptin is transported to the hypothalamus through the circulation, where it binds to the leptin receptor. This interaction regulates energy balance by affecting food intake and energy expenditure. Leptin decreases secretion of neuropeptide Y. In addition, through neuronal pathways, the activation of leptin receptor in the hypothalamus increases the release of norepinephrine from sympathetic nerve terminals that innervate adipose tissue leading to increased metabolism of fatty acids and dissipation of the energy as heat. (Modified from Scott J: New chapter for the fat controller. Nature 379:113, 1996. Reprinted with permission from Nature. Copyright 1996 Macmillan Magazines Limited.)

accounts for most instances of human obesity, although it is possible that polymorphisms in these genes cause subtle alterations resulting in obesity. It is clear that genetic influences play an important role in weight control.

Obesity increases the risk for a number of conditions, including the following:

- *Diabetes*: Obesity is associated with insulin resistance and hyperinsulinemia found in non–insulin-dependent, or type II, diabetes (Chapter 20).
- *Cardiovascular disorders*: Hypertension, hypertriglyceridemia, and low HDL cholesterol all increase the risk of coronary artery disease.
- *Cholelithiasis* (gallstones): Gallstones are six times more common in obese than in lean individuals.
- *Hypoventilation or pickwickian syndrome*: This is a group of respiratory abnormalities in obese individuals. It is associated with hypersomnolence, polycythemia, and right-sided heart failure.
- *Osteoarthritis*: Osteoarthritis is due to the cumulative effects of added wear and tear on the joints.

The relationships between *obesity and stroke* and between *obesity and cancer* are controversial.

Diet and Systemic Diseases (p. 455)

The composition of the diet can make a substantial contribution to the initiation and progression of disease.

- *Atherogenesis*: Reduction in the consumption of cholesterol and saturated animal fats (e.g., eggs, butter, beef) may reduce serum cholesterol levels and delay the development of atherosclerosis and coronary artery disease. Lowering the level of saturated fatty acids in the diet by substituting vegetable or fish oils for animal fat decreases serum cholesterol. People who consume diets that contain fresh fruits and vegetables, with a limited intake of meats and processed foods, have a lower risk of myocardial infarction.
- *Hypertension*: Hypertension is beneficially affected by restricting sodium intake.
- *Diverticulosis*: Dietary fiber increases fecal bulk and may have a preventive effect against diverticulosis.
- *Colon cancer*: High animal fat combined with low fiber intake has been implicated in the development of colon cancer.

Calorie restriction has been demonstrated to increase life span in experimental animals (Chapter 2).

Chemoprevention of Cancer (p. 455)

Populations that consume large quantities of fruits and vegetables in their diets have a lower risk of some types of cancer. Although the mechanism for this effect is uncertain, it has been suggested that carotenoids, which are converted to vitamin A in the liver and intestine, may be important in the primary chemoprevention of cancer. The anticarcinogenic effect of the fruits and vegetables may be the result of the ability of retinoic acids to promote differentiation of some mucus-secreting epithelial tissue, provide an oxidant that prevents DNA damage, and enhance immune responses. Despite the many trends and proclamations, to date there is no definite proof that diet can cause or protect against cancer.

Diseases of Infancy and Childhood

In general, the conditions that afflict infants and children fall into one (and sometimes more) of four main categories:

1. Those that are primarily a consequence of the immaturity of an organ or system (e.g., hyaline membrane disease)
2. Those related to the unique susceptibility of the fetus or infant to external or environmental factors (some malformations, infections)
3. Those that are due to particular genetic or inherited defects
4. Tumors and tumor-like conditions

INTRAUTERINE GROWTH RETARDATION

(p. 461)

The majority of infants who suffer intrauterine growth retardation (IUGR) are also *small for gestational age*. Factors known to result in IUGR can be divided into three main categories:

1. *Fetal*: Chromosomal disorders (most commonly trisomy 13, 18, and 21; live-born monosomy X; and triploidy); congenital anomalies; and congenital infections (most commonly cytomegalovirus, rubella, syphilis, and toxoplasmosis) occur.
2. *Placental*: Conditions include abruptio placentae, placenta previa, placental thrombosis and infarctions, placental infections, umbilical-placental vascular anomalies, and multiple gestations. *Confined placental mosaicism* is another cause of IUGR. Two genetic populations of cells (usually one normal and one abnormal—i.e., trisomic) are present in the placenta or fetus, depending on when during gestation and in which cell population the genetic error occurs. The resultant phenotype may vary depending on whether the maternal or paternal copy of the gene or chromosome is involved *(genomic imprinting)*.
3. *Maternal* (most common): The underlying mechanism is decreased blood flow to the placenta. This decrease can be caused by toxemia of pregnancy, chronic hypertension, nutritional status, maternal narcotic abuse, alcohol intake, heavy cigarette smoking, and intake of certain drugs (which may also be teratogens), such as phenytoin (Dilantin).

IMMATURITY OF ORGAN SYSTEMS
(p. 462)

Structural and functional immaturity of organ systems is a major cause of morbidity and mortality in preterm infants, particularly those who are small for gestational age.

Morphology

- *Lungs*: Findings include thick-walled alveolar septa with large amounts of interlobular and intralobular connective tissue resulting in a separation of the vascular supply from alveolar spaces, hindering oxygenation. Alveolar spaces frequently contain eosinophilic proteinaceous precipitate and occasional squamous epithelial cells. Development of alveoli continues after birth, with the full complement of alveoli reached at approximately 8 years of age.
- *Kidneys*: Primitive glomeruli and tubules are often present in the subcapsular zone (nephrogenic zone). Deeper glomeruli and tubules are well formed, however, and function is usually adequate, even in the premature infant.
- *Brain*: Grossly the external surface of the brain is relatively smooth, with markedly simplified to absent convolutions (sulci and gyri). Both cell migration and myelination are incomplete, so the brain is soft and gelatinous, and there is poor demarcation of white and gray matter structures. Vital brain centers are well developed enough to sustain normal function even in the very premature infant, although maintenance of homeostasis (temperature, respiration) is imperfect.
- *Liver*: The liver is large relative to the size of the preterm infant, partially as a result of the presence of *extramedullary hematopoiesis*. Many liver enzymes are not well developed, including those responsible for biliary excretion, partly explaining the frequent presence of physiologic jaundice in premature infants.

APGAR SCORE (p. 463)

The Apgar score is a measure of the physiologic condition and responsiveness of the newborn infant, having some correlation with survival. It is calculated at 1 and 5 minutes of life based on heart rate, respiratory effort, muscle tone, response to noxious stimulus, and skin color, each scored 0, 1, or 2. The higher the score, the better the outlook.

BIRTH INJURIES (p. 464)

The risk and type of birth injury vary with the gestational age and size of the infant, with injuries most commonly involving the head, skeletal system, liver, adrenal glands, and peripheral nerves.

- *Intracranial hemorrhage* is the most common important birth injury. Predisposing factors include prolonged labor, hypoxia, hemorrhagic disorders, and intracranial vascular anomalies. Consequences of intracranial hemorrhage include increases in intracranial pressure, damage to brain substance, and herniation of the medulla or base of the brain into the foramen magnum, with depression of function of the vital medullary centers.
- *Caput succedaneum* is an accumulation of interstitial fluid in

the soft tissue of the scalp, resulting in a circular area of edema, congestion, and swelling at the site where the head begins to enter the lower uterine canal. If there is accompanying hemorrhage, it is referred to as a *cephalohematoma*. Both caput succedaneum and cephalohematoma are of little clinical significance unless associated with an underlying skull fracture.

CONGENITAL MALFORMATIONS (p. 464)

Congenital malformations are defined as morphologic defects present at birth, although they may not become apparent until later in life. About 3% of newborn infants have a major malformation. These malformations represent a major cause of infant mortality and a significant cause of illness, disability, and death in the early years of life.

DEFINITIONS

Malformations   Intrinsic abnormalities occurring relatively early during the developmental process. They may involve single or multiple organ systems. Risk of recurrence varies.

Deformations   These arise relatively late in fetal life as a result of mechanical factors. They usually manifest as abnormalities in shape, form, or position of the body (e.g., clubfeet). Most are associated with a much lower risk of recurrence in subsequent siblings than are malformations. *The most common underlying factor is uterine constraint.* Predisposing factors are both maternal (e.g., first pregnancy, uterine leiomyomas) and fetal/placental (e.g., oligohydramnios, multiple fetuses, abnormal fetal presentation).

Disruptions   These result from secondary destruction or interference with an organ or body region that was previously normal in development. Disruptions may be caused by either external or internal interferences (e.g., amniotic bands). They are not heritable.

Sequence   A series of multiple congenital anomalies resulting from a single localized aberration in organogenesis leading to secondary effects in other organs. The primary abnormality may be a malformation, deformation, or disruption. A good example is the *oligohydramnios (Potter) sequence*: Diverse factors, such as renal agenesis or an amniotic leak, result in decreased amniotic fluid (oligohydramnios), compression of the fetus, and a classic phenotype in the newborn infant, including flattened facies and positional abnormalities of the hands and feet (Fig. 11–6 in *Robbins Pathologic Basis of Disease*).

Syndrome   Several defects are present that are thought to be pathogenetically related but cannot be explained on the basis of a single, localized initiating anomaly. They are most often caused by a single etiologic agent (e.g., viral infection or chromosomal abnormality) that simultaneously affects several tissues. When the underlying cause of a syndrome is known, such as neurofibromatosis in a child with café-au-lait spots and numerous soft tissue masses, the syndrome is referred to as a *disease*.

In contrast to the above-listed global definitions, *organ-specific terms* include the following:

Agenesis   Complete absence of an organ and its associated primordium.

Aplasia   Absence of an organ because of failure of the developmental anlage to develop.

Atresia   Absence of an opening, usually of a hollow visceral organ, such as the trachea or intestine.

Hypoplasia   Incomplete development or underdevelopment of an organ, with decreased numbers of cells (less severe form of aplasia).

Hyperplasia   Overdevelopment of an organ associated with increased numbers of cells.

Hypertrophy   Increase in organ size or function related to an increase in the size of individual cells.

Hypotrophy   Decrease in organ size or function related to a decrease in the size of individual cells.

Dysplasia   In the context of malformations, refers to abnormal organization of individual cells.

Causes of Malformations

The exact cause of a malformation is known in approximately half of cases.

GENETIC CAUSES

- *Karyotypic abnormalities*: Present in approximately 10 to 15% of live-born infants with congenital malformations; trisomy 21 is most common, followed by Klinefelter syndrome (47,XXY), Turner syndrome (45,XO), and trisomy 13. Most cytogenetic aberrations arise as defects in gametogenesis and so are not familial.
- *Single-gene mutations* of large effect: Relatively uncommon but follow mendelian patterns of inheritance.
- *Multifactorial*: Interaction of two or more genes of small effect with environmental factors.

ENVIRONMENTAL CAUSES

The presence and nature of malformations resulting from environmental factors are related to the timing of the intrauterine exposure and the differential susceptibility of various organ systems (Fig. 11–7, p. 468, in *Robbins Pathologic Basis of Disease*).

- *Viruses*
  - *Cytomegalovirus* (most common fetal viral infection): Highest risk for malformations occurs with infection in second trimester when organogenesis is largely complete; most commonly affects the central nervous system resulting in mental retardation, microcephaly, and deafness.
  - *Rubella*: Infection before 16 weeks' gestation may result in cataracts, heart defects, and deafness.
  - *Herpes simplex*

- *Drugs and chemicals*: Probably cause less than 1% of congenital malformations; agents suspected to be teratogenic include thalidomide, folate antagonists, androgenic hormones, alcohol, anticonvulsants, and 13-*cis*-retinoic acid.
- *Radiation*: Exposure to heavy doses during organogenesis can result in malformations, including microcephaly, blindness, skull defects, and spina bifida.

Mechanisms of Malformations

The pathogenesis of many congenital malformations is complex and poorly understood. The following principles are important:

- The *timing* of the prenatal teratogenic insult has an important impact on the occurrence and type of malformation produced—a given agent may produce different malformations if exposure occurs at different times of gestation.
- Teratogens and genetic defects *may act at several levels*, including cell proliferation, cell migration, differentiation, and damage to formed differentiated organs.
- Genetic defects *may cause malformations either directly or by influencing other genes*; an example of the latter is the group of morphogenesis genes, in particular, the *homeobox genes* and the *paired box* or *PAX genes*, which have proximal regulatory influences and distal target genes.

PERINATAL INFECTIONS (p. 470)

Specific infections are discussed in Chapter 8.

Transcervical or Ascending Infections
(p. 470)

Most bacterial and a few viral infections are acquired via the cervicovaginal route. They may be acquired either in utero by *inhalation* into the lungs of infected amniotic fluid or around the time of birth by passing through an infected birth canal. *Chorioamnionitis* of the placental membranes and *funisitis* (inflammation of the umbilical cord) are usually present. Pneumonia, sepsis, and frequently meningitis are the most common sequelae.

Transplacental or Hematologic Infections
(p. 470)

Most parasites and viral infections and a few bacterial infections gain access to the fetal bloodstream via the chorionic villi. Infection may occur at any time during gestation or, occasionally, at the time of delivery via maternal-to-fetal transfusion. Sequelae are highly variable, depending on the gestational timing and microorganism.

NEONATAL RESPIRATORY DISTRESS SYNDROME (p. 471)

Neonatal respiratory distress syndrome (RDS) may have many causes, including aspiration during birth of blood and amniotic fluid, brain injury with failure of central respiratory centers, asphyxiating coils of umbilical cord around the neck of the infant, and excessive maternal sedation. *Idiopathic RDS*, also known as *hyaline membrane disease*, is most important.

Etiology and Pathogenesis

RDS occurs primarily in the immature lung—60% incidence in infants born at less than 28 weeks' gestation and less than 5% incidence in infants born at greater than 37 weeks' gestation. RDS is associated with a deficiency of pulmonary surfactant, which is synthesized by type II pneumocytes, most abundant after 35 weeks' gestation (Chapter 15). Decreased surfactant results in increased alveolar surface tension with progressive atelectasis of alveoli and a higher inspiratory pressure required to expand the alveolus (hence respiratory distress). Hypoxemia results in acidosis, pulmonary vasoconstriction, pulmonary hypoperfusion, capillary endothelial and alveolar epithelial damage, and leak of plasma into the alveolus, which combines with fibrin and necrotic alveolar pneumocytes to form hyaline membranes. Corticosteroids help prevent RDS; they induce the formation of surfactant lipids and apoprotein in fetal lung.

Morphology

Grossly, lungs are solid, airless, and reddish purple. Microscopically, alveoli are poorly developed and frequently collapsed, and pink hyaline membranes line respiratory bronchioles, alveolar ducts, and random alveoli.

Clinical Presentation

The typical infant with RDS is preterm but appropriate for gestational age. The condition is associated with maternal diabetes (surfactant synthesis may be suppressed by high blood levels of insulin) and cesarean section delivery.

Before delivery, assessment of amniotic fluid phospholipids (lecithin/sphingomyelin ratio) is often performed in preterm infants as an indicator of the fetal level of surfactant synthesis. When the surfactant level is low, glucocorticoids may be administered in an attempt to induce surfactant synthesis. At birth, the infant may need to be resuscitated but quickly establishes spontaneous rhythmic breathing and normal color for a short period of time; shortly thereafter, respiratory distress ensues, the infant becomes cyanotic, and diffuse reticulogranular densities radiographically (ground-glass appearance) characterize the lungs. Oxygen therapy may alleviate the symptoms, but in some cases respiratory distress persists; cyanosis increases; and the infant becomes flaccid, unresponsive, and apneic. Surfactant replacement is often administered while ventilatory assistance is provided. In uncomplicated cases, recovery begins in 3 to 4 days. Infants who recover are at risk for developing *retinopathy of prematurity* (Chapter 29), *retrolental fibroplasia*, and *bronchopulmonary dysplasia* as a direct consequence of high-concentration oxygen therapy. Infants are also at risk for developing patent ductus arteriosus, intraventricular hemorrhage, and necrotizing enterocolitis.

ERYTHROBLASTOSIS FETALIS (HEMOLYTIC DISEASE OF THE NEWBORN) (p. 473)

Hemolytic disease of the newborn occurs as a consequence of blood group incompatibility between mother and fetus.

Etiology and Pathogenesis

The fetus inherits red blood cell antigens from the father (i.e., the D antigen of the Rh group), which the mother lacks. A small transplacental (fetal/maternal) bleed (usually occurring at the time of delivery) allows fetal red blood cells to enter the maternal circulation and to elicit an immune response with maternal antibody production in response to this *foreign* antigen (only a minority of foreign blood group antigens are immunogenic). The first exposure to the specific antigenic stimulus elicits primarily production of IgM antibodies that do not cross the placenta; however, the mother is now *sensitized* to this antigen. Subsequent exposures to even small amounts of the same antigen (usually small transplacental bleeds occurring in subsequent pregnancies) elicit maternal production of IgG antibodies that *do* cross the placenta and bind to fetal red blood cells, resulting in red blood cell lysis.

Of the numerous Rh antigens, the D antigen is the major cause of Rh incompatibility (D antigen positive is referred to as *Rh-positive*; D antigen negative is referred to as *Rh-negative*). In Rh-negative mothers, immunoprophylaxis with anti-D immunoglobulin prevents sensitization and hemolytic disease of the newborn in the majority of cases. Although ABO incompatibility is more common than Rh incompatibility, hemolytic disease severe enough to require treatment is rare; this is primarily because

1. Most anti-A and anti-B antibodies are of the IgM type and do not cross the placenta.
2. Neonatal red cells express blood group antigens A and B poorly.
3. Many cells in addition to red cells express A and B antigens and therefore *sop up* some of the antibody that does gain access to the fetal bloodstream.

ABO hemolytic disease occurs almost exclusively in infants born to group O mothers, and there is no effective protection. Depending on the amount of IgG production and therefore fetal red blood cell lysis in erythroblastosis fetalis, the main consequences are anemia and the accumulation of bilirubin (jaundice). If hemolysis is mild, extramedullary hematopoiesis in the liver and spleen may suffice to maintain normal red cell levels. If hemolysis is marked, the presence of unconjugated bilirubin occurs; unconjugated bilirubin is water insoluble and has an affinity for lipids, binding to lipids in the brain and causing central nervous system damage referred to as *kernicterus*. If anemia is marked, hypoxic injury to the heart and liver may result in circulatory and hepatic failure and edema; when generalized edema and anasarca are present, the condition is referred to as *hydrops fetalis* (this is only one of many causes of hydrops fetalis (Table 11–5, p. 474, in *Robbins Pathologic Basis of Disease*).

Morphology

The morphologic findings vary with the severity of the hemolytic process. In general, there is evidence of abnormally increased erythropoietic activity. The red cell series in the bone marrow is hyperplastic, and there is extramedullary hematopoiesis in the liver, spleen, and frequently other tissues, such as lymph nodes, kidneys, lungs, and even heart. In jaundiced infants, the unconjugated bilirubin appears to be particularly toxic to the central nervous system. The brain is heavy and edematous, and there is bright yellow staining (*kernicterus*) localized particularly to the basal ganglia, thalamus, cerebellum, cerebral gray matter, and spinal cord. Although neural damage rarely occurs if the serum bilirubin concentration is less than 20 mg/dl, damage may occur at lower levels if the infant is premature. The gross presence of hydrops fetalis correlates with extensive subcutaneous and visceral edema, along with fluid in the peritoneal, pleural, and pericardial cavities.

INBORN ERRORS OF METABOLISM AND OTHER GENETIC DISORDERS (p. 475)

Only a few representative diseases occurring in the neonatal and childhood period are discussed in this chapter.

Phenylketonuria (p. 475)

Approximately 50% of dietary phenylalanine is required for protein synthesis; the remainder is converted into tyrosine by the phenylalanine hydroxylase system. Homozygotes for one of several different mutations in the *phenylalanine hydroxylase gene* display variable degrees of phenylalanine hydroxylase deficiency and hyperphenylalaninemia, accounting for several clinical variants. The most common mutation, *classic phenylketonuria (PKU)*, is relatively common in people of Scandinavian descent and uncommon in blacks and Jews.

Affected infants are relatively normal at birth but develop rising plasma phenylalanine levels within the first few weeks of life, resulting in impairment of brain development and mental retardation. Screens at birth for abnormally elevated levels of various phenylalanine metabolites in the urine result in early diagnosis of PKU; dietary restriction of phenylalanine can alleviate most of the clinical sequelae. Phenylalanine and its metabolites are teratogenic—most heterozygous infants born to mothers with PKU and high phenylalanine levels are microcephalic and mentally retarded *(maternal PKU)*.

Some mutations in the phenylalanine hydroxylase gene result in only a partial deficiency of phenylalanine hydroxylase and only moderately elevated serum levels of phenylalanine; these patients suffer no neurologic sequelae—the condition is referred to as *benign hyperphenylalaninemia. Other variants of PKU result from deficiencies in enzymes in the phenylalanine hydroxylase system other than phenylalanine hydroxylase; these patients have problems metabolizing other amino acids in addition to phenylalanine (such as tyrosine and tryptophan) and need to be diagnosed because restriction of dietary phenylalanine is not sufficient treatment.*

Galactosemia (p. 476)

Dietary lactose, present in milk, is split into glucose and galactose in the intestinal mucosa by lactase; galactose is then converted to glucose by three additional enzymes. The most common and clinically significant form of galactosemia is an autosomal recessive condition resulting from a homozygously inherited mutation in galactose-1-phosphate uridyl transferase (GALT) and subsequent accumulation of galactose-1-phosphate.

The clinical picture of galactosemia is variable, probably corresponding to several different mutations in GALT, but infants fail to thrive at birth and develop vomiting and diarrhea within a few days of milk ingestion. Liver, eyes, and brain are most severely affected, and the spectrum of morphologic changes includes early fatty change in the liver and hepatomegaly, which is followed by cirrhosis, cataracts, and nonspecific alterations in the central nervous system (the last-mentioned resulting in mental retardation).

Urinary screening tests at birth reveal the presence of an abnormal reducing sugar, and antenatal diagnosis is possible. Removal of dietary galactose for at least the first 2 years of life prevents most of the clinical and morphologic sequelae. Older patients, however, are frequently affected by a speech disorder and gonadal failure, possibly related to elevated levels of galactitol and galactonate that tend to persist despite dietary compliance.

Cystic Fibrosis (p. 477)

Cystic fibrosis is the most common lethal genetic disease that affects white populations, with an incidence of approximately 1 in 2000 live births. This widespread disorder occurs in the secretory process of all exocrine glands, affecting both mucus-secreting and eccrine sweat glands throughout the body.

ETIOLOGY AND PATHOGENESIS

The cystic fibrosis gene on *chromosome 7* encodes a protein named *CFTR* (cystic fibrosis transmembrane conductance regulator) that serves as a *chloride channel*. Various mutations in this gene disrupt epithelial chloride transport because normal duct epithelia require chloride channels for resorption of chloride and, conversely, normal airway epithelium requires chloride channels for secretion of chloride. The inability of the sweat gland ducts to resorb chloride results in an *increased sweat chloride concentration* (forming the basis of the clinical *sweat chloride* test used in the diagnosis of cystic fibrosis). The inability of airway epithelia to secrete chloride into the lumen, combined with a decrease in active sodium absorption, results in increased water reabsorption from the lumen; dehydration of the mucus layer coating the mucosal cells; defective mucociliary action; and the ultimate accumulation of hyperconcentrated, viscid secretions that obstruct the airways and predispose to recurrent pulmonary infections. In addition, there is evidence that the changes in secretions interface with antibacterial moieties produced by epithelial cells.

CFTR has two transmembrane domains, two nucleotide-binding domains, and a regulatory domain that contains protein kinase phosphorylation sites. Various mutations in the cystic fibrosis gene affect different regions of CFTR, resulting in different functional consequences that ultimately manifest as differences in the severity of clinical sequelae. At least 550 mutations of the cystic fibrosis gene have been identified, with the most common being the deletion of three nucleotides coding for phenylalanine at position 508, known as *delta F508*; this results in defective processing of the CFTR protein and its degradation before it reaches the cell surface. Virtual absence of CFTR results in severe clinical disease, including early pancreatic insufficiency and various degrees of pulmonary damage. Other mutations may be involved with milder disease and some with male sterility only. For most mutations, reliable prediction of clinical outcome based on genotype is not possible, although there is a correlation between the percentage of normal residual CFTR function and the presence of disease in various organs.

MORPHOLOGY

Morphologic findings are highly variable depending on which glands are affected and the severity of involvement.

- *Pancreas*: Abnormalities are present in approximately 90% of patients; changes range from accumulation of mucus in small ducts and mild dilation of exocrine glands to total atrophy of the exocrine glands and ducts, leaving only the islets within a fibrofatty stroma. Absence of pancreatic exocrine secretions impairs fat absorption, and there is resulting avitaminosis A, which may be partially responsible for squamous metaplasia frequently observed in ductal structures.
- *Intestine*: Thick viscid plugs of mucus may cause small intestinal obstruction in 5 to 10% of infants with cystic fibrosis, a condition known as *meconium ileus*.
- *Liver*: Plugging of bile canaliculi by mucinous material occurs; in approximately 5% of patients, this ultimately results in cirrhosis.
- *Salivary glands*: Salivary glands are frequently involved; progressive dilation of ducts, squamous metaplasia of ductal epithelium, and glandular atrophy occur.
- *Lungs*: Changes are seen in most cases and are the most serious complication of cystic fibrosis. There is hyperplasia of mucus-secreting cells, and thick secretions block and dilate bronchioles. Superimposed infections and even pulmonary abscesses are common, frequently resulting from *Staphylococcus aureus* or *Pseudomonas aeruginosa* or both; *Pseudomonas cepacia* infections have been associated with fulminant illness.
- *Epididymis and vas deferens*: Obstruction by thick secretions is responsible for azoospermia and infertility in 95% of males surviving to adulthood.

CLINICAL COURSE

The molecular variability and complexity, including secondary pathogenetic mechanisms, that underlie cystic fibrosis result in highly variable clinical manifestations, with symptoms ranging from mild to severe and onset occurring at birth to years later. Manifestations of malabsorption include large, foul-smelling stools; abdominal distention; and poor weight gain and usually appear during the first year of life. Faulty fat absorption results in deficiencies of the fat-soluble vitamins A, D, and K. Persistent pulmonary infections account for 80 to 90% of deaths; other pulmonary problems include obstructive pulmonary disease, chronic cough, and cor pulmonale; cystic fibrosis is the most common underlying diagnosis in children and adolescents undergoing bilateral lung transplantation. Median life expectancy is approximately 26 years, but this may be modified by gene therapy (transfer of the CFTR gene to correct the chloride defect in cells) in the future.

SUDDEN INFANT DEATH SYNDROME
(p. 481)

Sudden infant death syndrome (SIDS) is officially defined as the *"sudden death of an infant under 1 year of age which remains unexplained after a thorough case investigation, including performance of a complete autopsy, examination of the death scene, and review of the clinical history."* Moreover, most SIDS deaths occur between 2 and 4 months of life; the infant usually dies while asleep, and there is no evidence of distress or a struggle.

Most SIDS victims have had symptoms of minor upper respiratory infection. The pathogenesis remains poorly understood, and SIDS is most likely a heterogeneous, multifactorial disorder; approximately 10% of cases may be due to an underlying inborn error in metabolism. Potential risk factors include infant sleeping in a prone position, prematurity and low birth weight, infant not firstborn or product of a multiple gestation mother, SIDS in a prior sibling, young or unmarried mother, low socioeconomic status, short intergestational interval, and maternal smoking or drug abuse. Current work suggests developmental *immaturity* of critical hypothalamic centers involved in cardiopulmonary function may play a role.

Autopsy findings are usually subtle and of uncertain significance. They include astrogliosis of the brain stem, thymic and epicardial petechiae, and, frequently, evidence of a mild recent respiratory infection.

TUMORS AND TUMOR-LIKE LESIONS OF INFANCY AND CHILDHOOD (p. 482)

Benign tumors are much more common than malignant tumors, but cancer is the leading cause of death from disease in U.S. children between the ages of 4 and 14 years.

Benign Tumors and Tumor-Like Lesions
(p. 483)

It is frequently difficult to distinguish between true tumors and tumor-like lesions in the infant and child because displaced cells and masses of tissue may be present from birth that are histologically normal in appearance but nonetheless grow at approximately the same rate as the fetus and infant.

- *Heterotopia* is defined as microscopically normal cells or tissues that are present in abnormal locations; these cells are usually of little significance but may be clinically confused with true neoplasms.
- *Hamartomas* are excessive (but focal) overgrowth of cells and tissues native to the organ or site in which they occur; these can be thought of as the linkage between malformations and neoplasms.

HEMANGIOMAS

Hemangiomas are the most common tumors of infancy; they rarely become malignant. Most are located in the skin, particularly the face and scalp. They may enlarge along with the growth of the child, but commonly they spontaneously regress. Hemangiomas may represent one facet of a hereditary disorder such as *von Hippel-Lindau disease* (Chapter 29).

LYMPHANGIOMAS

Lymphangiomas may occur on the skin but also occur in the deeper regions of the neck, axilla, mediastinum, and retroperitoneal tissue. They tend to increase in size after birth and, depending on the location, become clinically significant if they encroach on vital structures. Histologically, lymphangiomas are composed of cystic and cavernous lymphatic spaces, with variable numbers of lymphocytes in the adjacent soft tissue.

FIBROUS TUMORS

Histologically, fibrous tumors range from sparsely cellular proliferations (fibromatosis) to richly cellular lesions indistinguishable from fibrosarcomas occurring in adults. In contrast to fibrous tumors occurring in adults, histology does not predict the biology of an individual tumor (e.g., *infantile fibrosarcoma* may spontaneously regress).

TERATOMAS

The incidence of teratoma has two peaks: one at 2 years of age and one in late adolescence. Most of those occurring in infancy and childhood arise in the sacrococcygeal region.

- Approximately 10% of sacrococcygeal teratomas are associated with congenital anomalies, primarily defects of the hindgut and cloacal region and other midline defects.
- Sacrococcygeal teratomas are histologically similar to other teratomas (Chapter 24 in *Robbins Pathologic Basis of Disease*) in that mesodermal, endodermal, and ectodermal elements are present. Approximately 75% contain mature tissues only and are benign; approximately half of the remainder are mixed with other germ cell malignancies (e.g., endodermal sinus tumor) and are malignant; the rest, designated *immature teratomas*, contain mature and immature tissue, and the malignant potential correlates with the amount of immature tissue elements present.

Malignant Tumors (p. 484)

Malignant tumors not discussed in this section are discussed in the organ system chapter from which they arise. Childhood malignancies differ biologically and histologically from their counterparts occurring later in life.

- There is a close relationship between abnormal development (teratogenesis) and tumor induction (oncogenesis).
- There is a greater prevalence of an underlying familial or genetic germ line aberration.
- There is a tendency for some histologic *malignancies* occurring in the fetal or neonatal period to regress spontaneously or cytodifferentiate.

The most frequent childhood cancers arise in the hematopoietic system (leukemia, some lymphomas), central nervous system (astrocytoma, medulloblastoma, ependymoma), adrenal medulla (neuroblastoma), retina (retinoblastoma), soft tissue (rhabdomyosarcoma), bone (Ewing sarcoma, osteogenetic sarcoma), and kidney (Wilms tumor). Leukemia accounts for more deaths in children younger than 15 years of age than all other tumors combined.

Histologically, many pediatric cancers tend to have a more primitive (embryonal) rather than anaplastic/pleomorphic appearance, frequently exhibiting features of organogenesis specific to the site of tumor origin. Some pediatric tumors with a primitive appearance are collectively referred to as *small, round blue cell tumors*—neuroblastoma, lymphoma, rhabdomyosarcoma, Ewing sarcoma/peripheral neuroectodermal tumor (PNET).

NEUROBLASTOMA AND GANGLIONEUROMA (p. 485)

The vast majority of neuroblastomas and ganglioneuromas occur in children younger than 5 years of age. They arise in the adrenal medulla or various ganglia and are made up of sheets of small, round blue cells within a neurofibrillary background and the presence of (Homer-Wright) pseudorosettes. Some tumors and tumor cells display variable amounts of differentiation toward ganglion cells, and, depending on the degree of differentiation, they are called *ganglioneuroblastomas* or *ganglioneuromas.*

Depending on the pattern of metastases, tumors are staged I (confined to the organ of origin) through IV (disseminated metastases). Stage IV/S tumors are unique; they usually occur in young infants or neonates, and there is a small adrenal tumor, a markedly enlarged liver from extensive liver metastases, and tumor nodules within the skin and bone marrow (without causing bony destruction). Infants with these disseminated tumors have a greater than 80% 5-year survival with minimal to no therapy.

In addition to higher stage (except IV/S) and older age, a worse prognosis is associated with near-diploid or near-tetraploid overall DNA content, deletions of the distal short arm of chromosome 1 (implying loss of tumor-suppressor gene function), and amplification of the n-*myc* oncogene. Expression of high levels of *Trk A* may also be associated with a more favorable outcome.

WILMS TUMOR (p. 487)

Wilms tumor is a tumor of the kidney that is usually diagnosed between 2 and 5 years of age. Although it is malignant, overall survival rate is greater than 90%. In addition to the many *sporadic* cases, there are associations with at least three groups of malformation syndromes, all involving aberrations in chromosome 11p:

1. *WAGR* (*W*ilms tumor, *a*niridia, *g*enital anomalies, mental *r*etardation): Patients with this syndrome have a 33% chance of developing Wilms tumor; WAGR involves *deletion on chromosome 11p band 13 of the Wilms tumor 1 (WT-1) gene* and also the *aniridia gene*, which is just distal to this locus (transgenic mice lacking both copies of the WT-1 locus have renal agenesis).

2. *Denys-Drash syndrome*: Patients have gonadal dysgenesis and nephropathy leading to renal failure, and most develop Wilms tumors; the genetic abnormality is a *dominant negative mutation in the WT-1 gene* that affects its DNA binding properties.

3. *Beckwith-Wiedemann syndrome*: Patients have enlargement of body organs, hemihypertrophy, renal medullary cysts, adrenal cytomegaly, and a predisposition to developing Wilms tumors and other primitive tumors; genetic abnormality (probably a deletion) is localized to *chromosome 11 band p15.5 (the Wilms tumor 2 [WT-2] gene)*; the function of the gene is unknown, but there may be a role for genomic imprinting in the pathogenesis of these cases because there is selected loss of maternal alleles in the group of Wilms tumors.

Morphologically the tumors are soft, frequently large, well-circumscribed renal masses characterized by triphasic histologic features of (1) blastema, (2) immature stroma, and (3) tubules—an attempt to recapitulate nephrogenesis. The histologic presence of *anaplasia*, observed in approximately 5% of tumors, is associated with a worse prognosis. *Nephroblastomatosis* is a *premalignant* or precursor lesion observed in the kidney. As noted, the prognosis with appropriate chemotherapy is now excellent, with long-term survival in greater than 90% of patients.

Diseases of the Blood Vessels

Pathologic changes in blood vessels most frequently have the following consequences:

- Narrowing or completely obstructing the lumens of vessels, either slowly (e.g., by atherosclerosis) or precipitously (e.g., by thrombosis or embolism), and thus restricting blood flow to a tissue or organ. The restriction of blood flow may induce atrophy or infarction in the tissue supplied by the narrowed vessel depending on the rate of development and severity of the narrowing.
- Weakening of the walls of vessels, leading to dilation, dissection, or rupture.

CONGENITAL ANOMALIES (p. 498)

Congenital anomalies include the following conditions:

- *Anomalous (e.g., aberrant, reduplicated) vessels* are principally of interest to surgeons.
- *Berry aneurysms* are outpouchings of vessels as a result of congenital focal wall weakness. They occur exclusively in cerebral vessels and occasionally rupture catastrophically.
- *Arteriovenous fistula* is an abnormal communication between artery and vein. It may be congenital or secondary to trauma, inflammation, or healed ruptured aneurysm. Fistulas may cause left-to-right vascular shunts, increasing venous return and predisposing to heart failure.

ARTERIOSCLEROSIS (p. 498)

Arteriosclerosis denotes thickening and loss of elasticity of arterial walls. The three types of arteriosclerosis are

1. Atherosclerosis
2. Monckeberg arteriosclerosis
3. Arteriolosclerosis (the latter primarily associated with hypertension and discussed in that context)

Atherosclerosis (p. 498)

Atherosclerosis is a slowly progressive disease of arteries, marked by elevated *fibrofatty intimal plaques*, formed by lipid deposition, smooth muscle cell proliferation, and synthesis of extracellular matrix in the intima. Large to medium-sized muscular and large elastic arteries are involved, principally in the abdominal aorta, coronary arteries, popliteal arteries, descending thoracic aorta, internal carotid arteries, and circle of Willis (in descending order of frequency). Lesions initially tend to be focal, only partially involving the vessel circumference, and are patchy along its length.

Atherosclerosis may begin in childhood but typically manifests in middle age or later life either as the vessel lumen is compromised, predisposing to thrombosis, or as the underlying media is thinned, predisposing to aneurysm formation. Fifty percent of all deaths in the United States are attributed to atherosclerosis, half resulting from myocardial infarction or sudden death in ischemic heart disease and the remainder from cerebrovascular accidents (stroke), aneurysm rupture, mesenteric occlusion, and gangrene of the extremities.

EPIDEMIOLOGY

Risk of the development of atherosclerosis increases with age, family history, hypertension, cigarette smoking, hypercholesterolemia, and diabetes—the last four often called the *major risk factors.*

The risk is correlated with the level of serum low-density lipoprotein (LDL), formed from the catabolism of very-low-density lipoprotein (VLDL). LDL carries 70% of the total serum cholesterol. Risk is *inversely* related to high-density lipoprotein (HDL) levels, perhaps because HDL helps clear cholesterol from vessel wall lesions. Hereditary defects involving the LDL receptor (e.g., in familial hypercholesterolemia) or LDL apoproteins cause elevated LDL, hypercholesterolemia, and accelerated atherosclerosis. Lesser or unquantified influences on the risk of atherosclerosis include obesity, sedentary or high-stress life style, type A personality, and the other factors listed in Table 12–1.

Table 12–1.   RISK FACTORS FOR ATHEROSCLEROSIS

Major
Nonmodifiable
  Increasing age
  Male gender
  Family history
Potentially controllable
  Hyperlipidemia (hypercholesterolemia, hypertriglyceridemia)
  Hypertension
  Cigarette smoking
  Diabetes

Lesser or Yet Uncertain Significance
Obesity
Low HDL
Physical inactivity
Stress (*type A* personality)
Postmenopausal estrogen deficiency
High carbohydrate intake
Alcohol
Homocysteine
Lipoprotein(a)
Impaired fibrinolysis
Chronic inflammation
Hardened (trans) unsaturated fat intake
Chlamydia pneumoniae or other infection

MORPHOLOGY

The characteristic atheromatous plaque *(atheroma)* is a raised white-yellow intimal lesion, protruding into the vessel lumen. *Histologically* the typical atheroma (also called *fibrofatty plaque*) is composed of a superficial *fibrous cap*, containing smooth muscle cells, leukocytes, and dense connective tissue extracellular matrix overlying a *necrotic core*, containing dead cells, lipid, cholesterol clefts, lipid-laden foam cells (macrophages and smooth muscle cells), and plasma proteins. In the periphery are proliferating small blood vessels. In addition, two common variants are as follows:

- *Fatty streaks*: Intimal collections of lipid-laden macrophages and smooth muscle cells, occurring in patients as young as 1 year of age. A causal relationship of fatty streaks to subsequent atheromatous plaques is suspected but has not been proven.
- *Complicated plaques*: Calcified, hemorrhagic, fissured, or ulcerated atheromas, predisposing to local thrombosis, medial thinning, cholesterol microemboli, and aneurysmal dilation.

PATHOGENESIS

The cause of atherosclerosis remains unknown, but most theories invoke some damage to the endothelium or underlying media. The causes of endothelial cell injury include hyperlipidemia, hemodynamic disturbances (such as disturbed flow), smoking, hypertension, toxins, and potentially infectious agents. The most important consequences of endothelial injury are increased endothelial permeability, adhesion of white cells and platelets, and activation of coagulation. This is followed by release or activation of chemical mediators, such as growth factors, and migration and subsequent proliferation of smooth muscle cells in the intima to produce the atheroma.

The contemporary view of the pathogenesis of atherosclerosis, called the *response to injury hypothesis, considers atherosclerosis to be a chronic inflammatory response of the arterial wall initiated by some form of injury to the endothelium* (Fig. 12–1). Central to this thesis are the following events:

- The development of focal regions of chronic endothelial injury, usually subtle, with resultant endothelial dysfunction, such as increased endothelial permeability and increased leukocyte adhesion (via cell adhesion molecules, such as vascular cell adhesion molecule 1)
- Adhesion of blood monocytes and other leukocytes to foci of injured endothelium
- Migration of monocytes into the intima and their transformation into macrophages, which accumulate lipid and become foam cells
- Insudation of lipoproteins into the vessel wall at foci of endothelial injury, mainly LDL with its high cholesterol content and VLDL
- Oxidation of such lipoproteins by the accumulated macrophages
- Adhesion of platelets to focal areas of endothelial injury or denudation (when present) or to other leukocytes
- Release of factors such as platelet-derived growth factor from activated platelets, macrophages, or vascular cells that cause migration of smooth muscle cells from media into the intima
- Proliferation of smooth muscle cells in the intima and elaboration of extracellular matrix, leading to accumulation of collagen and proteoglycans

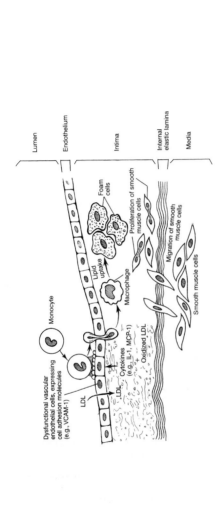

Figure 12-1

Schematic diagram of hypothetical sequence of events and cellular interactions in atherosclerosis. Hyperlipidemia, as well as other risk factors, is thought to cause endothelial injury resulting in adhesion of platelets and monocytes and release of growth factors, including platelet-derived growth factor (PDGF), which lead to smooth muscle cell migration and proliferation. Smooth muscle cells produce large amounts of collagen and proteoglycans, contributing to the atheromatous plaque. Foam cells of atheromatous plaques are derived from both macrophages and smooth muscle cells. Extracellular lipid is derived from insudation from the lumen, particularly in the presence of hypercholesterolemia, and from degenerating foam cells. Cholesterol accumulation in the plaque should be viewed as reflecting an imbalance between influx and efflux, and it is possible that high-density lipoprotein (HDL) helps clear cholesterol from these accumulations. (Modified from Libby P: Do vascular wall cytokines promote atherogenesis? Hosp Pract Oct. 15, 1992, p. 51.)

- Enhanced accumulation of lipids both within cells (macrophages and smooth muscle cells) and extracellularly

CLINICAL FEATURES

Atherosclerosis is asymptomatic for decades until it causes disease by the following mechanisms:

- Insidious narrowing of vascular lumens (e.g., gangrene of the lower leg because of stenosing atherosclerosis in the popliteal artery)
- Plaque rupture followed by superimposed thrombus causing sudden occlusion of the lumen (e.g., myocardial infarction precipitated by thrombotic occlusion of disrupted coronary arterial atheroma)
- Providing a source of embolic debris, known as *atheroembolism* (e.g., renal infarction resulting from cholesterol emboli originating in an ulcerated atherosclerotic aortic plaque)
- Weakening the wall of a vessel followed by aneurysm formation and possibly rupture (e.g., an abdominal aortic aneurysm)

Symptomatic atherosclerotic disease most often affects the heart, brain, kidneys, lower extremities, and small intestine.

Monckeberg Arteriosclerosis (Medial Calcific Sclerosis) (p. 498)

Monckeberg arteriosclerosis is characterized by focal calcifications in the *media* of small to medium-sized muscular arteries, without associated inflammation, largely sparing the intima and adventitia. The femoral, tibial, radial, and ulnar arteries and arteries of the genitalia are involved, typically after age 50. The process is unrelated to atherosclerosis but may occur concurrently. The pathogenesis is unknown. The calcific deposits are nonobstructive and otherwise of little clinical significance, but they may be visualized as vascular calcifications on radiographs of the extremities of older individuals.

HYPERTENSIVE VASCULAR DISEASE AND ARTERIOLOSCLEROSIS (p. 510)

Hypertension is the single most important risk factor in both coronary heart disease and cerebrovascular accidents; it may also lead directly to congestive heart failure (hypertensive heart disease), renal failure, and aortic dissection. When defined as diastolic blood pressure greater than 90 mm Hg and systolic blood pressure greater than 140 mm Hg, the prevalence of hypertension in the United States is about 25%.

About 90% of hypertension is primary and idiopathic (essential); the remaining is secondary and mostly related to renal disease or (less often) to renal artery stenosis (renovascular), endocrine abnormalities, vascular malformations, or neurogenic disorders. Causes and factors in the pathogenesis of essential and secondary hypertension are summarized in Table 12–2.

Regulation of Normal Blood Pressure (p. 511)

Blood pressure is a complex trait that is determined by the interaction of multiple genetic and environmental factors that

---

Table 12-2.   TYPES OF HYPERTENSION (SYSTOLIC
AND DIASTOLIC)

Primary, essential, or idiopathic hypertension
Secondary hypertension
   Renal
      Acute glomerulonephritis
      Chronic renal disease
      Polycystic disease
      Renal artery stenosis
      Renal vasculitis
      Renin-producing tumors
   Endocrine
      Adrenocortical hyperfunction (Cushing syndrome, primary
        aldosteronism, congenital adrenal hyperplasia)
      Estrogen hormones (glucocorticoids, estrogen [including pregnancy
        and oral contraceptive], sympathomimetics, tyramine-containing
        foods, monamine oxidase inhibitors)
      Pheochromocytoma
      Acromegaly
      Myxedema
      Thyrotoxicosis
   Cardiovascular
      Coartation of aorta
      Polyarteritis nodosa
      Aortic insufficiency
      Increased intravascular volume
      Increased cardiac output
      Rigidity of the aorta
   Neurologic
      Psychogenic
      Increased intracranial pressure
      Sleep apnea
      Acute stress, including surgery

---

*regulate the relationship between cardiac output and total periph-
eral resistance.*

- *Vasoconstriction increases vascular resistance.* Vasoconstrictors
  include angiotensin II, catecholamines, thromboxane, leukotrienes, and endothelin.
- Vasodilators include kinins, prostaglandins, nitric oxide, and
  adenosine.
- Regional *autoregulation* is also important, wherein increased
  blood flow leads to vasoconstriction and vice versa.
- Cardiac output is regulated by blood volume (affected by sodium load, mineralocorticoids, and natriuretic factors), heart
  rate, stroke volume, and contractility.

Mechanisms of Essential Hypertension

(p. 513)

Although unknown, the cause of essential hypertension at the
most elemental level must be related to a primary increase in
cardiac output (e.g., reduced renal sodium excretion) or to an
increase in peripheral resistance (e.g., owing to increased release of
vasoconstrictor agents, to increased sensitivity of vascular smooth
muscle cells, or to behavioral or neurogenic factors), or both
(i.e., an increase in cardiac output and an increase in peripheral
resistance). In most patients, multiple defects probably contribute.

Abnormalities in the renal mechanisms that regulate blood pressure also may contribute to essential hypertension, including

1. The renin-angiotensin system.
2. Sodium homeostasis.
3. Production of vasodepressor substances implicated in the pathogenesis of hypertension in unilateral renal artery stenosis and renal disease. For example, studies have suggested a propensity toward hypertension in individuals with specific molecular variants of the gene-encoding *angiotensinogen*, the physiologic substrate for renin.

Vascular Pathology in Hypertension (p. 514)

Hypertension accelerates atherogenesis and causes vascular structural changes that potentiate both aortic dissection and cerebrovascular hemorrhage. In addition, hypertension is associated with small vessel disease, primarily affecting arterioles and small arteries. The two basic types of arteriolosclerosis, *hyaline* and *hyperplastic*, are characterized by diffuse arteriolar wall thickening, luminal narrowing, and resultant ischemia of distal tissue.

HYALINE ARTERIOLOSCLEROSIS

Hyaline arteriolosclerosis occurs typically in elderly patients, particularly those with mild hypertension and mild diabetes. The lesion is thought to reflect endothelial injury, with subsequent leakage of plasma components into arteriolar walls and synthesis of extracellular matrix by smooth muscle cells. Microscopically, there is diffuse, pink, hyaline thickening of arteriolar walls. Hyaline arteriolosclerosis is the major microscopic feature of benign nephrosclerosis (p. 514).

HYPERPLASTIC ARTERIOLOSCLEROSIS

Hyperplastic arteriolosclerosis is characteristic of malignant hypertension (acute, severe elevations in blood pressure, p. 514). There is concentric laminated *(onionskin)* arteriolar thickening with reduplicated basement membrane and smooth muscle proliferation, frequently associated with fibrin deposition and wall necrosis—*necrotizing arteriolitis*.

INFLAMMATORY DISEASES: THE VASCULITIDES (p. 515)

Vasculitis (i.e., vascular inflammatory injury, often with necrosis) may be localized, as a result of direct injury (e.g., infection, trauma, toxins), or systemic, characterized by multifocal necrosis *(necrotizing vasculitis)* and thrombosis. Most systemic varieties of vasculitis are thought to have an immune origin, secondary to deposition of circulating antigen-antibody complexes (e.g., acute arteritis in serum sickness and systemic lupus erythematosus) (p. 516) or antibody to fixed tissue antigens (e.g., Goodpasture syndrome and Kawasaki disease) or delayed-type hypersensitivity reactions, especially in lesions with granulomas (e.g., temporal arteritis).

In many patients with vasculitis, the serum reacts with cytoplasmic antigens in neutrophils (by immunofluorescence and immunochemical assays), indicating the presence of *antineutrophilic cytoplasmic autoantibodies (ANCA)*. The pattern observed is either perinuclear (called *P-ANCA*), in which the major antigen is *myeloperoxidase*, or cytoplasmic (called *C-ANCA*), in which the leukocyte antigen is *proteinase 3*. Either ANCA specificity may occur in a patient with ANCA-associated vasculitis, but C-ANCA is most characteristic of Wegener granulomatosis, and P-ANCA is found in most cases of microscopic polyangiitis and Churg-Strauss syndrome. Approximately 10% of patients with these disorders do not demonstrate ANCA by typical assays, and moreover P-ANCA and C-ANCA can be found in other vasculitides as well. The close association between ANCA titers and disease activity, particularly C-ANCA in Wegener granulomatosis, suggests that they may be important in the pathogenesis of this disease, but the precise mechanisms by which ANCA induce injury are unknown. Classification of localized and systemic vasculitis reflects the pathogenesis, size, and site of the vessels involved, the histologic characteristics of the lesions, and the clinical manifestations (Fig. 12–2 and Table 12–2).

Giant Cell (Temporal) Arteritis (p. 516)

The most common form of vasculitis, giant cell (temporal) arteritis, is characterized by focal granulomatous inflammation of medium and small arteries, chiefly cranial vessels and most commonly the temporal arteries in elderly people. It may rarely involve the aortic arch *(giant cell aortitis)*. The cause is unknown.

Temporal arteritis typically presents with headache and facial pain; 50% of patients have systemic symptoms, including flulike syndrome with myalgias, arthralgias, and fever, called *polymyalgia rheumatica*. It may cause visual disturbances and even blindness (an acute emergency).

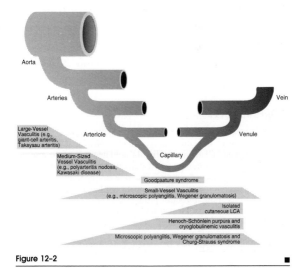

Figure 12–2 ∎

Diagrammatic representation of the parts of the vasculature involved by the major forms of systemic vasculitis. (From Jennette JC, Falk RJ: Small-vessel vasculitis. N Engl J Med *337*:1512, 1997.)

Morphologically, there may be one of three general appearances:

1. Granulomatous vasculitis with fragmented internal elastic lamina and a giant cell reaction to these fragments (two thirds of cases)
2. Nonspecific leukocytic infiltration by neutrophils, eosinophils, and lymphocytes of vessel walls
3. Intimal fibrosis with thickening of the walls and narrowing of lumens

These three patterns may represent stages in a continuum. There often is associated thrombosis.

Biopsy may be negative in one third of patients, presumably owing to the focality of the lesion. The disease responds well to steroids.

Takayasu Arteritis (p. 519)

Takayasu arteritis is a form of granulomatous vasculitis of medium to large arteries, characterized by fibrous thickening of the aortic arch with virtual obliteration of the mouths of the great vessels. The cause and pathogenesis remain unknown. This disease results in ocular disturbances, neurologic deficits, and markedly diminished upper extremity pulses. Occasionally (one third of cases), the disease involves the remainder of the aorta and its branches, and hypertension may occur with renal artery involvement. Another variant causes proximal aortic dilation with aortic valvular insufficiency. The condition is most common in Asia, in women 15 to 45 years of age.

Grossly, Takayasu arteritis produces irregular thickening of the aortic wall with intimal wrinkling. *Microscopically*, early stages show an adventitial perivascular (vasa vasorum) mononuclear cell infiltrate, followed in later stages by medial fibrosis, occasionally with granulomas and acellular intimal thickening. The morphologic changes may be indistinguishable from those of giant cell (temporal) arteritis.

Polyarteritis Nodosa (p. 520)

Polyarteritis nodosa (PAN) is a systemic disease characterized by necrotizing inflammation throughout the wall of various small to medium-sized arterial beds.

MORPHOLOGY

PAN lesions are sharply demarcated and often induce thrombosis, causing distal ischemic injury. *Microscopically*, acute lesions are segmental and characterized by fibrinoid necrosis of the arterial wall with an accompanying pan-vascular neutrophilic infiltrate that may extend into the adventitia. The process is sharply circumscribed and may not involve the entire circumference of the vessel. Healing lesions show fibroblast proliferation superimposed on ongoing fibrinoid necrosis. Healed lesions show only marked fibrotic thickening of the arterial wall, with associated elastic lamina fragmentation and sometimes aneurysmal dilation. Lesions at different histologic stages may be present concurrently.

CLINICAL FEATURES

Characteristically, PAN is a disease of young adults, with protean and nonspecific clinical signs and symptoms related to whatever tissue is involved (e.g., hematuria, albuminuria, and hypertension [kidneys]; abdominal pain and melena [gastrointestinal tract]; diffuse myalgias; and peripheral neuritis. The most common systemic manifestations include fever, malaise, and weight loss. PAN may be associated with *hepatitis B antigen*, and deposited immune complexes may play a role in pathogenesis.

The diagnosis is made by biopsy of affected arterial segments. Untreated, the disease is generally fatal, but a 90% cure or remission rate is achieved with immunosuppressive therapy.

Kawasaki Disease (Mucocutaneous Lymph Node Syndrome) (p. 521)

Kawasaki disease is an acute illness of infants and children characterized by fever; lymphadenopathy; skin rash; oral or conjunctival erythema; and (in 20% of cases) coronary arteritis, often with associated aneurysms. It is endemic in Japan but considerably less common in the United States.

Patients have numerous immunoregulatory disturbances, including T-cell activation, autoantibodies to endothelial cells, and circulating immune complexes, but the cause is unknown.

Morphologically the lesions resemble those of PAN. The disease typically is self-limited but rarely is fatal owing to coronary arteritis with subsequent aneurysm formation, thrombosis, or rupture leading to myocardial infarction. Aspirin and intravenous gamma globulin are thought to be helpful in reducing the long-term sequelae.

Microscopic Polyangiitis (Microscopic Polyarteritis, Leukocytoclastic Angiitis) (p. 521)

Microscopic polyangiitis may be distinguished from PAN by its involvement of smaller vessels (arterioles, capillaries, and venules), with lesions typically all synchronized to the same stage. This synchronization suggests an acute inciting agent (e.g., drugs, microorganisms, heterologous protein) forming immune complexes in a previously sensitized host. In general, the disease responds to removal of the offending agent.

Lesions may be confined to skin (cutaneous vasculitis) or may involve other sites, including lung, brain, heart, and kidneys. Fibrinoid necrosis often occurs, but affected vessels may reveal only fragmented neutrophilic nuclei within vessel walls and perivascularly *(leukocytoclastic angiitis)*.

A variant is *allergic granulomatosis and angiitis (Churg-Strauss syndrome)*, characterized by eosinophilia and bronchial asthma, with pulmonary and splenic vessel involvement and intravascular and extravascular granulomas. Specific syndromes with systemic hypersensitivity angiitis include Henoch-Schönlein purpura, essential mixed cryoglobulinemia, and vasculitis of malignancy (typically lymphoproliferative disorders). There is a strong association of disease activity with ANCA, particularly P-ANCA.

Wegener Granulomatosis (p. 522)

Wegener granulomatosis consists of the following triad:

1. Focal necrotizing vasculitis of the lung and upper airway
2. Necrotizing granulomas of the upper and lower respiratory tract
3. Necrotizing glomerulitis

The vascular lesions resemble those of acute PAN but are frequently accompanied by granuloma formation.

Peak incidence is in the forties. Without treatment, 80% of patients die within 1 year; in contrast, 90% respond to immunosuppression, particularly with cyclophosphamide.

Although immune complexes are occasionally seen in lesional tissue, no causative agent has been identified. Antineutrophilic cytoplasmic autoantibodies of the C-ANCA type, present in more than 90% of patients with active disease, are a good marker of disease activity.

Thromboangiitis Obliterans (Buerger Disease) (p. 523)

Typically encountered in heavy smokers, often before the age of 35 years, thromboangiitis obliterans is marked by segmental, thrombosing, acute, and chronic inflammation of intermediate and small *arteries and veins* in the extremities. It begins with nodular phlebitis, followed by Raynaud-like cold sensitivity and leg claudication.

Acute lesions consist of neutrophilic infiltration of the arterial wall, with mural or occlusive thrombi containing microabscesses, often with giant cell formation and secondary involvement of the adjacent vein and nerve. Late lesions show organization and recanalization. The cause is unknown. The vascular insufficiency can lead to excruciating pain and ultimately gangrene of the extremities.

Raynaud Disease (p. 524)

Raynaud disease and Raynaud phenomenon can be distinguished as follows:

- *Raynaud disease* refers to paroxysmal pallor or cyanosis of the digits of the hands or feet and infrequently the tips of the nose or ears (acral parts), caused by intense vasospasm of local small arteries or arterioles, principally of young, otherwise healthy women. Of uncertain etiology, Raynaud disease reflects an exaggeration of normal central and local vasomotor responses to cold or emotion.
- In contrast, *Raynaud phenomenon* refers to arterial insufficiency of the extremities *secondary to the arterial narrowing induced by various conditions, including atherosclerosis, systemic lupus erythematosus, systemic sclerosis (scleroderma), and Buerger disease.*

ANEURYSMS AND DISSECTION (p. 524)

Aneurysms are localized abnormal dilations of vessels. A *true aneurysm* is bounded by generally complete but often attenuated arterial wall components. Most common (and significant) are abdominal aortic aneurysms, but the iliac and other large arteries are sometimes involved. In contrast, a *false aneurysm* (also called *pseudoaneurysm* or *pulsating hematoma*) is an extravascular hematoma that communicates with the intravascular space; part of the vessel wall is missing. Morbidity and mortality of aneurysms are secondary to

- Rupture
- Impingement on adjacent structures

- Occlusion of proximate vessels by either extrinsic pressure or superimposed thrombosis
- Embolism from mural thrombosis

Causes of aneurysms include atherosclerosis and cystic medial degeneration (the two most common causes), syphilis, trauma, PAN, congenital defects, and infections (called *mycotic aneurysms*).

Atherosclerosis causes arterial wall thinning through medial destruction secondary to intimal plaque. *Atherosclerotic aneurysms usually occur in the abdominal aorta, most frequently between the renal arteries and the iliac bifurcation or in the common iliac arteries.* The arch and descending parts of the thoracic aorta can be involved as well as arteries other than the aorta.

Abdominal Aortic Aneurysms (p. 525)

Abdominal aortic aneurysms are typically found in men older than age 50. The risk of rupture increases with the maximal diameter of the bulge: minimal risk if less than 5 cm but a risk of 5 to 10% per year when more than 5 cm. Operative mortality is 5% for unruptured aneurysm but more than 50% after rupture. Because atherosclerotic peripheral (aortic) vascular disease is usually accompanied by severe coronary atherosclerosis, patients with abdominal aortic aneurysms have a high incidence of ischemic heart disease.

Syphilitic (Luetic) Aneurysms (p. 526)

A syphilitic aneurysm is an aneurysm appearing in the tertiary stage of syphilis, typically confined to the ascending aorta and arch. These aneurysms may extend retrograde to the aortic valve ring with dilation, causing commissural widening and narrowing and rolling of leaflets, leading to valvular insufficiency. With time, chronic left ventricular overload produces massive cardiac hypertrophy (often to 1000 gm), called *cor bovinum.*

Syphilitic aortitis begins as adventitial inflammation, especially involving the vasa vasorum, with resultant obliterative endarteritis. Narrowing of the lumens causes aortic medial ischemia and results in patchy elastic fiber and smooth muscle loss, with weakening of the wall and inflammatory scarring. Affected vasa vasorum have hyperplastic thickening of the walls and a perivascular infiltrate of lymphocytes and plasma cells.

Symptoms occur via

1. The development of luetic heart disease
2. Impingement of aortic aneurysm on surrounding thoracic organs
3. Rarely, rupture

Aortic Dissection (Dissecting Hematoma)
(p. 526)

Dissection of blood along the laminar planes of the aortic media, with the formation of an intramural blood-filled channel, is an ominous event. It often ruptures, causing massive hemorrhage that may produce sudden death. Aortic dissection is not usually associated with preexisting marked dilation of the aorta. It occurs principally in two groups:

1. Men 40 to 60 years of age, in whom hypertension is almost invariably an antecedent (>90% of dissections)
2. In younger individuals with a localized or systemic abnormality of connective tissue that affects the aorta (e.g., cystic medial degeneration in Marfan syndrome)

Dissection also can be a complication of therapeutic or diagnostic arterial cannulation or other trauma.

Hypertensive patients have nonspecific degenerative histologic changes of variable degree that include mild to moderate elastic fragmentation and excess amorphous interstitial material. More dramatic medial pathology frequently accompanies Marfan syndrome, consisting of the following:

1. Elastic tissue fragmentation and disruption
2. Focal separation of the elastic and fibromuscular elements by small, cleftlike or cystic spaces filled with material resembling amorphous extracellular matrix of connective tissue without inflammation, often called *cystic medial degeneration*

The defect in Marfan syndrome is now known to be due to a genetic decrease or loss of *microfibrillary protein* of elastic tissue.

The risk and nature of serious complications of dissection depend strongly on the level of the aorta affected. Complications include rupture of the dissection into a body cavity, extension into the great arteries of the neck or other major branches of the aorta, or retrograde dissection that disrupts the aortic valve. Thus, aortic dissections are generally classified into two types:

1. The more common (and dangerous) *proximal* lesions, involving the ascending aorta (types I and II of DeBakey's classification, often collectively called *type A*)
2. *Distal lesions not involving the ascending part* and usually beginning distal to the subclavian artery (DeBakey type III, often called *type B*)

The classic clinical symptom of aortic dissection is the sudden onset of excruciating pain, usually beginning in the anterior chest, radiating to the back, and moving downward as the dissection progresses. There is an intimal tear (a portal of entry of blood) in the ascending aorta, within 10 cm of the aortic valve, in 90% of patients with type A dissection. When an intimal portal of entry is not present, rupture of an intramural vasa vasorum is thought to be the source of the hemorrhage.

VEINS AND LYMPHATICS (p. 528)

Disorders of veins are common clinical problems, 90% of which comprise *varicose veins* or *phlebothrombosis*.

Varicose Veins (p. 529)

Varicose veins are abnormally dilated, tortuous veins (typically the superficial veins of the lower extremities) resulting from chronic increased intraluminal pressure. The walls of varicose veins are markedly thinned at points of maximal dilation. Although there is frequent intraluminal thrombosis, varicosities in the superficial veins are rarely a source of clinically significant emboli.

Varicose veins occur in 10 to 20% of the general population and in women more often than men, presumably secondary to venous stasis occurring in pregnancy. Other pathogenetic influences include hereditary defects in venous wall development, obesity, prolonged dependent position of the legs, proximal intravascular thrombosis, and compressive tumor masses.

Vein dilation or deformation renders the valves incompetent, with consequent stasis, persistent edema, and trophic skin changes, ultimately resulting in stasis dermatitis and ulceration (varicose ulcers). Affected tissues have impaired circulation and thus are vulnerable to injury and the formation of varicose ulcers, which heal poorly.

Thrombophlebitis and Phlebothrombosis

(p. 530)

The terms *thrombophlebitis* and *phlebothrombosis* designate the same entity. Thrombosis within a vein *(phlebothrombosis)* incites inflammation within the vein wall *(thrombophlebitis)*. Predisposing factors for thrombosis include congestive heart failure, neoplasia, pregnancy, postoperative state, prolonged immobilization, or local infection. Ninety percent occur in the deep leg veins. Other sites include the periprostatic plexus in men and ovarian and pelvic veins in women. *In contrast to thromboses in superficial leg veins, those in deep veins are common sources of emboli.*

Migratory thrombophlebitis (Trousseau syndrome) consists of multiple venous thrombi appearing in one place then disappearing to crop up elsewhere. It is attributed to hypercoagulability associated with cancer, particularly visceral adenocarcinomas, and may be associated with nonbacterial thrombotic endocarditis.

Obstruction of Superior or Inferior Vena Cava (Superior or Inferior Vena Caval Syndromes) (p. 530)

The superior vena caval syndrome is usually caused by neoplasms that compress or invade the superior vena cava, most commonly a primary bronchogenic carcinoma or mediastinal lymphoma. Regardless of the cause, the consequent obstruction produces a distinctive clinical complex manifested by dusky cyanosis and marked dilation of the veins of the head, neck, and arms.

Analogous to the superior vena caval syndrome, the inferior vena caval syndrome may be caused by many of the same processes. Moreover, certain neoplasms, particularly hepatocellular carcinoma and renal cell carcinoma, show a striking tendency to grow within the lumens of the veins, extending into the inferior vena cava and occasionally extending to the heart. Obstruction to the inferior vena cava induces marked edema of the legs; distention of the superficial collateral veins of the lower abdomen; and, when the renal veins are involved, massive proteinuria.

Lymphangitis and Lymphedema (p. 530)

Lymphangitis denotes infection involving the lymphatics draining a locus of inflammation, frequently (but not exclusively) resulting from β-hemolytic streptococci. Lymphangitis presents as a cluster of painful subcutaneous red streaks along involved lymph channels, with regional lymphadenopathy.

Morphologically, dilated lymphatics are filled with neutrophils and histiocytes. Inflammation frequently extends into the perilymphatic tissue and may develop into cellulitis or frank abscess.

It is occasionally associated with involvement of lymph nodes *(acute lymphadenitis)* and may lead to septicemia.

Lymphedema is lymphatic obstruction with lymphatic dilation and abnormal accumulation of interstitial fluid in the affected drainage site.

- When prolonged, lymphedema causes interstitial fibrosis. In skin and subcutaneous tissue, it gives rise to a *peau d'orange* (orange peel) appearance of skin, with associated ulcers and brawny induration.
- Chylous accumulations in any body cavity may occur secondary to rupture of obstructed, dilated lymphatics.
- The most common causes of obstruction are
  - Malignancy
  - Surgical resection of regional lymph nodes
  - Postradiation fibrosis
  - Filariasis
  - Postinflammatory thrombosis with lymphatic scarring

TUMORS (p. 531)

Tumors of the blood and lymphatic vessels constitute a spectrum from benign hemangiomas (some of which are regarded as hamartomatous); to intermediate lesions that are locally aggressive but infrequently metastasize; to relatively rare, highly malignant angiosarcomas. In addition, congenital or developmental malformations (e.g., Sturge-Weber syndrome) and non-neoplastic reactive vascular proliferations (e.g., *bacillary angiomatosis*) may present as tumor-like lesions.

Classically, benign vascular neoplasms are composed of *well-formed vascular channels lined by endothelial cells,* which may be confirmed by immunohistochemistry. Frankly malignant tumors show few or poorly developed vascular channels with solid, cellular, anaplastic endothelial proliferation. A few entities fall into an intermediate group.

Benign Tumors and Tumor-like Conditions
(p. 532)

HEMANGIOMA (p. 532)

Hemangiomas are common lesions, especially in childhood, making up 7% of all benign tumors. They encompass several histologic and clinical variants.

- *Capillary hemangiomas* usually occur in skin or mucous membranes but also in viscera. The tumors range from 1 to 2 mm to several centimeters in diameter. All are well-defined, unencapsulated lesions composed of closely packed aggregates of capillary-sized, thin-walled vessels. They may be partially or completely thrombosed.
- *Juvenile capillary (strawberry) hemangiomas* comprise a specific variant, are present at birth, grow rapidly for a few months, and begin regressing at age 1 to 3 years. Eighty percent disappear by age 7.
- *Cavernous hemangiomas* are distinguished by the formation of *large, cavernous vascular channels,* typically forming unencapsulated but discrete lesions, usually 1 to 2 cm in diameter (with rare giant forms). They have the same distribution as capillary

hemangiomas but are particularly common in the liver, where they may be discovered by computed tomography scan as a small tumor. They may also involve the central nervous system and other viscera. Cavernous hemangiomas in the cerebellum, brain stem, or eye grounds are associated with similar angiomatous or cystic neoplasms in pancreas and liver in *von Hippel–Lindau disease.*

■ *Pyogenic granulomas (lobular capillary hemangiomas)* are an ulcerated polypoid variant of capillary hemangiomas on skin or oral mucosa, often occurring secondary to trauma. They consist of proliferating capillaries with significant interspersed edema and inflammatory infiltrates, resembling exuberant granulation tissue. Pregnancy tumor *(granuloma gravidarum)* is essentially the same lesion, occurring in the gingiva in 1 to 5% of pregnant women, which regresses after delivery.

GLOMUS TUMOR (GLOMANGIOMA)
(p. 533)

Glomus tumor is a benign, extremely painful tumor of modified smooth muscle cells arising from the glomus body, a temperature-sensitive neuromyoarterial receptor that regulates arteriolar flow. Receptors and their tumors are most commonly found in the distal phalanges, especially beneath nail beds.

Grossly the tumors are less than 1 cm in diameter and may be pinpoint. *Histologically,* they consist of branching vascular channels separated by a stroma dominated by aggregates, nests, and masses of specialized glomus cells that resemble smooth muscle cells on electron microscopy.

VASCULAR ECTASIAS (p. 534)

Vascular ectasias are an aggregation of abnormally prominent capillaries, venules, and arterioles in skin or mucous membranes, which are acquired exaggerations of existing vessels.

■ *Nevus flammeus* is the term used for an ordinary birthmark. It consists of a macular cutaneous lesion that histologically shows only dermal vessel dilation. A special variety is the *port-wine stain* of the face and neck, which persists and grows along with the child, thickening the involved skin. Most eventually regress. Facial port-wine nevi with associated leptomeningeal angiomatous masses, mental retardation, seizures, hemiplegia, and skull radiopacities characterize the *Sturge-Weber syndrome.*

■ *Spider telangiectasias* are minute focal or subcutaneous arterioles, often pulsatile, arranged in radial fashion around a central core. They typically occur above the waist and are associated with hyperestrogenic states, such as pregnancy and cirrhosis.

■ *Hereditary hemorrhagic telangiectasia (Osler-Weber-Rendu disease)* is a rare, mendelian dominant disorder characterized by multiple small (<5 mm) aneurysmal lesions or telangiectasia on skin and mucous membranes. The syndrome typically presents with epistaxis, hemoptysis, or gastrointestinal or genitourinary bleeding, becoming more serious with advancing age.

BACILLARY ANGIOMATOSIS (p. 534)

Bacillary angiomatosis is a potentially fatal infectious disease caused by a rickettsia-like bacteria *(Bartonella henselae)* that induces a distinct non-neoplastic proliferation of small blood vessels in the skin, lymph nodes, and visceral organs of immunocompromised patients, especially those with human immunodeficiency virus (HIV) infections, such as acquired immunodeficiency syndrome (AIDS). Grossly, skin lesions have one or more red papules and nodular subcutaneous masses histologically resembling a tumor-like capillary proliferation with atypical endothelial cells with mitoses. In contrast to pyogenic granuloma, Kaposi sarcoma, or angiosarcoma, however, there are numerous neutrophils, nuclear dust, and purplish granular material (the bacteria). Treatment with erythromycin cures the condition.

SIMPLE (CAPILLARY) LYMPHANGIOMA
(p. 533)

Simple lymphangioma occurs typically in the head, neck, and axillary subcutaneous tissue but also on the trunk and within connective tissue of viscera. *Grossly*, the tumors are 1- to 2-cm cutaneous nodules or pedunculated lesions or well-demarcated, compressible gray-pink visceral masses. *Microscopically*, they are made up of a network of endothelium-lined spaces, identifiable as lymphatics only by the absence of blood cells. Variants include *lymphangiomyomas*, which have smooth muscle in the vessel walls.

CAVERNOUS LYMPHANGIOMA (CYSTIC HYGROMA) (p. 533)

Cavernous lymphangioma is analogous to the cavernous hemangiomas. The masses, however, tend to be much larger (up to 15 cm), typically in the neck or axilla of children. They are difficult to resect, owing to a lack of discrete margins or encapsulation, and so tend to recur. *Microscopically*, they are composed of hugely dilated cystic spaces lined by endothelium with scant stroma.

Intermediate-Grade Tumors (p. 535)
HEMANGIOENDOTHELIOMA (p. 537)

Hemangioendotheliomas are neoplasms that lie in the interface between benign and malignant and must be distinguished from the much more aggressive angiosarcomas. Most lesions are cured by excision, although up to 40% may recur, and 20% eventually metastasize.

Microscopically, vascular channels may be evident or inconspicuous, with dominant masses and sheets of somewhat pleomorphic, spindle-shaped to large, plump cells (especially in the *epithelioid* variant) of endothelial origin. Differential diagnosis includes metastatic carcinoma, melanoma, and sarcomas that can assume an epithelioid appearance.

KAPOSI SARCOMA (p. 535)

Four forms of Kaposi sarcoma are recognized, based on epidemiology:

1. *Chronic/classic/European Kaposi sarcoma* occurs typically in elderly men of Eastern European (especially Ashkenazi Jews) or Mediterranean descent. The lesions consist of multiple red-to-purple cutaneous plaques and nodules on the lower extremities,

with unusual visceral involvement. This form rarely causes death but is marked by an erratic course of relapses and remissions.

2. *Lymphadenopathic/African Kaposi sarcoma* is clinically similar to the classic form but occurs in younger men in equatorial Africa, where it makes up approximately 10% of all tumors. This disease is largely restricted to the lymph nodes and is aggressive.

3. *Transplant-associated Kaposi sarcoma* occurs in patients undergoing immunosuppressive therapy. There is both cutaneous and visceral systemic involvement. Lesions may regress when immunosuppression is discontinued.

4. *Acquired immunodeficiency syndrome (AIDS)—associated (epidemic) Kaposi sarcoma* occurs more commonly in homosexuals than in other risk groups of AIDS patients. Lesions may occur anywhere in the skin and mucous membranes, lymph nodes, gastrointestinal tract, or viscera. Wide visceral dissemination occurs early and frequently, but lesions respond to cytotoxic chemotherapy or α-interferon.

Microscopically the characteristic lesions consist of sheets of plump, spindle-shaped cells creating slitlike vascular spaces filled with red blood cells, intermingled with vascular channels lined by recognizable endothelium. There are also scattered microhemorrhages and hemosiderin deposits. The origin of the tumor cells remains uncertain, but current evidence favors a viral-associated (if not viral-caused by HIV or human herpesvirus 8) neoplasm of endothelial cells whose course is influenced by immune status.

Malignant Tumors (p. 537)

ANGIOSARCOMA (HEMANGIOSARCOMA OR LYMPHANGIOSARCOMA) (p. 537)

Among vascular tumors, angiosarcomas are the most malignant. Hepatic angiosarcomas are associated with arsenicals (in some pesticides), polyvinylchloride (used in plastic manufacture), and Thorotrast (radiocontrast material used from 1928 to 1950) and in these settings are often multicentric, concomitantly arising in the spleen.

These neoplasms tend to arise in skin, soft tissue, breast, liver, and spleen. They begin as small, well-demarcated red nodules evolving into large, fleshy, gray-white, soft tissue masses. *Microscopically*, all degrees of differentiation are found, from the highly vascular variety with plump, anaplastic endothelial cells to quite undifferentiated lesions without vascular lumens and with marked cellular atypia, including giant cells. Angiosarcomas metastasize widely and are frequently fatal.

Angiosarcomas may also arise in the setting of lymphedema, most typically approximately 10 years after radical mastectomy for breast cancer. In such cases, the tumor presumably arises from dilated lymphatic vessels (*lymphangiosarcomas*). Clinically the edematous arm may undergo acute swelling followed by the appearance of subcutaneous nodules, hemorrhage, and skin ulceration. Angiosarcomas may also be induced by radiation in the absence of lymphedema and have also been associated with foreign material introduced into the body either iatrogenically or accidentally.

HEMANGIOPERICYTOMA (p. 538)

Hemangiopericytoma is a tumor of pericytes that most commonly arises on the lower extremities or in the retroperitoneum.

Most are small, but they may be as large as 8 cm. *Microscopically,* they are composed of numerous capillary channels encased by nests and masses of spindle-shaped to round cells extrinsic to the endothelial basement membrane (resembling pericytes). Fifty percent metastasize.

PATHOLOGY OF THERAPEUTIC INTERVENTIONS IN VASCULAR DISEASE (p. 538)

Balloon Angioplasty and Related Techniques (p. 538)

Balloon angioplasty is dilation of an atheromatous stenosis of an artery by a balloon catheter. This approach is most commonly used to dilate a stenosed coronary artery. Balloon dilation of an atherosclerotic vessel characteristically causes plaque fracture, medial dissection, and stretching of the media of the dissected segment. The complications of balloon angioplasty and related techniques include abrupt reclosure in a small percentage of patients and proliferative restenosis in approximately one third of patients within the first 4 to 6 months.

Vascular Replacement (p. 539)

Large-diameter (>10 cm) Dacron grafts in the aorta perform well. In contrast, small-diameter fabric vascular grafts (<6 to 8 mm) perform less well. Failure of small-diameter vascular prostheses of autologous saphenous vein or expanded polytetrafluoroethylene is due most frequently to thrombotic occlusion or intimal fibrous hyperplasia, either generalized (in vein graft) or anastomotic only (in synthetic graft).

The long-term patency of saphenous veins used as coronary artery bypass grafts is 60% or less at 10 years, owing to pathologic changes, including thrombosis (usually early), intimal thickening (several months to several years), and atherosclerosis (>2 to 3 years postoperatively). Internal mammary arteries are also used with a greater than 90% patency at 10 years. Late symptom recurrence results most frequently from either graft occlusion or progression of atherosclerosis in the native vessels distal to the grafts.

Diseases of The Heart

Heart disease is the predominant cause of morbidity and mortality in industrialized nations, accounting for 40% of all deaths in the United States.

- Eighty percent of cardiac deaths are attributable to *ischemic heart disease.*
- An additional 5 to 10% are attributable to the following:
  - Hypertensive heart disease (including cor pulmonale)
  - Congenital heart disease
  - The common valvular diseases (calcific aortic valvular stenosis, mitral valve prolapse, rheumatic heart disease, and infective endocarditis)

Abnormal circulatory function usually results from one or more of the following mechanisms:

- Disruption of the continuity of circulation (e.g., rupture of a major vessel, such as the aorta) with significant loss of blood volume
- A disorder of cardiac conduction (e.g., heart block) or other arrhythmia (e.g., ventricular fibrillation) that leads to uncoordinated contractions of the muscular walls
- A lesion preventing valve opening or narrowing the lumen of a vessel (e.g., aortic valvular stenosis or coarctation) that obstructs blood flow and overworks the pump behind the obstruction
- Regurgitant flow (e.g., mitral or aortic regurgitation) that causes some of the output from each contraction to be directed backward, so that the pump repeatedly expels the same blood
- Failure of the pump itself (congestive heart failure [CHF])

CHF is the potential common end point of many forms of serious heart disease.

CONGESTIVE HEART FAILURE (p. 546)

CHF is the pathophysiologic state resulting from impaired cardiac function that renders the heart unable to maintain an output sufficient for the metabolic requirements of the tissues and organs of the body. Most instances of heart failure are the consequence of progressive deterioration of myocardial contractile function *(systolic dysfunction),* as often occurs with ischemic injury, pressure or volume overload, or dilated cardiomyopathy. The damaged muscle contracts weakly or inadequately, and the chambers cannot empty properly. Sometimes, however, failure results from an inability of the heart chambers to relax sufficiently during diastole to fill the ventricle properly *(diastolic dysfunction).* This situation can occur with massive left ventricular hypertrophy, myocardial fibrosis, deposition of amyloid, or constrictive pericarditis. Regardless of the underlying mechanism, CHF is characterized by diminished cardiac output *(forward failure)* or damming back of blood in the venous system *(backward failure)*, or both.

With the exception of frank myocyte death, the mechanisms of myocardial decompensation in CHF are not well understood. Because adult myocytes cannot replicate, pressure or volume stress induces hypertrophy (i.e., increased heart size, primarily as a result of increased myocyte size). The mechanism translating physical stress into cellular changes is uncertain. Hypertrophy is initially adaptive but can make myocytes especially vulnerable to injury.

Other compensatory changes include

- Ventricular dilation (to improve contraction by stretching of myofibers according to the Frank-Starling law).
- Blood volume expansion by salt and water retention
- Tachycardia

These compensatory changes ultimately constitute further burdens on cardiac function. They combine with both the primary cardiac disease and the secondary hypertrophy to induce dilation in excess of the optimal tension-generating point, leading to progressive CHF.

Left-Sided Heart Failure (p. 549)

The major causes of left-sided heart failure are ischemic heart disease, hypertension, aortic and mitral valve disease, and myocardial disease. It is manifested most commonly by *pulmonary congestion and edema* secondary to impairment of lung vascular outflow.

- Reduced cardiac output also causes reduced renal perfusion, leading to
  - Further salt and water retention
  - Ischemic acute tubular necrosis
  - Impairment of waste excretion, causing prerenal azotemia
- Central nervous system perfusion is reduced, often resulting in *hypoxic encephalopathy*, with symptoms ranging from irritability to coma.

Right-Sided Heart Failure (p. 549)

Right-sided heart failure is typically a consequence of left-sided failure. Pure right-sided heart failure may be caused by intrinsic disease of the lungs or pulmonary vasculature causing functional right ventricular outflow obstruction *(cor pulmonale)* or tricuspid or pulmonary valvular disease.

The major manifestations are as follows:

- Portal, systemic, and dependent peripheral (e.g., feet, ankles, sacrum) congestion and edema and effusions (pleural and peritoneal [*ascites*]).
- *Hepatomegaly* with centrilobular congestion and atrophy of central hepatocytes, producing a *nutmeg* appearance *(chronic passive congestion).*
  - With severe hypoxia, *centrilobular necrosis* can occur, and with high right-sided pressure, sinusoidal rupture causes *central hemorrhagic necrosis.*
  - Subsequent central fibrosis creates *cardiac sclerosis.*

- *Congestive splenomegaly* with sinusoidal dilation, focal hemorrhages, and later hemosiderin deposits and fibrosis.
- *Renal congestion*, hypoxic injury, and acute tubular necrosis, more marked in right-sided than in left-sided CHF.

ISCHEMIC HEART DISEASE (p. 550)

Ischemic heart disease is the generic designation for a group of closely related syndromes resulting from *ischemia*—an imbalance between the supply and demand of the heart for oxygenated blood. Ischemia results in not only insufficiency of oxygen *(hypoxia, anoxia)*, but also reduced availability of nutrient substrates and inadequate removal of metabolites.

Ischemia can be caused by the following mechanisms:

- *Reduced coronary blood flow* (the cause in >90%); often a combination of coronary atherosclerosis with vasospasm, thrombosis, or both. Uncommon causes of inadequate coronary flow are arteritis, emboli, cocaine-induced vasospasm, and shock with systemic hypotension.
- *Increased myocardial demand* (e.g., tachycardia, hypertrophy) exceeding vascular supply.

Hypoxemia as a result of diminished oxygen transport, owing to severe anemia, advanced lung disease, cyanotic congenital heart disease, carbon monoxide poisoning, or cigarette smoking is far less deleterious as a cause of ischemic heart disease but may contribute to damage if superimposed on decreased blood supply or increased demand.

There are four overlapping ischemic syndromes, differing largely in rate of onset and ultimate severity of ischemia:

1. *Angina pectoris* is marked by paroxysmal substernal or precordial pain or discomfort resulting from ischemia *without frank infarction*. Three somewhat distinctive patterns of angina have been delineated—stable, Prinzmetal, and unstable. They are differentiated clinically on the basis of the provocation and severity of the pain. The underlying coronary arterial pathology typically is characterized by greater than 75% stenoses in major coronary arteries with stable angina, vasospasm in Prinzmetal angina, and plaque disruption with variable mural thromboses in unstable angina.

2. *Myocardial infarction* is marked by death of cardiac muscle cells (see later).

3. *Chronic ischemic heart disease* is seen typically in elderly patients with moderate to severe multivessel coronary atherosclerosis who insidiously develop CHF; it may result from postinfarction cardiac decompensation or slow ischemic myocyte degeneration.

  ❏ *Microscopically* the myocardium has variable myocyte atrophy with perinuclear deposition of lipofuscin, myocytolysis of single cells or clusters, diffuse perivascular and interstitial fibrosis, and patchy to confluent replacement fibrosis.

  ❏ The diagnosis requires exclusion of other causes of CHF in elderly patients. Death may be precipitated by slowly progressive CHF, be due to a superimposed acute myocardial infarction (MI) or an arrhythmic event, or be secondary to unrelated causes.

4. *Sudden cardiac death* is defined as unexpected cardiac death

within 1 hour of symptom onset. There are 300,000 to 400,000 cases of sudden cardiac death annually in the United States. It is predominantly caused by ischemic heart disease; 75 to 95% of victims have marked atherosclerotic stenoses, often with acute disruption of plaque in one or more coronary arteries. In rescued patients, only about 25–50% develop MI. Infrequently, it is a consequence of aortic valvular stenosis, hereditary or acquired conduction system abnormalities, electrolyte derangements, mitral valve prolapse, dilated or hypertrophic cardiomyopathy, myocardial deposition, myocarditis, or intrinsic electrical instability.

The ultimate mechanism of death is a fatal arrhythmia (e.g., asystole or ventricular fibrillation), presumably triggered in most cases by conduction system scarring, acute ischemic injury, or electrical instability resulting from an ischemic focus or electrolytic imbalance.

Myocardial Infarction (p. 554)

There are two interrelated types of MI, with different morphology, pathogenesis, and clinical significance:

1. *Transmural infarct*: Infarction of the full thickness of the ventricular wall, usually caused by severe coronary atherosclerosis worsened by acute plaque disruption and superimposed occlusive thrombosis

2. *Subendocardial infarct*: Limited to the inner one third to one half of the ventricular wall (an area normally of diminished perfusion)

PATHOGENESIS

At least 90% of *transmural infarcts* are a consequence of coronary atherosclerosis with one or more stenosing and subsequently disrupted plaques. Significant plaques typically occur in the proximal 2 cm of the left anterior descending and left circumflex coronary arteries and in the proximal and distal thirds of the right coronary artery. In a few cases, vasospasm, platelet aggregation, or both induce an MI without atherosclerotic stenosis. Complete vessel occlusion, however, may not necessarily cause MI, owing to collateral blood flow.

- Nearly all transmural MIs affect the left ventricle; 15% simultaneously involve the right ventricle, particularly in posterior-inferior left ventricle infarcts. Isolated right ventricle infarction occurs in 1 to 3% of cases.
- The initial event in most transmural MIs is erosion, ulceration, fissuring, rupture, or hemorrhagic expansion (collectively called *acute plaque change* or *disruption*) of a partially stenosing atheroma, presumably precipitated by vasospasm or hemodynamic stresses.
- The most vulnerable plaques tend to have a relatively soft core of lipids (largely cholesterol and its esters with a high concentration of macrophages) separated from the lumen by a thin fibrous cap.
- Thrombosis follows the acute plaque change.
- The time interval between onset of complete myocardial ischemia and the initiation of irreversible injury is 20 to 40 minutes.
- In the absence of sudden death, thrombi may lyse spontaneously or with fibrinolytic treatment, or vasospasm may relax, thereby re-establishing flow and thus sparing some myocardium from necrosis.

- Reflow to *(reperfusion of)* precariously injured cells may restore viability but leave the cells poorly contractile *(stunned)* for up to 1 to 2 days.

Subendocardial infarcts are usually caused either 1) by diffuse coronary atherosclerosis and global borderline perfusion made transiently critical by increased demand, vasospasm, or hypotension but without superimposed thrombosis or 2) by a disrupted plaque with overlying thrombus, which spontaneously lyses, thereby limiting the extent of myocardial injury. Myocardial injury is usually less than in a transmural infarct and often multifocal. The pathogenesis of irreversible ischemic myocardial injury is summarized in Figure 13–1.

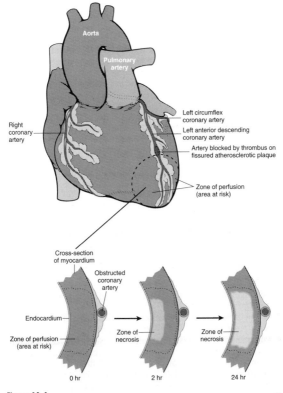

Figure 13-1 ∎

Schematic representation of the progression of myocardial necrosis after coronary artery occlusion. Necrosis begins in a small zone of the myocardium under the endocardial surface in the center of the ischemic zone that depends on the occluded vessel for perfusion. This entire region *(shaded)* is the area at risk. A narrow zone of myocardium immediately beneath the endocardium is spared from necrosis because it can be oxygenated by diffusion from the ventricle. (From Kumar V, Cotran RS, and Robbins SL: Basic Pathology, 6th ed. Philadelphia, WB Saunders, 1997.)

MORPHOLOGY

A myocardial infarct undergoes a characteristic sequence of gross and microscopic changes.

Grossly,

- Before 6 to 12 hours, the lesion is usually inapparent; however, in as early as 3 to 6 hours, changes may be accentuated by use of histochemical techniques (e.g., triphenyl tetrazolium chloride staining for dehydrogenases; it colors viable myocardium red-brown but leaves nonviable areas pale).
- By 18 to 24 hours, infarcted tissue is usually readily apparent—pale to cyanotic.
- In the first week, the lesion becomes progressively more sharply defined, yellow, and softened.
- A circumferential rim of hyperemic granulation tissue appears by 7 to 10 days and progressively expands.
- White fibrous scar is usually well established by 6 weeks.

Microscopically,

- Within 1 hour of ischemic injury, there is intercellular edema, and myocytes at the edge of the infarct may become wavy and buckled, attributable to stretching of these noncontractile dead fibers by adjacent viable contracting myocytes. At this stage, typical coagulative necrosis is not yet evident.
- From 12 to 72 hours postinfarction, there is neutrophilic infiltration into the necrotic tissue, with progressive evolution of characteristic myocyte coagulative necrosis. The dead myocytes become hypereosinophilic with loss of nuclei.
- Between 3 and 7 days after onset, dead myocytes begin to disintegrate and are resorbed by macrophages and enzyme proteolysis.
- After 7 to 10 days, granulation tissue progressively replaces necrotic tissue, ultimately generating a dense fibrous scar.

CLINICAL FEATURES

Diagnosis is based mainly on symptoms (chest pain, nausea, diaphoresis, dyspnea), electrocardiographic changes, and serum elevation of myocardial enzymes (creatine kinase-MB isoenzyme) or other proteins (troponin I, troponin T, or myoglobin) that leak out of dead cells.

- Angiography, echocardiography, and perfusion scintigraphy are adjunctive.
- About 25% of patients experience sudden death after infarction, most presumably secondary to a fatal arrhythmia.
- Of patients who survive the acute event, 80 to 90% subsequently develop complications (cited below); the early mortality rate is approximately 10%. Early restoration of flow through the occluded vessel responsible for the infarct by thrombolysis or balloon angioplasty provides a generally better prognosis.

Complications, which depend on the size and location of the necrosis as well as the reserve of functional myocardium, consist of the following:

- *Arrhythmias*
- *Congestive heart failure*
- *Cardiogenic shock* (usually seen with >40% of left ventricle infarcted)

- *Ventricular rupture* within the first 10 days (median, 4 to 5 days)—rupture of the free wall causing pericardial hemorrhage and tamponade and rupture of the septum producing a left-to-right shunt with right-sided heart volume overload
- Rarely, *papillary muscle infarction* with or without rupture, often causing mitral valve dysfunction
- *Fibrinous-to-hemorrhagic pericarditis*, common 2 to 3 days postinfarction (usually not clinically significant)
- *Mural thrombosis* in a noncontractile area, with risk of *peripheral embolization*
- Deformation of a large area of transmural infarction (*expansion*), which may heal into a *ventricular aneurysm*, both of which are prone to mural thrombosis
- Repetitive infarction (*extension*)

Overall mortality in the first year is 30% and thereafter 5 to 10% per year.

HYPERTENSIVE HEART DISEASE (p. 564)

Systemic (Left-Sided) Hypertensive Heart Disease (p. 564)

Diagnostic criteria are as follows:

- *Left ventricle hypertrophy*, typically concentric
- A history or extracardiac anatomic evidence of hypertension
- Absence of other lesions that might induce cardiac hypertrophy (e.g., aortic valve stenosis, coarctation of aorta)

PATHOGENESIS

Pathogenesis involves myocyte hypertrophic enlargement as a response to the increased work, whereby the cells augment contractile and other proteins but cannot divide. Thickened myocardium reduces left ventricle compliance, impairing diastolic filling while increasing oxygen demand. Individual myocyte hypertrophy increases the distance for oxygen and nutrient diffusion from adjacent capillaries. Coronary atherosclerosis accompanying hypertension adds the element of ischemia.

MORPHOLOGY

Grossly, there is a thickened left ventricle wall with increased heart weight (usually >2 cm wall thickness, heart weight >500 gm).

- Myocytes and nuclei are enlarged.
- In the long-term, diffuse interstitial fibrosis and focal myocyte atrophy and degeneration may develop, with left ventricle chamber dilation and wall thinning.

CLINICAL FEATURES

CHF is the cause of death in one third of hypertensive patients; hypertensive hypertrophy also increases the risk of sudden cardiac death. The remainder die of renal disease, stroke, or unrelated causes. Therapeutic control of pressure may, in time, lead to regression of the myocyte hypertrophy and diminution of heart size.

Pulmonary (Right-Sided) Heart Disease (Cor Pulmonale) (p. 565)

Cor pulmonale is the right-sided counterpart to systemic hypertensive heart disease; basically, right ventricle hypertrophy or dilation is secondary to pulmonary hypertension caused by disorders affecting lung structure or function. Excluded is right ventricle enlargement resulting from congenital heart disease or left ventricle pathology.

- *Acute cor pulmonale* refers to right ventricle dilation after massive pulmonary embolization.
- *Chronic cor pulmonale* is the result of chronic right ventricle pressure overload. Vasoconstriction in the pulmonary vascular beds incident to hypoxemia and acidosis (as would be expected with any significant pulmonary parenchymal or primary vascular pathology) exacerbates baseline pulmonary hypertension.

MORPHOLOGY

Right ventricle hypertrophy, often to 1 cm or more thickness; dilation; or both are present.

- Right ventricle dilation may lead to tricuspid regurgitation.
- Pulmonary arteriolar wall thickening and often pulmonary arterial atherosclerosis reflect the increased right-sided pressure.
- The left side of the heart is essentially normal.

CLINICAL FEATURES

Chronic cor pulmonale, common because chronic obstructive pulmonary disease is widespread, is responsible for some hospital admissions for cardiac decompensation. Cardiac symptoms may be masked by those of underlying lung disease.

VALVULAR HEART DISEASE (p. 566)

Valvular heart disease in adults is caused most commonly by degeneration (e.g., calcific aortic stenosis with or without a bicuspid valve, mitral annular calcification, mitral valve prolapse), immunologic-inflammatory processes (e.g., rheumatic heart disease), or infection (e.g., infective endocarditis).

Degenerative Calcific Aortic Valve Stenosis (p. 567)

Degenerative calcific aortic valve stenoses are common age-related lesions that generally become clinically important in patients in their seventies and eighties. The remainder are congenitally bicuspid valves (occurring in 1 to 2% of the population), often becoming calcified earlier (in patients in their fifties and sixties).

MORPHOLOGY

Grossly, heaped-up subendothelial rigid calcific masses within sinuses of Valsalva cause thickening and immobility of the valve cusps with narrowing of orifice. In contrast to rheumatic aortic stenosis, there is no commissural fusion. There is usually concentric left ventricle hypertrophy from chronic pressure overload.

CLINICAL FEATURES

The need for surgical intervention is heralded by angina (hampered microcirculatory perfusion in hypertrophied myocardium), syncope (with increased risk of sudden death), or CHF.

Mitral Annular Calcification (p. 568)

Mitral annular calcifications are degenerative, noninflammatory, calcific deposits within the mitral annulus, usually in the elderly.

- Regurgitation may occur owing to inadequate systolic contraction of the mitral valve ring.
- The leaflets may be unable to open over bulky deposits, causing stenosis.
- Nodular calcific deposits may cause arrhythmias by impinging on the conduction pathways.
- They rarely are a focus of infective endocarditis.

Mitral Valve Prolapse (Myxomatous Degeneration of the Mitral Valve) (p. 568)

One or both mitral valve leaflets are enlarged, myxomatous, and floppy, and they balloon back (prolapse) into the left atrium during systole, causing midsystolic click and mitral valve insufficiency. The disease occurs in 5 to 10% of the U.S. population, typically those between 20 and 40 years of age. It is of uncertain etiology, but a developmental anomaly is suspected, perhaps affecting all connective tissues because it is common in Marfan syndrome.

MORPHOLOGY

Grossly, there is interchordal ballooning (>4 mm) of the mitral valve leaflets and elongated, attenuated, or occasionally ruptured chordae tendineae. There is no commissural fusion.

Microscopically, there is thinning and degeneration of the *fibrosa* layer (on which the strength of the leaflet depends), with myxomatous thickening of the *spongiosa*. Similar changes can be seen in the chordae.

Secondary changes are due to injury incident to the billowing leaflets and include

- Fibrous thickening of valve leaflets, especially at points of contact
- Thickened left ventricle endocardium at sites of friction from the prolapsing leaflets or elongated chordae
- Atrial thrombosis behind the ballooning cusps
- Calcification of the mitral annulus

CLINICAL FEATURES

Some patients have coincidental aortic, tricuspid, or pulmonary valve involvement. Mitral valve prolapse is generally asymptomatic and discovered only as a midsystolic click on auscultation. It may be associated with atypical chest pain, dyspnea, fatigue, or psychiatric manifestations (e.g., depression, anxiety). Patients have an increased risk of

- Infective endocarditis
- Slow, progressive mitral valvular insufficiency that may produce CHF
- Atrial and ventricular arrhythmias
- Sudden death

Rheumatic Fever and Rheumatic Heart Disease (p. 570)

Rheumatic fever is an acute, recurrent inflammatory disease that typically occurs 1 to 5 weeks after a group A streptococcal infection (usually sore throat). It occurs mainly in children (ages 5 to 15 years), but adults may suffer the first attack. Most evidence suggests it is secondary to host antistreptococcal antibodies that are cross-reactive to cardiac antigens.

Diagnosis rests on the clinical history and the presence of two of five major (Jones) criteria, as follows:

1. *Erythema marginatum*: Macular skin lesions with erythematous rims and central clearing, typically in a *bathing suit* distribution
2. *Sydenham chorea*: A neurologic disorder with rapid, involuntary, purposeless movements
3. *Carditis*: Noted in 50 to 75% of children and 35% of adults; usually involves myocardium, endocardium, and pericardium (a *pancarditis*)
4. *Subcutaneous nodules*
5. *Migratory large joint polyarthritis*: Seen in 90% of adults; less common in children

Minor criteria include

- Fever
- Arthralgia
- Leukocytosis

During acute rheumatic fever, death is rare and most frequently secondary to myocarditis. Typically, myocarditis and arthritis are transient and largely resolve without complications, but the valvular involvement may lead to deformation and scarring with permanent dysfunction (*chronic rheumatic heart disease*) and subsequent CHF.

Chronic rheumatic heart disease is more likely to occur

1. When the first attack is in early childhood
2. When the first bout of rheumatic fever is severe
3. With recurrent attacks

MORPHOLOGY

Characteristic features are as follows:

- *Aschoff bodies* are pathognomonic foci of fibrinoid necrosis found in many sites, most often the myocardium. Initially surrounded by lymphocytes, macrophages, and a few plasma cells, they are slowly replaced by fibrous scar.
- Transient fibrinous pericarditis in the acute phase may contain Aschoff bodies.
- Inflammatory valvulitis induces formation of beady fibrinous vegetations (*verrucae*) acutely. Aschoff bodies may be present in the inflamed valves.

- The chronic (or healed) valve shows
  1. Fibrous thickening of leaflets
  2. Bridging fibrosis across the commissures *(commissural fusion)*, generating *fishmouth* or *buttonhole* stenoses
  3. Thickened, fused, and shortened mitral valve chordae
- Calcification can occur deep in the fibrous leaflets.
- Solitary mitral involvement occurs in 65 to 70% of cases and combined aortic and mitral involvement in 20 to 25%; the tricuspid and pulmonic valves are less frequently affected.

Subendocardial collections of Aschoff nodules, usually in the left atrium, induce thickenings called *MacCallum plaques*.

CLINICAL FEATURES

Changes secondary to tight mitral stenosis include

- Left atrial hypertrophy and enlargement, occasionally with mural thrombi
- Chronic congestive changes in the lungs
- Right ventricle hypertrophy
- CHF

Other complications include

- Increased risk of developing infective endocarditis
- Atrial fibrillation secondary to atrial dilation

VEGETATIVE ENDOCARDITIS (p. 571)

A few cardiac disorders are marked mainly by vegetations on the valves. The major examples are

1. Infective endocarditis
2. Nonbacterial thrombotic endocarditis
3. Endocarditis associated with lupus erythematosus

Infective Endocarditis (p. 572)

Colonization of heart valves with microbiologic organisms leads to the formation of friable, infected vegetations and frequently valve injury, termed *infective endocarditis*. Traditionally, *acute* and *subacute* forms have been distinguished.

ACUTE INFECTIVE ENDOCARDITIS

Acute infective endocarditis is caused by highly virulent organisms (e.g., *Staphylococcus aureus*), often seeding a previously normal valve and producing a necrotizing, ulcerative, and invasive infection. It typically presents as a rapidly developing fever with rigors, malaise, and weakness. The larger vegetations in acute infective endocarditis often cause embolic complications, and there frequently is splenomegaly. Even with treatment, death occurs in days to weeks in 50 to 60% of patients.

SUBACUTE INFECTIVE ENDOCARDITIS

Subacute infective endocarditis is typically caused by an organism of moderate to low virulence (most frequently *Streptocccus viridans*) seeding an abnormal or previously injured valve, causing less valvular destruction than acute infective endocarditis. This pattern of infective endocarditis has an insidious onset with nonspecific malaise, low-grade fever, weight loss, and a flulike syndrome. The vegetations tend to be smaller than in acute infective endocarditis, and so embolic complications are less frequent than with acute infective endocarditis. The disease tends to have a protracted course even without treatment and is less often fatal than acute infective endocarditis.

PATHOGENESIS

Blood-borne bacteria (bacteremia) are prerequisites for infective endocarditis, acute or subacute. They may derive from an infection elsewhere in the body; intravenous drug abuse; dental or surgical procedures; or microinjuries to gut, urinary tract, oropharynx, or skin.

- Cardiac congenital anomalies are common subsoil for infective endocarditis, particularly the subacute variety, including tight shunts (e.g., ventricular septal defect [VSD]) or stenoses with jet streams. Chronic rheumatic heart disease is increasingly less common. Other risk factors include
  - Mitral valve prolapse
  - Degenerative calcific stenosis
  - Bicuspid aortic valve
  - Prosthetic valves
  - Indwelling catheters
- Contributory conditions include
  - Neutropenia
  - Immunosuppressed states
  - Intravenous drug abuse

MORPHOLOGY

Friable, 0.5- to 2.0-cm, microbe-laden vegetations are apparent on one or more valves.

- Acute infective endocarditis is commonly associated with bulky (1–2 cm) vegetations that cause erosions or perforations of leaflets, invading adjacent myocardium or aortic wall to produce abscess cavities.
- Subacute infective endocarditis has smaller vegetations that rarely erode or penetrate the leaflets.
- With nonvalvular infections, vegetations are typically on the downstream margin of a jet lesion.
- With prosthetic valves, ring abscess is almost always present.
- With intravenous drug abuse, vegetations are often acute and on right-sided valves, but left-sided valves are also frequently involved. The organism is most often *S. aureus*.

CLINICAL CONSEQUENCES

Clinical consequences of infective endocarditis include the following:

- Direct injury to valves (insufficiency or stenosis with CHF) or myocardium and aorta (ring abscess, perforation)
- Emboli to spleen, kidneys, heart, and brain with infarction or metastatic infection
- Renal injury, including embolic infarction or infection and antigen-antibody complex–mediated glomerulonephritis, which can result in nephrotic syndrome, renal failure, or both

Diagnosis is confirmed by blood cultures (with adequate sampling, positive in 80 to 95% of cases).

Nonbacterial Thrombotic Endocarditis
(p. 576)

Nonbacterial thrombotic endocarditis is characterized as follows:

- Previously called *marantic endocarditis*
- Small (1- to 5-mm), sterile, bland fibrin and platelet thrombi (vegetations) loosely adherent to valve leaflets (most often mitral) along the lines of closure and without significant inflammation or valve damage; attributed to systemic hypercoagulability
- May embolize to brain, heart, or elsewhere
- Characteristically (although not always) occurs in settings of cancer (particularly visceral adenocarcinomas or prolonged debilitating illness (e.g., renal failure, chronic sepsis), attributed to disseminated intravascular coagulation or other hypercoagulable state

Endocarditis Associated With Systemic Lupus Erythematosus (Libman-Sacks Endocarditis) (p. 577)

Valvulitis of uncertain pathogenesis may appear in systemic lupus erythematosus and in antiphospholipid syndrome. The mitral and tricuspid valves are most often affected with fibrinoid necrosis; mucoid degeneration; and subsequent development of small, fibrinous, sterile vegetations on *either* side of the valve leaflets. Valve deformations may result from healing of the vegetations.

Carcinoid Heart Disease (p. 577)

One feature of the carcinoid syndrome (p. 577) is related to elaboration by argentaffinomas of bioactive products, including serotonin, kallikrein, bradykinins, histamine, prostaglandins, and tachykinins P and K. The precise agent responsible for the cardiac lesions is uncertain, although it presumably is rapidly metabolized in passage through the lung, causing predominantly right-sided heart lesions.

MORPHOLOGY

Plaquelike intimal thickenings of the endocardium of the tricuspid valve, right ventricular flow tract, and pulmonic valve are superimposed on the unaltered endocardium. The left side of the heart is usually unaffected.

Left-sided but similar valve lesions have been reported to complicate the use of fenfluramine and phentermine (fen-phen), appetite suppressants used for the treatment of obesity, which may affect systemic serotonin metabolism.

Complications of Artificial Valves (p. 578)

Prosthetic valves are of two basic types: mechanical (rigid, synthetic) and bioprosthetic (glutaraldehyde-pretreated animal valves). Complications include the following:

- *Paravalvular leak*: Separation of the sewing ring from the valve annulus.

- *Thrombosis, thromboembolism*, or both: A major cause of morbidity and mortality in 1 to 4% of patients per year by hindering valve function or embolizing. This complication is more common with mechanical valves. Hemorrhage can occur secondary to long-term anticoagulation therapy used to prevent thrombosis.
- *Infective endocarditis*: 5% of patients within 5 years of valve replacement. This complication is difficult to cure without surgery.
- *Structural deterioration*: An uncommon problem with most mechanical valves, but 20 to 30% of bioprosthetic valves require replacement for degeneration within 10 years.
- *Others*: Occlusion as a result of tissue overgrowth and hemolysis from mechanical trauma to erythrocytes.

MYOCARDIAL DISEASE (p. 578)

Although myocardial dysfunction occurs secondarily in ischemic, valvular, hypertensive, and other heart diseases, the term *myocardial diseases* implies myocardial dysfunction as the major cause of heart disease. It includes

- Inflammatory disorders *(myocarditis)*
- Immunologic and systemic metabolic disorders
- Genetic abnormalities in cardiac muscle cells

When the cardiac abnormality is primary in and localized to the myocardium, the condition is called *cardiomyopathy*. Cardiomyopathy is not synonymous with CHF because the latter is a late stage of many significant forms of cardiac disease.

Endomyocardial biopsy obtained via a percutaneously inserted catheter threaded pervenously into the right ventricle allows pathologic examination of cardiac tissue.

Cardiomyopathy (p. 579)

Cardiomyopathy can be divided into three categories (Table 13–1), as follows:

1. Dilated
2. Hypertrophic
3. Restrictive based on the resultant pathophysiology

DILATED CARDIOMYOPATHY (p. 579)

Dilated cardiomyopathy is characterized by gradual four-chamber hypertrophy and dilation. Dilated cardiomyopathy may occur at any age as slow, progressive CHF. Only 25% of patients survive beyond 5 years. Although the cause in a specific case is unknown, certain pathogenetic pathways are suspected to contribute to many, as follows:

- *Genetic defect*: Often with a family history. To date, few definite biochemical or structural abnormalities have been established.
- *Alcohol toxicity*: Attributed to direct toxicity of alcohol or a metabolite (especially acetaldehyde), which has a direct toxic effect on the myocardium. No morphologic features distinguish alcohol-induced cardiac damage from idiopathic dilated cardiomyopathy or associated chronic thiamine deficiency (e.g., analogous to beriberi).

Table 13-1. CARDIOMYOPATHY AND INDIRECT MYOCARDIAL DYSFUNCTION: FUNCTIONAL PATTERNS AND CAUSES

Functional Pattern	Left Ventricular Ejection Fraction	Mechanisms of Heart Failure	Causes	Indirect Myocardial Dysfunction (Not Cardiomyopathy)
Dilated	<40%	Impairment of contractility (systolic dysfunction)	Idiopathic; alcohol; peripartum; genetic; myocarditis; hemochromatosis; chronic anemia; doxorubicin (Adriamycin); sarcoidosis	Ischemic heart disease; valvular heart disease; hypertensive heart disease; congenital heart disease
Hypertrophic	50–80%	Impairment of compliance (diastolic dysfunction)	Idiopathic; genetic; Friedreich ataxia; storage disease; infants of diabetic mothers	Hypertensive heart disease; aortic stenosis
Restrictive	45–90%	Impairment of compliance (diastolic dysfunction)	Idiopathic; amyloidosis; radiation-induced fibrosis	Pericardial constriction

- *Peripartum cardiomyopathy*: The designation given to a glob-ally dilated heart discovered within several months before or after delivery. Although the mechanism behind this relationship is uncertain, pregnancy invokes the possibilities of hypertension, volume overload, nutritional deficiency, other metabolic de-rangement, or an as yet poorly characterized immunologic reac-tion.
- *Postviral myocarditis* (see later): Supported mostly by occa-sional cases in which endomyocardial biopsy specimens have documented the progression of myocarditis to dilated cardiomy-opathy.

Morphology

Morphologic characteristics are as follows:

- Cardiomegaly (up to 900 gm) is present, but wall thickness measurement may not reflect the degree of hypertrophy owing to dilation. The heart is flabby.
- Poor contractile function and stasis can lead to mural thrombi.
- Valves and coronary arteries are generally usual for age.
- *Microscopic changes* are often subtle and entirely nonspecific:
  • 25% have no significant alterations.
  • The remainder have diffuse myocyte hypertrophy and variable interstitial myocardial fibrosis.
- Mild to moderate focal endocardial thickening is sometimes seen, especially in the ventricles.

Arrhythmogenic right ventricular cardiomyopathy *(arrhythmo-genic right ventricular dysplasia)* is a sometimes familial disorder most commonly associated with right-sided and sometimes left-sided heart failure and various rhythm disturbances, particularly ventricular tachycardia, and sudden death. Morphologically the right ventricular wall is severely thinned, with extensive fatty infiltration, loss of myocytes, and interstitial fibrosis. Death occurs (unless the patient receives a transplant) secondary to progressive CHF, embolism of mural thrombi, or fatal arrhythmias.

HYPERTROPHIC CARDIOMYOPATHY (p. 581)

Hypertrophic cardiomyopathy is also termed *idiopathic hyper-trophic subaortic stenosis* and *hypertrophic obstructive cardiomy-opathy.*

- Hypertrophic cardiomyopathy is characterized by a heavy, mus-cular, *hypercontractile*, poorly compliant heart with poor dia-stolic relaxation.
- More than half of cases are transmitted by autosomal dominant inheritance.
- Symptomatic disease presents usually in young adults with dyspnea, angina, near-syncope, and CHF, but the condition may be asymptomatic.
- There is an increased risk of sudden death.

Morphology

There is no discernible difference between familial and sporadic cases of hypertrophic cardiomyopathy. All are characterized by marked cardiomegaly owing to hypertrophy, left ventricle more than right ventricle, often with atrial dilation.

- Classically, there is disproportionate thickening of the septum versus left ventricle free wall (asymmetric septal hypertrophy).

Some cases, however, show concentric or symmetric hypertrophy.

- The left ventricle cavity is compressed into a *banana-like configuration* by the asymmetrically bulging interventricular septum.
- If the basal septum is thickened at the level of the mitral valve, left ventricle–systolic outflow may be compromised by contact of the anterior mitral leaflet with the septum (systolic anterior motion), giving rise to *obstructive hypertrophic cardiomyopathy*, reflected by a fibrous plaque on the septum.
- *Microscopically*, in addition to marked myofiber hypertrophy, 25 to 50% of the septum usually shows helter-skelter *myocyte disarray*, accompanied by myofilament disorganization within muscle cells.
- Other findings include patchy replacement fibrosis, presumably as a result of focal ischemic injury and abnormal thick-walled arteries of uncertain origin.

Pathogenesis

Families with hypertrophic cardiomyopathy have been shown to have various mutations of the gene for the myosin heavy chain or other contractile proteins. The pathogenetic link between abnormal contractile proteins and the hypertrophic cardiomyopathy phenotype, however, remains uncertain.

Clinical Features

The course of hypertrophic cardiomyopathy is highly variable, but certain mutations have a characteristic favorable or unfavorable prognosis. Most patients remain unchanged for years, but some progressively worsen. Major complications include

- Atrial fibrillation with mural thrombus
- Embolization
- Infective endocarditis
- CHF
- Sudden death

Outflow obstruction is seldom a major problem.

RESTRICTIVE CARDIOMYOPATHY (p. 583)

Restrictive cardiomyopathy is a rarity of diverse origins, all marked by a restriction of ventricular filling and thus reduced cardiac output. Interstitial myocardial fibrosis or the following are usually present.

- *Endomyocardial fibrosis*: Endomyocardial fibrosis is found typically in children and young adults in Africa. It is characterized by ventricular subendocardial fibrosis extending from the apex to the inflow tract of one or both ventricles, often with mural thrombus formation; the atrioventricular valves may be involved. Restrictive physiology occurs from reduced ventricular chamber volume. The basic cause is unknown.
- *Loeffler endocarditis*: Loeffler endocarditis is characterized by endomyocardial fibrosis with large mural thrombi, similar to that described previously but found in temperate zones. The two conditions of endomyocardial fibrosis, however, have many overlaps. Both are frequently associated with the following:

  1. Peripheral eosinophilia.
  2. Eosinophilic infiltration of multiple organs, including the heart.

3. A rapidly fatal course. The cardiac changes are probably due to toxic products of eosinophils.

- *Endocardial fibroelastosis*: Endocardial fibroelastosis is an uncommon disorder of obscure etiology and possibly the end point of diverse disorders, characterized by focal-to-diffuse, cartilage-like fibroelastic thickening of the endocardium, left ventricle more often than right ventricle. It can occur at all ages but is most common in patients younger than 2 years old. Congenital cardiac anomalies are present in one third of cases.

Myocarditis (p. 584)

Myocarditis is characterized as follows:

- Myocardial inflammation is the principal feature.
- The clinical spectrum is broad, from entirely asymptomatic to abrupt onset of arrhythmia, CHF, or even sudden death; most patients recover quickly and without sequelae.
- Causes include virtually all types of microbiologic agents and immune-mediated injury (Table 13–2).
- Most cases are thought to be of viral origin (e.g., coxsackievirus A and B, echovirus). Cardiac involvement occurs days to a few weeks after a primary viral infection at another site.
- Rarely cases are of bacterial origin secondary to bacteremia (e.g., staphylococcal, tuberculous).
- *Trypanosoma cruzi*, the organism that causes Chagas disease, is associated with myocarditis in up to 50% of the population in endemic areas of South America.
- Noninfectious myocarditis may be immune mediated (e.g., associated with rheumatic fever, systemic lupus erythematosus, or drug allergies).
- In many cases, the cause is unknown (e.g., sarcoidosis, giant cell myocarditis, and Fiedler myocarditis; the latter two are often fatal), or the microbe is unidentifiable.

Table 13–2. MAJOR CAUSES OF MYOCARDITIS

Infections

Viruses (e.g., coxsackievirus, ECHO, influenza, HIV, cytomegalovirus)
Chlamydia (e.g., *C. psittaci*)
Rickettsia (e.g., *R. typhi* [typhus fever])
Bacteria (e.g., *Corynebacterium* [diphtheria], *Neisseria* [meningococcus], *Borrelia* [Lyme disease])
Fungi (e.g., *Candida*)
Protozoa (e.g., *Trypanosoma* [Chagas disease]), toxoplasmosis)
Helminths (e.g., trichinosis)

Immune-Mediated Reactions

Postviral
Poststreptococcal (rheumatic fever)
Systemic lupus erythematosus
Drug hypersensitivity (e.g., methyldopa, sulfonamides)
Transplant rejection

Unknown

Sarcoidosis
Giant cell myocarditis

ECHO, enteric cytopathogenic human orphan virus; HIV, human immunodeficiency virus.

MORPHOLOGY

Gross manifestations of myocarditis include a flabby ventricular myocardium often with four-chamber dilation and patchy, diffuse hemorrhagic mottling.

- Often mural thrombi arise in dilated chambers.
- Endocardium and valves are unaffected.
- After the acute stage, there may be residual dilation or hypertrophy with small interstitial foci of fibrosis.

Microscopically, there is a myocardial inflammatory infiltrate with associated myocyte necrosis or degeneration. Lesions are typically focal (and may or may not be seen on endomyocardial biopsy). In myocarditis associated with *viral* infections, there usually is isolated myofiber necrosis with interstitial edema and a mononuclear cell infiltrate. After the acute stage, inflammatory lesions may resolve, leaving either no residua or variable interstitial and focal fibrosis. It may present later as dilated cardiomyopathy.

- *Bacteria and other larger parasites* produce reactions characteristic of the lesions they induce in other tissues (e.g., neutrophilic infiltrate, abscesses, granulomas).
- Myocarditis occurs in approximately two thirds of patients with Lyme disease; myocardial spirochetes can be demonstrated in some. *Lyme myocarditis* is usually mild and reversible but occasionally requires a temporary pacemaker for atrioventricular block.
- In *Chagas disease*, trypanosomes parasitize myocytes and produce acute and chronic inflammation, including eosinophils.
- In *hypersensitivity reactions*, there are predominantly perivascular mononuclear and eosinophilic infiltrates, occasionally with acute vasculitis and spotty myofiber necrosis. This variant is often induced by therapeutic drugs.
- In *idiopathic giant cell myocarditis*, there is focal myocyte necrosis associated with granulomatous inflammation, including multinucleated giant cells. This variant has a poor prognosis.

Other Specific Heart Muscle Diseases
(p. 586)

Common morphologic changes with cardiotoxic agents include myofiber swelling, fatty change, and individual cell lysis. Electron microscopy shows mitochondrial abnormalities, smooth endoplasmic reticulum swelling and fragmentation, and myofibril lysis. With time, delicate interstitial fibrosis and focal replacement scarring occur.

The anthracycline chemotherapeutic agents doxorubicin (Adriamycin) and daunorubicin induce a dose-dependent cardiotoxicity (usually total dose >500 mg/m^2), attributed primarily to lipid peroxidation of myofiber membranes. Both the physiologic and the morphologic patterns are indistinguishable from those of idiopathic dilated cardiomyopathy.

Iron overload with hemosiderin deposits in myofibers can occur in hereditary hemochromatosis and hemosiderosis from multiple blood transfusions. Patients with iron storage disease present most commonly with a dilated pattern.

Amyloidosis is seen as patchy and perivascular hyaline deposits. It may occur as part of systemic amyloidosis (p. 251) or may be isolated (e.g., senile cardiac amyloidosis, occurring to some extent in 50% of individuals more than 70 years old). Often, cardiac involvement is incidental, but it may induce arrhythmias or restrictive physiology.

Catecholamines, either administered exogenously (e.g., epinephrine) or produced endogenously (i.e., pheochromocytomas), induce tachycardia and vasomotor constriction (with superimposed platelet aggregation), resulting in diffuse but patchy ischemic necrosis. *Cocaine* may have a similar effect by blocking catecholamine reuptake at adrenergic nerve terminals.

PERICARDIAL DISEASE (p. 587)

Pericardial disease is unusually primary; generally, it is secondary to diseases of adjacent structures or part of a systemic disorder.

Pericardial Effusion (p. 587)

The normal pericardial sac contains 30 to 50 ml of serous, typically *noninflammatory* fluid. Accumulations rarely exceed 500 ml.

- *Serous*: This is the most common form. Serosa is smooth and glistening. Fluid accumulates slowly and therefore is well tolerated until a large volume compromises diastolic filling. The most common causes are CHF and hypoproteinemia.
- *Serosanguineous*: This form is usually the result of blunt chest trauma (e.g., cardiopulmonary resuscitation). The serosanguineous form is rarely clinically significant.
- *Chylous*: This form is caused by lymphatic obstruction (benign or malignant). It is rarely clinically significant.

Hemopericardium (p. 587)

Hemipericardium refers to accumulation of pure, often clotted blood in the pericardium without an inflammatory component. It is usually due to traumatic perforation, myocardial rupture after a transmural MI, rupture of the intrapericardial aorta, or hemorrhage from an abscess or tumor metastasis. Escaping blood rapidly fills the sac under high pressure, and as little as 200 to 300 ml may cause tamponade.

Pericarditis (p. 587)

Pericarditis is usually secondary to disorders involving the heart or adjacent mediastinal structures (e.g., MI, surgery, trauma, radiation, tumors, infections) or, less frequently, systemic abnormalities (e.g., uremia, autoimmune diseases). Acute pericarditis is most often of viral origin. Chronic reactions also can occur (e.g., with tuberculosis and fungi), and healing may lead to damaging adhesions.

ACUTE PERICARDITIS (p. 587)

Acute pericarditis occurs in several forms.

- *Serous pericarditis*: This form usually consists of 50 to 200 ml of slowly accumulating exudate characteristically produced by nonbacterial involvements, including rheumatic fever, systemic lupus erythematosus, tumors, uremia, and primary viral infections (e.g., Coxsackie). Frequently the cause is unknown. Microscopically, there is a scant epicardial and pericardial acute and chronic inflammatory infiltration (mostly lymphocytes). The fluid resorbs if the underlying disease remits, rarely leaving any residuals.

- *Fibrinous and serofibrinous pericarditis*: This is the most common clinical form, seen with MI, associated with a pericardial friction rub. It may also be caused by any of the aforementioned etiologies. Exudate may be completely resolved or be organized, leaving typically delicate, stringy adhesions *(adhesive pericarditis)* or plaquelike thickening, both usually inconsequential.
- *Purulent (suppurative) pericarditis*: This form usually signifies bacterial, fungal, or parasitic infection, which has reached the pericardium by direct extension, by hematogenous or lymphatic spread, or during cardiotomy. Most common causative organisms are gram-positive staphylococci, streptococci, and pneumococci. Purulent pericarditis is typically composed of 400 to 500 ml of a thin-to-creamy pus with erythematous, granular serosal surfaces. It presents with prominent fever, rigors, and a friction rub. It usually organizes and may produce mediastinopericarditis or *constrictive pericarditis* (see later).
- *Hemorrhagic pericarditis*: Hemorrhagic pericarditis denotes an exudate of blood admixed with fibrinous-to-suppurative effusion. Most commonly, it follows cardiac surgery or is associated with tuberculosis or malignancy. It usually organizes with or without calcification.
- *Caseous pericarditis*: This form is due to tuberculosis (typically by direct extension from neighboring lymph nodes) or, less commonly, mycotic infection. This pattern is the most frequent antecedent to fibrocalcific constrictive pericarditis.

CHRONIC OR HEALED PERICARDITIS (p. 589)

Healing of acute lesions can lead to resolution or pericardial fibrosis ranging from a thick, pearly, nonadherent epicardial plaque *(soldier's plaque)*; to thin, delicate adhesions; to massive adhesions, as described next.

- *Adhesive mediastinopericarditis* is clinically significant—the pericardial sac is obliterated, and the parietal layer is tethered to mediastinal tissue. The heart thus contracts against all the surrounding attached structures, with subsequent hypertrophy and dilation.
- Usual antecedents are tuberculous or purulent pericarditis.
- *Constrictive pericarditis* is clinically significant—marked by thick (up to 1-cm), dense, fibrous obliteration, often with calcification of the pericardial sac that encases the heart, limiting diastolic expansion and restricting cardiac output. Tuberculosis is the most common cause.

Rheumatoid Heart Disease (p. 589)

Rheumatoid arthritis involves the heart in 20 to 40% of severe chronic cases. The typical finding is pericarditis, marked by a mixture of fibrin and necrotic debris derived from pericardial rheumatoid granulomas. This may progress to form dense, fibrous, and potentially restrictive adhesions. Less frequently, granulomatous rheumatoid nodules occur in the myocardium, endocardium, aortic root, or valves, where they are particularly damaging. Rheumatoid valvulitis can produce changes similar to those seen in rheumatic heart disease but classically without commissural fusion.

TUMORS (p. 589)

Primary heart tumors are rare, but cardiac metastases (usually hematogenous) occur in some patients who die of cancer. Metastases involve the pericardium or penetrate into the myocardium, or both. The spectrum of cardiac effects of noncardiac tumors is summarized in Table 13–3. The following are potential primary cardiac tumors:

- *Myxomas*: *Myxomas are the most common primary cardiac tumor in adults.* Usually single, 90% arise in the atria in the region of the fossa ovale; the left-to-right ratio is 4:1. *Grossly* 1 to 10 cm in diameter, they are sessile to pedunculated and vary from globular and hard to papillary or villous and myxoid. *They may cause symptoms by physical obstruction or wrecking-ball trauma to the atrioventricular valves or by peripheral embolization. Histologically*, they are composed of stellate or globular multipotential mesenchymal myxoma cells, admixed with endothelial cells, smooth muscle cells, and inflammatory cells, all in an acid mucopolysaccharide matrix. The weight of evidence supports a hamartomatous origin.
- *Lipomas*: Lipomas are circumscribed but poorly encapsulated, often subendocardial large polypoid accumulations of adipose tissue, more commonly in the left ventricle, right atrium, or septum. Symptoms depend on location and on encroachment on valve function or conduction pathways. These are probably hamartomas.
- *Papillary fibroelastomas*: Papillary fibroelastomas may cause emboli but are usually an incidental finding at autopsy. They are characteristically found on right-sided valves in children and left-sided valves in adults. They are composed of clusters of 2- to 5-mm hairlike projections. *Microscopically*, filaments have a core of myxoid connective tissue with smooth muscle cells and fibroblasts, covered by endothelium. They probably derive from organized thrombi.
- *Rhabdomyomas*: Rhabdomyomas are much less common than myxomas but are the most common primary heart tumor in children. Rhabdomyomas may cause valvular or outflow tract obstruction. *Grossly,* they may be left-sided or right-sided gray-

Table 13–3. CARDIOVASCULAR EFFECTS OF NONCARDIAC NEOPLASMS

Direct Consequences of Tumor
Pericardial and myocardial metastases
Large vessel obstruction
Pulmonary tumor emboli
Indirect Consequences of Tumor
Complications of circulating mediators
    Nonbacterial thrombotic endocarditis
    Carcinoid heart disease
    Pheochromocytoma-associated heart disease
    Myeloma-associated amyloidosis
Effects of tumor therapy
    Chemotherapy
    Radiation therapy

Modified from Schoen FJ, et al: Cardiac effects of non-cardiac neoplasms. Cardiol Clin 2:657, 1984.

white ventricular wall masses up to several centimeters in diameter. *Microscopically*, they are composed of large, rounded, or polygonal cells rich in glycogen and containing myofibrils. Cytoplasmic strands radiating from the central nucleus to plasma membrane create *spider cells*. Rhabdomyomas are probably hamartomas; some are associated with tuberous sclerosis.

- *Angiosarcomas and rhabdomyosarcomas*: These malignant neoplasms resemble their counterparts in other locations.

CONGENITAL HEART DISEASE (p. 591)

Some cardiac abnormalities are incompatible with intrauterine survival; others manifest shortly after birth as the circulation changes from fetal to postnatal configuration; still others cause cardiac malfunction only in adult life; and some are entirely inconsequential.

Twelve anomalies (Table 13–4) account for about 85% of cases. Bicuspid aortic valve and mitral valve prolapse are not included because they are generally not significant in childhood (and have been previously discussed in the context of valvular diseases).

Etiology

The causes of congenital heart disease are unknown in 90% of cases; they are likely multifactorial with genetic and environmental inputs. There is a 2-fold to 10-fold increase in the incidence of congenital heart disease in siblings of an affected child.

Causative single gene abnormalities have recently been recognized. Five percent of cases are associated with well-known multisystem syndromes based on chromosomal abnormalities (e.g., trisomy 21 [Down syndrome]). *Fewer than 1% of congenital*

Table 13–4. RELATIVE FREQUENCY AND GENDER DISTRIBUTION OF 12 MOST COMMONLY ENCOUNTERED CONGENITAL CARDIAC MALFORMATIONS

Malformation	Relative Frequency (%)	Male-to-Female Ratio
Ventricular septal defect	32	1:1
Atrial septal defect	8	1:2
Patent ductus arteriosus	8	1:2
Tetralogy of Fallot	8	1:1
Pulmonary stenosis	8	1:1
Aortic stenosis or atresia	8	3:1
Coarctation of aorta	6	2:1
Transposition of great arteries	5	2:1
Atrioventricular septal defect	4	1:1
Tricuspid atresia	2	1:1
Total anomalous pulmonary venous connection	2	1:1
Truncus arteriosus	1	1:1
Other	8	—

Modified from Edwards WD: Congenital heart disease. In Damjanov I, Linder J (eds): Anderson's Pathology, 10th ed. St. Louis, Mosby, 1996, pp 1339–1396.

defects are clearly environmental, the best documented being maternal rubella in the first trimester, which causes patent ductus arteriosus (PDA), pulmonic and aortic stenosis, tetralogy of Fallot, and other defects. Thalidomide, excessive alcohol consumption, and excessive cigarette smoking also have been strongly implicated. The most critical juncture is embryologic cardiac development in gestational weeks 3 through 8.

Clinical Consequences

Children with significant congenital anomalies have not only direct hemodynamic sequelae, but also failure to thrive and have retarded development or cyanosis. They also are at increased risk of chronic or recurrent illness and of infective endocarditis (owing to abnormal valves or to endocardial injury from jet lesions). The various congenital anomalies are of two types: shunts or obstructions.

SHUNTS

A *shunt* denotes abnormal communication between heart chambers, between vessels, or between chambers and vessels. Depending on pressure relationships, blood may be shunted from left to right (more common) or right to left.

- *Right-to-left shunts (cyanotic congenital heart disease)* cause cyanosis from the outset as poorly oxygenated blood passes into the systemic circulation. They also permit emboli from venous sources to pass directly into the systemic circulation *(paradoxic embolism)*.
- *Left-to-right shunts* induce chronic right-sided heart overload with secondary pulmonary hypertension and right ventricle hypertrophy, but eventually right-sided pressure exceeds left-sided pressure, and the shunt becomes right to left. Hence, cyanosis appears late. Once significant pulmonary hypertension develops, the structural defects of congenital heart disease are considered irreversible.

  Secondary findings in long-standing cyanotic heart disease include

- Clubbing of the fingers and toes
- Hypertrophic osteoarthropathy
- Polycythemia

OBSTRUCTIONS

Obstructions are typically coarctation, valvular stenoses, or atresias. These do not cause cyanosis.

Left-to-Right Shunts: Late Cyanosis (p. 593)

The major anomalies in left-to-right shunts

- Atrial septal defect (ASD)
- VSD
- PDA

ATRIAL SEPTAL DEFECT (p. 593)

ASD denotes an abnormal opening in the atrial septum that allows free communication of blood. ASD is the most common congenital cardiac anomaly presenting in adults and falls into three categories:

1. *Primum type*: Represents 5% of ASDs and common in Down syndrome. It occurs low in the atrial septum, occasionally in association with mitral valve deformities.

2. *Secundum type*: Represents 90% of ASDs and occurs at the foramen ovale. The aperture may be of any size (generating a single atrial chamber if large) and may be single, multiple, or fenestrated. It is usually isolated but sometimes associated with other anomalies.

3. *Sinus venosus type*: Represents 5% of ASDs and occurs high in the septum near the superior vena cava entrance. It is sometimes associated with anomalous right pulmonary venous drainage into the superior vena cava or right atrium.

- Even large ASDs are usually asymptomatic until adulthood, when either right-sided heart failure occurs or gradually increasing right-sided hypertrophy and pulmonary artery pressure finally induce right-to-left shunting with cyanosis.
- Surgical correction early in life is advocated to prevent pulmonary vascular changes and paradoxic embolism.

VENTRICULAR SEPTAL DEFECT (p. 594)

An abnormal opening in the ventricular septum that allows free communication between left and right ventricles, VSD is the most common congenital cardiac anomaly.

- VSD is frequently associated with other structural anomalies, particularly tetralogy of Fallot, but 30% are isolated. Ninety percent involve the membranous septum (membranous VSD) near the aortic valve; the remainder are muscular.
- Depending on the size of the defect, the clinical picture ranges (in decreasing order of importance) from fulminant CHF to late cyanosis, to asymptomatic holosystolic murmurs, to spontaneous closure (50% of those <0.5 cm in diameter).
- With a small to moderate-sized VSD, patients are at increased risk of infective endocarditis.
- Surgical correction is desirable before right-sided heart overload and pulmonary vascular disease develop.

PATENT DUCTUS ARTERIOSUS (p. 594)

- In the fetus, the ductus arteriosus permits blood flow between the aorta (distal to the left subclavian artery) and the pulmonary artery.
- At term, and under the influence of relatively high oxygen tension and reduced local prostaglandin E synthesis, muscular contraction closes the ductus within 1 to 2 days of life. Persistent patency beyond that point is generally permanent.
- About 85 to 90% of PDAs occur as isolated defects. The length and diameter (up to 1 cm) are variable. There is associated left ventricle hypertrophy and pulmonary artery dilation.
- Although initially asymptomatic and notable only for a prominent heart murmur (described as *machinery-like*), long-standing PDA induces pulmonary hypertension with subsequent right ventricle hypertrophy and finally right-to-left shunting to produce late cyanosis.
- Early closure of a PDA (either surgically or with prostaglandin administration in otherwise normal infants) is advocated.

Right-to-Left Shunts: Early Cyanosis (p. 595)

The major anomalies among right-to-left shunts are

1. Tetralogy of Fallot
2. Transposition of the great vessels
3. Truncus arteriosus

TETRALOGY OF FALLOT (p. 595)

The four cardinal features of tetralogy of Fallot, owing to embryologic anterosuperior displacement of the infundibular septum, are

1. VSD
2. Dextroposed aorta overriding the VSD
3. Pulmonary stenosis with right ventricle outflow obstruction
4. Right ventricle hypertrophy.

Additional cardiac anomalies may be present. Cyanosis is present from birth or soon after.

- The severity of symptoms is directly related to the extent of right ventricle outflow obstruction. With a large VSD and mild pulmonary valvular stenosis, there is a mild left-to-right shunt without cyanosis. More severe pulmonary stenosis produces a cyanotic right-to-left shunt.
- With complete pulmonary obstruction, survival is permitted only by flow through a patent ductus arteriosus (PDA) or dilated bronchial arteries.
- It is reasonable to delay surgical correction, provided that the child can tolerate the level of oxygenation. Pulmonary valvular stenosis protects the lung from volume and pressure overload, and right ventricle failure is rare owing to decompression into the left ventricle or aorta.

TRANSPOSITION OF GREAT ARTERIES (p. 595)

The aorta arises from the right ventricle and the pulmonary artery from the left.

- Fetal development occurs as a result of mixing venous and systemic blood through the PDA and a patent foramen ovale. Therefore, postnatal life critically depends on continued patency of the ductus as well as a VSD, ASD, or patent foramen ovale.
- Prognosis depends on the severity of tissue hypoxia and the ability of the right ventricle to maintain aortic flow. Untreated, most children die within the first few months.
- Particularly common in children of diabetic mothers, this malformation causes cyanosis.

TRUNCUS ARTERIOSUS (p. 596)

Associated with numerous concomitant cardiac defects, truncus arteriosus is basically a developmental failure of the aorta and pulmonary artery to separate. It results in an infundibular VSD with a single vessel receiving blood from both right ventricle and left ventricle.

Patients present with early cyanosis as a result of right-to-left shunting. Eventually the flow reverses, and they develop right ventricle hypertrophy with pulmonary vascular hypertension. The anomaly carries a poor prognosis.

Obstructive Congenital Anomalies (p. 596)

COARCTATION OF AORTA (p. 596)

- Coarctation of the aorta represents a constriction of the aorta; 50% occur as isolated defects, the remainder with multiple other anomalies.
- In most cases, cardiomegaly (chronic pressure overload hypertrophy) occurs.
- Clinical manifestations depend on the location and severity of the constriction. Most occur just distal to the ductus or ligamentum arteriosus *(postductal).*
- *Preductal* coarctation manifests early in life and may be rapidly fatal. Survival depends on the ability of the ductus arteriosus to sustain blood flow to the distal aorta and lower body adequately. Even then, there tends to be lower body cyanosis. This form usually involves a 1- to 5-cm segment of the aortic root and is often associated with fetal right ventricle hypertrophy and early right-sided heart failure.
- *Postductal* coarctation is generally asymptomatic unless severe. It usually leads to upper extremity hypertension but low flow and hypotension in the lower extremities, causing arterial insufficiency (claudication, cold sensitivity). Collateral flow around the coarctation generally develops, with intercostal rib notching (noted on x-ray views) and internal mammary and axillary artery dilation.
- Untreated, the mean life span is 40 years, with death secondary to CHF, aortic dissection proximal to the coarctation, intracranial hemorrhage, or infective endoaortitis at the site of narrowing.

PULMONARY VALVE STENOSIS OR ATRESIA WITH INTACT INTERVENTRICULAR SEPTUM (p. 597)

- Pulmonary valve stenosis or atresia with intact interventricular septum occurs in isolation or in association with other anomalies (e.g., transposition or tetralogy).
- With *complete pulmonic atresia*, there is virtually always a hypoplastic right ventricle and an ASD with blood entering the lungs via a PDA.
- *Pulmonary stenosis*, generally caused by cuspal fusion, may vary from mild to severe.
- Pulmonary outflow obstructions may also be subvalvular or supravalvular and even multiple.
- Mild stenosis is generally asymptomatic. Progressively more severe stenoses cause increasing cyanosis with earlier onset.

AORTIC VALVE STENOSIS AND ATRESIA (p. 597)

- *Congenital complete aortic atresia* is rare and incompatible with neonatal survival. Survival with congenital *aortic valvular stenosis* (two types—valvular and subvalvular) depends on the severity of the lesion.
- Rare single-cusp aortic valves are also seen.
- Consequences include infective endocarditis, left ventricle hypertrophy (pressure overload), poststenotic dilation of the aortic root, and (rarely) sudden death.

■ Bicuspid aortic valve is a common anomaly but is generally functionally unimportant throughout early life. It is prone to calcific degeneration (described earlier), however, and can increase risk of infective endocarditis.

CARDIAC TRANSPLANTATION (p. 598)

Transplantation of cardiac allografts is now frequently performed, most commonly for dilated cardiomyopathy and ischemic heart disease. The 1-year survival is 70 to 80%, and 5-year survival is greater than 60%.

Allograft rejection is a major postoperative problem, characterized by interstitial lymphocytic inflammation that damages adjacent myocytes. More severe stages are accompanied by extensive myocyte necrosis and frequently inflammatory vascular injury. Other postoperative problems include infection and development of malignancies in the immunosuppressed patient, particularly lymphomas (generally related to Epstein-Barr virus). The major current limitation to the long-term success of cardiac transplantation is late, progressive, diffuse intimal proliferation of the coronary arteries *(graft arteriosclerosis),* which causes downstream myocardial ischemia and its consequences.

Diseases of Red Cells

ANEMIAS (p. 604)

Anemia is a reduction in the oxygen transport capacity of blood, usually as a result of a reduction below normal limits of the total circulating red cell mass. This reduction is reflected by lower than normal hematocrit and hemoglobin concentrations. In most anemias, erythropoietin production and erythropoiesis are increased, causing erythroid marrow hyperplasia. Increased erythropoiesis can also occur in the spleen and liver of infants (extramedullary hematopoiesis). Classification of anemias here is based on the mechanism of production (Table 14–1). Anemias can also be classified on the basis of red cell indices, such as mean cell volume, mean cell hemoglobin concentration, and mean cell hemoglobin.

Anemias of Blood Loss (p. 605)

Clinical and morphologic reactions to blood loss depend on the rate of hemorrhage (acute versus chronic):

- *Acute blood loss:* Alterations reflect principally the loss of blood volume (which may lead to shock and death). After several days, if the acute episode is survived, marrow compensation is evidenced by an increase in reticulocytes.
- *Chronic blood loss:* Anemia usually results when iron reserves are depleted, giving rise to iron deficiency anemia. Marrow is active (erythropoiesis) as iron becomes available.

Hemolytic Anemias (p. 606)

Hemolytic anemias are characterized by

1. Premature destruction of red cells
2. Accumulation of the products of hemoglobin catabolism (e.g., bilirubin)
3. Marked increase in erythropoiesis within the marrow and associated reticulocytosis

Hemolysis may occur predominantly intravascularly or extravascularly:

- *Intravascular hemolysis* occurs when red cells are damaged by mechanical injury (e.g., microangiopathic hemolytic anemia, described later) or by complement-mediated lysis (e.g., antibody-coated mismatched blood transfusion). It is manifested by
  • Hemoglobinemia and hemoglobinuria
  • Hemosiderinuria

Table 14-1. CLASSIFICATION OF ANEMIA
ACCORDING TO MECHANISM OF
PRODUCTION

Blood Loss
Acute: trauma
Chronic: lesions of gastrointestinal tract, gynecologic disturbances
Increased Rate of Destruction (Hemolytic Anemias)
Intrinsic (intracorpuscular) abnormalities of red cells
  Hereditary
    Red cell membrane disorders, e.g., disorders of membrane
      cytoskeleton: spherocytosis, elliptocytosis
    Red cell enzyme deficiencies, e.g., enzymes of hexose
      monophosphate shunt: G6PD, glutathione synthetase
    Disorders of hemoglobin synthesis
      Deficient globin synthesis: thalassemia syndromes
      Structurally abnormal globin synthesis (hemoglobinopathies): sickle
        cell anemia, unstable hemoglobins
  Acquired
    Membrane defect: paroxysmal nocturnal hemoglobinuria
Extrinsic (extracorpuscular) abnormalities
  Antibody mediated
  Mechanical trauma to red cells, e.g., microangiopathic hemolytic
    anemias, thrombotic thrombocytopenia purpura, DIC
  Infections: malaria
  Chemical injury: lead poisoning
  Sequestration in mononuclear phagocyte system: hypersplenism
Impaired Red Cell Production
Disturbance of proliferation and differentiation of stem cells: aplastic
  anemia, pure red cell aplasia, anemia of renal failure
Disturbance of proliferation and maturation of erythroblasts
  Defective DNA synthesis: deficiency or impaired use of vitamin B_{12} and
    folic acid (megaloblastic anemias)
  Defective hemoglobin synthesis, e.g., deficient heme synthesis: iron
    deficiency

G6PD, glucose-6-phosphate dehydrogenase; DIC, disseminated intravascular coagulation.

- Jaundice (conjugated hyperbilirubinemia)
- Reduction in serum haptoglobin (a protein that binds free hemoglobin)
- *Extravascular hemolysis* occurs within the mononuclear phagocytic cells of the spleen and other organs. Predisposing factors are injury to the red cell membrane, reduced deformability, or opsonization of the red cells. The manifestations of extravascular hemolysis are similar to those of intravascular hemolysis except for the absence of hemoglobinemia and hemoglobinuria.

HEREDITARY SPHEROCYTOSIS (p. 607)

Approximately 75% are autosomal dominant disorders characterized by defects in the red cell membrane that render erythrocytes spheroidal, less deformable, and vulnerable to splenic sequestration and destruction.

Pathophysiology

Proteins that form the skeleton of the red cell membrane are either reduced in amount or defective in structure. A deficiency of spectrin is the most common abnormality. Spectrin-deficient red cells have unstable cell membranes, pieces of which are lost spontaneously. The resulting reduction in the cell surface causes the red cells to assume a spheroidal shape. Spherocytic red cells have reduced membrane flexibility and hence are trapped and destroyed in the splenic cords.

Morphology

Morphologic findings are as follows:

■ Many red cells appear abnormally small and lack central pallor (spherocytes).
■ Splenic cords of Billroth are markedly congested and exhibit prominent erythrophagocytosis.
■ Marrow shows normoblastic hyperplasia.

Clinical Features

Although there is significant clinical variability, anemia, moderate splenomegaly, and jaundice are characteristic. Intercurrent infections may trigger two types of crises:

1. Hemolytic crisis associated with massive hemolysis
2. An aplastic crisis characterized by a temporary suppression of erythropoiesis, usually triggered by intercurrent, often parvovirus, infections

Forty percent to 50% of adults develop gallstones as a result of chronic hyperbilirubinemia.

Diagnosis of hereditary spherocytosis depends on family history, hematologic findings, and laboratory evidence of spherocytosis shown by examination of peripheral smears and increased red cell osmotic fragility. Most patients have increased mean cell hemoglobin concentration as a result of cellular dehydration.

GLUCOSE-6-PHOSPHATE DEHYDROGENASE DEFICIENCY (p. 610)

Glucose-6-phosphate dehydrogenase (G6PD) is an enzyme in the hexose monophosphate shunt that produces reduced glutathione, which is necessary to protect red cells from oxidative injuries. When G6PD-deficient cells are subjected to oxidant stresses in the form of infections or exposure to certain drugs, hemoglobin is oxidized and denatured. The altered hemoglobin precipitates within the cells in the form of Heinz bodies, which attach to the cell membrane and reduce its flexibility. Inclusion-bearing cells are susceptible to destruction by the splenic macrophages. In addition, Heinz bodies can also damage cell membranes directly; thus, the hemolysis in G6PD deficiency is both extravascular and intravascular.

Inheritance of the mutant G6PD gene is X-linked. There are several G6PD variants; only two, G6PD A$^-$ and G6PD Mediterranean, lead to clinically significant hemolysis. A$^-$ is present in about 10% of American blacks. It is associated with progressive loss of G6PD in older red cells, which undergo hemolysis on exposure to oxidant drugs, principally the antimalarials. Because younger red cells are unaffected, hemolytic episodes are self-limited. In the Mediterranean form, the level of G6PD is much lower, and thus hemolytic anemia is more severe. Patients with

G6PD deficiency may also develop hemolysis after ingestion of fava beans (*favism*) because these legumes generate oxidants.

SICKLE CELL DISEASE (p. 611)

Sickle cell disease, a hereditary hemoglobinopathy resulting from a point mutation of the globin gene, is associated with substitution of valine for glutamic acid at the sixth position of the β-globin chain. This change transforms hemoglobin A (HbA) to hemoglobin S (HbS). Approximately 8% of American blacks are heterozygous for HbS.

Sickling Phenomenon

On deoxygenation, HbS molecules undergo aggregation and polymerization, leading to sickling of the red cells. In the homozygous state, irreversibly sickled cells can be identified in the peripheral blood. Many factors influence sickling of the red cells, as follows:

- The amount of HbS and its interaction with other hemoglobin chains in the cell (the most important factor). In heterozygotes, approximately 40% of hemoglobin is HbS; the rest is HbA, which interacts only weakly with HbS during the processes of aggregation. Therefore, the heterozygote has little tendency to sickle and is said to have *sickle cell trait*. In contrast, *the homozygote has all HbS and full-blown sickle cell anemia*. β-globin chains other than HbA also influence the sickling process. For example, fetal hemoglobin (HbF) with its γ-globin chains also fails to interact with HbS, and hence newborns do not manifest the vaso-occlusive complications of the disease until they are 5 to 6 months old, when the amount of HbF in the cells begins to approach adult levels. HbC, another mutant hemoglobin, has a greater tendency to aggregate with HbS than does HbA, hence those who inherit HbS and HbC (double heterozygotes for HbS and HbC) have a more severe disease (HbSC) than do patients with the sickle cell trait.
- The mean corpuscular hemoglobin concentration (MCHC) per cell. The higher the HbS concentration within the cell, the greater the chances of contact and interaction between HbS molecules. Thus, dehydration, which increases the MCHC, greatly facilitates sickling and may trigger occlusion of small blood vessels. Conversely the coexistence of α-thalassemia reduces the MCHC and therefore the severity of sickling.

Consequences of Sickling

Consequences of sickling include the following conditions:

- *Chronic hemolytic state*: Sickle cells have rigid and nondeformable cell membranes and are therefore prone to sequestration and destruction. The average red cell survival is shortened to approximately 20 days and correlates with the percentage of irreversibly sickled cells in circulation.
- *Microvascular occlusions*: Because of their inelasticity and propensity to adhere to the capillary endothelium, sickle cells tend to occlude small blood vessels. The resultant hypoxic injury (infarction) is a clinically important and the most debilitating component of sickle cell anemia.

Morphology

Morphologic findings are as follows:

- The *spleen* is commonly enlarged in early phases of disease owing to trapping of sickled cells in the splenic cords. Late in the course, repeated episodes of vaso-occlusion lead to progressive scarring and shrinkage in size *(autosplenectomy)*.
- *Bone marrow* shows normoblastic hyperplasia. Expansion of the marrow when severe may cause resorption of bone.
- *Microvascular occlusions* produce tissue damage in several organs.

Clinical Features

Sickle cell disease is characterized by the following:

- Chronic hemolytic anemia with its associated features (e.g., chronic hyperbilirubinemia and propensity to develop gallstones).
- Vaso-occlusive crises representing painful episodes of ischemic necroses, affecting most commonly bones, lungs, liver, brain, penis, and spleen. In children, a painful crisis affecting bones may mimic osteomyelitis.
- Aplastic crisis representing temporary marrow suppression of erythropoiesis triggered by parvovirus infections; some cases may be caused by folate deficiency.
- Increased susceptibility to infections, particularly *Salmonella* osteomyelitis, and others caused by encapsulated organisms such as *Streptococcus pneumoniae* and *Haemophilus influenzae.* Progressive splenic fibrosis and impairment of the alternate complement pathway are believed to predispose to infections.

Diagnosis

Diagnosis of sickle cell disease is based on clinical findings, the appearance of sickle cells in the peripheral blood smear, and detection of HbS by hemoglobin electrophoresis. Prenatal detection of heterozygotes and homozygotes is possible through analysis of fetal DNA.

THALASSEMIA SYNDROMES (p. 615)

Thalassemia syndromes are a heterogeneous group of mendelian disorders, characterized by a lack of or decreased synthesis of either the normal α-globin or the normal β-globin chain of hemoglobin A ($\alpha_2\beta_2$). β chains are encoded by two genes on chromosome 11 and α chains by two pairs of genes on chromosome 16.

Genetic Defects

- *β-Thalassemia syndromes* are characterized by deficient synthesis of the β-globin chain:
  - In β°-thalassemia, there is total absence of β-globin chains in the homozygous state.
  - In β^+-thalassemia, there is reduced (but detectable) β-globin synthesis in the homozygous state.
  - Several different point mutations that affect transcription, processing, or translation of β-globin mRNA have been found to cause β°-thalassemia and β^+-thalassemia; mutations that cause aberrant splicing of mRNA are most common.
- *α-Thalassemia* is characterized by reduced synthesis of α-globin

chains because of deletion of one to all four of the normally present α-globin genes.

Pathophysiology

The hematologic consequences of diminished synthesis of one globin chain derive from both low intracellular hemoglobin (hypochromia) and a relative excess of the other chain.

- β-*Thalassemia*: With a decrease in the synthesis of β-globin, most of the α chains produced cannot find complementary β chains to bind. The free α chains form highly unstable aggregates that produce a variety of untoward effects, the most important being cell membrane damage, leading to a loss of K^+ and impaired DNA synthesis. These changes cause destruction of red cell precursors within the marrow (ineffective erythropoiesis) and hemolysis of the abnormal red cells in the spleen (hemolytic state). The resulting anemia, if severe, causes marked compensatory expansion of the erythropoietic marrow, which may encroach on the cortical bone and cause skeletal abnormalities in growing children. Ineffective erythropoiesis is also associated with excessive absorption of dietary iron, which along with repeated blood transfusions (needed by some patients) leads to severe iron overload.
- α-*Thalassemia*: α-thalassemia is associated with an imbalance in the synthesis of α chains and non-α chains (β, γ, or δ). The unpaired non-α chains form unstable aggregates that damage red cells and their precursors.

Clinical Classification

β-Thalassemia. Classification of β-thalassemia is based on the severity of anemia, which, in turn, is based on the type of genetic defect ($β^+$ or $β°$) as well as gene dosage (homozygous or heterozygous).

- *Thalassemia major*: This is most common in Mediterranean countries and parts of Africa and Southeast Asia. Individuals homozygous for β-thalassemia genes have severe, transfusion-dependent anemia. Hemoglobin levels range between 3 and 6 gm/dl. Peripheral blood smear shows severe abnormalities, including marked anisocytosis with many small and virtually colorless (microcytic, hypochromic) red cells, target cells, stippled red cells, and fragmented red cells. The clinical course of β-thalassemia major is generally brief because, unless the patient is supported by transfusions, death occurs at an early age from the profound effects of anemia. Blood transfusions lessen the anemia and suppress secondary features (bone deformities) related to excessive erythropoiesis. In multiply transfused patients, cardiac failure resulting from progressive iron overload and secondary hemochromatosis is an important cause of morbidity and mortality.
- *Thalassemia minor*: The presence of one normal gene in the heterozygote allows enough β-globin chain synthesis, so that affected individuals are usually asymptomatic. This form is more common than thalassemia major and affects the same ethnic groups. Peripheral blood smear usually shows some minor abnormalities, including hypochromia, microcytosis, basophilic stippling, and target cells. A characteristic finding on hemoglobin electrophoresis is an increase in HbA_2, which may constitute 4 to 8% of the total hemoglobin. Recognition of β-

thalassemia trait is important for genetic counseling and because it may mimic the hypochromic microcytic anemia of iron deficiency.

■ *Thalassemia intermedia*: This is characterized by clinical features and severity that are intermediate between the major and minor forms. These patients, as alluded to in the previous discussion, are genetically heterogeneous.

α-Thalassemia. Classification of α-thalassemia is made on the basis of the number of α-globin genes deleted, which, in turn, determines the severity of anemia.

■ *Silent carrier state*: This state results from the deletion of a single α-globin gene; reduction in α-globin chain synthesis is barely detectable. The silent carrier state is completely asymptomatic.
■ *α-Thalassemia trait*: Deletion of two α-globin genes occurs either from the same chromosome or from each of the two chromosomes. Both genetic patterns are identical clinically, but the position of deleted genes makes a difference in the likelihood of severe α-thalassemia (HbH disease or hydrops fetalis) in the offspring. The clinical picture is identical to that described for β-thalassemia minor.
■ *Hemoglobin H (HbH) disease*: Deletion of three of the four α-globin genes occurs. Synthesis of α chains is markedly suppressed, and unstable tetramers of excess β-globin (HbH) are formed. Clinically, HbH disease resembles β-thalassemia intermedia.
■ *Hydrops fetalis*: Deletion of all four α-globin genes occurs. In the fetus, excess γ-globin chains form tetramers (Hb Barts) that have extremely high oxygen affinity but are unable to deliver the oxygen to tissues. This form is not compatible with life.

The clinical and genetic features of thalassemia are summarized in Table 14–2.

PAROXYSMAL NOCTURNAL HEMOGLOBINURIA (p. 619)

Paroxysmal nocturnal hemoglobinuria is a rare disorder, characterized by chronic intravascular hemolysis. This is the only hemolytic anemia resulting from a membrane defect that is not inherited. Red cells have increased sensitivity to complement-mediated lysis owing to deficiency of a family of membrane proteins that are anchored into the cell membrane through glycosylphosphatidylinositol. A mutation in phosphatidylinositol glycan prevents the synthesis of glycosylphosphatidylinositol and hence causes paroxysmal nocturnal hemoglobinuria. Among the glycosylphosphatidylinositol-linked proteins are several that regulate complement activation. These are decay-accelerating factor (CD55), membrane inhibitor of reactive lysis (CD59), and C8-binding protein. A deficiency of these proteins causes spontaneous in vivo activation of the alternative complement pathway. Because platelets and granulocytes also have reduced activity of these proteins, their functions are affected as well; therefore, in addition to hemolysis, these patients are predisposed to infections and thrombosis, the latter involving especially the portal, cerebral, and hepatic veins.

Paroxysmal nocturnal hemoglobinuria is a clonal disorder of multipotent stem cells that sometimes transforms into other stem cell disorders, such as aplastic anemia and acute leukemia. In the absence of such transformation, paroxysmal nocturnal hemoglo-

Table 14–2. CLINICAL AND GENETIC CLASSIFICATION OF THALASSEMIAS

Clinical Nomenclature	Genotype	Disease	Molecular Genetics
β-Thalassemias			
Thalassemia major	Homozygous β^0-thalassemia (β^0/β^0)	Severe, requires blood transfusions regularly	Rare gene deletions in β^0/β^0. Defects in transcription, processing, or translation of β-globin mRNA
	Homozygous β^+-thalassemia (β^+/β^+)	Severe but does not require regular blood transfusions	
Thalassemia intermedia	β^0/β	Asymptomatic, with mild or absent anemia; red cell abnormalities seen	
	β^+/β^+		
	β^0/β		
Thalassemia minor	β^+/β		
α-Thalassemias			
Silent carrier	$-\alpha/\alpha\alpha$	Asymptomatic; no red cell abnormality	Gene deletions mainly
α-Thalassemia trait	$--/\alpha\alpha$ (Asian)	Asymptomatic, similar to β-thalassemia minor	
	$-\alpha/-\alpha$ (black African)		
HbH disease	$--/-\alpha$	Severe, resembles β-thalassemia intermedia	
Hydrops fetalis	$--/--$	Lethal in utero	

DISEASES OF RED CELLS

binuria is usually a chronic disease with a median survival of 10 years.

IMMUNOHEMOLYTIC ANEMIAS (p. 620)

Hemolysis in immunohemolytic anemias is related to emergence of anti–red cell antibodies. The major diagnostic criterion is the Coombs antiglobulin test, which detects antibodies on the surface of red cells. Classification is based on the nature of the antibodies and the presence or absence of an underlying disorder (Table 14–3).

Warm Antibody Hemolytic Anemia

Warm antibody hemolytic anemia is idiopathic in 60% of cases. The IgG anti–red cell antibodies coat the red cells but are not complement fixing. Opsonized red cells assume a spheroidal shape owing to partial loss of red cell membrane in the process of phagocytosis by splenic macrophages. Spherocytes are eventually sequestered and destroyed in the spleen; thus, splenomegaly is characteristic.

The mechanism of antibody formation is best understood in drug-induced hemolytic anemias:

- *Hapten model*: Drugs (e.g., penicillin, cephalosporins, and quinidine) may act as a hapten and combine with the drug or the red cell–drug complex.
- *Autoantibody model*: The drug (e.g., the antihypertensive agent α-methyldopa) in some manner initiates production of antibodies directed against intrinsic red cell antigens.

Table 14–3. CLASSIFICATION OF IMMUNE HEMOLYTIC ANEMIAS

Warm Antibody Type

The antibody is of the IgG type, does not usually fix complement, and is active at 37°C

Primary or idiopathic
Secondary to:
  Lymphomas and leukemias
  Other neoplastic diseases
  Autoimmune disorder (particularly SLE)
  Drugs

Cold Agglutinin Type

The antibodies are IgM and are most active in vitro at 0–4°C. Antibodies dissociate at ≥30°C. The antibody fixes complement at warmer temperatures, but agglutination of cells by IgM and complement occurs only in the peripheral cool parts of the body

Acute (mycoplasmal infection, infectious mononucleosis)
Chronic
  Idiopathic
  Associated with lymphoma

Cold Hemolysins (Paroxysmal Cold Hemoglobinuria)

IgG antibodies bind to red cells at low temperature, fix complement, and cause hemolysis when the temperature is raised to 30°C

SLE, systemic lupus erythematosus.

Cold Agglutinin Immune Hemolytic Anemia

Cold agglutinin immune hemolytic anemia is caused by IgM antibodies that agglutinate red cells at low temperatures.

- *Acute*: This form occurs during the recovery phase of certain infectious disorders (e.g., *Mycoplasma* pneumonia and infectious mononucleosis). This form of agglutinin immune hemolytic anemia is self-limited and rarely induces manifestations of hemolysis.
- *Chronic*: This form occurs with lymphoproliferative disorders and as an idiopathic condition. Clinical symptoms result from agglutination of red cells and fixation of complement in distal body parts, where the temperature may drop below 30°C. The hemolytic anemia usually is of variable severity; vascular obstruction by agglutinated red cells results in pallor, cyanosis of the body parts exposed to cold temperatures, and Raynaud phenomenon.

Cold Hemolysin Hemolytic Anemia

Cold hemolysin hemolytic anemia is characteristic of the disease paroxysmal cold hemoglobinuria, which manifests as acute intermittent massive intravascular hemolysis after exposure to cold. Autoantibodies are IgG in nature (Donath-Landsteiner antibody) and are directed against the P blood group antigen. They attach to the red cells and bind complement at low temperatures; when the temperature is elevated, hemolysis occurs. Most cases follow infections (e.g., *Mycoplasma* pneumonia, measles, mumps, and some ill-defined viral and influenza syndromes).

HEMOLYTIC ANEMIA RESULTING FROM TRAUMA TO RED CELLS (MICROANGIOPATHIC ANEMIA) (p. 621)

Significant trauma to the red cells resulting in their fragmentation in the circulation can produce intravascular hemolysis. Underlying conditions are as follows:

- Prosthetic heart valves that create turbulent flow and shearing forces.
- Diffuse narrowing of the microvasculature owing to deposition of fibrin, as occurs in disseminated intravascular coagulation (DIC).

The peripheral blood reveals fragmented erythrocytes in the form of burr cells, helmet cells, and triangular cells.

Anemias of Diminished Erythropoiesis (p. 621)

Impaired red cell production may be caused by a variety of disorders, such as deficiency of some vital substrate (iron, vitamin B_{12}, and folate) or stem cell failure.

MEGALOBLASTIC ANEMIAS (p. 621)

Megaloblastic anemias, caused most commonly by a deficiency of vitamin B_{12} or folate, have the following features in common:

- Abnormally large erythroid precursors (megaloblasts) whose nuclear maturation lags behind the cytoplasmic maturation; nuclear changes, such as pyknosis, that are normally associated with maturation of erythroblasts are delayed or fail to occur.

- Ineffective erythropoiesis (death of megaloblasts in the marrow) associated with compensatory megaloblastic hyperplasia.
- Prominent anisocytosis (variability in cell size), a reflection of the abnormal erythropoiesis, including abnormally large and oval red cells (macro-ovalocytes) with a mean corpuscular volume in excess of 100 m^3.
- Abnormal granulopoiesis yielding giant metamyelocytes and hypersegmented neutrophils.

Pathophysiology

Vitamin B$_{12}$ and folic acid are essential coenzymes in the DNA synthetic pathway. A deficiency of these nutrients results in deranged or inadequate synthesis of DNA, but the synthesis of RNA and proteins is unaffected. Therefore, cytoplasmic enlargement and maturation occur without concomitant nuclear maturation. In addition to affecting red cell precursors, a deficiency of vitamin B$_{12}$ and folate affects all rapidly dividing cells, including all myeloid cells and the mucosal epithelium of the gastrointestinal tract. The anemia results from

- Ineffective erythropoiesis
- Production of abnormal erythrocytes that are susceptible to accelerated hemolysis, by poorly defined mechanisms

Ineffective granulopoiesis and thrombopoiesis as well as premature destruction may also affect granulocyte and platelet precursors, giving rise to pancytopenia.

Many pathways may lead to a vitamin B$_{12}$ deficiency. The ultimate source of this vitamin is dietary animal products. Absorption of vitamin B$_{12}$ occurs as follows:

- Peptic digestion releases dietary vitamin B$_{12}$, which is then bound to salivary vitamin B$_{12}$–binding proteins called *R binders*.
- R-B$_{12}$ complexes transported to the duodenum are split by pancreatic proteases, and the released vitamin B$_{12}$ attaches to intrinsic factor (IF), secreted by the parietal cells of the gastric fundic mucosa.
- IF-B$_{12}$ complex passes to the distal ileum, where it attaches to the epithelial IF receptors, followed by absorption of vitamin B$_{12}$, which is then transported to the tissues by transcobalamin II.

A deficiency of vitamin B$_{12}$ may result from impaired absorption because of

- Achlorhydria (in elderly individuals), which impairs release of vitamin B$_{12}$ from the protein-bound form
- Gastrectomy, which leads to loss of IF
- Pernicious anemia, an autoimmune disorder that damages gastric parietal cells and the production of IF
- Resection of the ileum (preventing absorption of IF-B$_{12}$ complex)
- Malabsorption syndromes
- Increased requirements (e.g., pregnancy)
- Inadequate diet, uncommon because the body has large reserves of vitamin B$_{12}$

PERNICIOUS ANEMIA (p. 623)

Pernicious anemia is caused by a lack of IF production as a result of chronic atrophic gastritis. The gastric mucosal atrophy is marked by a loss of parietal cells.

Pernicious anemia in all likelihood results from an autoimmune reaction against gastric parietal cells. In favor of this concept are the following:

- Autoantibodies are present in the serum and gastric juice of most patients with pernicious anemia:
  - Type I antibodies, which block binding of vitamin B_{12} to IF (blocking antibodies)
  - Type II antibodies, which prevent binding of IF or IF-B_{12} complex to its ileal receptor (binding antibodies)
  - Antibodies directed against the gastric proton pump, which bind to the parietal cells (parietal canalicular antibodies)
- Autoimmune gastritis is induced by CD4+ T cells in animal models. In humans also, the gastric injury is believed to be initiated by autoreactive T cells; the autoantibodies are formed secondarily and cause further gastric mucosal injury.
- There is a significant association of pernicious anemia with autoimmune disorders of the adrenal and thyroid glands.

Morphology

Characteristic changes are found in the marrow, alimentary tract, and central nervous system:

- *Bone marrow*: Megaloblastic erythroid hyperplasia; giant myelocytes and metamyelocytes with hypersegmented polymorphs; large multilobed nuclei in megakaryocytes.
- *Alimentary canal*: Atrophic glossitis—the tongue is shiny, glazed, and red; gastric fundal atrophy with virtual absence of parietal cells; atrophic gastric mucosa replaced by mucus-secreting goblet cells (intestinalization).
- *Central nervous system*: Lesions found in 75% of cases; characterized by demyelination of the dorsal and lateral tracts of the spinal cord leading to spastic paresis and sensory ataxia. The basis of central nervous system changes is obscure and possibly distinct from hematologic effects (folate deficiency produces megaloblastic anemia, but neurologic changes are absent).

Clinical Features

Onset is insidious; patients are in their forties and fifties. Symptoms are those of anemia and involvement of the posterolateral spinal tracts. There is increased risk of gastric cancer. Diagnosis is based on measurement of serum vitamin B_{12} levels and hematologic response (reticulocytosis) after parenteral administration of the vitamin.

ANEMIA OF FOLATE DEFICIENCY (p. 626)

Folic acid deficiency induces a megaloblastic anemia that is clinically and hematologically indistinguishable from that encountered in vitamin B_{12} deficiency. The neurologic changes seen in the latter, however, do not occur, and gastric atrophy is absent. Deficiency of folic acid may result from

- Inadequate intake, usually encountered in those who live on marginal diets (e.g., chronic alcoholics, the elderly, and the indigent)
- Malabsorption syndromes, such as tropical and nontropical sprue
- Increased demand, as in pregnancy, infancy, and disseminated cancer

■ Administration of folate antagonists, such as methotrexate, used in cancer chemotherapy

Diagnosis of folate deficiency requires demonstration of decreased folate levels in serum or red cells.

IRON DEFICIENCY ANEMIA (p. 627)

Deficiency of iron is an extremely common cause of anemia worldwide.

Iron Metabolism

The normal Western diet contains approximately 10 to 20 mg of iron per day, most of which is in the form of heme contained in animal products. The remainder is inorganic iron found in vegetables. About 20% of heme iron (in contrast to 1 to 2% of nonheme iron) is absorbable. The duodenum is the primary site of absorption. Dietary heme iron enters the mucosal cells directly, whereas nonheme iron is transported into the cell by luminal mucins, a membrane-associated iron transport protein (called *Nramp2*), and cytosolic mobilferrin. A fraction of the absorbed iron is rapidly delivered to plasma transferrin. The remainder is bound to mucosal ferritin, some to be transferred more slowly to plasma transferrin and some to be lost with exfoliation of mucosal cells. When the body is replete with iron, most of the iron that enters the duodenal epithelium is bound to ferritin and lost with exfoliation; in iron deficiency, transfer to plasma transferrin is enhanced.

Total body iron content is in the range of 2 gm for women and 6 gm for men. Approximately 80% of functional body iron is found in hemoglobin, myoglobin, and iron-containing enzymes (e.g., catalase and cytochromes). The iron storage pool, represented by hemosiderin and ferritin-bound iron, contains approximately 15 to 20% of total body iron. It is found in all tissues but particularly in liver, spleen, bone marrow, and skeletal muscle. Because serum ferritin is largely derived from the storage pool of iron, its level is a good indicator of the adequacy of body iron stores.

Etiology

Negative iron balance and consequent anemia may result from low dietary intake, malabsorption, excessive demand, and chronic blood loss.

■ *Low dietary intake* alone is rarely the cause of iron deficiency in the United States because the average daily dietary intake of 10 to 20 mg is more than enough for men and nearly adequate for women.
■ *Malabsorption* may occur with sprue and celiac disease or after gastrectomy.
■ *Increased demands* not met by normal dietary intake may occur in pregnancy and infancy.
■ *Chronic blood loss* is the most important cause of iron deficiency anemia in the Western world; this loss may occur from the gastrointestinal tract (e.g., peptic ulcers, colonic cancer, hemorrhoids, hookworm disease) or the female genital tract (e.g., menorrhagia, metrorrhagia, cancers).

Clinical Features

Clinical features are as follows:

- *Peripheral blood*: Red blood cells are pale (hypochromic) and smaller than normal (microcytic).
- *Marrow*: There is mild hyperplasia of normoblasts, associated with loss of sideroblasts and absence of stainable iron in the reticuloendothelial cells.
- *Other organs*: In severe iron deficiency, depletion of essential iron-containing enzymes gives rise to changes such as alopecia, koilonychia, and atrophy of the tongue and gastric mucosa. Esophageal webs may appear, completing the *Plummer-Vinson triad* of hypochromic microcytic anemia, atrophic glossitis, and esophageal webs.

Diagnosis

Diagnosis rests on clinical and hematologic features along with

- Low serum iron and ferritin
- Increased total plasma iron-binding capacity
- Reduced plasma transferrin saturation

ANEMIA OF CHRONIC DISEASE (p. 630)

Chronic disease is a common cause of anemia in hospitalized patients and may occur in association with chronic microbial infections (e.g., tuberculosis, osteomyelitis), chronic immunologic disorders (e.g., regional enteritis, rheumatoid arthritis), or neoplasms (e.g., carcinomas of breast, lung). Serum iron levels and total plasma iron-binding capacity are reduced, but there is abundant storage iron. This combination suggests that there is a defect in the reutilization of iron as a result of some impediment in transfer of iron from the reticuloendothelial (storage) system to the erythroid precursors. The major cause, however, seems to be marrow hypoproliferation resulting from reduced renal erythropoietin generation, caused probably by the action of cytokines such as interleukin-1, tumor necrosis factor-α, and interferon-γ. The anemia is normocytic, normochromic or microcytic, hypochromic. Treatment of the underlying condition or administration of erythropoietin corrects the anemia.

APLASTIC ANEMIA (p. 630)

Aplastic anemia is characterized by failure or suppression of multipotent myeloid stem cells and resultant neutropenia, anemia, and thrombocytopenia (pancytopenia).

Etiology

Aplastic anemia may be idiopathic (in 65% of cases) or caused by the following:

- Myelotoxic drugs or chemicals, the most common cause of secondary aplastic anemia. Damage to the marrow may be dose related, predictable, and reversible or may be idiosyncratic, affecting only some of the exposed individuals and in an unpredictable manner. Best documented as predictable myelotoxins are benzene, alkylating agents, and antimetabolites (vincristine, busulfan); idiosyncratic reactions are caused by chloramphenicol, chlorpromazine, and streptomycin.

- Irradiation, when the whole body is exposed.
- Infections (e.g., non-A, non-B, non-C, and non-G hepatitis).
- Inherited diseases (e.g., Fanconi anemia, associated with multiple congenital anomalies).

Pathogenesis

In idiopathic cases, stem cell failure may be due to the following:

- A primary defect in the number or function of stem cells, resulting in some cases from a somatic mutation affecting stem cells. Genetically damaged stem cells may, in rare cases, be transformed to leukemias.
- Suppression of antigenically altered stem cells by immune (T cell-mediated) mechanisms. Stem cell alterations may be secondary to environmental insults, drug exposure, or infections.

Morphology

Morphologic findings are as follows:

- Hypocellular marrow (hematopoietic cells replaced by fat cells)
- Secondary effects of granulocytopenia (infections) and thrombocytopenia (bleeding)

Clinical Features

Onset is insidious with symptoms related to a paucity of red cells, neutrophils, and platelets. Splenomegaly is characteristically absent. In cases resulting from chemical or drug exposure, withdrawal of the inciting agent may lead to recovery. Treatment with bone marrow transplantation or immunosuppressive therapy is also of value.

PURE RED CELL APLASIA (p. 632)

Pure red cell aplasia is a rare form of marrow failure that results from absence or near-absence of red cell precursors. The acute form may be drug or virus induced or may occur as an *aplastic crisis* in chronic hemolytic states. Pure red cell aplasia may also appear insidiously in patients with thymomas; in this setting, the anemia is cured by resection of the tumor.

OTHER FORMS OF MARROW FAILURE (p. 632)

Other forms of marrow failure are as follows:

- *Myelophthisic anemia*: This is caused by space-occupying lesions that destroy or distort marrow architecture and depress its productive capacity. Myelophthisic anemia is associated with a paucity of all blood elements and, in many cases, the presence of white and red cell precursors in the blood. The most common cause is metastatic cancer.
- *Diffuse liver disease* (toxic, infectious, or cirrhotic): The anemia is attributed to bone marrow failure, although other factors, such as bleeding from varices and folate deficiency, may also contribute.
- *Chronic renal failure*: Chronic renal failure is almost invariably associated with anemia. The basis is multifactorial, including reduced red cell production because of inadequate production

of erythropoietin. Administration of recombinant erythropoietin is associated with significant improvement in the majority of cases.

POLYCYTHEMIA (p. 632)

Polycythemia is an increased concentration of red cells that may be relative or absolute.

- *Relative*, owing to decreased plasma volume and associated with
  - Dehydration (e.g., deprivation of water or prolonged vomiting)
  - Stress polycythemia, an obscure condition of unknown cause also called *Gaisböck syndrome*
- *Absolute*
  - *Primary*: Increase in red cell mass as a result of intrinsic abnormality of myeloid stem cells; related to myeloproliferative syndrome (p. 679)
  - *Secondary*: Increase in red cell mass in response to increased levels of erythropoietin, which may be
    1. Appropriate (lung disease, high-altitude living, cyanotic heart disease)
    2. Inappropriate (erythropoietin-secreting tumors, such as renal cell carcinoma, hepatocellular carcinoma, cerebellar hemangioblastoma)

BLEEDING DISORDERS (p. 633)

Hemorrhagic diatheses may be caused by increased fragility of blood vessels, disorders of platelets, defects in coagulation, or a combination of these. Evaluation of bleeding disorders requires laboratory tests, as follows:

- Bleeding time
- Platelet counts
- Prothrombin time
- Partial thromboplastin time
- Other specialized tests (e.g., clotting factor levels)

Increased Vascular Fragility (p. 634)

Disorders of increased vascular fragility are relatively common but usually do not cause serious bleeding. Most often, they induce petechial and purpuric hemorrhages. Platelet count and coagulation time are usually normal; bleeding time is variable. Conditions include the following:

- *Infections*, especially meningococcemia and rickettsioses: Underlying mechanisms are vasculitis or DIC (discussed later).
- *Drug reactions*: Reactions are often mediated by the deposition of immune complexes in the vessel walls with production of a hypersensitivity vasculitis.
- *Poor vascular support*: This results from
  1. Impaired formation of collagen, as occurs in scurvy and Ehlers-Danlos syndrome
  2. Loss of perivascular supporting tissue, associated with Cushing syndrome
- *Henoch-Schönlein purpura*: This is a systemic hypersensitivity reaction of unknown cause characterized by a purpuric rash, colicky abdominal pain, polyarthralgia, and acute glomerulone-

phritis. It is associated with vascular and glomerular mesangial deposition of immune complexes.

Thrombocytopenia (p. 634)

Thrombocytopenia is a decrease in platelet number, characterized principally by petechial bleeding, most often from small vessels of the skin and mucous membranes. Thrombocytopenia must be severe, to levels of 10,000 to 20,000 platelets per mm^3 (reference range, 150,000 to 300,000 per mm^3), before the bleeding tendency becomes clinically evident.

Causes of thrombocytopenia are many and can be classified into five major categories:

1. *Decreased production of platelets*: This occurs in generalized diseases of the bone marrow that compromise the number of megakaryocytes (e.g., aplastic anemia, disseminated cancer) as well as in ineffective megakaryopoiesis (e.g., megaloblastic states).

2. *Decreased platelet survival*: Decreased survival usually results from immunologically mediated destruction of platelets; it may follow drug ingestion (e.g., quinine, quinidine, methyldopa) or infections (particularly human immunodeficiency virus [HIV] infection, see subsequently). There is usually a compensatory megakaryocytic marrow hyperplasia. Platelet destruction can also result from mechanical injury in a manner similar to red cell fragmentation in microangiopathic hemolytic anemias.

3. *Sequestration*: Sequestration may occur in the presence of splenomegaly. In these instances, splenectomy can cure the thrombocytopenia.

4. *Dilutional*: Massive transfusions may cause a relative reduction in the number of circulating platelets because blood stored for longer than 24 hours contains virtually no viable platelets.

5. *HIV-associated*: This is multifactorial because of immune complex injury, antiplatelet antibodies, and HIV-induced suppression of megakaryocytes.

The more common forms of thrombocytopenia are described.

IDIOPATHIC THROMBOCYTOPENIC PURPURA (p. 635)

Idiopathic thrombocytopenic purpura is associated with immunologically mediated destruction of platelets. Two forms are recognized:

1. *Acute idiopathic thrombocytopenic purpura*: This self-limited disorder is seen most often in children after a viral infection (e.g., rubella, cytomegalovirus infection, viral hepatitis, infectious mononucleosis). Platelet destruction is probably related to formation of antiplatelet autoantibodies.

2. *Chronic idiopathic thrombocytopenic purpura*: Destruction of platelets results from the presence of platelet autoantibodies directed toward two platelet antigens—the platelet membrane glycoprotein complexes IIb/IIIa and Ib/IX. These antibodies can be demonstrated in the plasma as well as bound to platelet surface (PAIgG) in approximately 80% of patients. Destruction of antibody-coated platelets occurs in the spleen, which is also the major site of autoantibody synthesis. Splenectomy is beneficial in 75 to 80% of patients.

Clinical Features

Chronic idiopathic thrombocytopenic purpura most often occurs in adults, particularly women of childbearing age. Most commonly, there is a long history of easy bruising or nosebleeds. Sometimes the onset is sudden, with a shower of petechial hemorrhages or internal bleeding (melena, hematuria). Subarachnoid or intracerebral hemorrhage is a rare but serious consequence. The idiopathic form must be distinguished from that secondary to other immunologically mediated thrombocytopenias that accompany systemic lupus erythematosus, acquired immunodeficiency syndrome (AIDS), and drug injury.

Morphology

The spleen is normal in size, but histologically there is congestion of the sinusoids, and splenic follicles may show prominent germinal centers. An increased number of megakaryocytes are usually seen in the bone marrow.

Diagnosis

Diagnosis is suggested by clinical features such as petechial hemorrhages and thrombocytopenia and must be supported by demonstration of increased megakaryocytes in the marrow. As would be expected based on the low platelet count, the bleeding time is prolonged, but prothrombin time and partial thromboplastin time are normal. Tests for antiplatelet antibody are not routinely performed. Splenomegaly and lymphadenopathy are extremely uncommon.

THROMBOTIC THROMBOCYTOPENIC PURPURA AND HEMOLYTIC UREMIC SYNDROME (p. 636)

Thrombotic thrombocytopenic purpura and hemolytic uremic syndrome are two related disorders within the spectrum of *thrombotic microangiopathies*. They are characterized by thrombocytopenia, microangiopathic hemolytic anemia, fever, transient neurologic deficits (thrombotic thrombocytopenic purpura) or renal failure (hemolytic uremic syndrome). In some patients, however, there is overlap in symptoms. Most of these clinical manifestations are caused by *widespread hyaline microthrombi* (composed of dense aggregates of platelets and fibrin) that are found in arterioles and capillaries.

Pathophysiology

The fundamental defect in all cases is endothelial injury due to a variety of causes. Hemolytic uremic syndrome most commonly follows verotoxin-producing *Escherichia coli*. Although the inciting agent in thrombotic thrombocytopenic purpura has not been identified, a preceding influenza-like illness is frequently reported, suggesting a viral cause. Although thrombotic microangiopathies and DIC are similar with respect to some clinical features, in contrast to DIC, activation of the clotting system is not present.

Clinical Features

Thrombotic thrombocytopenic purpura typically affects women, whereas hemolytic uremic syndrome usually occurs in children, but these distinctions are not absolute. These are serious illnesses that can be managed effectively, and 80% survival can be expected.

Hemorrhagic Disorders Related to Defective Platelet Functions (p. 637)

Hemorrhagic disorders related to defective platelet functions are characterized by prolonged bleeding time in association with normal platelet count. Disorders may be congenital or acquired.

- *Congenital*:
    1. *Defective platelet adhesion*: Defective platelet adhesion is exemplified by the autosomal recessive Bernard-Soulier syndrome, which is caused by a deficiency of a platelet membrane glycoprotein complex (GpIb/IX), the platelet receptor for von Willebrand factor (vWF). This is necessary for platelet-collagen adhesion.
    2. *Defective platelet aggregation*: Defective platelet aggregation is exemplified by thrombasthenia, an autosomal recessive disorder resulting from a deficiency of platelet membrane glycoprotein (GpIIb/ GpIIIa), involved in binding fibrinogen.
    3. *Disorders of platelet secretion*: In this group of disorders, initial platelet aggregation with collagen or adenosine diphosphate (ADP) is normal, but subsequent platelet responses, such as secretion of prostaglandins and granule-bound ADP, are impaired.
- *Acquired*: Of the many conditions associated with acquired defects, two are clinically significant:
    1. *Aspirin ingestion*: Aspirin is a potent inhibitor of the enzyme cyclooxygenase and can suppress the synthesis of thromboxane A_2, which is necessary for platelet aggregation. The antiplatelet effect of aspirin forms the basis of its use in the prevention of myocardial infarction.
    2. *Uremia*: The pathogenesis of bleeding in uremic patients is complex and includes platelet function defects.

Hemorrhagic Diatheses Related to Abnormalities in Clotting Factors (p. 637)

Bleeding seen in patients with abnormalities of the clotting factors differs somewhat from that encountered in patients with platelet deficiencies:

- The spontaneous appearance of petechiae or purpura is uncommon; more often, the bleeding manifests as the development of large ecchymoses or hematomas after an injury or as prolonged bleeding after a laceration or any form of surgical procedure.
- Bleeding into the gastrointestinal and urinary tracts, and particularly into weight-bearing joints, is common.

Clotting abnormalities may occur as acquired defects or may be hereditary in origin.

ACQUIRED DEFICIENCIES

Acquired deficiencies are usually characterized by multiple clotting abnormalities. Vitamin K deficiency results in depressed synthesis of factors II, VII, IX, and X and protein C. Because the liver makes virtually all the clotting factors, severe parenchymal liver disease may be associated with a hemorrhagic diathesis. DIC produces a deficiency of multiple coagulation factors.

HEREDITARY DEFICIENCIES

Hereditary deficiencies typically affect a single clotting factor. The most common inherited disorders are hemophilia (A and B) and von Willebrand disease. A review of the structure and function of factor VIII-vWF complex aids in understanding of these disorders.

Plasma factor VIII-vWF is a complex made up of two separate proteins (factor VIII and vWF) that can be distinguished by functional, biochemical, and immunologic criteria. One component required for activation of factor X in the intrinsic coagulation pathway is called *factor VIII procoagulant protein* or factor VIII. Deficiency of factor VIII gives rise to classic hemophilia (hemophilia A). Factor VIII is linked to vWF, which forms approximately 99% of the complex and exists in the form of a series of multimers ranging in size from 4×10^3 to 12×10^6 daltons. vWF is necessary for adhesion of platelets to subendothelial collagen. Glycoprotein Ib serves as the major platelet membrane receptor, and it is believed that it is through this receptor that vWF bridges collagen and platelets. Ristocetin binds to platelets in vitro and induces aggregation by activating vWF receptors on their surface. vWF also acts as a carrier for factor VIII.

The two components of factor VIII-vWF complex are coded by separate genes and synthesized by different cells. vWF is produced by endothelial cells and megakaryocytes. Hepatocytes are the major source of factor VIII.

VON WILLEBRAND DISEASE (p. 638)

Von Willebrand disease is an extremely common disorder that can be grouped into two categories:

- Type 1 and type 3 von Willebrand disease are associated with reduced quantity of vWF. Type 1 is an autosomal dominant disorder and is the most common form. Clinically, it is quite mild. Type 3 is an autosomal recessive variant that is severe but uncommon.
- Type 2 disease is an autosomal dominant disorder in which the assembly of vWF multimer is defective, and hence the intermediate and large multimers (the most active forms of vWF) are reduced.

Levels of factor VIII may be reduced in von Willebrand disease because vWF stabilizes factor VIII in circulation. Therefore, patients have a compound defect involving platelet function and the coagulation pathway. This compound defect is reflected in the laboratory by a prolonged bleeding time in the presence of a normal platelet count and prolonged partial thromboplastin time. Except in the most severely affected patients, however, effects of factor VIII deficiency, such as bleeding into the joints, which characterize hemophilia, are uncommon. Clinically, von Willebrand disease presents with spontaneous bleeding from mucous membranes, excessive bleeding from wounds, and menorrhagia.

FACTOR VIII DEFICIENCY (HEMOPHILIA A)
(p. 639)

Hemophilia A is characterized by a reduced amount or activity of factor VIII. This disorder is inherited as an X-linked recessive trait that primarily affects males. Clinical features develop only in the presence of severe deficiency (factor VIII levels <1% of normal). Mild or moderate degrees of deficiency (levels between 1% and 50% of normal) are asymptomatic, although post-traumatic bleeding may be excessive. The variable degrees of deficiency in the level of factor VIII procoagulant protein result from different types of mutations in the factor VIII gene. Clinically, hemophilia is associated with the following:

- Massive hemorrhage after trauma or operative procedures
- *Spontaneous* hemorrhages in regions of the body normally subject to trauma, particularly the joints (hemarthroses), with recurrent bleeding into joints leading to progressive, crippling deformities
- Absence of petechiae
- Prolonged partial thromboplastin time and normal bleeding time

Diagnosis is possible only by assay for factor VIII. The cloning of the factor VIII gene has permitted antenatal diagnosis of hemophilia A.

Treatment consists of replacement therapy with factor VIII concentrates, which carries the risk of transmission of viral hepatitis. Before the routine screening of blood for HIV antibodies, transmission of HIV led to the development of AIDS in many hemophiliacs. With the current practice of using heat-treated factor VIII concentrates derived from the blood of HIV-seronegative donors, the risk of HIV transmission has been virtually eliminated.

FACTOR IX DEFICIENCY (CHRISTMAS DISEASE, HEMOPHILIA B) (p. 639)

Christmas disease, or hemophilia B, is clinically indistinguishable from hemophilia A. Inherited as an X-linked recessive trait, it may occur asymptomatically or with associated hemorrhage. Identification of Christmas disease is possible only by assay of factor IX levels.

Disseminated Intravascular Coagulation

(p. 640)

DIC is an acute, subacute, or chronic thrombohemorrhagic disorder occurring as a *secondary complication in a variety of diseases* (Table 14–4). DIC is characterized by activation of the coagulation sequence, leading to the formation of microthrombi throughout the microcirculation. As a consequence of the thrombotic diathesis, there is consumption of platelets, fibrin, and coagulation factors and, secondarily, activation of fibrinolytic mechanisms. Thus, DIC may present with

- **Signs and symptoms relating to infarction caused by microthrombi**
- A hemorrhagic diathesis resulting from depletion of the elements required for hemostasis and activation of the fibrinolytic mechanisms

PATHOGENESIS

There are two major mechanisms by which DIC may be triggered (Fig. 14–1):

1. Release of tissue factor or thromboplastic substances into the circulation
2. Widespread injury to the endothelial cells

Table 14–4. MAJOR DISORDERS ASSOCIATED WITH DISSEMINATED INTRAVASCULAR COAGULATION

Obstetric complications
  Abruptio placentae
  Retained dead fetus
  Septic abortion
  Amniotic fluid embolism
  Toxemia
Infections
  Gram-negative sepsis
  Meningococcemia
  Rocky Mountain spotted fever
  Histoplasmosis
  Aspergillosis
  Malaria
Neoplasms
  Carcinoma of pancreas, prostate, lung, and stomach
  Acute promyelocytic leukemia
Massive tissue injury
  Traumatic
  Burns
  Extensive surgery
Miscellaneous
  Acute intravascular hemolysis, snakebite, giant hemangioma, shock, heat-stroke, vasculitis, aortic aneurysm, liver disease

The *tissue factor or thromboplastic substances released into the circulation* may be derived from a variety of sources (e.g., placenta in obstetric complications and granules of leukemic cells in acute promyelocytic leukemia). Mucus released from certain adenocarcinomas can also act as a thromboplastic substance. In gram-negative sepsis, bacterial endotoxins can cause release of thromboplastic substances contained within endothelial cells and the lysosomes of granulocytes and monocytes. Furthermore, activated monocytes release interleukin-1 and tumor necrosis factor-α, both of which increase the expression of tissue factor on endothelial cell membranes and simultaneously decrease the expression of thrombomodulin. This results in both activation of the clotting system and inhibition of coagulation control.

Endothelial injury can initiate DIC by causing release of tissue factor from endothelial cells and by promoting platelet aggregation and activation of the intrinsic coagulation pathway as a result of exposure of subendothelial connective tissue. Widespread endothelial injury may be produced by deposition of antigen-antibody complexes (e.g., systemic lupus erythematosus), temperature extremes (e.g., heatstroke, burns), or microorganisms (e.g., meningococci, rickettsiae).

MORPHOLOGY

Microthrombi, with infarctions and, in some cases, hemorrhages, are found in many organs and tissues. Clinically significant changes are encountered in the following organs:

- *Kidneys*: Thrombi are found in renal glomeruli; they may be associated with microinfarcts or bilateral renal cortical necrosis.
- *Lungs*: Microthrombi are found in alveolar capillaries; some-

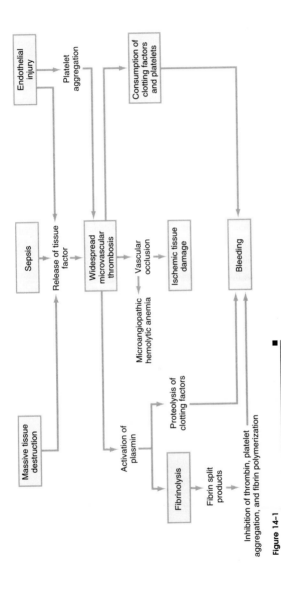

Figure 14-1

Pathophysiology of disseminated intravascular coagulation (DIC).

times they are associated with a histologic picture resembling acute respiratory distress syndrome.

- *Brain*: Microinfarcts and fresh hemorrhages may be seen.
- *Adrenals*: Massive hemorrhages give rise to the Waterhouse-Friderichsen syndrome seen in meningococcemia.
- *Placenta*: Widespread thrombi are noted, associated with atrophy of cytotrophoblast and syncytiotrophoblast.

CLINICAL FEATURES

About 50% of individuals with DIC are obstetric patients having complications of pregnancy; 33% have carcinomatosis. Sepsis and major trauma are responsible for most of the remaining cases. The onset may be fulminating, as in endotoxic shock or amniotic fluid embolism, or insidious, as in cases of carcinomatosis or retention of a dead fetus. There are numerous clinical manifestations. A few common patterns are as follows:

- A microangiopathic hemolytic anemia resulting from widespread microvascular occlusion
- Respiratory symptoms (e.g., dyspnea, cyanosis, or extreme respiratory difficulty)
- Neurologic signs and symptoms, including convulsions and coma
- Oliguria and acute renal failure
- Circulatory failure and shock

In general, acute DIC, associated, for example, with obstetric complications or major trauma, is dominated by bleeding diatheses, whereas chronic DIC, such as may occur in a patient with cancer, tends to present initially with thrombotic complications.

The prognosis is highly variable and depends, to a considerable extent, on the underlying disorder; each patient must be treated individually. Depending on the clinical picture, potent anticoagulants, such as heparin and antithrombin III, or coagulants in the form of fresh-frozen plasma may be administered.

Diseases of White Cells

Disorders of white cells may be associated with a deficiency of leukocytes (leukopenias) or proliferations that may be reactive or neoplastic.

LEUKOPENIA (p. 646)

Leukopenia may occur because of decreased numbers of any one of the specific types of leukocytes but most often involves the neutrophils (neutropenia, granulocytopenia). Lymphopenia is less common; in addition to rare congenital immunodeficiency diseases, it is observed in specific settings (e.g., advanced human immunodeficiency virus [HIV] infection, after therapy with glucocorticoids or cytotoxic drugs, autoimmune disorders, malnutrition, certain acute viral infections).

Neutropenia (Agranulocytosis) (p. 646)

Clinically relevant neutropenia occurs when neutrophil counts fall below 1000 cells/mm³, and counts less than 500/mm³ greatly increase the risk of severe bacterial and fungal infections. When counts are very low (>200 to 300/mm³), the condition is of such magnitude that it is referred to as *agranulocytosis*.

The half-life of a neutrophil is only 6 to 7 hours. As a result, an insult that impairs granulopoiesis can quickly produce neutropenia. Mechanisms include the following:

- *Inadequate or ineffective granulopoiesis*, as is observed with
  - Suppression of myeloid stem cells, as occurs in aplastic anemia (Chapter 14) and a variety of infiltrative marrow disorders (tumors, granulomatous disease)
  - Suppression of the committed granulocytic precursors, which occurs after exposure to certain drugs
  - Disease states characterized by ineffective granulopoiesis (e.g., megaloblastic anemias [owing to vitamin B₁₂ or folate deficiency] and myelodysplastic syndromes)
  - Rare inherited conditions (such as Kostmann syndrome)
- *Accelerated removal or destruction of neutrophils*, as in
  - Injury to the neutrophils caused by immunologic disorders (e.g., systemic lupus erythematosus) or exposure to drugs
  - Splenic sequestration
  - Increased peripheral utilization in overwhelming bacterial, fungal, or rickettsial infections

The most significant neutropenias (agranulocytoses) are produced by drugs. These may be

- *Dose-related*, meaning that agranulocytosis occurs in a predictable fashion (many chemotherapeutic cancer drugs, such as alkylating agents and antimetabolites, produce this type of neutropenia).
- *Idiosyncratic and unpredictable* (implicated drugs include aminopyrine, chloramphenicol, sulfonamides, chlorpromazine, thiouracil, and phenylbutazone).

MORPHOLOGY

Anatomic alterations in bone marrow depend on the underlying basis of the neutropenia:

- *Marrow hypercellularity* with increased numbers of granulocytic precursors, seen when the neutropenia is caused by increased destruction of mature neutrophils, or with ineffective granulopoiesis, as occurs in megaloblastic anemias and myelodysplastic syndromes.
- *Marrow hypocellularity*, noted when agranulocytosis is caused by agents that destroy or suppress committed granulocytic progenitor cells. In isolated neutropenia, only the granulocytic lineage is affected. If the insult also impairs erythroid and megakaryocytic progenitors, pancytopenia and aplastic anemia (empty marrow) may result.

CLINICAL COURSE

Symptoms and signs are related to bacterial or fungal infections and include malaise, chills, and fever, often followed by marked weakness and fatigability. Ulcerating necrotizing lesions of the gingiva, floor of the mouth, buccal mucosa, pharynx, or anywhere within the oral cavity (agranulocytic angina) are quite characteristic. All these sites often show massive growth of microorganisms with relatively poor leukocytic response.

PROGNOSIS

The prognosis is unpredictable. Infections in this setting are often fulminant; neutropenic patients are commonly treated with broad-spectrum antibiotics at first sign of infection. Granulocyte-colony stimulating factor may be used to decrease the duration and severity of the granulocytic nadir caused by chemotherapeutic drugs.

REACTIVE (INFLAMMATORY) PROLIFERATIONS OF WHITE CELLS AND NODES (p. 647)

Leukocytosis (p. 647)

Leukocytosis is a common reaction in a variety of inflammatory states. The particular white cell series affected varies with the underlying cause:

- *Polymorphonuclear leukocytosis* (neutrophilic granulocytosis, neutrophilia) accompanies acute inflammation associated with infection or other stimuli, such as tissue necrosis.

- *Eosinophilic leukocytosis* (eosinophilia) is seen in
  1. Allergic disorders (such as asthma, hay fever, allergic skin diseases)
  2. Parasitic infestations
  3. Drug reactions
  4. Certain malignancies (e.g., Hodgkin disease [HD] and some non-Hodgkin lymphomas [NHLs])
  5. Collagen vascular disorders and some vasculitides
  6. Atheroembolic disease transiently
- *Basophilic leukocytosis* is rare, often indicative of a myeloproliferative disease (e.g., chronic myelogenous leukemia).
- *Monocytosis* may be seen in
  1. Chronic infections (e.g., tuberculosis, bacterial endocarditis, rickettsiosis, and malaria)
  2. Collagen vascular diseases (e.g., systemic lupus erythematosus)
  3. Inflammatory bowel diseases (e.g., ulcerative colitis)
- *Lymphocytosis* accompanies monocytosis in many disorders associated with chronic immunologic stimulation (e.g., tuberculosis, brucellosis). It is also seen in viral infections (e.g., hepatitis A, cytomegalovirus, Epstein-Barr virus) and in *Bordetella pertussis* infection.

PATHOGENESIS

Elevation of the peripheral blood neutrophil count, the most common form of leukocytosis, can occur through a variety of mechanisms, as follows:

- *Expansion of the marrow neutrophilic progenitor cell and storage pools* occurs over hours to days in response to increased levels of colony-stimulating factors released from marrow stromal elements. Important pathophysiologic stimulants of colony-stimulating factor production include sustained elevations of interleukin-1 (IL-1) and tumor necrosis factor (TNF), as seen with infections and inflammatory disorders.
- *Increased release of mature neutrophils from the bone marrow storage pool* occurs rapidly in response to elevated levels of IL-1 and TNF, as seen in acute infection.
- *Increased demargination of peripheral blood neutrophils* is seen in acute stress and in response to elevations of glucocorticoids.
- *Decreased extravasation of neutrophils into tissues* is seen in patients treated with glucocorticoids.

Other factors induce different forms of leukocytosis through analogous mechanisms. For example, IL-5 causes eosinophilic leukocytosis by enhancing the differentiation of eosinophilic precursor cells, whereas the c-kit ligand and IL-7 stimulate lymphopoiesis and lymphocytosis.

TOXIC CHANGES IN NEUTROPHILS

Sepsis or severe inflammatory disorders may cause the appearance of

1. Abnormally coarse, dark neutrophilic granules (toxic granulations)
2. Blue cytoplasmic patches representing dilated endoplasmic reticulum (Döhle bodies)
3. Cytoplasmic vacuoles

LEUKEMOID REACTIONS

Differentiation of reactive leukocytosis from neoplastic leukocytosis (leukemia) is usually not difficult, but problems may arise in two settings:

1. In childhood acute viral infections, in which atypical lymphocytes resembling the cells of acute lymphoblastic leukemia (ALL) may appear in the peripheral blood or bone marrow
2. In severe inflammatory states, in which many immature granulocytes sometimes appear in the blood, simulating a picture of myelogenous leukemia

ACUTE NONSPECIFIC LYMPHADENITIS

Acute nonspecific lymphadenitis can be localized or systemic.

- The *localized* form is commonly caused by direct microbiologic drainage; it is seen most frequently in the cervical area in association with infections of the teeth or tonsils.
- The *systemic* form is characteristic of viral infections and bacteremia, particularly in children.

MORPHOLOGY

Macroscopically the nodes become swollen, gray-red, and engorged. Histologically, there are large germinal centers containing numerous mitotic figures. When pyogenic organisms are the cause of the reaction, a neutrophilic infiltrate is seen about the follicles and within the lymphoid sinuses; centers of the follicles may undergo necrosis.

CLINICAL FEATURES

Affected nodes are enlarged; tender; and, when abscess formation is extensive, fluctuant. The overlying skin is frequently red, and sometimes penetration of the infection to the skin surface may produce draining sinuses. With control of the infection, the lymph nodes may revert to their normal appearance; scarring may follow destructive, suppurative inflammatory reactions.

Chronic Nonspecific Lymphadenitis (p. 649)

Chronic nonspecific lymphadenitis may occur in the following patterns:

- *Follicular hyperplasia*:
  - This pattern is caused by inflammatory processes that activate B cells. It is distinguished by the prominence of large, round or oblong germinal centers (secondary follicles) containing two distinct regions:
    1. A dark zone containing proliferating blastlike B cells (centroblasts)
    2. A light zone composed of B cells with irregular or cleaved nuclear contours (centrocytes)
  - Causes include rheumatoid arthritis, toxoplasmosis, and early stages of HIV infection. It may be accompanied by *marginal zone B-cell hyperplasia*, particularly in immune reactions caused by toxoplasmosis and early HIV infection.
  - Follicular hyperplasia may be confused morphologically with

follicular lymphomas. Favoring a diagnosis of follicular hyperplasia are

1. Preservation of the lymph node architecture, including interfollicular T-cell zones and the sinusoids
2. Marked variation in the shape and size of lymphoid nodules
3. The presence of frequent mitotic figures, phagocytic macrophages, and recognizable light and dark zones, all of which tend to be absent from neoplastic follicles.

- *Paracortical lymphoid hyperplasia*: This pattern is characterized by reactive changes within the T-cell regions of the lymph node. Activated parafollicular T cells (immunoblasts three to four times the size of resting lymphocytes) proliferate and may partially efface B-cell follicles. It is seen in immunologic reactions induced by drugs (especially phenytoin [Dilantin]), in acute viral infections (particularly infectious mononucleosis), and after vaccination against certain viral diseases.

- *Sinus histiocytosis* (also called *reticular hyperplasia*): This pattern is characterized by distention and prominence of the lymphatic sinusoids resulting from marked hypertrophy of lining endothelial cells and infiltration with histiocytes. This is often observed in lymph nodes draining areas involved by cancers; it may represent an immunologic response to tumor antigens.

NEOPLASTIC PROLIFERATIONS OF WHITE CELLS (p. 650)

White cell neoplasms can be organized into three broad categories of disease:

1. *Lymphoid neoplasms*, encompassing a diverse group of tumors of B-cell, T-cell, or natural killer (NK) cell origin
2. *Myeloid neoplasms*, which originate from transformed hematopoietic stem cells that normally give rise to cells of the myeloid (i.e., erythroid, granulocytic, or thrombocytic) lineage.
3. *Histiocytoses*, which represent proliferative lesions of histiocytes, including Langerhans cells.

Lymphoid Neoplasms (p. 651)

DEFINITIONS

Two descriptive terms are often applied to lymphoid neoplasms.

- *Leukemias*: Usually present with widespread involvement of the bone marrow, often accompanied by the presence of large numbers of tumor cells in the peripheral blood.
- *Lymphomas*: Describes proliferations arising as discrete tissue masses (e.g., within lymph nodes, the spleen, or within extranodal tissues).

Among the *lymphomas*, two broad categories of disease are recognized:

- *HD* (Hodgkin lymphoma), segregated because of important clinical and histologic distinctions
- *NHL* (non-Hodgkin lymphomas), comprising all forms besides HD.

Table 15-1. SUMMARY OF THE LYMPHOID NEOPLASMS OF THE REAL CLASSIFICATION

	Salient Features
Tumors of Precursor B Lymphocytes	
Precursor B-cell acute lymphoblastic leukemia/lymphoma	Aggressive neoplasm of immature TdT + B cells that is most common in childhood; usually presents with extensive marrow and peripheral blood involvement. Genetically heterogeneous
Tumors of Precursor T Lymphocytes	
Precursor T-cell acute lymphoblastic leukemia/lymphoma	Agressive neoplasm of immature TdT + T cells that is most common in adolescent boys; often presents as a mediastinal mass. Genetically heterogeneous
Tumors of Mature B Cells	
Small lymphocytic lymphoma/chronic lymphocytic leukemia	Indolent CD5 + /CD23 + B-cell tumor of older adults; most commonly presents within bone marrow and peripheral blood; nodal and splenic enlargement also frequently observed
Mantle cell lymphoma	Moderately aggressive tumor of CD5 + / CD23 − B cells. Presents in older adults within lymph nodes or at extranodal sites. Associated with rearrangements of the *BCL1* gene
Follicular lymphoma	CD10 + B-cell tumor of older adults associated with *BCL2* gene rearrangements; usually presents in lymph nodes. Usually indolent
Burkitt lymphoma	Aggressive B-cell tumor of adolescents and young adults. Often appears at extranodal sites. Uniformly associated with rearrangements of the *c-myc* gene.
Diffuse large B-cell lymphoma	Aggressive B-cell tumor; occurs at all ages but most common in adults. May appear at extranodal sites or within lymph nodes. Morphologically and genetically heterogeneous
Marginal zone lymphoma	CD5 − /CD10 − B-cell tumor of adults that arises at extranodal sites of chronic inflammatory or autoimmune reactions. Often indolent, spreads late in its course
Hairy cell leukemia	CD5 − /CD10 − B-cell tumor of older adults that presents in bone marrow and spleen; nodal disease almost never seen. Generally good prognosis
Lymphoplasmacytic lymphoma	CD5 − /CD10 − tumor of mature B cells that show partial differentiation to IgM-producing plasma cells; presents in marrow, liver, and spleen. Older patients; often associated with symptoms of serum hyperviscosity
Multiple myeloma/ solitary plasmacytoma	Tumor of terminally differentiated B cells (plasma cells); presents in older adults as destructive bony lesions. Tumor cells usually secrete a complete or partial immunoglobulin. Poor prognosis

Table 15–1.   SUMMARY OF THE LYMPHOID
NEOPLASMS OF THE REAL
CLASSIFICATION *Continued*

	Salient Features
Tumors of Mature T Cells and NK Cells	
Peripheral T-cell lymphoma	Histologically and genetically heterogeneous tumors of mature T cells. Usually present in adults within lymph nodes. Generally aggressive course
Adult T-cell leukemia/ lymphoma	Tumors of CD4 + mature T cells that present in adults in marrow, skin, and lymph nodes. Associated with HTLV-1 infection. Poor prognosis
Mycosis fungoides/ Sezary syndrome	Tumor of CD4 + epidermotropic mature T cells. Occurs in adults; generally indolent course
Large granular lymphocytic leukemia	Indolent tumor of mature T cells or (less commonly) NK cells; presents in adults with marrow and peripheral blood involvement. Often complicated by anemia or neutropenia
Angiocentric lymphoma	Presents in adults as locally destructive masses, often in the sinonasal area. Tumor cells usually express NK cell markers and contain Epstein-Barr virus genomes. Generally aggressive

REAL, Revised European-American classification of lymphoid neoplasms; TdT, terminal deoxytransferase; NK, natural killer cell; HTLV, human T-cell lymphotropic virus.

Another group of lymphoid tumors with distinctive features are the *plasma cell neoplasms*, tumors composed of terminally differentiated B cells.

CLASSIFICATIONS

Multiple classification schemes of lymphoid neoplasms have been published, each with its own merits. Currently favored is the *Revised European-American Classification of Lymphoid Neoplasms (REAL)*, which defines distinct entities based on clinical features, morphology, immunophenotype, and genotype. It includes the lymphocytic leukemias, NHLs, and plasma cell neoplasms, which are sorted into four broad categories, based on immunophenotype:

1. *Precursor B-cell neoplasms* (neoplasms of immature B cells)
2. *Peripheral B-cell neoplasms* (neoplasms of mature B cells)
3. *Precursor T-cell neoplasms* (neoplasms of immature T cells)
4. *Peripheral T-cell and NK cell neoplasms* (neoplasms of mature T cells and NK cells)

The salient features of the most common or most pathogenetically interesting entities of the REAL classification are summarized in Table 15–1. Before discussing these specific entities, it is helpful to consider some general principles relevant to lymphoid neoplasms.

- Diagnosis requires histologic examination of lymph nodes or other involved tissues.

- Although traditionally considered to be malignant, lymphoid neoplasms display a wide range of behavior, from seemingly benign to rapidly fatal.
- The vast majority of lymphoid neoplasms (80 to 85%) are of B-cell origin, with most of the remainder being T-cell tumors; only rarely are tumors of NK cell origin. A few are histiocytic.
- All lymphoid neoplasms are derived from a single transformed cell and are therefore monoclonal. In most lymphoid neoplasms, antigen receptor gene rearrangement precedes transformation; hence daughter cells derived from the malignant progenitor share the same antigen receptor gene configuration and sequence and synthesize identical antigen receptor proteins (either immunoglobulins or T-cell receptors).
- Neoplastic B and T cells usually circulate widely but tend to home to and grow in areas where their normal counterparts reside.
- As tumors of the immune system, lymphoid neoplasms tend to disrupt normal regulatory mechanisms, leading to frequent immune abnormalities.

SPECIFIC ENTITIES OF THE REAL CLASSIFICATION (p. 654)

Precursor B-Cell and T-Cell Neoplasms

Acute Lymphoblastic Leukemia/Lymphoma. ALL are a group of neoplasms composed of immature, precursor B (pre-B) or precursor T (pre-T) lymphocytes *(lymphoblasts)*.

- *Most (approximately 85%) are pre-B tumors manifesting as childhood acute leukemias* with extensive bone marrow and peripheral blood involvement.
- The less common *pre-T ALLs tend to present in adolescent boys as lymphomas, often with mediastinal masses.*

Morphology. Lymphoblasts in Wright-Giemsa stains have relatively condensed chromatin; lack conspicuous nucleoli; and have scant, agranular cytoplasm that contains periodic acid–Schiff (PAS)–positive material. Pre-B and pre-T lymphoblasts are morphologically identical. Leukemic blasts are typically analyzed for expression of myeloid and lymphoid surface markers to

1. Distinguish ALL from acute myelogenous leukemia with certainty
2. Subclassify ALL

Immunophenotypic Subtypes. Immunostaining for terminal deoxytransferase (TdT), a specialized DNA polymerase expressed only by pre-B and pre-T lymphoblasts, is positive in greater than 95% of cases. Subclassification is based on the origin of the lymphoblasts and their stage of differentiation (detailed in Table 15–2 and summarized here):

- Pre-B ALL cells are arrested at stages preceding surface expression of immunoglobulin. The leukemic blasts of almost every patient with pre-B ALL express the pan B-cell antigen CD19.
- Pre-T ALL cells are arrested at early intrathymic stages of maturation. They express CD1a and show variable expression of other T-cell markers.

Table 15-2. IMMUNOLOGIC CLASSIFICATION OF ACUTE LYMPHOCYTIC LEUKEMIA

| | B-Lineage Markers | | | | T-Lineage Markers | | | Frequency (%) |
Category	Tdt	CD19	Cd10	Cm	Slg	CD7	CD3	CD2	
Very early pre-B	+	+	–	–	–	–	–	–	5–10
B									
Early pre-B	+	+	+	–	–	–	–	–	50–60
Pre-B	+	+	+	+	–	–	–	–	20
T-lineage	+	–	–	–	–	+	+*	+	15

TdT, terminal deoxytransferase; Cm, cytoplasmic IgM heavy chain; Slg, surface immunoglobulin.
*CD3 staining may be cytoplasmic or membranous.

Cytogenetics and Molecular Genetics. Approximately 90% of ALL have numerical or structural chromosomal changes. Prognostically important chromosomal aberrations include the following:

- *Hyperdiploidy (51 to 60 chromosomes)*: Associated with pre-B cell phenotype and relatively good prognosis.
- *t(12;21)*: Associated with early pre-B cell phenotype and good prognosis.
- *t(9;22), the Philadelphia chromosome*: Found in 5% of childhood pre-B ALL but in up to 25% of adult cases. Associated with poor prognosis.
- *Translocations involving chromosome 11 at band q23 (MLL gene)*: Associated with presentation at ages younger than 2 years, early pre-B phenotype, and poor prognosis.

Pre-B and pre-T ALL are associated with distinctive recurrent chromosomal translocations, indicating that different molecular mechanisms underlie their pathogenesis.

Clinical Features. Approximately 2500 new cases of ALL are diagnosed each year in the United States, with a peak incidence at approximately 4 years of age. ALL and acute myelogenous leukemia are immunophenotypically and genotypically distinct but have similar clinical features stemming from accumulation of neoplastic *blast* cells in the bone marrow. The major clinical features of both ALL and acute myelogenous leukemia as well as those features that are somewhat more characteristic of ALL are as follows:

- *Abrupt stormy onset*: Most patients present within days to a few weeks of the onset of symptoms.
- *Symptoms related to depression of normal marrow function*: Symptoms include fatigue mainly as a result of anemia; fever, reflecting an infection owing to absence of mature leukocytes; and bleeding (petechiae, ecchymoses, epistaxis, gum bleeding) secondary to thrombocytopenia.
- *Bone pain and tenderness*, resulting from marrow expansion with infiltration of the subperiosteum.
- *Generalized lymphadenopathy, splenomegaly,* and *hepatomegaly* caused by neoplastic infiltration: Each is more common in ALL than in acute myelogenous leukemia. In patients with pre-T cell ALL with thymic involvement, invasion of large vessels and airways may occur. Testicular involvement is relatively common in ALL.
- *Central nervous system manifestations*, such as headache, vomiting, and nerve palsies resulting from meningeal spread: These manifestations are also more common in ALL than acute myelogenous leukemia.

Prognosis. With aggressive chemotherapy (given together with prophylactic treatment of the central nervous system), more than 90% of children with ALL achieve complete remission, and at least two thirds are cured. Three factors are associated with a worse prognosis:

1. Age younger than 2 years, possibly because of the strong association of infantile ALL with translocations involving the *MLL* gene on chromosome 11
2. Presentation in adolescence or adulthood
3. The presence of the t(9;22) (the Philadelphia chromosome)

The high incidence of the t(9;22) in adult cases may partially explain the poor outcome in older patients, only a minority of whom remain disease-free 5 years after diagnosis.

Peripheral B-Cell Neoplasms

Chronic Lymphocytic Leukemia/Small Lymphocytic Lymphoma. Chronic lymphocytic leukemia/small lymphocytic lymphoma (CLL/SLL) are morphologically, phenotypically, and genotypically indistinguishable, differing only in the degree of peripheral blood lymphocytosis.

Morphology. Lymph node architecture is diffusely effaced by small lymphocytes of 6 to 12 μ containing round to slightly irregular nuclei mixed with variable numbers of larger cells called *prolymphocytes*. Prolymphocytes often gather together focally to form loose aggregates referred to as *proliferation centers*, which are pathognomonic for CLL/SLL. In CLL, the peripheral blood contains increased small, round lymphocytes with scant cytoplasm that are frequently disrupted, producing so-called *smudge cells*. Involvement of the bone marrow, spleen, and liver is common in CLL/SLL.

Immunophenotype. CLL/SLL express the pan-B cell markers (CD19 and CD20) and characteristically coexpress CD5, a marker that is found on a small subset of normal B cells. Low-level surface expression of immunoglobulin (usually IgM) is typical.

Chromosomal Abnormalities and Molecular Genetics. The reported incidence of chromosomal abnormalities varies from 25 to 67%. Most common are

1. Trisomy 12
2. Deletions of 13q12-14
3. Deletions of 11q

Each abnormality is seen in 20 to 30% of cases. Trisomy 12 and deletions of 11q correlate with higher-stage disease and portend a worse prognosis.

Clinical Features. CLL (defined as absolute lymphocyte count >4000/mm^3) is the most common leukemia of adults in the Western world. A small minority of patients present without lymphocytosis and are classified as having SLL, which constitutes approximately 4% of NHLs. Characteristic features include

- Presentation at ages older than 50 years (median age, 60)
- Male predominance (male-female, 2:1)
- Nonspecific symptoms at presentation (easy fatigability, weight loss, and anorexia)
- Generalized lymphadenopathy and hepatosplenomegaly (50 to 60% of the cases)
- Lymphocytosis in CLL, with counts as high as 200,000 per mm^3
- Immune abnormalities, including hypogammaglobulinemia (common) and autoantibodies against red blood cells or platelets producing autoimmune hemolytic anemia or thrombocytopenia (10 to 15% of cases)

Prognosis. The prognosis is extremely variable, depending primarily on the clinical stage. Overall, median survival is 4 to 6 years, but patients with minimal tumor burden often survive 10 years or more. Hypogammaglobulinemia leads to increased susceptibility to bacterial infection. CLL/SLL tends to *transform* to more aggressive histologies:

- *Prolymphocytic transformation* (15 to 30% of patients) is marked by worsening cytopenias, increasing splenomegaly, and the appearance of large numbers of *prolymphocytes* (cells with a large nucleus containing a single, prominent, centrally placed nucleolus) in the peripheral blood.

- *Transformation to diffuse large B-cell lymphoma* (so-called *Richter syndrome,* seen in about 10% of patients) usually presents as a rapidly enlarging mass within a lymph node or the spleen.

Both prolymphocytic and large cell transformation are ominous events, with most patients surviving less than 1 year.

Follicular Lymphoma. Follicular lymphoma is the most common form of NHL in the United States (45% of adult lymphomas).

Morphology. In lymph nodes, a nodular or nodular and diffuse growth pattern comprises two principal cell types:

1. *Centrocytes,* small cells with irregular or cleaved nuclear contours and scant cytoplasm (small cleaved cells)
2. *Centroblasts,* larger cells with open nuclear chromatin, several nucleoli, and modest amounts of cytoplasm.

Centrocytes predominate in most tumors. Involvement of spleen, liver, and bone marrow is common; peripheral blood involvement is seen in 10% of cases.

Immunophenotype. The neoplastic cells resemble normal follicular center B cells (CD19+, CD20+, CD10+, surface Ig+). Tumor cells also consistently express BCL-2 protein (normal follicular center B cells are BCL-2 negative).

Cytogenetics and Molecular Genetics. A (14;18) translocation that juxtaposes the *IgH* locus on chromosome 14 and the *BCL-2* locus on chromosome 18 is characteristic (70% of cases) and leads to overexpression of BCL-2 protein, which blocks apoptosis and promotes tumor cell survival.

Clinical Features. Follicular lymphoma tends to present with painless, generalized lymphadenopathy in middle-aged adults. It often follows an indolent waxing and waning course; the overall median survival is 7 to 9 years. Follicular lymphoma is incurable with conventional chemotherapy. Histologic transformation to diffuse large B-cell lymphoma occurs sometime during the course of the disease in 30 to 50% of cases. After transformation, median survival is less than 1 year.

Diffuse Large B-Cell Lymphoma. Diffuse large B-cell lymphoma comprises a heterogeneous group of tumors constituting about 20% of NHLs and 60 to 70% of aggressive lymphoid neoplasms.

Morphology. All variants share a relatively large cell size (usually four to five times the diameter of a small lymphocyte) and a diffuse pattern of growth obliterating the underlying architecture. The nucleus of the tumor cells may be round, oval, folded, or even multilobulated; is vesicular in appearance; and contains one to three prominent nucleoli. Cytoplasm is moderately abundant and may be pale or basophilic.

Immunophenotype. Mature B-cell tumors express the pan-B cell markers CD19 and CD20.

Cytogenetics and Molecular Genetics. Two chromosomal rearrangements are relatively common:

- *About 30% of tumors have the t(14;18) translocation* characteristic of follicular lymphoma. These tumors are considered to be of follicular center cell origin. Sometimes they are associated with the presence of typical follicular lymphoma at other sites (e.g., bone marrow), suggesting that they represent *transformed* follicular lymphomas.
- *An additional 20 to 30% of tumors contain various translocations that have in common a breakpoint involving the BCL-*

6 locus on chromosome 3. This gene encodes a zinc-finger transcription factor normally expressed in germinal centers, consistent with a role in control of B-cell differentiation.

Special Subtypes. Several distinctive subtypes of large B-cell lymphoma have been described. Only two that occur in the setting of immunodeficiency states, including acquired immunodeficiency syndrome (AIDS), are of sufficient pathogenetic interest to merit a brief discussion.

■ *Immunodeficiency-associated large B-cell lymphoma*: These tumors arise in the setting of severe T-cell immunodeficiency. The neoplastic cells are often latently infected with Epstein-Barr virus, which is thought to play a critical pathogenic role. Restoration of T-cell immunity may lead to regression of such Epstein-Barr virus–positive proliferations.

■ *Body cavity–based large cell lymphoma*: These arise as malignant pleural or ascitic effusions. They are mostly seen in patients with advanced HIV infection but also occasionally in HIV-negative elderly adults. The tumor cells are infected with human herpesvirus 8 (HHV8), which is believed to play a causal role in tumorigenesis.

Clinical Features. Diffuse large B-cell lymphoma may occur at any age but most frequently occur in older adults (median age of approximately 60). Patients often present with a rapidly enlarging, symptomatic mass at a single nodal or extranodal site. Waldeyer ring, the oropharyngeal lymphoid tissues that include the tonsils and adenoids, is commonly involved. Extranodal presentation (e.g., in the gastrointestinal tract, skin, bone, or brain) is relatively frequent. Involvement of liver, spleen, and bone marrow occurs but usually only late in the course.

Prognosis. Diffuse large B-cell lymphomas are aggressive tumors that are rapidly fatal if untreated. With intensive combination chemotherapy, complete remission is achieved in 60 to 80% of the patients; approximately 50% appear to be cured. Patients with limited disease fare better than patients with widespread disease or a large bulky tumor mass. Tumors with *BCL-6* rearrangements appear to have a better prognosis, whereas the presence of *p53* mutations correlates with a worse outcome.

Burkitt Lymphoma. Within the category of Burkitt lymphoma fall

1. African (endemic) Burkitt lymphoma
2. Sporadic (nonendemic) Burkitt lymphoma
3. A subset of aggressive lymphomas occurring in patients infected with HIV

Burkitt lymphomas occurring in these settings are histologically identical, but clinical, genotypic, and virologic differences exist.

Morphology. Involved tissues are diffusely effaced by intermediate-sized tumor cells, 10 to 25 μ in diameter, containing round or oval nuclei with coarse chromatin, several nucleoli, and a moderate amount of faintly basophilic or amphophilic cytoplasm. A high mitotic index is typical, as is apoptotic tumor cell death. These apoptotic cells are devoured by scattered large, pale phagocytic macrophages, producing the characteristic *starry sky* appearance. Occasionally, patients with Burkitt lymphoma present with a leukemic picture. In such cases, the tumor cells in marrow aspirates have slightly clumped nuclear chromatin; two to five distinct nucleoli; and royal blue cytoplasm containing multiple, clear cytoplasmic vacuoles.

Immunophenotype. These are tumors of relatively mature B cells expressing surface IgM; monotypic κ or λ light chain; and CD19, CD20, and CD10.

Cytogenetic and Molecular Genetic Features. *All forms of Burkitt lymphoma are highly associated with translocations of the c-MYC gene on chromosome 8.* The partner is usually the IgH locus (t(8;14)) but may also be the k (t(2;8)) or l (t(8;22)) light chain locus. *Essentially all African tumors are latently infected with Epstein-Barr virus, which is also present in about 25% of HIV-associated tumors and in a minority of sporadic cases.* Molecular analysis has shown that the configuration of the viral DNA is identical in all tumor cells within individual cases, indicating that infection precedes cellular transformation.

Clinical Features. Both the African and the sporadic cases of BL are found largely in children or young adults, accounting for approximately 30% of childhood NHLs in the United States. Most present at extranodal sites as a rapidly growing mass; endemic African Burkitt lymphoma often presents as a mandibular mass, whereas nonendemic Burkitt lymphoma most commonly presents as an abdominal mass involving the ileocecum and peritoneum.

Prognosis. Burkitt lymphoma is aggressive but responds well to short-term, high-dose chemotherapy, with many patients appearing to be cured.

Plasma Cell Neoplasms and Related Entities

Plasma cell neoplasms and related entities are a group of neoplasms of terminally differentiated B cells that have in common the expansion of a single clone of immunoglobulin-secreting plasma cells and a resultant increase in serum levels of a single homogeneous immunoglobulin or its fragments, hence the synonym *monoclonal gammopathies.* The monoclonal immunoglobulin identified in the blood or urine is referred to as an *M component* in reference to *my*eloma. The M component is usually a complete immunoglobulin, which, in some cases, is secreted along with excess free light (L) or heavy (H) chains. Occasionally, only L or H chains are produced, without complete immunoglobulin. Because of their small size, free L chains are excreted in the urine.

A variety of clinicopathologic entities are associated with monoclonal gammopathies:

- Multiple myeloma (plasma cell myeloma)
- Solitary plasmacytoma
- Monoclonal gammopathy of undetermined significance
- Waldenström macroglobulinemia, most commonly seen in patients with lymphoplasmacytic lymphoma
- Heavy-chain disease, a rare disorder characterized by the appearance of free heavy chains in the blood; most commonly associated with unusual small bowel lymphomas that occur in Middle Eastern populations (so-called Mediterranean lymphoma)
- Primary or immunocyte-associated amyloidosis, most commonly associated with multiple myeloma; occasionally occurs in patients without an overt plasma cell neoplasm

Multiple Myeloma. Multiple myeloma, the most common of the malignant gammopathies, is a plasma cell neoplasm of older adults characterized by destructive bony lesions at multiple sites.

Etiology and Pathogenesis. Cells with mature plasma cell morphology and function accumulate within lesions; however, small lymphoid cells within the peripheral blood have been shown to express immunoglobulin identical to that of neoplastic plasma cells, suggesting that they represent a progenitor cell population.

- The proliferation and survival of myeloma cells seem to depend on several cytokines, most notably IL-6.
- A variety of cytokines produced by the tumor cells, particularly IL-1b and IL-6, act as osteoclast-activating factors and likely contribute to the characteristic bony destruction.
- Up to 30% of cases have a balanced translocation, t(4;14)(p16.3;q32), that places the *FGFR3* (fibroblast growth factor receptor 3) gene under the control of IgH promoter elements.

Morphology. Morphologic findings are as follows:

- Bony lesions typically in the skull have a sharply defined, punched-out appearance when viewed radiologically. Less commonly, generalized osteoporosis may be seen. Although any bone may be affected, vertebral column, ribs, skull, pelvis, and femur are most commonly involved.
- Microscopic examination of the bone marrow reveals an increased number of plasma cells, often with abnormal features, which usually constitute greater than 30% of all cells. These cells may diffusely infiltrate the marrow or be present in sheet-like masses that completely replace normal elements.
- Significant renal disease is seen in a majority of patients. Several microscopic changes may be seen singly or in combination:
  - *Protein casts* consisting of immunoglobulins, albumin, and Tamm-Horsfall protein in the distal convoluted tubule and collecting ducts, often surrounded by multinucleated giant cells (so-called *myeloma kidney*)
  - *Metastatic calcifications* secondary to hypercalcemia
  - *Pyelonephritis,* owing to predisposition to bacterial infections
  - *Amyloid deposition* of the AL type, most notably within glomeruli; most commonly associated with λ light-chain disease; usually associated with systemic amyloidosis, which appears in 10% of patients
  - *Nonamyloidotic light-chain deposition* (glomerular and peritubular hyaline deposits that do not stain with Congo red); most common with κ light-chain disease
  - *Interstitial infiltrates of abnormal plasma cells or chronic inflammatory cells*
- In advanced disease, plasma cell infiltrates may be observed in many sites, including spleen, liver, lymph nodes, skin, and nerve roots.

Laboratory Findings. In 99% of patients, electrophoretic analysis reveals increased levels of a single immunoglobulin in the blood or light chains (Bence Jones proteins) in the urine. The most common serum *M protein* is IgG (55% of cases), followed by IgA (25% of cases). Myelomas expressing IgM, IgD, or IgE are rare. In approximately 20% of patients, Bence Jones proteinuria is present as an isolated finding. In addition, *the levels of normal serum immunoglobulins are characteristically decreased.*

Clinical Features and Complications. The peak age incidence of multiple myeloma is between 50 and 60 years. The principal clinical features stem from the following:

1. Infiltration of organs, particularly bones, by the neoplastic plasma cells

2. The production of excessive immunoglobulins, which often have abnormal physicochemical properties
3. The suppression of normal humoral immunity

Complications are as follows:

- *Bone infiltration* is manifested by pain and pathologic fractures. Hypercalcemia resulting from bone resorption may give rise to neurologic manifestations, such as confusion, weakness, lethargy, constipation, and polyuria, and also contributes to renal disease.
- *Recurrent infections* with bacteria, such as *Streptococcus pneumoniae*, *Staphylococcus aureus*, and *E. coli*, result from decreased production of normal immunoglobulins.
- Excessive production and aggregation of M proteins (usually IgA or IgG$_3$) leads to the *hyperviscosity syndrome* (described under lymphoplasmacytic lymphoma) in approximately 7% of patients.
- *Renal insufficiency*, occurring in up to 50% of patients, is multifactorial. The most important factor appears to be Bence Jones proteinuria because the excreted light chains are often toxic to the tubular epithelial cells. Hypercalcemia, pyelonephritis, and amyloidosis and other forms of light-chain deposition also contribute to renal dysfunction.
- *Extensive marrow involvement* gives rise to a normocytic, normochromic anemia, sometimes accompanied by moderate leukopenia and thrombocytopenia.

Prognosis. The prognosis depends on the stage of advancement at diagnosis. Patients with multiple bony lesions, increasing levels of M protein in the serum, and high levels of urine Bence-Jones protein have a grave prognosis. Chemotherapy induces remission in 50 to 70% of patients, but the median survival is still only 3 years. Infection and renal failure are the two most common causes of death.

Solitary Myeloma (Plasmacytoma). About 3 to 5% of plasma cell neoplasms present as a solitary lesion of either bone or soft tissue. Modest elevations of M proteins in the blood or urine may be found in a minority of patients.

- The solitary bony lesions tend to occur in the same locations as in multiple myeloma and progress to multiple myeloma in most cases over 5 to 10 years.
- Extraosseous lesions are often located in the lungs, oronasopharynx, or nasal sinuses; only rarely disseminate; and can often be cured by local resection.

Monoclonal Gammopathy of Uncertain Significance. M proteins can be identified in the serum of 1% of asymptomatic healthy persons older than 50 years of age and in 3% older than 70 years of age.

- In general, such asymptomatic individuals have less than 3 gm/dl of monoclonal protein in the serum and no Bence Jones proteinuria. Other forms of monoclonal gammopathy, particularly indolent multiple myeloma, must be carefully excluded.
- Most patients follow a completely benign clinical course. Unpredictably, however, approximately 20% of patients develop a malignant plasma cell neoplasm (usually multiple myeloma) over a period of 10 to 15 years.

Lymphoplasmacytic Lymphoma. Lymphoplasmacytic lymphoma is a B-cell neoplasm of older adults that usually secretes monoclonal IgM, often in amounts sufficient to cause a hyperviscosity syndrome known as *Waldenström macroglobulinemia.*

Morphology. Typically, there is a diffuse marrow infiltrate of neoplastic lymphocytes, plasma cells, and intermediate plasmacytoid lymphocytes (so-called *plymphocytes*), mixed with reactive mast cells. A similar polymorphous infiltrate may be present in the lymph nodes, spleen, or liver in patients having disseminated disease.

Clinical Features. Lymphoplasmacytic lymphoma tends to present after age 50 with nonspecific complaints, such as weakness, fatigue, and weight loss. Approximately half the patients have lymphadenopathy, hepatomegaly, and splenomegaly. Anemia caused by marrow infiltration is often present and may be exacerbated by autoimmune hemolysis caused by cold agglutinins of the IgM type (seen in about 10% of patients). IgM-secreting tumors cause additional complaints that stem from the physicochemical properties of macroglobulin. Because of its large size and increased concentration in blood, IgM tends to increase the viscosity of the blood greatly, giving rise to a hyperviscosity syndrome characterized by the following:

- *Visual impairment* results from the striking tortuosity and distention of retinal veins, which often assume a *sausage-link* appearance at points of arteriovenous crossings; retinal hemorrhages and exudates may also be seen.
- *Neurologic problems*, such as headaches, dizziness, deafness, and stupor, stem from sluggish blood flow and sludging.
- *Bleeding* is related to the formation of complexes between macroglobulins and clotting factors as well as interference with platelet functions.
- *Cryoglobulinemia* results from precipitation of macroglobulins at low temperatures, producing symptoms such as Raynaud phenomenon and cold urticaria.

Prognosis. Lymphoplasmacytic lymphoma is an incurable progressive disease with a median survival of about 4 years. Because it is mostly intravascular, symptoms related to IgM (such as hyperviscosity and hemolysis) can be alleviated by plasmapheresis.

Mantle Cell Lymphoma. Mantle cell lymphoma comprises about 3% of NHLs in the United States and a somewhat higher fraction of NHLs in Europe (7 to 9%).

Morphology. Morphologic features are as follows:

- Within lymph nodes, tumor cells may either accumulate about normal germinal centers or diffusely efface normal architecture. The proliferation consists of a homogeneous population of small lymphocytes with round to irregular to occasionally deeply clefted (cleaved) nuclear contours, condensed nuclear chromatin, inconspicuous nucleoli, and scant cytoplasm.
- Peripheral blood lymphocytosis, usually less than 20,000 mm^3, is seen in 20 to 40% of patients.
- Bone marrow and splenic involvement are frequently observed.
- Extranodal disease is relatively common and often takes the form of multifocal mucosal involvement of the small bowel and colon (*lymphomatoid polyposis*).

Immunophenotype. Mantle cell lymphoma is a CD5+ B-cell neoplasm that *characteristically overexpresses cyclin D1*, a protein involved in regulation of G1 to S phase progression during the cell cycle.

Cytogenetic Abnormalities and Molecular Genetics. A distinctive t(11;14), detected in about 70% of cases by cytogenetics and an even higher fraction of tumors analyzed by fluorescent in-situ hybridization, results in juxtaposition of the *BCL-1* locus and the *IgH* locus. This rearrangement leads to dysregulated expression of *BCL-1*, which encodes the cyclin D1 protein.

Clinical Features. Most patients are men aged older than 50 years presenting with generalized lymphadenopathy and bone marrow and liver involvement. Splenomegaly is present in about 50% of patients. B symptoms (fever and weight loss) are observed in a minority of patients.

Prognosis. The prognosis is poor, with a median survival of only 3 to 4 years. Most patients succumb to complications of organ dysfunction caused by tumor infiltration.

Marginal Zone Lymphomas. Marginal zone lymphomas encompass a heterogeneous group of B-cell tumors that may primarily arise within the lymph nodes, spleen, or extranodal tissues. Because the extranodal tumors were initially recognized at mucosal sites, they have been referred to as tumors of *m*ucosa-*a*ssociated *l*ymphoid *t*issues (or MALToma).

Notable clinicopathologic characteristics shared by the extranodal marginal zone lymphomas include the following:

- At sites of involvement, *chronic autoimmune reactions* (e.g., the salivary gland in Sjögren disease and the thyroid gland in Hashimoto thyroiditis) or *infections* (e.g., the stomach in *Helicobacter pylori*) occur.
- *Lymphomas remain localized at sites of origin for long periods*, spreading systemically only late in their course.
- Lymphomas are composed of cells at various stages of B lymphoid differentiation, often including terminally differentiated plasma cells. In most cases, however, *the predominant tumor cell population resembles normal marginal zone B cells*.
- Molecular analyses have shown that these are monoclonal (and therefore neoplastic) proliferations, and increased clinical follow-up has shown a predilection for dissemination and transformation to large B-cell lymphomas.

Pathogenesis. Stepwise progression from a polyclonal immune response to a monoclonal neoplasm has been proposed.

- The process begins as a reactive, polyclonal immune reaction, sometimes triggered by an environmental agent (e.g., *Helicobacter* gastritis).
- Over time, a monoclonal B-cell neoplasm emerges, probably as a result of acquired genetic changes, that is still dependent on local factors (e.g., factors produced by reactive T-helper cells) for growth and survival.
- With further clonal evolution, spread to distant sites and transformation to diffuse large B-cell lymphoma occurs.

Prognosis. The prognosis before dissemination is extremely good, with many patients being cured with local therapy directed at the tumor cells or the inciting factor (e.g., *Helicobacter*).

Hairy Cell Leukemia. Hairy cell leukemia is a rare but distinctive B-cell neoplasm of uncertain origin.

Morphology. Morphologic findings are as follows:

- Hairy cell leukemia derives its name from fine hairlike projections on the tumor cells (seen with phase-contrast microscopy). On routine peripheral smears, tumor cells have round, oblong, or reniform nuclei and modest amounts of pale blue cytoplasm, often with threadlike or bleblike extensions.

- Marrow biopsy specimens contain a diffuse interstitial infiltrate of cells with oblong or reniform nuclei, condensed chromatin, and abundant pale cytoplasm. Because of trapping in an extracellular matrix composed of reticulin fibrils, tumor cells are frequently absent from marrow aspirate smears.
- Splenic red pulp is preferentially infiltrated, leading to a beefy red gross appearance and obliteration of white pulp.
- Hepatic portal triads are frequently infiltrated.

Histochemistry and Immunophenotype. Hairy cells express B-cell markers, surface immunoglobulin, CD11c (an adhesion molecule), CD25 (the IL-2 receptor), and plasma cell–associated antigen-1 (PCA-1). A characteristic cytochemical feature is the presence of tartrate-resistant acid phosphatase.

Clinical Features. Hairy cell leukemia constitutes about 2% of all leukemias; it is predominantly a disease of middle-aged white men (male:female ratio, 4:1). Clinical manifestations largely result from infiltration of bone marrow, liver, and spleen.

- *Splenomegaly*, often massive, is the most common and sometimes the only abnormal physical finding.
- *Hepatomegaly* is less common and not as marked, and lymphadenopathy is distinctly rare.
- *Pancytopenia*, resulting from marrow infiltration and splenic sequestration, is seen in more than half the cases.
- *Infections* are the presenting feature in one third of cases. Frequent monocytopenia may contribute to a high incidence of atypical mycobacterial infection, possibly related to monocytopenia.

Prognosis. Hairy cell leukemia is an indolent disorder with a good prognosis. It is exceptionally sensitive to particular chemotherapeutic regimens, which produce long-lasting remissions in a majority of patients.

Peripheral T-Cell and Natural Killer Cell Neoplasms

Peripheral T-cell and NK cell neoplasms include a heterogeneous group of neoplasms having phenotypes resembling mature T cells or NK cells. Peripheral T-cell tumors comprise about 15% of NHLs in the United States and Europe, whereas NK cell tumors are rare in the Westen hemisphere. Both types of tumors are more common in Asia. Only relatively common entities are mentioned.

Peripheral T-Cell Lymphoma, Unspecified. Peripheral T-cell lymphomas as a group are heterogeneous and not easily categorized. Most fall into a wastebasket diagnostic category, *peripheral T-cell lymphoma, unspecified.*

Morphology. Certain findings are characteristic, but none are reliably predictive of T-cell phenotype. The tumors diffusely efface the lymph nodes and are most commonly composed of a pleomorphic mixture of small-sized, intermediate-sized, and large-sized malignant T cells. A prominent infiltrate of reactive cells, such as eosinophils and macrophages, probably attracted by T cell–derived cytokines, or a proliferation of small vessels, may often be observed.

Immunophenotyping. By definition, all peripheral T-cell lymphomas have a mature T-cell phenotype; they lack TdT and CD1 and express pan-T cell markers (e.g., CD2, CD3) and either T cell alpha beta ($\alpha\beta$) or delta gamma ($\delta\gamma$) receptors.

Clinical Features and Prognosis. Most patients present with generalized lymphadenopathy, sometimes accompanied by eosinophilia, pruritus, fever, and weight loss. Although cures have been reported, the prognosis appears worse than with aggressive mature B-cell neoplasms (e.g., diffuse large B-cell lymphoma).

Adult T-Cell Leukemia/Lymphoma. Adult T-cell leukemia/lymphoma is observed in patients infected by *human T-cell leukemia virus type 1 (HTLV-1)*; it is thus most frequent in regions where HTLV-1 is endemic (southern Japan and the Caribbean basin). The tumor cells express CD4 and contain clonal HTLV-1 provirus, compatible with direct pathogenic involvement of the virus in this neoplasm. The appearance of the tumor cells is highly variable; *cells with multilobular nuclei, described as cloverleaf or flower cells, are most characteristic.*

Commonly observed clinical findings include

1. Skin involvement
2. Generalized lymphadenopathy and hepatosplenomegaly
3. Peripheral blood lymphocytosis
4. Hypercalcemia

This is an extremely aggressive disease that is refractory to treatment in most cases, with a median survival of about 8 months.

Mycosis Fungoides and Sezary Syndrome. Mycosis fungoides and Sezary syndrome are different manifestations of closely related T-cell tumors characterized by involvement of the skin (cutaneous T-cell lymphomas).

Morphology. Mycosis fungoides presents with an inflammatory *premycotic phase* and progresses through a *plaque phase* to a *tumor phase.* Histologically, there is infiltration of the epidermis and upper dermis by neoplastic T cells, which often have a cerebriform nucleus, characterized by marked infolding of the nuclear membrane. Disease progression is marked by extracutaneous spread, most commonly to lymph nodes and bone marrow. *Sezary syndrome* is a variant in which skin involvement is manifested as a generalized exfoliative erythroderma and in which there is an associated leukemia of *Sezary* cells that also have a cerebriform appearance. Circulating tumor cells can also be identified in up to 25% of cases of mycosis fungoides in the plaque or tumor phase.

Immunophenotype. In the vast majority of patients, tumor is composed of CD4+ peripheral T cells.

Prognosis. Median survival is 8 to 9 years.

Large Granular Lymphocytic Leukemia. Large granular lymphocytic leukemia is a rare neoplasm that has gone by a variety of names, including *Tg lymphoproliferative disease, CD8 lymphocytosis,* and *CD8+ T-CLL.*

Morphology. The cytologic hallmark is the presence of lymphocytes in the peripheral blood and bone marrow with abundant cytoplasm containing scattered coarse *azurophilic granules.* Marrow involvement is usually focal, without physical displacement of normal hematopoietic elements. The splenic red pulp and hepatic sinusoids are also usually infiltrated.

Immunophenotype. Two variants are recognized:

1. T-cell tumors that usually express surface CD3 and CD8
2. NK cell tumors that express CD16 and CD56

Clinical Features. Patients usually present with mild to moderate lymphocytosis and variable splenomegaly, neutropenia, and anemia.

- *Neutropenia* is more common and associated with arrested maturation of progenitor cells in the marrow through unknown mechanisms.
- *Pure red cell aplasia* occurs in a small minority of patients, stemming from a direct suppressive effect of the tumor cells on erythroid progenitors.
- There is also associated an increased incidence of *rheumatologic disorders*; some patients present with Felty syndrome, characterized by the triad of rheumatoid arthritis, splenomegaly, and neutropenia.

Prognosis. The course is variable, being largely dependent on the severity of the cytopenias.

Angiocentric Lymphoma. Angiocentric lymphoma (previously called *lethal midline granuloma* and *midline malignant reticulosis*) is rare in the United States and Europe but constitutes up to 3% of NHLs in Asia.

Morphology. Most commonly presenting as a destructive midline mass involving the nasopharynx or, less commonly, the skin, the tumor cell infiltrate typically surrounds and invades small vessels, leading to extensive ischemic necrosis. The histologic appearance is variable; on touch preparations, the tumor cells often contain large *azurophilic granules* resembling those observed in normal NK cells.

Immunophenotype and Genotype. Most tumors express NK cell markers and lack T-cell receptor rearrangements, supporting an NK cell origin. *Additionally the tumor cells are latently infected with Epstein-Barr virus in most cases.*

Prognosis. Although some cases follow an indolent course, most are aggressive neoplasms that are poorly responsive to therapy.

HODGKIN DISEASE (p. 670)

HD, a category of lymphoid neoplasia, is one of the most common forms of malignancy in young adults, with an average age at diagnosis of 32 years. Differences from NHL are as follows:

- Characterized morphologically by the presence of scattered distinctive neoplastic giant cells called *Reed-Sternberg (RS) cells*, within a predominant background of reactive lymphocytes, histiocytes, and granulocytes
- Often associated with somewhat distinctive clinical features (Table 15–3)

Table 15–3. CLINICAL DIFFERENCES BETWEEN HODGKIN DISEASE AND NON-HODGKIN LYMPHOMA

Hodgkin Disease	Non-Hodgkin Lymphoma
More often localized to a single axial group of nodes (cervical, mediastinal, para-aortic)	More frequent involvement of multiple peripheral nodes
Orderly spread by contiguity	Noncontiguous spread
Mesenteric nodes and Waldeyer ring rarely involved	Waldeyer ring and mesenteric nodes commonly involved
Extranodal involvement uncommon	Extranodal involvement common

- Origin of the neoplastic cell in the more common forms still uncertain
- Immunophenotypically unique from other lymphoid neoplasms

Staging

Because HD spreads predictably from its site of origin to contiguous lymphoid groups, patients with limited disease can be cured with local radiotherapy. For this reason, the *staging of HD* is not only prognostically important, but also guides therapy. It requires careful physical examination and several investigative procedures, including computed tomography of the abdomen and pelvis, chest radiography, and biopsy of the bone marrow. Because radiologic imaging does not reliably detect splenic disease, staging laparotomy (during which abdominal lymph nodes are sampled and the spleen is removed for histologic evaluation) is still used in patients being considered for treatment with radiotherapy alone.

Morphology of Reed-Sternberg Cells and Variants

Reed-Sternberg cells and their variants are the neoplastic element, and their identification is essential for the histologic diagnosis.

- *Classic, diagnostic Reed-Sternberg cells* are quite large (15 to 45 μ in diameter) and may have either a single bilobed nucleus or multiple nuclei. Each nucleus or nuclear lobe contains a large, inclusion-like nucleolus, generally surrounded by a clear halo, that is about the size of a small lymphocyte (5 to 7 μ in diameter).
- *Mononuclear variants* contain only a single round or oblong nucleus with a large inclusion-like nucleolus.
- *Lacunar cells* have more delicate folded or multilobate nuclei surrounded by abundant pale cytoplasm that is often retracted during tissue processing, leaving the nucleus in an empty hole (the lacune).
- *Lymphocytic and histiocytic variants (L + H cells)* have polypoid nuclei resembling popcorn kernels, inconspicuous nucleoli, and moderately abundant cytoplasm.

Cells similar or identical in appearance to Reed-Sternberg cells occur in other conditions, such as infectious mononucleosis, solid tissue cancers, and NHL. Thus, Reed-Sternberg cells must be present in an appropriate background of non-neoplastic inflammatory cells (lymphocytes, plasma cells, eosinophils) for the diagnosis to be made.

Immunophenotype of Reed-Sternberg Cells and Variants

Classic Reed-Sternberg cells, mononuclear variants, and lacunar variants usually have a similar phenotype, being negative for B-cell and T-cell markers and *positive for CD15 and CD30.* L + H cells mark in a distinctive fashion, as they are usually positive for pan-B cell markers (such as CD20) and negative for CD15 and CD30. Immunophenotyping is often helpful in subtyping of HD and distinguishing HD from NHL and other conditions in which Reed-Sternberg–like cells may be seen.

Four subtypes of HD (in the Rye classification) are described next.

Hodgkin Disease, Nodular Sclerosis Type. The most common form of HD, constituting 65% to 75% of cases, this type is characterized by the presence of

1. A particular variant of the Reed-Sternberg cell, the *lacunar cell*

2. *Collagen bands* that divide the lymphoid tissue into circumscribed nodules

Neoplastic cells are found in a polymorphous background of small T lymphocytes, eosinophils, plasma cells, and macrophages. Classic Reed-Sternberg cells are uncommon but can be found. This is the only form of HD that is more common in women and strikes adolescents or young adults. It has a propensity to involve the lower cervical, supraclavicular, and mediastinal lymph nodes. The prognosis is excellent.

Hodgkin Disease, Mixed Cellularity Type. This form of HD constitutes about 25% of cases. It is rendered distinctive by diffuse effacement of lymph nodes by a heterogeneous cellular infiltrate, which includes small lymphocytes, eosinophils, plasma cells, and benign macrophages admixed with the neoplastic cells. *Classic Reed-Sternberg cells and mononuclear variants are usually plentiful.* This form of HD is more common in men. Compared with the lymphocyte predominance and nodular sclerosis subtypes, it is more likely to be associated with older age, so-called B symptoms (fever and weight loss), and advanced tumor stage. Nonetheless, the overall prognosis is good.

Hodgkin Disease, Lymphocyte Predominance Type. This uncommon variant accounts for approximately 6% of all cases. It is characterized by nodal effacement by a vaguely nodular infiltrate of small lymphocytes admixed with variable numbers of benign histiocytes and *L + H Reed-Sternberg cell variants.* Classic Reed-Sternberg cells are extremely difficult to find. Other cells, such as eosinophils, neutrophils, and plasma cells, are scanty or absent, and there is little evidence of necrosis or fibrosis.

A majority of patients with lymphocyte predominance HD are men, usually younger than 35 years old, with isolated cervical or axillary lymphadenopathy. The overall prognosis is excellent.

Etiology and Pathogenesis

It is now widely accepted that HD is a clonal neoplastic disorder and that the Reed-Sternberg cells and variants represent the transformed cells. The histologic pattern is partly influenced by cytokines secreted by the Reed-Sternberg cells and the reactive background cells:

- IL-5 synthesis by Reed-Sternberg cells correlates with eosinophil accumulation (a feature of mixed cellularity and nodular sclerosis subtypes).
- Transforming growth factor (TGF)-β, a fibrogenic cytokine, is found almost exclusively in the nodular sclerosis variant, in which it is produced by eosinophils.

Cytokines released from Reed-Sternberg cells likely induce the accumulation of reactive cells, which may, in turn, support the growth and survival of tumor cells.

Origin of Reed-Sternberg Cells. In the specific case of the lymphocyte predominance subtype, the evidence for a B-cell origin is fairly convincing. In the mixed cellularity and nodular sclerosis subtypes of HD, the origin remains uncertain but also tends to point toward a B-cell origin.

Pathogenesis. *Substantial evidence exists that implicates*

Epstein-Barr virus infection, which may be one of several steps involved in the pathogenesis of some HD subtypes.

- Patients with a history of infectious mononucleosis or with elevated titers of antibodies against Epstein-Barr virus antigens incur a slightly higher risk of HD.
- Epstein-Barr virus genomes and Epstein-Barr virus–specific RNA transcripts can be identified in Reed-Sternberg cells in 40% of cases of nodular sclerosis HD and 60 to 70% of cases of mixed cellularity HD but are not seen in the lymphocyte predominance type.
- The configuration of the Epstein-Barr virus DNA is the same in all tumor cells within a given case, indicating that infection occurred before cellular transformation.
- Epstein-Barr virus–positive tumor cells express latent membrane protein-1, a protein encoded by the Epstein-Barr virus genome that has been shown to have transforming activity.

Clinical Features

HD usually presents with a painless enlargement of lymph nodes. Involvement of extranodal sites, lymphoid tissue of Waldeyer ring, or mesenteric lymph nodes is unusual and suggests the diagnosis of NHL. The anatomic stage is of clinical importance (Table 15–4). Younger patients with the more favorable histologic types tend to present in clinical stage I or II without systemic manifestations. Patients with disseminated disease (stages III and IV) and the mixed cellularity or lymphocyte depletion subtypes are more likely to present with B symptoms (fever, weight loss).

Prognosis

Tumor burden (i.e., stage) rather than histologic type is the most important prognostic variable. Currently the 5-year survival rate of patients with stages I and IIA is close to 90%, and many

---

Table 15–4. CLINICAL STAGING OF HODGKIN DISEASE AND NON-HODGKIN LYMPHOMAS (ANN ARBOR CLASSIFICATION)

Stage*	Distribution of Disease
I	Involvement of a single lymph node region (I) or involvement of a single extralymphatic organ or site (I_E)
II	Involvement of two or more lymph node regions on the same side of the diaphragm alone (II) or with involvement of limited contiguous extralymphatic organ or tissue (II_E)
III	Involvement of lymph node regions on both sides of the diaphragm (III), which may include the spleen (III_S) or limited contiguous extralymphatic organ or site (III_E, III_{ES}).
IV	Multiple or disseminated foci or involvement of one or more extralymphatic organs or tissues with or without lymphatic involvement.

*All stages are further divided on the basis of the absence *(A)* or presence *(B)* of the following systemic symptoms: significant fever, night sweats, or unexplained weight loss of >10% or normal body weight.

From Carbone PT, et al: Symposium (Ann Arbor): Staging in Hodgkin's disease. Cancer Res 31:1707, 1971.

appeared to be cured. Even with advanced disease (stages IVA and IVB), 60 to 70% 5-year disease-free survival can be achieved.

Complications of Therapy

Long-term HD survivors treated with chemotherapy and radiotherapy have an increased risk of developing second hematologic cancers (myelodysplastic syndromes, acute myelogenous leukemia, NHL) or solid cancers of the lung, breast, stomach, skin, or soft tissues. Non-neoplastic complications of radiotherapy have included pulmonary fibrosis and accelerated atherosclerosis. New combinations of chemotherapeutic drugs and more judicious use of radiotherapy may alleviate these complications.

Myeloid Neoplasms (p. 675)

The common feature that unites myeloid neoplasms is an origin in a progenitor cell that normally gives rise to terminally differentiated cells of the myeloid series (erythrocytes, granulocytes, monocytes, and platelets). These diseases almost always primarily involve the bone marrow and to a lesser degree the secondary hematopoietic organs (the spleen, liver, and lymph nodes) and present with altered hematopoiesis. They can be segregated into three groups:

- *Acute myelogenous leukemia*, characterized by accumulation of immature myeloid cells in the bone marrow
- The *myelodysplastic syndromes*, associated with ineffective hematopoiesis and associated cytopenias
- The *chronic myeloproliferative disorders*, usually associated with an increased production of terminally differentiated myeloid cells

ACUTE MYELOGENOUS LEUKEMIA (p. 675)

Acute myelogenous leukemia is a heterogeneous group of disorders; in all forms, relatively undifferentiated myeloid progenitor cells (blasts) accumulate in the marrow.

Pathophysiology

Acute myelogenous leukemia is associated with acquired (or, rarely, inherited) genetic alterations that act to inhibit terminal differentiation (commitment). Myeloid cells normally die through differentiation; hence, this block in differentiation leads to the build-up in the marrow of immature neoplastic myeloid cells (blasts). These blasts suppress remaining normal hematopoietic progenitor cells by physical replacement as well as by other unknown mechanisms, leading to hematopoietic failure. Therapy is directed at killing of blasts (through treatment with cytotoxic drugs) or, in the specific case of acute promyelocytic leukemia, at overcoming the block in differentiation.

Classification

In the revised French-American-British (FAB) classification (Table 15-5), acute myelogenous leukemia is divided into eight categories (M0 to M7), taking into account both the degree of maturation (M0 to M3) and the lineage of the leukemic blasts (M4 to M7). Histochemical stains (for peroxidase, specific esterase, and nonspecific esterase) play an important role in classifying these

Table 15-5. REVISED FAB CLASSIFICATION OF ACUTE MYELOGENOUS LEUKEMIAS (AMLs)

	Class	Incidence (% of AML)	Marrow Morphology/Comments
M0	Minimally differentiated AML	2–3	Blasts lack definitive cytologic and cytochemical markers of myeloblasts (e.g., myeloperoxidase negative) but express myeloid lineage antigens and resemble myeloblasts ultrastructurally
M1	AML, without differentiation	20	Immature but ≥3% are peroxidase positive. Few granules or Auer rods and little maturation beyond the myeloblast stage
M2	AML with maturation	30–40	Full range of myeloid maturation through granulocytes. Auer rods present in most cases. Presence of t(8;21) defines a prognostically favorable subgroup
M3	Acute promyelocytic leukemia	5–10	Majority of cells are hypergranular promyelocytes, often with many Auer rods per cell. Patients are younger (median age, 35–40 y) and often develop DIC. The t(15;17) translocation is characteristic
M4	Acute myelomonocytic leukemia	15–20	Myelocytic and monocytic differentiation evident. Myeloid elements resemble M2 AML. Monoblasts are positive for nonspecific esterases. Presence of chromosome 16 abnormalities defines a subset (M4eo) with marrow eosinophilia and excellent prognosis
M5	Acute monocytic leukemia	10	In M5a subtype, monoblasts (peroxidase-negative, nonspecific esterase-positive) and promonocytes predominate in marrow and blood. In M5b subtype, mature monocytes predominate in the peripheral blood. M5a and M5b occur in older patients. Characterized by high incidence of organomegaly, lymphadenopathy, and tissue infiltration
M6	Acute erythroleukemia	5	Dysplastic erythroid precursors (some megaloblastoid, others with giant or multiple nuclei) predominate, and within the nonerythroid cells, >30% are myeloblasts; seen in advanced age; makes up 1% of de novo AML, and 20% of therapy-related AML
M7	Acute megakaryocytic leukemia	1	Blasts of megakaryocytic lineage predominate. Blasts react with platelet-specific antibodies directed against glycoprotein IIb/IIIa or vWF. Myelofibrosis or increased marrow reticulin seen in most cases

DIC, disseminated intravascular coagulation; vWF, von Willebrand factor.

tumors. Monoclonal antibodies that recognize common and lineage-specific determinants on myeloid cells are also useful.

Morphology

The diagnosis of acute myelogenous leukemia is based on finding greater than 30% myeloid blasts or, in the case of acute promyelocytic leukemia, greater than 30% blasts and promyelocytes, in the bone marrow. The following types of immature myeloid cells are observed in various acute myelogenous leukemia subtypes:

- *Myeloblasts* have delicate nuclear chromatin; two to four nucleoli; and voluminous cytoplasm that often contains fine, azurophilic, peroxidase-positive granules or distinctive red-staining, peroxidase-positive, needle-like structures called *Auer rods*. When present, Auer rods are taken to be definitive evidence of myeloid differentiation.
- *Monoblasts* often have folded or lobulated nuclei, lack Auer rods, and usually do not express peroxidase but can be identified by staining for nonspecific esterase.
- Neoplastic *progranulocytes*, which predominate in the M3 subtype, often have bilobed nuclei and usually contain abundant, abnormally coarse azurophilic granules that are intensely peroxidase positive. Multiple Auer rods are also often present in these cells.
- *Erythroblasts*, which predominate in the M6 subtype, often have intensely basophilic cytoplasm and a round nucleus containing a single bar-shaped nucleolus.
- *Megakaryoblasts* are often difficult to recognize morphologically; detection of thrombocyte-specific markers is usually required to document their presence.

The number of acute myelogenous leukemia cells in the peripheral blood is highly variable, sometimes being more than 100,000 cells per microliter but being under 10,000 cells per microliter in about 50% of the patients. Occasionally the peripheral smear may not contain any blasts (aleukemic leukemia).

Chromosomal Abnormalities

Special high-resolution banding techniques have revealed chromosomal abnormalities in approximately 90% of all acute myelogenous leukemia patients. In 50 to 70% of the cases, the karyotypic changes can be detected by standard cytogenetic techniques. Several associations have emerged:

- Acute myelogenous leukemia arising de novo in patients with no risk factors is often associated with balanced chromosomal translocations.
- Acute myelogenous leukemias that follow a myelodysplastic syndrome or that occur after exposure to DNA-damaging agents (such as chemotherapy or radiation therapy) are commonly associated with deletions or monosomies involving chromosomes 5 and 7 and usually lack chromosomal translocations.
- Acute myelogenous leukemias specifically occurring after treatment with chemotherapeutic drugs that inhibit the enzyme topoisomerase II are often associated with translocations involving the *MLL* gene on chromosome 11 at band q23.

The t(15;17) translocation characteristic of acute promyelocytic leukemia (M3) is of particular pathogenetic and therapeutic interest.

- It results in the fusion of a truncated retinoic acid receptor-α

(RAR-α) gene on chromosome 17 to the PML (for *promyelocytic leukemia*) gene on chromosome 15.

- The fusion gene encodes an abnormal retinoic acid receptor that blocks myeloid cell differentiation, probably by interfering with the function of other retinoid receptors.
- The block in differentiation is overcome in vitro and in vivo by pharmacologic doses of the vitamin A derivative *all-trans-retinoic acid*, causing neoplastic promyelocytes to differentiate into neutrophils, which rapidly die. *Death by differentiation* clears the marrow of neoplastic cells and allows for resumption of normal hematopoiesis.

Clinical Features

Acute myelogenous leukemias affect primarily adults, peaking in incidence between the ages of 15 and 39 years, but also constitute 20% of childhood leukemias. The clinical findings in acute myelogenous leukemia are similar to ALL.

- Most patients present within weeks or a few months of the onset of symptoms with findings related to *anemia, neutropenia,* and *thrombocytopenia,* most notably fatigue, fever, and spontaneous mucosal and cutaneous bleeding.
- The *bleeding diathesis* caused by the thrombocytopenia is often the most striking clinical and anatomic feature of the disease, leading to petechiae and ecchymoses in the skin and hemorrhages into serosal linings, the gingivae, the gastrointestinal tract, and the urinary tract.
- *Procoagulants* released by leukemic cells, especially in acute promyelocytic leukemia (M3), may produce *disseminated intravascular coagulation.*
- *Neutropenia leads to infections,* particularly in the oral cavity, skin, lungs, kidneys, urinary bladder, and colon, often caused by *opportunists,* such as fungi, *Pseudomonas,* and commensals.

Signs and symptoms related to infiltration of tissues are generally less striking than in ALL.

- Mild lymphadenopathy and organomegaly may occur.
- In monocytic tumors (M4 and M5), infiltration of the skin (leukemia cutis) and the gingiva may be observed.
- Central nervous system spread is less common than in ALL but is still seen.
- Rarely, patients present with localized masses composed of myeloblasts known variously as *myeloblastomas, granulocytic sarcomas,* or *chloromas.* These inevitably progress to a typical acute myelogenous leukemia picture over a period of up to several years.

Prognosis

The prognosis is variable, depending on the underlying molecular pathogenesis. Overall, 60% of patients achieve complete remission with chemotherapy, but only 15 to 30% of these remain free from disease for 5 years. The prognosis is especially dismal for patients with acute myelogenous leukemia arising out of a myelodysplastic syndrome or after genotoxic therapy, possibly because *normal* hematopoietic stem cells in such patients have been damaged.

MYELODYSPLASTIC SYNDROMES (p. 678)

Myelodysplastic syndromes are a group of clonal stem cell disorders characterized by ineffective hematopoiesis and an increased risk of transformation to acute myelogenous leukemia. The bone marrow is partly or wholly replaced by the clonal progeny of a mutant multipotent stem cell that retains the capacity to differentiate into red cells, granulocytes, and platelets but in a manner that is both ineffective and disordered. The marrow is usually hypercellular or normocellular, but the peripheral blood shows pancytopenia.

Myelodysplastic syndrome arises in two distinct settings:

1. *Idiopathic or primary myelodysplastic syndrome*, occurring mainly in patients older than age 50, often develops insidiously.

2. *Therapy-related myelodysplastic syndrome* is a complication of previous myelosuppressive drug therapy or radiation therapy, usually appearing from 2 to 8 years after treatment.

All forms of myelodysplastic syndrome can transform to acute myelogenous leukemia; transformation occurs most rapidly and with highest frequency in patients with therapy-related myelodysplastic syndrome. Characteristic morphologic changes are typically seen in the marrow and the peripheral blood. Cytogenetic analysis is helpful in confirming the diagnosis.

Pathogenesis

The pathogenesis is unknown. Myelodysplastic syndrome may arise out of a background of stem cell damage. Both primary myelodysplastic syndrome and therapy-related myelodysplastic syndrome occurring after exposure to radiation or alkylating chemotherapeutic drugs are associated with similar clonal chromosomal abnormalities, including monosomy 5 and monosomy 7, deletions of 5q and 7q, trisomy 8, and deletions of 20q.

Morphology

The most characteristic finding is disordered (dysplastic) differentiation affecting all three lineages (erythroid, myeloid, and megakaryocytic). Common abnormalities include the following:

- *Erythroid*:
  1. Ringed sideroblasts, erythroblasts with iron-laden mitochondria that are visible as perinuclear granules with the Prussian blue stain.
  2. Megaloblastoid maturation, resembling that seen in vitamin B_{12} and folate deficiency.
  3. Nuclear budding abnormalities, recognized as nuclei with misshapened, often polypoid outlines.
- *Granulocytic*:
  1. Neutrophils with decreased numbers of secondary granules, toxic granulations, or Döhle bodies.
  2. Pseudo-Pelger-Huet cells, neutrophils with only two nuclear lobes. Myeloblasts may be increased, but by definition comprise less than 30% of the overall marrow cellularity.
- *Megakaryocytic*: Megakaryocytes with single nuclear lobes or multiple separate nuclei (pawn ball megakaryocytes) are also characteristic.
- *Peripheral blood*: The peripheral blood often contains pseudo-Pelger-Huet cells, giant platelets, macrocytes, poikilocytes, and a relative or absolute monocytosis. Myeloblasts usually comprise less than 10% of the peripheral leukocytes.

Clinical Course

Primary myelodysplastic syndrome affects primarily individuals older than 60 years of age. Approximately half are asymptomatic at presentation, with the disease being discovered after incidental blood tests. The course is dominated by symptoms stemming from cytopenias, particularly thrombocytopenia. Progression to acute myelogenous leukemia occurs in 10 to 40% of individuals and is often accompanied by the appearance of additional clonal cytogenetic changes.

Prognosis

The median survival varies from 9 to 29 months, but some individuals may live for 5 years or more. Factors portending a worse outcome include the following:

- Development after cytotoxic therapy: Therapy-related myelodysplastic syndrome patients have more severe cytopenias, often progress rapidly to acute myelogenous leukemia, and have an overall median survival of only 4 to 8 months.
- Increased numbers of blasts in the marrow or peripheral blood.
- Multiple clonal chromosomal abnormalities.
- Severe thrombocytopenia.

CHRONIC MYELOPROLIFERATIVE DISORDERS
(p. 679)

Four chronic myeloproliferative disorders (MPDs) are recognized:

1. *Chronic myelogenous leukemia*
2. *Polycythemia vera*
3. *Essential thrombocytosis*
4. *Myelofibrosis with myeloid metaplasia*

In the latter three disorders, the target of neoplastic transformation is a multipotent progenitor cell capable of giving rise to mature erythrocytes, platelets, granulocytes, and monocytes. In chronic myelogenous leukemia, the pluripotent stem cell that can give rise to lymphoid and myeloid cells seems to be affected.

Chronic MPDs differ from acute myelogenous leukemia in that, although the neoplastic cells and their offspring flood the bone marrow and suppress residual normal progenitor cells, terminal differentiation is initially unaffected. This combination leads to marrow hypercellularity, increased hematopoiesis, and (often) elevated peripheral blood counts. Certain features are common to each of the four chronic MPDs:

- Circulation and homing of neoplastic stem cells to secondary hematopoietic organs, particularly the spleen. Resultant *extramedullary hematopoiesis* leads to splenomegaly.
- Termination in a spent phase characterized by *marrow fibrosis* and peripheral blood cytopenias.
- *Progression over time to acute leukemia*. This invariably occurs only with chronic myelogenous leukemia.

The pathologic findings in the chronic MPDs are not specific, having considerable degree of overlap with one another and some reactive conditions. Diagnosis and classification requires correlation of morphologic findings with other clinical and laboratory findings, particularly cytogenetics.

Chronic Myelogenous Leukemia

Chronic myelogenous leukemia is a neoplasm arising in pluripotent hematopoietic stem cells that leads to preferential proliferation of granulocytic progenitors.

Pathophysiology. Chronic myelogenous leukemia is distinguished from other chronic MPDs by the presence of the t(9;22), the Philadelphia chromosome (Ph[1]).

- The translocation leads to fusion of portions of the *BCR* gene from chromosome 22 and the *ABL* gene from chromosome 9.
- The resultant *BCR-ABL* fusion gene directs the synthesis of a 210-kD fusion protein with tyrosine kinase activity.
- Expression of the BCR-ABL fusion protein in murine hematopoietic progenitor cells gives rise to a syndrome resembling human chronic myelogenous leukemia, suggesting a critical role in stem cell transformation.
- In human chronic myelogenous leukemia and murine models, there is a marked increase in neoplastic granulocytic precursors in the marrow, which coexist with a smaller number of *BCR-ABL*-negative (normal) progenitor cells. The basis for preferential proliferation of granulocytic precursors is not known.

Morphology. Chronic myelogenous leukemia marrow specimens are usually 100% cellular, with most of the increased cellularity being composed of maturing granulocytic precursors. Peripheral blood examination reveals increased granulocytes, often exceeding 100,000 cells per mm[3]. A mixture of neutrophils, metamyelocytes, and myelocytes, with less than 10% myeloblasts, is typical. Peripheral blood eosinophilia, basophilia, and thrombocytosis are also common. Extramedullary hematopoiesis within the splenic red pulp produces marked splenomegaly, often complicated by focal infarction.

Laboratory Findings. Chronic myelogenous leukemia is best differentiated from other chronic MPDs by detection of the *BCR-ABL* fusion gene, either through chromosomal analysis or polymerase chain reaction–based molecular tests.

- In greater than 90% of cases, karyotyping reveals the Ph[1].
- In 5 to 10% of cases, the rearrangement is complex or cytogenetically cryptic; in such cases, other methods, such as fluorescent in-situ hybridization or the reverse transcriptase polymerase chain reaction, must be used to detect the *BCR-ABL* fusion gene or transcript.
- The absence of leukocyte alkaline phosphatase in chronic myelogenous leukemia is also helpful because leukemoid reactions and other chronic MPDs are associated with an elevated leukocyte alkaline phosphatase.

Clinical Features. Chronic myelogenous leukemia primarily occurs in adults between the ages of 25 and 60 years, with the peak incidence in the thirties and forties. The onset of chronic myelogenous leukemia is insidious; initial symptoms are often caused by mild to moderate anemia or by hypermetabolism owing to increased cell turnover and include fatigability, weakness, weight loss, and anorexia. Others present with symptoms related to splenomegaly or splenic infarction.

The course of chronic myelogenous leukemia is one of slow progression.

- After a variable *stable phase* period averaging 3 years, approximately 50% of patients enter an *accelerated phase* marked by worsening anemia and thrombocytopenia, increased basophilia, and refractoriness to treatment. Additional clonal cytogenetic abnormalities, such as trisomy 8, isochromosome 17q, or duplication of the Ph[1], may appear.
- Within 6 to 12 months, the accelerated phase terminates in acute leukemia (*blast crisis*).

- In the remaining 50%, blast crises occur abruptly without an intermediate accelerated phase.
- In 70% of patients, the blasts have the morphologic and cytochemical features of myeloblasts, whereas in about 30% of patients, the blasts contain the enzyme TdT and express early B-lineage antigens, such as CD10 and CD19. Rarely the blasts resemble precursor T cells.
- Less commonly, patients may progress to a phase of diffuse marrow fibrosis.

Prognosis. Chronic myelogenous leukemia is curable with allogeneic bone marrow transplantation performed during the stable phase.

Polycythemia Vera

Polycythemia vera arises in a transformed multipotent myeloid stem cell and is characterized by increased proliferation and production of erythroid, granulocytic, and megakaryocytic elements. Increased marrow production is reflected in the peripheral blood by erythrocytosis (polycythemia), granulocytosis, and thrombocytosis, but *the absolute increase in red cell mass is responsible for most of the clinical symptoms.*

Pathophysiology. The pathophysiology is largely unknown. Polycythemia vera progenitor cells have a decreased requirement for erythropoietin and other hematopoietic growth factors. The growth factor independence of polycythemia vera cells may be caused by mutations in a factor or factors common to multiple hematopoietic growth factor signaling pathways.

Morphology. Early in the course, characteristic findings include

- *Bone marrow hypercellularity* as a result of an increase in progenitors of all lineages (erythroid, granulocytic, and megakaryocytic)
- Peripheral blood *basophilia and neutrophilia*
- The presence of *giant platelets* and *megakaryocytic fragments* in peripheral smears
- *Mild organomegaly*

Late in the course of some patients, the character of the disease changes:

- Marrow fibrosis may become prominent *(spent phase)*, leading to displacement of hematopoietic cells (15 to 20% of patients).
- Marrow fibrosis results in increased *extramedullary hematopoiesis* in the spleen and liver, producing more prominent organomegaly.
- Transformation to acute myelogenous leukemia occurs in 2% of patients treated with phlebotomy.

Laboratory Findings. Polycythemia vera is associated with a constellation of findings that help to establish the diagnosis, as follows:

- The hemoglobin concentration ranges from 14 to 28 gm/dl with hematocrit values of 60% or more.
- The white cell count is typically elevated, ranging between 12,000 and 50,000 cells per mm^3, and the platelet count is often greater than 500,000 cells per mm^3.
- Leukocyte alkaline phosphatase levels are above normal and the Ph[1] is absent.
- Platelets show defects in functional aggregation studies.

Clinical Course. Polycythemia vera appears insidiously, usually in late middle age (median age at onset, 60 years). Symptoms are related to the following factors:

- *Erythrocytosis*: Increased red cell mass and accompanying increase in total blood volume leads to abnormal blood flow, vascular distention, and vascular stasis. These cause ruddy red appearance (plethora), cyanosis, and hypertension (70% of patients).
- *Basophilia*: Release of histamine may underlie gastrointestinal symptoms, increased tendency to peptic ulceration, and intense pruritus.
- *High cell turnover*: High turnover gives rise to hyperuricemia and symptomatic gout (5 to 10% of cases).
- *Platelet dysfunction*: Together with abnormal blood flow, platelet dysfunction leads to increased risk of both major bleeding and thrombotic episodes. About 25% of patients first come to clinical attention with thrombotic episodes, whereas life-threatening hemorrhages occur in 5 to 10% of cases.

Prognosis. With no treatment, death from bleeding or thrombosis occurs within months. With simple phlebotomy to maintain hematocrit within normal range, median survival is about 10 years.

Essential Thrombocytosis

In essential thrombocytosis, an MPD arising in multipotent stem cells, increased proliferation and production are largely confined to the megakaryocytic elements.

Pathogenesis. Pathogenesis is largely unknown. Essential thrombocytosis resembles polycythemia vera in that the cells of the megakaryocytic series have a diminished requirement for growth factors. Dysfunctions of platelets derived from the neoplastic clone probably contribute to the major clinical features of bleeding and thrombosis.

Morphology. Bone marrow cellularity is usually mildly to moderately increased; megakaryocytes are often markedly increased in number and include abnormally large forms. Peripheral smears usually reveal thrombocytosis (usually >600,000 mm^3) and abnormally large platelets, frequently accompanied by mild leukocytosis. Neoplastic extramedullary hematopoiesis may produce mild organomegaly (50% of cases). Uncommonly, essential thrombocytosis may evolve to a spent phase of marrow fibrosis or transform to acute myelogenous leukemia.

Clinical Features. Essential thrombocytosis is the rarest of the chronic MPDs; it usually occurs past the age of 60 but is also seen in young adults. Qualitative and quantitative abnormalities in platelets underlie the major clinical manifestations of thrombosis and hemorrhage. *Erythromelalgia*, the throbbing and burning of hands and feet caused by occlusion of small arterioles by platelet aggregates, is a characteristic symptom.

Prognosis. Essential thrombocytosis has an indolent course; long asymptomatic periods are punctuated by thrombotic or hemorrhagic crises. Median survival time is 12 to 15 years.

Myelofibrosis with Myeloid Metaplasia

Myelofibrosis with myeloid metaplasia also arises from a transformed multipotent myeloid stem cell but differs in that progression to marrow fibrosis (myelofibrosis) histologically identical to the spent phase of the other chronic MPDs occurs early in the course.

Pathophysiology. The pathologic features of myelofibrosis with myeloid metaplasia stem from extensive collagen deposition in the marrow by non-neoplastic fibroblasts, inexorably displacing hematopoietic elements, including stem cells. Marrow obliteration leads to extensive extramedullary hematopoiesis in spleen, liver, and sometimes lymph nodes. Fibrosis appears to be caused by the inappropriate release of two fibroblast mitogens, platelet-derived growth factor and TGF-β, from neoplastic megakaryocytes.

Morphology. Morphologic features include the following:

- Early, the marrow is often hypercellular and contains large, dysplastic, and abnormally clustered megakaryocytes. With progression, diffuse marrow fibrosis appears that displaces hematopoietic elements. Late in the course, the fibrotic marrow space may be largely converted to bone (osteosclerosis).
- Myelofibrotic obliteration of the marrow space leads to extensive extramedullary hematopoiesis, principally in the spleen, which may enlarge to weights of 4000 gm or more, and to a lesser degree in the liver and the lymph nodes.
- Nucleated erythroid progenitors and early granulocytes are inappropriately released from the fibrotic marrow and sites of extramedullary hematopoiesis; their appearance in the peripheral blood is termed *leukoerythroblastosis*. Other frequent peripheral blood findings include tear-drop erythrocytes (dacryocytes), increased basophils, and abnormally large platelets.

Laboratory Findings. Moderate to severe normochromic, normocytic anemia is common. The white cell count is usually normal or reduced but may be markedly elevated (80,000 to 100,000 cells per mm^3) during the early cellular marrow phase. Thrombocytopenia, often of a severe degree, appears with disease progression.

Clinical Features. Myelofibrosis with myeloid metaplasia is uncommon in individuals younger than 60 years of age. The disorder comes to attention because of progressive anemia or marked splenic enlargement. Nonspecific symptoms, such as fatigue, weight loss, and night sweats, result from increased metabolism associated with the expanded mass of hematopoietic cells. Owing to high cell turnover, hyperuricemia and secondary gout may complicate the picture.

Prognosis. The prognosis is variable, with median survival time of 1 to 5 years. Threats to life are intercurrent infections; thrombotic episodes or bleeding related to platelet abnormalities; and, in 5 to 20% of cases, transformation to acute myelogenous leukemia.

Langerhans Cell Histiocytosis (p. 685)

There are three types of histiocytoses:

1. *True histiocytic lymphomas* (rare)
2. *Benign, reactive histiocytoses*
3. *Langerhans cell histiocytoses*

The Langerhans cell histiocytoses (also referred to as *histiocytosis X*) represent clonal proliferations of these antigen-presenting dendritic cells, which are normally found in many organs.

MORPHOLOGY AND IMMUNOPHENOTYPE

The tumor cells have abundant, often vacuolated cytoplasm, with vesicular oval or indented nuclei; expression of HLA-DR, Fc receptors, and CD1a is characteristic. Under the electron microscope *cytoplasmic structures known as HX bodies (Birbeck granules)* are seen, which sometimes have a periodicity and a dilated terminal end that produces an appearance resembling a tennis racquet. A prominent infiltrate of reactive cells, including plasma cells, macrophages, and eosinophils (which may be scant or numerous), is usually mixed with the neoplastic histiocytes.

CLINICAL FEATURES AND PROGNOSIS

Three patterns of disease are recognized, each with a different course and prognosis:

1. *Unifocal Langerhans cell histiocytosis (unifocal eosinophilic granuloma)*: Usually affects the skeletal system as an erosive, expanding accumulation of Langerhans cells within calvarium, ribs, or femur; may also occur in skin, lungs, or stomach. Lesions may be asymptomatic or painful; pathologic fractures may occur. This is an indolent disorder of children and young adults, especially men. It may remit spontaneously or be cured by local excision or irradiation.

2. *Multifocal Langerhans cell histiocytosis*: Usually affects children, who present with fever; diffuse eruptions, particularly on the scalp and in the ear canals; frequent bouts of otitis media, mastoiditis, and upper respiratory tract infections; bone lesions; and mild lymphadenopathy, hepatomegaly, and splenomegaly. In about 50% of patients, the posterior pituitary stalk of the hypothalamus is involved, leading to diabetes insipidus. The combination of calvarial bone defects, diabetes insipidus, and exophthalmos is referred to as the *Hand-Schüller-Christian triad*. Spontaneous regression may be seen; persistent disease is treated with chemotherapy.

3. *Acute disseminated Langerhans cell histiocytosis (Letterer-Siwe disease)*: Occurs most frequently before 2 years of age. This is an aggressive systemic disorder in which Langerhans histiocytes infiltrate and proliferate within skin, spleen, liver, lung, and bone marrow. Anemia and destructive bony lesions are seen. Letterer-Siwe disease is rapidly fatal if untreated. With intensive chemotherapy, 5-year survival is about 50%.

Etiologic and Pathogenetic Factors in White Cell Neoplasia: Summary and Perspectives

A number of common themes pertain to the etiology and pathogenetic mechanisms underlying white cell neoplasia.

CHROMOSOMAL TRANSLOCATIONS AND ONCOGENES

- Nonrandom karyotypic abnormalities, most commonly translocations, are present in the majority of white cell neoplasms. These may lead to inappropriate expression of an unaltered protein or to the synthesis of an entirely novel fusion oncoprotein.
- Some translocations are seen only in one type of tumor and are therefore diagnostic of that disease (e.g., the t(15;17) is seen only in acute promyelocytic leukemia). In other cases, translocations are seen in multiple neoplasms, perhaps because of more general effects on hematopoietic and lymphoid progenitors. An example is the t(9;22), the Ph[1] chromosome, which can be seen

in ALL, acute myelogenous leukemia, and chronic myelogenous leukemia.
- Expression of oncoproteins in the bone marrow of mice often produces diseases resembling their human counterparts, demonstrating that they have a central role in tumorigenesis. Examples include the products of the t(15;17) or the t(9;22) fusion genes, which produce murine tumors resembling acute promyelocytic leukemia and chronic myelogenous leukemia.

INHERITED GENETIC FACTORS

- Genetic diseases that promote genomic instability, such as Bloom syndrome, Fanconi anemia, and ataxia telangiectasia, are at increased risk for development of acute leukemia. In addition, Down syndrome (trisomy 21) and neurofibromatosis type I are both associated with an increased incidence of childhood leukemia.

VIRUSES AND ENVIRONMENTAL AGENTS

- Three viruses, HTLV-1, Epstein-Barr virus, and HHV8, have been implicated. Clonal episomal Epstein-Barr virus genomes are found in the tumor cells of African Burkitt lymphoma, in 30 to 40% of cases of HD, in many diffuse large B-cell lymphomas occurring in the setting of T-cell immunodeficiency, and in angiocentric lymphoma. HTLV-1 is associated with ALL. HHV8 is associated with an unusual subset of large B-cell lymphomas presenting as lymphomatous effusions.
- Several environmental agents that lead to chronic immune stimulation predispose to lymphoid neoplasia. The most clear-cut associations are *H. pylori* infection with gastric marginal zone lymphoma and gluten-sensitive enteropathy and intestinal T-cell lymphoma.

IATROGENIC FACTORS

Radiotherapy and certain forms of chemotherapy used to treat cancer increase the risk of subsequent hematolymphoid neoplasms, including myelodysplastic syndrome, acute myelogenous leukemia, and NHL.

SPLENOMEGALY (p. 688)

The spleen may be enlarged in a variety of conditions (Table 15–6). Splenic enlargement is often a feature of hematolymphoid disorders.

Hypersplenism (p. 688)

Hypersplenism is observed in a minority of patients with splenic enlargement. It is characterized by

1. Splenomegaly
2. A reduction of one or more of the cellular elements of the blood, resulting from increased sequestration of cells and the consequent enhanced lysis by splenic macrophages
3. Correction of the cytopenias after splenectomy

Table 15–6. DISORDERS ASSOCIATED WITH SPLENOMEGALY

Infections
Nonspecific splenitis of various blood-borne infections
    (particularly infective endocarditis)
Infectious mononucleosis
Tuberculosis
Typhoid fever
Brucellosis
Cytomegalovirus
Syphilis
Malaria
Histoplasmosis
Toxoplasmosis
Kala-azar
Trypanosomiasis
Schistosomiasis
Leishmaniasis
Echinococcosis
Congestive States Related to Portal Hypertension
Cirrhosis of the liver
Portal or splenic vein thrombosis
Cardiac failure
Lymphohematogenous Disorders
Hodgkin disease
Non-Hodgkin lymphoma and lymphocytic leukemias
Multiple myeloma
Myeloproliferative disorders
Hemolytic anemias
Thrombocytopenic purpura
Immunologic-Inflammatory Conditions
Rheumatoid arthritis
Systemic lupus erythematosus
Storage Diseases
Gaucher disease
Niemann-Pick disease
Mucopolysaccharidoses
Miscellaneous
Amyloidosis
Primary neoplasms and cysts
Secondary neoplasms

Nonspecific Acute Splenitis (p. 688)

Nonspecific acute splenitis is associated with enlargement; it may occur with any blood-borne infection. Grossly the spleen is red and extremely soft. Microscopically the major change is acute congestion of the red pulp, which may efface the lymphoid follicles, accompanied by reticuloendothelial hyperplasia.

Congestive Splenomegaly (p. 689)

Passive chronic venous congestion and enlargement may result from the following:

- Systemic, or central venous, congestion, encountered in cardiac decompensation involving the right side of the heart
- Intrahepatic derangement of portal venous drainage, as occurs in various forms of cirrhosis of the liver

- Obstruction to the extrahepatic portal vein and splenic vein, as occurs in spontaneous portal vein thrombosis; inflammatory involvement of the portal vein *(pylephlebitis)*, such as follows intraperitoneal infections; and thrombosis of the splenic vein

In all of the aforementioned settings, there is moderate to severe enlargement of the spleen, which may weigh from 500 to more than 1000 gm. Microscopically the pulp is suffused with red cells during the early phases but becomes increasingly more fibrous and cellular with time. Organization of focal hemorrhages gives rise to areas of fibrosis containing deposits of iron and calcium salts encrusted on connective tissue and elastic fibers *(Gandy-Gamna nodules)*.

Splenic Neoplasms (p. 690)

Benign splenic tumors include fibromas, osteomas, chondromas, lymphangiomas, and hemangiomas. Malignant hematolymphoid neoplasms (e.g., lymphoid leukemias, Hodgkin and non-Hodgkin lymphomas, myeloproliferative disorders) often involve the spleen secondarily and much less commonly originate at this site. Rarely, hemangiosarcomas may arise primarily within the spleen. Metastasis of solid tumors to the spleen is not common and is usually observed only in advanced malignancies.

THYMIC DEVELOPMENTAL DISORDERS
(p. 691)

Thymic developmental disorders can be classified as follows:

- *Thymic hypoplasia or aplasia,* accompanied by parathyroid aplasia and variable defects involving the heart and great vessels, is seen in DiGeorge syndrome.
- *Thymic cysts* are uncommon lesions lined by stratified to columnar epithelium that are probably developmental in origin and generally of little clinical significance.

Thymic Hyperplasia (p. 691)

Thymic hyperplasia refers to the appearance of reactive B-cell lymphoid follicles within the thymus. This is seen in chronic inflammatory and immunologic states, particularly myasthenia gravis (65 to 75% of these cases).

Thymomas (p. 691)

Thymomas are neoplasms derived from cortical or medullary thymic epithelial cells.

MORPHOLOGY

Macroscopically, thymomas are usually lobulated, firm, gray-white masses up to 15 to 20 cm in longest dimension sometimes containing areas of cystic necrosis and calcification. In malignant tumors (20 to 25% of cases), there is invasion of adjacent structures; benign tumors are well encapsulated.

Microscopically, thymomas are composed of a mixture of neoplastic epithelial cells and variable numbers of reactive thymocytes. They are classified according to their appearance and pattern of growth:

- *Benign medullary thymoma*: This is composed of a proliferation of often elongated or spindle-shaped cells. This pattern often has few admixed thymocytes.
- *Benign cortical thymoma*: The neoplastic epithelial cells are plump, have abundant cytoplasm and rounded vesicular nuclei, and are often mixed with large numbers of reactive thymocytes.
- *Benign mixed thymoma*: This contains both the medullary and the cortical patterns.
- *Malignant thymoma type I*: This is a tumor that is cytologically benign but that invades local structures. Morphologically the tumor most commonly resembles a cortical thymoma.
- *Malignant thymoma type II*: Better thought of as *thymic carcinoma*, these are cytologically malignant, uncommon tumors (approximately 5% of thymomas). Macroscopically, they are usually fleshy and obviously invasive. Microscopically, they most commonly
  1. Resemble *squamous cell carcinoma*
  2. Are composed of cytologically anaplastic cortical-type epithelial cells scattered against a dense background of nonneoplastic thymocytes (so-called *lymphoepithelioma*).

The lymphoepithelioma type is more common in Asia and often contains clonal Epstein-Barr virus genomes.

CLINICAL COURSE

These are tumors of adults, many of which are discovered incidentally. About 40% present because of local pressure symptoms and 30 to 45% because of their association with *myasthenia gravis*. Thymomas are also associated with other paraneoplastic syndromes, such as acquired hypogammaglobulinemia, pure red cell aplasia, Graves disease, pernicious anemia, dermatomyositis-polymyositis, and Cushing syndrome.

PROGNOSIS

With minimal or no invasion, simple excision yields a greater than 90% 5-year survival. Extensive invasion is often accompanied by local metastasis and is associated with a less than 50% 5-year survival.

Diseases of the Respiratory System

CONGENITAL ANOMALIES (p. 699)

Congenital Cysts (p. 699)

Congenital cysts are formed by abnormal detachment of a fragment of primitive foregut. Bronchogenic cysts are most common and consist of cystic spaces lined by bronchial-type epithelium. Complications include infection, with suppuration, abscess formation, or both, and rupture into bronchi or the pleural cavity, causing hemorrhage or hemoptysis and pneumothorax.

Bronchopulmonary Sequestration (p. 699)

Bronchopulmonary sequestration refers to the presence of lung tissue (lobes or segments) *without* a normal connection to the airway system and with vascular supply derived from the aorta or its branches, not the pulmonary artery.

- *Extralobar sequestrations* are found most often in infants as abnormal mediastinal masses and in association with other congenital anomalies.
- *Intralobar sequestrations* are found *within the lung parenchyma*. They are more common in adults and are associated with recurrent infections.

ATELECTASIS (p. 699)

Atelectasis refers to incomplete expansion or collapse of parts of or a whole lung. There are *three* basic types, all of which are reversible:

1. *Resorption atelectasis*, which follows complete obstruction of an airway (e.g., excessive bronchial secretions as in bronchial asthma or chronic bronchitis, foreign body aspiration, or bronchial neoplasms)
2. *Compressive atelectasis*, when pleural space is expanded by fluid (e.g., effusions from cardiac failure or neoplasms, blood from rupture of a thoracic aneurysm) or by air (pneumothorax).
3. *Patchy atelectasis*, which develops when there is loss of pulmonary surfactant, as in neonatal respiratory distress syndrome (Chapter 11).

PULMONARY VASCULAR DISEASE (p. 700)

Pulmonary Edema (p. 700)

Hemodynamic disturbances or changes in microvascular permeability (see adult respiratory distress syndrome [ARDS] subsequently) can cause pulmonary edema (Table 16–1). Chronic edema predisposes to infection in addition to impairing normal respiratory function.

MORPHOLOGY

Regardless of the cause, the lungs become heavy, wet, and subcrepitant. Fluid accumulates, especially in the dependent, basal regions of the lower lobes.

Histologic findings include engorged capillaries and filling of the intra-alveolar airspaces by a granular pink precipitate. In chronic congestion and edema (such as in mitral stenosis), interstitial fibrosis may supervene, associated with numerous hemosiderin-laden macrophages *(brown induration).*

Adult Respiratory Distress Syndrome
(p. 700)

ARDS is characterized by diffuse alveolar capillary damage, leading to severe pulmonary edema, respiratory failure, and arte-

---

Table 16–1.   CLASSIFICATION AND CAUSES OF PULMONARY EDEMA

Hemodynamic Edema

Increased hydrostatic pressure
   Left-sided heart failure
   Mitral stenosis
   Volume overload
   Pulmonary vein obstruction
Decreased oncotic pressure
   Hypoalbuminemia
      Nephrotic syndrome
      Liver disease
      Protein-losing enteropathies
Lymphatic obstruction

Edema Due to Microvascular Injury

Infectious agents: viruses, *Mycoplasma,* other
Inhaled gases: oxygen, sulfur dioxide, cyanates, smoke
Liquid aspiration: gastric contents, near-drowning
Drugs and chemicals
   Chemotherapeutic agents: bleomycin, other
   Other medications: amphotericin B, colchicine, gold
   Other: heroin, kerosene, paraquat
Shock, trauma, and sepsis
Radiation
Miscellaneous
   Acute pancreatitis; extracorporeal circulation; massive fat, air, or
      amniotic fluid embolism; uremia; heat; diabetic ketoacidosis;
      thrombotic thrombocytopenic purpura; disseminated
      intravascular coagulation

Edema of Undetermined Origin

High altitude
Neurogenic

rial hypoxemia refractory to oxygen therapy. The major origins are listed as causes of microvascular injury and edema in Table 16–1. Respiratory failure, unresponsive to oxygen therapy, develops with diffuse bilateral infiltrates on x-ray and frequent superimposed infections, resulting in greater than 50% mortality.

PATHOGENESIS

The basic lesion is diffuse damage to the alveolar wall, initially involving the capillary endothelium but eventually the epithelium as well. Damage leads to the acute stage of ARDS with increased capillary permeability and edema, fibrin exudation, formation of hyaline membranes (composed of necrotic epithelial cell debris and exuded proteins), and septal inflammation. Mechanisms of injury include the following:

- *Oxygen-derived free radicals*, especially in the toxicity induced by prolonged exposure (e.g., in respirators) to high concentrations of oxygen or other toxins (e.g., paraquat).
- *Aggregation of activated neutrophils* in the pulmonary vasculature. These neutrophils damage epithelium by secreting several types of injurious factors, including oxygen-derived free radicals and lysosomal enzymes (proteases), as well as arachidonic acid metabolites that augment neutrophil aggregation.
- *Activation of lung macrophages*, which release oxidants, proteases, and proinflammatory cytokines (e.g., interleukin [IL]-8).
- *Loss or damage to surfactant*, contributing to atelectasis, which (in combination with pulmonary edema) results in the stiff lungs characteristic of ARDS.

MORPHOLOGY

Morphologic findings are as follows:

- In the *acute stage*, lungs are diffusely firm, red, boggy, and heavy with acute diffuse alveolar damage (edema, hyaline membranes, acute inflammation by histology).
- In the *proliferative/organizing stage*, there are patchy areas of interstitial fibrosis and type II epithelial proliferation, frequently in fatal cases with superimposed bacterial infection.

Pulmonary Embolism, Hemorrhage, and Infarction (p. 703)

Occlusions of pulmonary arteries are almost always embolic; in situ thromboses are rare, occurring only with pulmonary hypertension and pulmonary atherosclerosis. Thrombosis, however, may complete a partial embolic occlusion.

Greater than 95% of pulmonary emboli arise in deep veins of legs. The frequency of pulmonary embolism correlates with a predisposition to thrombosis in the legs. Occurrence at autopsy ranges from 1% in the general population to 30% in hospitalized patients with severe burns, trauma, or fractures.

Potential consequences are as follows:

- Large emboli (about 5%) impacting in the major pulmonary arteries or astride the bifurcation of the pulmonary artery (saddle embolus):
  - Emboli may cause instantaneous death.
  - Emboli may cause cardiovascular collapse (e.g., acute cor

pulmonale [right-sided heart failure]). A shower of, or repeated, small emboli may have the same effect.
  • Hemodynamic compromise is secondary not only to vascular obstruction, but also to reflex vasoconstriction caused by such agents as thromboxane A_2.
■ Small emboli (60 to 80%):
  • Emboli may be clinically silent in patients without cardiovascular failure.
  • Emboli may cause transient chest pain and sometimes hemoptysis owing to pulmonary hemorrhage (blood in the alveoli but no ischemic necrosis of the pulmonary parenchyma).
  • In patients with compromised pulmonary circulation (cardiac failure), emboli may give rise to infarctions, generally small, manifest pathologically as peripheral, wedge-shaped hemorrhagic areas.
■ Middle-sized emboli (about 20 to 35%) that occlude moderate-sized peripheral pulmonary branches:
  • Emboli usually induce infarction.
■ Uncommonly, overt or covert multiple small emboli produce right-sided heart strain (chronic cor pulmonale) and eventually pulmonary hypertension and vascular sclerosis.

CLINICAL SIGNIFICANCE

Diagnosis of pulmonary emboli is often difficult; almost two thirds, even when fatal, are not diagnosed before death. Many are silent; others are catastrophic; and although they may produce infarction, the diagnosis may not be evident clinically.

Even without treatment, there is usually improvement in perfusion within the first day owing to fibrinolysis and contraction of the thrombotic mass. The embolus may completely resolve or be reduced to fibrous mural plaque within weeks or months, and the infarct may be converted to a fibrous scar. With diagnosis and fibrinolytic agents, improvement is greatly speeded, and mortality rate may be reduced to 5 to 10%.

Pulmonary Hypertension (p. 704)

Elevated pulmonary artery pressure is caused by increased pulmonary vascular resistance. Most commonly, pulmonary hypertension is secondary to

■ Chronic obstructive or interstitial lung disease
■ Left-sided heart disease
■ Recurrent pulmonary emboli

Primary (or idiopathic) pulmonary hypertension is uncommon, seen in children or in women aged 20 to 40; it generally progresses to severe respiratory insufficiency, cor pulmonale, and death over several years. Therapies include vasodilators and occasionally heart-lung transplantation. The cause is unknown, but current hypotheses postulate that endothelial dysfunction and injury (which can be triggered by some chemical and dietary agents) lead to persistent vasoconstriction and subsequent intimal and medial hypertrophy and resultant increases in vascular resistance.

MORPHOLOGY

Vascular lesions seen in all types of pulmonary hypertension include

1. Atheroma in large elastic arteries
2. Intimal fibrosis or medial hypertrophy in medium-sized muscular arteries and smaller arterioles

The presence of numerous organized thrombi suggests recurrent pulmonary thromboembolism. So-called *plexogenic arteriopathy* (tufts within capillary channels creating a vascular plexus) is seen in severe primary pulmonary hypertension or with some congenital cardiovascular anomalies.

CHRONIC OBSTRUCTIVE PULMONARY DISEASE (p. 706)

Diffuse pulmonary disease is classified physiologically as

1. *Obstructive disease*, characterized by increased resistance to airflow
2. *Restrictive disease* (see interstitial lung disease subsequently), characterized by reduced expansion of lung parenchyma, with decreased total lung capacity

Chronic obstructive pulmonary disease (COPD) describes a spectrum of clinical diseases from pure emphysema to pure bronchitis (Table 16–2). Although there are certain differences between these two extremes, many individuals show overlapping features because of the common pathogenetic denominator, cigarette smoking.

Emphysema (p. 707)

Emphysema is defined morphologically as the abnormal enlargement of airspaces distal to the terminal bronchioles, with destruction of their walls. Emphysema is further classified according to the anatomic distribution of the lesion within the acinus.

CENTRIACINAR EMPHYSEMA

Centriacinar emphysema is characterized by

- Destruction and enlargement of the central or proximal parts of the respiratory unit—the acinus—sparing distal alveoli
- Predominant involvement of upper lobes and apices

Severe lesions are seen primarily in male smokers, often in association with chronic bronchitis.

PANACINAR EMPHYSEMA

Panacinar emphysema is characterized by

- Uniform destruction and enlargement of the acinus
- Predominance in lower basal zones
- Strong association with α_1-antitrypsin deficiency

PARASEPTAL EMPHYSEMA

Paraseptal emphysema involves mostly the distal acinus, sparing the proximal, and

- Is found near the pleura and adjacent to fibrosis or scars
- Is often the underlying lesion of spontaneous pneumothorax

Table 16-2. DISORDERS ASSOCIATED WITH AIRFLOW OBSTRUCTION: SPECTRUM OF CHRONIC OBSTRUCTIVE PULMONARY DISEASE

Clinical Term	Anatomic Site	Major Pathologic Changes	Cause	Signs and Symptoms
Chronic bronchitis	Bronchus	Mucous gland hyperplasia, hypersecretion	Tobacco smoke, air pollutants	Cough, sputum production
Bronchiectasis	Bronchus	Airway dilation and scarring	Persistent or severe infections	Cough, purulent sputum, fever
Asthma	Bronchus	Smooth muscle hyperplasia, excess mucus, inflammation	Immunologic or undefined causes	Episodic wheezing, cough, dyspnea
Emphysema	Acinus	Airspace enlargement; wall destruction	Tobacco smoke	Dyspnea
Small airway disease,* bronchiolitis	Bronchiole	Inflammatory scarring/obliteration	Tobacco smoke, air pollutants, miscellaneous	Cough, dyspnea

*A feature of chronic bronchitis (see text).

IRREGULAR EMPHYSEMA

Irregular emphysema refers to irregular involvement of the acinus and is associated with scarring. It is usually asymptomatic.

Other related entities are *bullous emphysema* (blebs or bullae >1 cm in diameter) and *interstitial emphysema* (entrance of air into the connective tissue of the lung, mediastinum, or subcutaneous tissue).

PATHOGENESIS

The protease-antiprotease hypothesis holds that destruction of alveolar walls in emphysema stems from an imbalance between proteases and their inhibitors in the lung. The evidence is as follows:

- Individuals with a hereditary deficiency of the major protease inhibitor, α_1-antitrypsin, invariably develop emphysema and at a younger age if they smoke.
- Pulmonary instillation of proteolytic enzymes, including neutrophil elastase, results in emphysema in experimental animals.

Tobacco smoking contributes to emphysema by

- Recruiting neutrophils into the lung by factors from smoke-activated alveolar macrophages
- Stimulating release of elastase from neutrophils
- Enhancing macrophage elastase activity
- Inactivation of α_1-antitrypsin by oxidants in tobacco smoke or free radicals released by activated neutrophils

Hence, *impaction of smoke particles in the small bronchioles leads to recruitment of inflammatory cells, increased elastase, and decreased α_1-antitrypsin, resulting in the centriacinar pattern of emphysema seen in smokers.*

MORPHOLOGY

With diffuse forms, lungs can become voluminous and pillowy. Microscopically, airspaces are enlarged, walls thinned, and septal capillaries compressed and bloodless. Rupture of walls may produce honeycombing.

Chronic Bronchitis (p. 711)

Chronic bronchitis is defined clinically as persistent cough with sputum production for at least 3 months in at least 2 consecutive years.

MORPHOLOGY

Chronic bronchitis is characterized by

- Hyperemia and edema of mucous membranes of the lung
- Mucinous secretions or casts filling airways
- Increase in size of the mucous glands
- Bronchial or bronchiolar mucous plugging, inflammation, and fibrosis
- Squamous metaplasia or dysplasia of bronchial epithelium

Chronic irritation of the airways by inhaled substances, especially tobacco smoke, is the dominant factor in the pathogenesis of chronic bronchitis. These irritants cause bronchitis by eliciting

- Hypersecretion of mucus
- Subsequent hypertrophy of mucous glands
- Goblet cell metaplasia in bronchiolar epithelium
- Bronchiolitis

Infections are a secondary factor that maintain and promote the injury initiated by smoking.

Bronchial Asthma (p. 712)

Bronchial asthma is a chronic relapsing inflammatory disorder, featuring increased responsiveness of the tracheobronchial tree to various stimuli, resulting in paroxysmal contraction of bronchial airways. Two major types are recognized:

1. Extrinsic atopic (allergen, reagin-mediated)
2. Intrinsic nonreaginic (idiopathic) or precipitated by various factors.

Atopic (allergic) asthma, the most common type, is triggered by environmental antigens (e.g., dust, pollen, food), often with a positive family history of atopy. It is a classic type I immunoglobulin E (IgE)-mediated hypersensitivity reaction having

- An acute phase with binding of antigen by IgE-coated mast cells causing release of primary mediators (e.g., leukotrienes) and secondary mediators (e.g., cytokines, neuropeptides). These acute-phase mediators result in bronchospasm, edema, mucus secretion, and recruitment of leukocytes.
- An ensuing late-phase reaction mediated by recruited leukocytes (e.g., eosinophils, lymphocytes, neutrophils, monocytes). The late phase is characterized by persistent bronchospasm and edema, leukocytic infiltration, and loss of damaged epithelial cells.

Nonatopic asthma (nonreaginic), the other common type of asthma, is often triggered by respiratory tract infections, chemical irritants, and drugs, usually without a family history and with little or no evidence of IgE-mediated hypersensitivity. The primary cause of increased airway reactivity is unknown.

MORPHOLOGY

The lungs are overinflated and show patchy atelectasis, with occlusion of airways by mucous plugs. *Microscopically* the lungs exhibit edema, an inflammatory infiltrate in bronchial walls with numerous eosinophils, hypertrophy of bronchial wall musculature and of submucosal mucous glands, whorled mucous plugs (Curschmann spirals), and crystalloid debris of eosinophil membranes (Charcot-Leyden crystals) within airways.

Bronchiectasis (p. 716)

Bronchiectasis represents a chronic necrotizing infection of bronchi and bronchioles leading to or associated with abnormal permanent dilation of these airways. Clinical features include cough, fever, and abundant purulent sputum. In severe cases, obstructive respiratory insufficiency may be seen. Complications include cor pulmonale, metastatic abscesses, and systemic amyloidosis.

Bronchiectasis is seen in association with

- Bronchial obstruction, such as by tumor or foreign bodies
- Congenital or hereditary conditions (e.g., cystic fibrosis, intralobar sequestrations)
- Immotile cilia syndromes (e.g., Kartagener syndrome)
- Necrotizing pneumonia

Persistent obstruction leads to atelectasis and diminished elastic forces holding airways taut, resulting in relaxation and dilation. These changes become irreversible if they occur during development or if added infection contributes further damage to the airway walls.

MORPHOLOGY

The most severe changes are seen in distal airways of lower lobes, with dilations of varying shapes (*cylindrical, fusiform, or saccular*). Histology shows a spectrum of mild to necrotizing acute and chronic inflammation of the airways. Fibrosis develops in chronic cases. Extension of bronchial infection may lead to abscess formation.

PULMONARY INFECTIONS (p. 717)

Pulmonary infections occur when normal lung or systemic defense mechanisms are impaired. Pulmonary defense mechanisms include nasal, tracheobronchial, and alveolar mechanisms to filter, neutralize, and clear inhaled organisms and particles. Important factors interfering with normal lung defenses are

- Loss of or decreased cough reflex leading to aspiration (seen in coma, anesthesia, drug effects)
- Injury to mucociliary apparatus (as with cigarette or other smoke or gaseous inhalations)
- Decreased phagocytic or bactericidal function of the alveolar macrophage (owing to alcohol, tobacco, oxygen toxicity)
- Edema or congestion (congestive heart failure)
- Accumulation of secretions

Bacterial Pneumonia (p. 717)

Bacterial infections occur in two frequently overlapping morphologic patterns (*bronchopneumonia and lobar pneumonia*) and can be caused by a variety of gram-positive and gram-negative organisms. Depending on bacterial virulence and host resistance, the same organism may in one instance cause bronchopneumonia and in another instance lobar pneumonia and sometimes intermediate involvements.

BRONCHOPNEUMONIA (p. 717)

Bronchopneumonia is marked by patchy exudative consolidation of lung parenchyma, caused most commonly by staphylococci, streptococci, pneumococci, *Haemophilus influenzae*, *Pseudomonas aeruginosa*, and coliform bacteria. Grossly the lungs show dispersed, elevated, focal areas of palpable consolidation and suppuration. Histologic features consist of an acute (neutrophilic) suppurative exudate filling airspaces and airways, usually about bronchi and bronchioles. Resolution of the exudate usually restores normal lung structure, but organization may occur and result in fibrous scarring in some cases, or aggressive disease may produce abscesses. A predominantly interstitial pattern of inflammation is seen in some pediatric infections, as with *Escherichia coli* or group B hemolytic streptococci.

LOBAR PNEUMONIA (p. 717)

Lobar pneumonia involves a large portion of or an entire lobe of lung. Most lobar pneumonias are caused by pneumococci, which enter the lungs via the airways. Occasionally, they are caused by other organisms (*Klebsiella pneumoniae*, staphylococci, streptococci, *H. influenzae*).

The following sequence of stages is *classic* but infrequently seen because of antibiotic therapy. The various stages portray the natural history of uncomplicated lobar pneumonia.

- *Congestion* predominates in the first 24 hours.
- *Red hepatization* (consolidation) describes lung tissue with confluent acute exudation containing neutrophils and red cells, giving a red, firm, liver-like gross appearance.
- *Gray hepatization* follows, as the red cells disintegrate and the remaining fibrinosuppurative exudate persists, giving a gray-brown gross appearance.
- *Resolution* is the favorable final stage in which consolidated exudate undergoes enzymatic and cellular degradation and clearance. Normal structure is restored.

Complications of lobar pneumonia, and sometimes bronchopneumonia, are

- Abscess formation
- Empyema (spread of infection to pleural cavity)
- Organization of exudate into fibrotic scar tissue
- Bacteremia and sepsis, with infection of other organs

Viral and Mycoplasmal (Primary, Atypical) Pneumonia (p. 721)

Infections by viruses (e.g., influenza A or B, respiratory syncytial virus, adenovirus, rhinovirus, herpes simplex, cytomegalovirus) or *Mycoplasma pneumoniae* result in varied clinical and pathologic patterns, ranging from relatively mild upper respiratory tract involvements (e.g., the common cold) to severe lower respiratory tract disease.

MORPHOLOGY

Patchy or lobar areas of congestion are seen *without* the consolidation of bacterial pneumonias (hence the term *atypical* pneumonia). Other findings include the following:

- A predominance of interstitial pneumonitis with widened, edematous alveolar walls containing a mononuclear inflammatory cell infiltrate
- The formation of *hyaline membranes*, reflecting diffuse alveolar damage
- Frequent superimposed bacterial infection

Certain viruses cause necrosis of bronchial or alveolar epithelium in severe infections (herpes simplex, adenovirus, varicella), and characteristic cytopathic changes are seen with some (e.g., cytomegaly and nuclear inclusions in cytomegalovirus infection).

LUNG ABSCESS (p. 722)

Lung abscess is marked by localized suppurative necrosis of lung tissue of infectious origin. Commonly involved are staphylococci, streptococci, numerous gram-negative species, and anaerobes. Mixed infections are frequent, reflecting aspiration of oral contents. These infections can be initiated by the following:

- Aspiration of infective material, as in oropharyngeal surgical procedures; dental sepsis; or aspiration secondary to diminished consciousness from coma, drugs, anesthesia, and seizures
- Antecedent primary bacterial infection
- Septic emboli from infected thrombi or cardiac valve vegetations
- Obstructive tumors
- Direct traumatic punctures
- Spread of infection from adjacent organs

Complications include extension into the pleural cavity, hemorrhage, septic embolization, and secondary amyloidosis.

MORPHOLOGY

Abscesses vary in number (single or multiple) and size (microscopic to many centimeters in diameter). Aspiration abscesses are more common on the right, reflecting the more vertical right bronchus. They contain variable mixtures of pus and air, depending on available drainage through airways. Chronic abscesses are often surrounded by a reactive fibrous wall.

TUBERCULOSIS (p. 722)

Tuberculosis is a chronic, communicable disease caused by *Mycobacterium tuberculosis* made distinctive by a necrotizing (caseating) granulomatous tissue response to seeded organisms. Transmission is usually by inhalation of infected droplets produced by the coughing or sneezing of infected individuals. Predisposing factors are any debilitating or immunosuppressive condition (e.g., diabetes, alcoholism, malnutrition, chronic lung disease).

PATHOGENESIS

The cell wall lipids and carbohydrates of *M. tuberculosis* appear to enhance virulence by interfering with phagolysosomal fusion. This interference allows the intracellular survival of mycobacteria.

Delayed hypersensitivity (type IV) to the tubercle bacillus develops in 2 to 4 weeks after initial infection. A sensitized individual shows increased induration (>5 mm) at the site of intradermal injection of purified protein derivative of *M. tuberculosis* (PPD test). A positive test result indicates sensitivity, however, not active disease.

Once sensitization appears during infection, the nonspecific inflammatory response becomes granulomatous (abundant *epithelioid histiocytes*, occasional giant cells, and peripheral mononuclear cells [Chapter 3]). There is often central, caseous necrosis of the granulomas. A concomitant increase in resistance—the ability to inhibit intracellular replication of bacilli—occurs. There are several forms of tuberculosis, depending on the individual's hypersensitivity and resistance.

PRIMARY PULMONARY TUBERCULOSIS
(p. 723)

Primary pulmonary tuberculosis occurs in individuals lacking previous contact with tubercle bacilli. It begins as a single granulomatous lesion, known as a *Ghon focus*, subjacent to the pleura in the inferior upper lobe or superior lower lobe regions. Tubercle bacilli can be demonstrated histologically with acid-fast stains in early lesions. Old scarred tubercles may have no visible organisms but contain infective organisms, sometimes for decades. The spread to draining ipsilateral bronchial or hilar lymph nodes results in a combination of lung and lymph node lesions called the *Ghon complex.*

In most cases, the infection does not progress and results in local scarring and calcification. Infrequently a progressive primary tuberculous pneumonia ensues. A further complication, miliary disseminated tuberculosis, may occur if tubercle bacilli gain access to the bloodstream.

SECONDARY PULMONARY TUBERCULOSIS
(p. 723)

Secondary pulmonary tuberculosis denotes active infection in a previously sensitized individual. Most cases represent reactivation of dormant bacilli from primary lesions. Occasionally, exogenous sources of tuberculosis cause secondary disease.

Secondary tuberculosis is generally found in the apices of the lungs, reflecting the preference of *M. tuberculosis* for high P_{O_2}. These lesions may progress to *cavitary fibrocaseous tuberculosis, tuberculous bronchopneumonia,* or *miliary tuberculosis.*

Clinical Features

Primary tuberculosis is usually asymptomatic. The secondary form more often causes insidious fever, night sweats, weight loss, productive cough with blood-streaked sputum, or hemoptysis. Diagnosis relies on culture of the organism or demonstration of acid-fast bacilli in sputum or biopsy tissue. Prognosis and course are variable, depending on the extent of disease, the underlying health of the individual, and other variables, but chemotherapy is effective in all but neglected cases and those caused by emerging, highly drug-resistant strains.

DISSEMINATED TUBERCULOSIS (p. 725)

Hematogenous spread of tubercle bacilli may produce

- *Miliary tuberculosis* with myriad minute foci of infection in many organs, particularly liver, bone marrow, spleen, and kidneys
- *Isolated organ tuberculosis* when disseminated organisms become established in only one or two organs, most often adrenals, kidneys, bone (tuberculous osteomyelitis), or female genital tract (salpingitis, endometritis).

INTERSTITIAL LUNG DISEASE (p. 726)

Interstitial lung disease comprises a heterogeneous group of diseases with similar clinical, radiologic, and pathologic changes.

- *Clinical*: Restrictive lung disease, including dyspnea, decreased lung volumes, and decreased compliance.
- *Radiologic*: Diffuse infiltrates, ground-glass shadows.
- *Pathologic*: Diffuse, chronic inflammation or fibrosis of alveolar interstitium. Most changes are nonspecific, but there are some characteristic features in certain diseases (e.g., asbestos bodies).

Pathogenesis

The pathogenetic sequence of events in this group of diseases involves initial, early, and late mechanisms.

- The *initial event* is injury to epithelium or endothelium via inhaled or blood-borne toxins or agents.
- The *early acute* changes of alveolitis follow, consisting of recruitment by chemotactic factors (e.g., IL-8) of activated inflammatory or immune cells. These cells release injurious (oxidants, cytokines) and fibrogenic (platelet-derived growth factor, fibroblast growth factor, IL-1) mediators.
- The *late effects* of the various bioactive substances result in interstitial fibrosis.

PNEUMOCONIOSES (p. 727)

Pneumoconioses are disorders caused by the inhalation of any aerosol, including mineral dusts, organic dusts, fumes, and vapors. The following factors determine the health effects of inhaled dusts:

- The amount of dust retained, in turn determined by the concentration, duration of exposure, and effectiveness of clearance mechanisms.
- The size, shape, and buoyancy of particles: Those greater than 5 mm in diameter are filtered in upper airways, and those less than 1 mm can remain suspended and be exhaled, leaving the 1- to 5-mm particles to settle in the alveoli as the most potentially dangerous particles.
- The physicochemical reactivity and solubility of particles. Quartz, for example, may injure cells directly via free radicals on the particle surface. Highly soluble particles may rapidly cause toxicity; other particles resist dissolution and may persist to invoke a chronic fibrotic reaction.

Carbon Dust-Coal Workers' Pneumoconiosis (p. 729)

The range of pulmonary effects of carbon dust includes the following:

- *Anthracosis*, the small harmless accumulations seen in the lungs of urban dwellers and smokers.
- *Simple coal workers' pneumoconiosis (CWP)*, with more prominent and numerous aggregates of coal dust–laden macrophages forming coal *macules*. Clinical features may include cough and blackish sputum, but no significant dysfunction is seen in uncomplicated cases.
- *Progressive massive fibrosis or complicated CWP*, manifested

by severe fibrosis and scarring in areas of dust accumulation. This pattern reflects a much heavier dust burden and results in disabling respiratory insufficiency.

- Factors involved in determining the progression of simple CWP to progressive massive fibrosis include duration and magnitude of exposure and secretion of fibrogenic factors by coal dust–laden macrophages.

MORPHOLOGY

Morphologic findings are as follows:

- In simple CWP, black coal macules composed of dust-filled macrophages 1 to 5 mm in diameter are present diffusely, especially in the upper zones of the upper and lower lobes.
- In complicated CWP, large, blackened scars replace substantial portions of the lung (black lung disease), especially in the upper zones.

Silicosis (p. 730)

Prolonged inhalation of silica particles produces a chronic, nodular, dense pulmonary fibrosis. Sources of silica exposure include

- Mining (gold, tin, copper, coal) and quarrying
- Sandblasting
- Metal grinding
- Manufacture of ceramics

PATHOGENESIS

Silicosis involves persistent inflammation and fibrosis by the interaction of silica particles and lung macrophages. Ingested silica leads to macrophage activation and release of oxidants, cytokines, and growth factors that ultimately cause fibroblast proliferation and collagen deposition. Injury also may be perpetuated by direct toxic effects on the macrophage, causing cell death and release of the silica—restarting the injury cycle.

MORPHOLOGY

Distinct collagenous nodules start as small lesions in the upper lung but grow larger and more diffuse as the disease progresses. Coalescence of lesions forms large areas of dense scar. Calcification or concomitant blackening by coal dust is often present.

Microscopically, hyalinized whorls of collagen are seen with scant inflammation. Polarized light often shows birefringent silica particles within nodules.

Asbestosis (p. 732)

Asbestos is a family of fibrous silicates including curled, flexible *serpentines* (e.g., chrysotile) and brittle straight *amphiboles* (e.g., crocidolite). Heavy occupational exposure causes diffuse interstitial fibrosis, which is morphologically nonspecific except for the presence of numerous asbestos bodies (described subsequently) within the scarred lung.

PATHOGENESIS

Inhaled fibers that reach the alveoli are ingested by alveolar macrophages, stimulating release of C5a and other chemoattractants. Amphiboles (straight, stiff) reach the deep lung more than serpentine fibers, accounting for greater pathogenicity. Most of the inhaled asbestos is cleared by the macrophages; the rest reaches the interstitium and lymphatics. *Some ingested fibers are coated by hemosiderin and glycoproteins to form characteristic, beaded, dumbbell-shaped asbestos bodies.*

Possible mechanisms for lung injury and progressive fibrosis include

- Release of enzymes or toxic free radicals by the macrophages or neutrophils recruited to sites of asbestos deposition
- Release of fibrogenic cytokines and growth factors by alveolar macrophages after phagocytosis of fibers
- Direct stimulation of fibroblast collagen synthesis by asbestos

In addition to pulmonary fibrosis, asbestos induces *pleural reactions,* manifested by

1. Benign effusions.
2. Fibrous pleural adhesions.
3. Dense fibrocalcific plaques, found on the pleura or diaphragm. The plaques may sometimes be calcified; they do not contain asbestos bodies.

Asbestos exposure is also associated with increased risk of *bronchogenic carcinoma* and malignant mesothelioma.

SARCOIDOSIS (p. 734)

Sarcoidosis is a relatively common disease of unknown etiology, characterized by noncaseating granulomas in virtually any tissue. Women are affected more frequently than men, and American blacks are affected 10 times more often than American whites. There are also geographic and other ethnic variations in prevalence.

Sarcoidosis may be entirely asymptomatic and discovered only incidentally at autopsy or as bilateral hilar adenopathy on a chest radiograph obtained for other reasons. Alternatively, it may present as isolated cutaneous or ocular lesions, peripheral lymphadenopathy, or hepatosplenomegaly; with the insidious onset of respiratory difficulties or constitutional symptoms (fever, night sweats, weight loss); or with an acute onset accompanied by fever, erythema nodosum, and polyarthritis.

Although elevated serum IgG and calcium, characteristic chest and phalangeal x-ray changes, and a typical clinical history may strongly suggest the diagnosis, *it can be definitively established only by biopsy (often liver or lymph node) to document noncaseating granulomas.* Other diseases (e.g., tuberculosis, berylliosis, fungal infections), however, may also show the same histologic features. Diagnosis of sarcoidosis is then one of exclusion.

Etiology

The distinctive granulomatous response suggests an immune-mediated phenomenon. Immune abnormalities include the following:

- Lymphocytic alveolitis, with numerous activated CD4 + T cells (increased IL-2 production, HLA-DR antigen proliferation), and similarly activated alveolar macrophages (increased IL-1, oxygen radical production).
- Cutaneous anergy to a wide variety of agents that normally induce a local cutaneous delayed hypersensitivity reaction (e.g., tuberculin).
- An absolute lymphopenia mainly caused by reduced circulating T cells. Circulating B cells are present in normal numbers and are hyperreactive.
- Activated helper T cells and their secreted cytokines account for the influx of monocytes and subsequent granulomas and cell-mediated injury in tissues.
- Elevated circulating γ-δ T cells (associated with mycobacterial disease) and (variably) positive polymerase chain reaction assays for mycobacterial DNA in sarcoidal tissue; the latter has revived interest in an infectious cause, but the cause of sarcoidosis remains unknown.

Morphology

Other than organomegaly (liver, spleen, lymph nodes), no macroscopic change is apparent in sarcoidosis. Characteristic are the microscopic granulomas composed of tightly clustered epithelioid histiocytes, often including multinucleated giant cells. There is rarely central necrosis. Also frequently present (60% of granulomas) are *Schaumann bodies* (laminated, calcified proteinaceous concretions) and *asteroid bodies* (stellate inclusions within giant cells).

LYMPH NODES

Lymph nodes are virtually always involved, most commonly in the hilar and mediastinal regions, but possibly any node. Tonsils are affected 25 to 33% of the time.

LUNGS

The lungs are a common site of involvement. Characteristically, diffuse, scattered granulomas (showing a reticulonodular pattern on x-rays) occur that are not grossly apparent except for foci of coalesced granulomas. Pulmonary lesions have a strong tendency to heal, so that only hyalinized scars may be seen microscopically.

SPLEEN AND LIVER

The spleen and liver are microscopically affected in up to 75% of patients. Splenomegaly occurs in only 18%. Hepatomegaly is less frequent.

SKIN

Cutaneous sarcoid occurs in 33 to 50% of patients, presenting in a variety of gross forms, including discrete subcutaneous nodules, erythematous scaling plaques, and lesions in the mucous membranes.

EYE

The eyes are affected in 20 to 50% of cases, as iritis, iridocyclitis, or choroid retinitis.

Clinical Features

Sarcoid may

- Be slowly progressive
- Pursue a remitting or resolving course
- Spontaneously resolve (with or without steroid therapy)

In 65 to 70% of patients, there are no or only minimal residual manifestations; 20% have permanent lung or ocular dysfunction; and 10% die, primarily from progressive pulmonary fibrosis and cor pulmonale.

IDIOPATHIC PULMONARY FIBROSIS
(p. 735)

Idiopathic pulmonary fibrosis is a poorly understood disorder of unknown cause *characterized by progressive pulmonary interstitial fibrosis that results in hypoxemia*. In some cases, immune complex deposition (the antigens are unknown) can be identified, but their role in causing the disorder is not established. The disease is most common between 30 and 50 years of age.

Morphology

Changes vary according to stage.

- In *early stages*, there is interstitial and intra-alveolar edema, interstitial infiltration by leukocytes, and type II pneumonocyte proliferation.
- Interstitial and intra-alveolar fibrosis are characteristic of *intermediate stages*.
- In the *end stages*, the lung consists of spaces lined by pneumocytes and separated by inflammatory fibrous tissue (honeycomb lung).

The disease is progressive in most cases, resulting in pulmonary insufficiency, cor pulmonale, and cardiac failure.

HYPERSENSITIVITY PNEUMONITIS (p. 737)

Hypersensitivity pneumonitis is an immunologically mediated disorder that is caused by inhaled dusts or antigens:

- Farmer's lung: spores of thermophilic actinomycetes in hay
- Pigeon breeder's lung: proteins from bird feathers or excreta
- Humidifier or air-conditioner lung: thermophilic bacteria

Histologic changes include interstitial pneumonitis and fibrosis and a variable number of noncaseating, loosely formed granulomas. Early cessation of exposure to the injurious agent prevents progression to serious chronic fibrosis. The clinical manifestations are varied and include cough, dyspnea, fever, diffuse and nodular radiographic densities, and a restrictive pattern of pulmonary dysfunction.

PULMONARY EOSINOPHILIA (p. 738)

Pulmonary eosinophilia refers to diverse clinicopathologic conditions characterized by infiltration of eosinophils in the pulmonary interstitial or alveolar spaces, including the following:

- *Simple pulmonary eosinophilia* (Loeffler syndrome): Of uncertain origin, transient, benign infiltrates with prominent eosinophilia in blood and lung
- *Tropical eosinophilia*: Caused by microfilariae
- *Secondary chronic pulmonary eosinophilia*: Induced by infections, hypersensitivity, asthma, and allergic bronchopulmonary aspergillosis
- *Idiopathic chronic eosinophilic pneumonia*: A disorder of unknown etiology, manifested by focal consolidation of lung with prominent lymphocytes and eosinophils

Idiopathic chronic eosinophilic pneumonia is generally steroid responsive.

BRONCHIOLITIS OBLITERANS–ORGANIZING PNEUMONIA
(p. 738)

Bronchiolitis obliterans–organizing pneumonia is a common response to infectious or inflammatory injury of the lungs.

- It is clinically associated with cough, dyspnea, and often a recent respiratory tract infection; other etiologic associations are inhaled toxins, drugs, collagen vascular disease, and graft-versus-host disease in bone marrow transplant recipients.
- Major pathologic findings include loose fibrous tissue plugs within bronchioles and organizing pneumonia.
- Many patients improve gradually or with steroid therapy.

DIFFUSE PULMONARY HEMORRHAGE
(p. 738)

Diffuse pulmonary hemorrhage is a serious complication of some interstitial lung diseases, particularly the so-called *pulmonary hemorrhage syndromes*, which include the following:

- *Goodpasture syndrome*: a necrotizing, hemorrhagic interstitial pneumonitis and progressive glomerulonephritis caused by antibodies against analogous basement membrane antigens in lungs and kidneys
- *Idiopathic pulmonary hemosiderosis*: a chronic, episodic hemorrhage of the lung, of unknown cause, resulting in prominent hemosiderin deposition and fibrosis
- *Vasculitis-associated hemorrhage*: seen with Wegener granulomatosis, systemic lupus erythematosus, and hypersensitivity angiitis

PULMONARY ALVEOLAR PROTEINOSIS
(p. 739)

Pulmonary alveolar proteinosis is a disease of obscure etiology and pathogenesis characterized *radiologically* by diffuse pulmonary opacification; *histologically* by accumulation of dense, amorphous, periodic acid–Schiff (PAS)–positive, lipid-laden material in intra-alveolar spaces; and *clinically* by respiratory difficulty, cough, and sputum-containing gelatinous material. The intra-alveolar exudate consists of surfactant-like material, necrotic alveolar macrophages, and type II epithelial cells.

The disease may occur after exposure to irritating dusts and chemicals and in immunosuppressed individuals. It is progressive in many patients, but some have a benign course with eventual resolution of the lesions.

COMPLICATIONS OF THERAPIES (p. 740)

Important complications of therapy include the following:

- *Drug-induced lung disease*, ranging from acute bronchospasm to chronic fibrosis.
- *Radiation-induced lung disease*, in which acute pneumonitis occurs 1 to 6 months after therapy (usually for thoracic tumors); pathology is that of diffuse alveolar damage. Chronic radiation fibrosis may follow.
- *Rejection of transplanted lungs*, including acute vascular and chronic airway forms.

TUMORS (p. 741)

Bronchogenic Carcinoma (p. 741)

Bronchogenic carcinoma constitutes 90 to 95% of lung tumors. It is the most common cause of cancer death in both men and women.

PATHOGENESIS

Tobacco smoking is well established as the most important and common etiologic factor in the development of lung cancer.

- *Statistically*, there is an unequivocal link between the frequency of lung cancer and the number of pack-years of smoking.
- *Clinically*, hyperplastic and atypical changes can be seen in the bronchial epithelium of smokers and in the vicinity of bronchial cancer.
- *Experimentally*, there are numerous known carcinogens in cigarette smoke (e.g., polycyclic aromatic hydrocarbons), but it has not been possible to induce bronchogenic cancers readily by inhalation in experimental animals.

Other etiologic factors include exposure to radiation (atomic bomb survivors, uranium miners), asbestos (especially combined with smoking), air pollution (radon, particulates), and miscellaneous occupational inhaled substances (e.g., nickel, chromates, arsenic). Genetic mechanisms implicated include dominant oncogenes (e.g., K-*ras* in adenocarcinomas) and loss of tumor-suppressor genes.

HISTOLOGIC TYPES

Bronchogenic carcinomas are classified by their predominant histologic appearance (Table 16–3).

- *Adenocarcinoma* is the most common lung cancer in women and men. It frequently presents as a peripheral mass. The

Table 16-3. HISTOLOGIC CLASSIFICATION OF BRONCHOGENIC CARCINOMA

Squamous cell (epidermoid) carcinoma
Adenocarcinoma
  Bronchial derived (acinar, papillary, solid)
  Bronchioloalveolar
Small cell carcinoma
  Oat cell (lymphocyte-like)
  Intermediate cell polygonal
  Combined (usually with squamous)
Large cell carcinoma (undifferentiated, giant cell, clear cell)
Combined squamous cell carcinoma and adenocarcinoma

characteristic microscopic features include gland formation, usually with mucin production. There is often an adjacent desmoplastic tissue response.

- *Squamous cell carcinoma* has the closest correlation with smoking. Most arise in or near the hilus of the lung. Microscopically, they vary from well-differentiated keratinizing neoplasms to anaplastic tumors with only focal differentiation.
- *Small cell carcinoma* is the most malignant of lung cancers and usually presents as a central or hilar tumor. It is strongly associated with cigarette smoking. The characteristic microscopic features include small, *oatlike* cells with little cytoplasm in nests or clusters, without squamous or glandular organization. Ultrastructurally the cancer cells may exhibit neurosecretory granules, and immunohistochemical cell stains are usually positive for neuroendocrine markers. These tumors most often produce paraneoplastic syndromes (described later).
- *Large cell carcinoma* probably represents poorly differentiated squamous cell carcinomas or adenocarcinomas. Occasionally, there are peculiar histologic elements (giant cell, clear cell, spindle cell variants).

CLINICAL FEATURES

Bronchogenic carcinomas usually present with cough, weight loss, chest pain, and dyspnea (Table 16–4). Overall 5-year survival is approximately 9%. Surgical resection of solitary (non–small cell) tumors offers some improved survival (30 to 40% 5-year survival) for a minority of patients with localized disease. Small cell carcinoma has almost always metastasized by the time of diagnosis, precluding surgical intervention. It is responsive to chemotherapy but ultimately recurs. Other types show disappointing responses to chemotherapy.

Paraneoplastic syndromes associated with bronchogenic carcinoma often stem from release of the following hormones:

- Antidiuretic hormone (syndrome of inappropriate antidiuretic hormone release)
- Adrenocorticotropic hormone (Cushing syndrome)
- Parathormone or prostaglandin E (hypercalcemia)
- Calcitonin (hypocalcemia)
- Gonadotropins (gynecomastia)
- Serotonin (carcinoid syndrome)

Other paraneoplastic syndromes include myopathy, peripheral neu-

Table 16-4. LOCAL EFFECTS OF LUNG TUMOR SPREAD

Clinical Feature	Pathologic Basis
Pneumonia, abscess, lobar collapse	Tumor obstruction of airway
Lipid pneumonia	Tumor obstruction; accumulation of cellular lipid in foamy macrophages
Pleural effusion	Hoarseness
Tumor spread into pleura	Recurrent laryngeal nerve invasion
Dysphagia	Diaphragm paralysis
Rib destruction	Superior vena caval syndrome
Esophageal invasion	Phrenic nerve invasion
Chest wall invasion	Superior vena caval compression by tumor
Horner syndrome*	Pericarditis, tamponade
Sympathetic ganglia invasion	Pericardial involvement

*Horner syndrome = enophthalmos, ptosis, miosis, and anhidrosis, unilateral.

ropathy, acanthosis nigricans, and hypertrophic pulmonary osteoarthropathy (e.g., clubbing of fingers).

Bronchioloalveolar Carcinoma (p. 747)

Bronchioloalveolar carcinoma is an uncommon form of adenocarcinoma arising in the terminal bronchioloalveolar regions, almost always in the lung periphery. Macroscopic forms include single or multiple nodules or a diffuse, pneumonic consolidation with tumor. Histologically the tumor is distinctive in that tall, columnar, often mucin-producing tumor cells line up along preserved alveolar septa, forming papillary projections within the spaces. Clinically, they occur in men and women equally and are not usually associated with smoking. Prognosis is relatively favorable after resection of a solitary nodule but dismal for those with diffuse involvement.

Bronchial Carcinoid (p. 747)

Bronchial carcinoid represents 1 to 5% of all lung tumors. The tumor is characterized by neuroendocrine differentiation. Surgical resection is curative in 90 to 95%. A minority (10%) are more aggressive, exhibiting local invasion or distant metastases.

Grossly the tumors are usually intrabronchial, highly vascular, polypoid masses less than 3 to 4 cm in diameter. Microscopically, they are composed of uniform, small, round cells in nests or cords *resembling intestinal carcinoids*. Occasionally, tumors show atypia, mitoses, or pleomorphism. Neurosecretory granules are seen ultrastructurally, and neuroendocrine differentiation is confirmed by immunostaining for neuron-specific enolase, serotonin, calcitonin, or bombesin.

Miscellaneous Tumors (p. 748)

Hamartomas are relatively common, benign, nodular neoplasms composed of cartilage and admixtures of other mesenchymal tissues (e.g., fat, blood vessels, fibrous tissue). *Mediastinal tumors*

Table 16–5. MEDIASTINAL TUMORS

Superior Mediastinum	*Posterior Mediastinum*
Lymphoma	Neurogenic tumors (schwannoma,
Thymoma	neurofibroma)
Thyroid lesions	Lymphoma
Metastatic carcinoma	Gastroenteric hernia
Parathyroid tumors	*Middle Mediastinum*
Anterior Mediastinum	Bronchogenic cysts
Thymoma	Pericardial cyst
Teratoma	Lymphoma
Lymphoma	
Thyroid lesions	
Parathyroid tumors	

arise from local structures or may represent metastatic disease (Table 16–5).

Secondary involvement of the lung by metastatic tumor is common. Spread to the lung can occur via direct extension from contiguous organs or lymphatics or hematogenous routes. Patterns of disease include discrete masses or nodules, growth within peribronchial lymphatics (lymphangitis carcinomatosa), and (rarely) multiple tumor microemboli.

DISEASES OF THE PLEURA (p. 749)

Most pleural lesions are secondary to underlying lung disease.

Pleural Effusions (p. 750)

Accumulations of transudate (hydrothorax) or serous exudate may appear with

- Increased hydrostatic pressure (e.g., heart failure)
- Increased vascular permeability (e.g., pneumonia)
- Decreased oncotic pressure (e.g., nephrotic syndrome)
- Increased negative intrapleural pressure (e.g., atelectasis)
- Decreased lymphatic drainage (e.g., carcinomatosis)

Pleuritis (p. 750)

The various patterns of inflammatory reaction include

1. Serofibrinous pleuritis, reflecting inflammatory processes in the lung (e.g., tuberculosis, pneumonia, infarcts, abscesses, or systemic diseases [such as rheumatoid arthritis, uremia])
2. *Suppurative pleuritis* or empyema, usually reflecting infection of the pleural space leading to accumulation of pus

Organization of these exudates with dense fibrous adhesions can affect lung expansion. *Hemorrhagic pleuritis* occurs with bleeding disorders, neoplastic involvement, and certain rickettsial diseases.

Other pleural fluid accumulations include hemothorax (a fatal complication of a ruptured aortic aneurysm) and chylothorax (a collection of milky lymph fluid, usually with neoplastic lymphatic obstruction).

Pneumothorax (p. 751)

Pneumothorax refers to air or gas in the pleural cavity. Pneumothorax can be traumatic (e.g., resulting from air escape from the lung after rib fractures) or spontaneous, occurring in young individuals after rupture of peripheral apical blebs. *Tension pneumothorax* occurs when lung and mediastinal structures are compressed by the collected air. It represents a serious, potentially fatal complication.

Pleural Tumors (p. 751)

The most common pleural tumors are metastatic from lung, breast, ovaries, or other organs. Metastases often cause a malignant effusion containing tumor cells that can be detected by cytopathologic examination.

Pleural Fibroma (p. 751)

Pleural fibroma is a localized, noninvasive, fibroblastic tumor *(benign mesothelioma)* composed of submesothelial fibroblasts in the pleural surfaces of the lungs. Resection is curative.

Malignant Mesothelioma (p. 751)

Malignant mesothelioma refers to an uncommon tumor of mesothelial cells. This tumor occurs most often on the pleura and rarely in the peritoneum or other organs. It is associated with occupational exposure to asbestos in 90% of cases, but only 20% of patients have actual pulmonary asbestosis. The lifetime risk in heavily exposed individuals is 7 to 10%, and the latent period between exposure and the development of mesothelioma is 25 to 45 years. Nevertheless, bronchogenic carcinoma remains the most common lung tumor found in asbestos workers.

CLINICAL FEATURES

Patients present with chest pain, dyspnea, and recurrent pleural effusions.

MORPHOLOGY

The tumor spreads diffusely over the surface of the lung and its fissures, forming a sheath of neoplastic tissue around the lung. It rarely is primary in the peritoneum.

Microscopically the tumor consists typically of biphasic patterns of growth:

- Sarcomatoid conformation consisting of malignant, spindle-shaped cells resembling fibrosarcoma.
- Epithelioid growth composed of epithelium-like cells that form tubules and papillary projections resembling adenocarcinomas. Antigenic (keratin positivity) and ultrastructural (microvilli) features present in mesotheliomas allow distinction from adenocarcinomas.
- Epithelioid pattern is most common (70%), followed by sarcomatoid (20%) and mixed (biphasic) (10%) tumors.

Mesotheliomas are highly malignant tumors that invade the lung and can metastasize widely. Few patients survive longer than 2 years.

Diseases of the Head and Neck

ORAL CAVITY (p. 756)
Oral Inflammations (p. 756)

Oral inflammations consist of infections as well as a number of reactive lesions. The major infections include the following:

- *Herpes simplex virus* (HSV) type I infections cause the common cold sores or, uncommonly in children, a severe form of inflammation called *acute herpetic gingivostomatitis*. The lesions consist of vesicles, large bullae, or shallow ulcerations. Histologically, there is intracellular and intercellular edema (acantholysis), eosinophilic intranuclear inclusions, and giant cells. Vesicles heal spontaneously within 3 to 4 weeks, but reactivation frequently occurs in the form of groups of small vesicles that dry up in 4 to 6 days.
- *Oral candidiasis* is manifested by superficial gray-to-white inflammatory membranes composed of organisms enmeshed in its fibrinosuppurative exudate. It occurs on a background of diabetes, neutropenia, or immunodeficiency, principally acquired immunodeficiency syndrome (AIDS).

Reactive lesions include the following:

- *Irritation fibroma* occurs at the gingivodental margin and consists of a mass of fibrous tissue covered by squamous mucosa.
- *Pyogenic granuloma* is a form of capillary hemangioma seen commonly in pregnant women (pregnancy tumor) (Chapter 12).
- *Peripheral giant cell granuloma* (giant cell epulis) is made up of a striking aggregation of multinucleated foreign body–like giant cells separated by fibroangiomatous stroma.

Oral Manifestations of Systemic Disease
(p. 758)

Oral manifestations of systemic disease occur in a variety of infections, such as scarlet fever, measles, and infectious mononucleosis; dermatologic conditions, such as lichen planus and erythema multiforme; hematologic disorders, such as the pancytopenias and leukemias, especially monocytic leukemia; and miscellaneous conditions, such as in the melanotic pigmentations of Addison disease and pregnancy, the fibrous gingival enlargement of chronic phenytoin (Dilantin) ingestion, and the telangiectases of Rendu-Osler-Weber syndrome.

Hairy leukoplakia is an oral lesion restricted to patients with AIDS. It presents as a white, confluent, fluffy, hyperkeratotic lesion. Epstein-Barr virus is the major cause of the condition, but human papillomavirus with its koilocytosis and human immunodeficiency virus (HIV) transcripts also have been occasionally found.

Tumors and Precancerous Lesions (p. 759)

LEUKOPLAKIA AND ERYTHROPLAKIA (p. 759)

Leukoplakia is defined as a white plaque on the oral mucous membranes that cannot be removed by scraping and cannot be classified clinically or microscopically as another disease entity. Thus defined, the lesions range from benign epithelial thickenings to highly atypical dysplastic changes that merge with carcinoma in situ. Thus, *leukoplakia* is a clinical term, and until proved otherwise, leukoplakia should be considered precancerous. *Erythroplakia* is less common but more ominous because the epithelial changes tend to be markedly atypical and incur a higher risk of malignant transformation.

Both leukoplakia and erythroplakia are intimately linked to the use of tobacco, particularly chewing tobacco and buccal pouches. Other potential influences are alcohol, bad teeth, and ill-fitting dentures. Human papillomavirus type 16 has been identified in tobacco-related lesions. The frequency over time of carcinoma in situ or overt cancerous changes in leukoplakia is 5 to 6% and in erythroplakia about 50%.

SQUAMOUS CELL CARCINOMA (p. 760)

Ninety-five percent of oral cancers are squamous cell carcinomas, most frequently diagnosed between the ages of 50 and 70. Tobacco and alcohol are the most common associations. Smokers have a 6-fold to 15-fold greater risk of cancer than matched controls. Human papillomavirus types 6, 16, and 18 are present in 10 to 15% of cases. Chewing of betel nuts and pan are important regional influences in India and parts of Asia. Genetic factors may also play a role because deletions in chromosomes 18q, 10p, 8p, and 3p are seen in some cases. Favored locations are the floor of the mouth, tongue, hard palate, and base of tongue. The lesions can be raised, firm, ulcerated, or verrucous and histologically are typical squamous carcinomas, either keratinizing or less well-differentiated. They tend to infiltrate locally before they metastasize to other sites, particularly mediastinal lymph nodes, lungs, liver, and bones. The prognosis is best with lip lesions and poorest with the tumors in the floor of the mouth and base of the tongue (20 to 30% 5-year survival).

NOSE (p. 762)

Inflammations (p. 762)

- *Infectious rhinitis*, or the common cold, is caused by adenoviruses, echoviruses, and rhinoviruses.
- *Allergic rhinitis* affects 20% of the U.S. population and is an IgE-mediated immune reaction with an early-phase and late-phase response.
- *Nasal polyps* occur after recurrent attacks of rhinitis. Polyps consist of edematous mucosa, having a loose stroma infiltrated by neutrophils, eosinophils, and plasma cells. When multiple

or large, they obstruct the airway and impair sinus drainage, necessitating removal.

■ *Sinusitis* is commonly preceded by acute or chronic rhinitis, but maxillary sinusitis may arise by extension of a periapical tooth infection through the bony floor of the sinus. The offending organisms are inhabitants of the oral cavity, commonly a mixed microbial flora. Severe chronic sinusitis may be caused by fungi (e.g., mucormycosis), especially in diabetics. In *Kartagener syndrome*, sinusitis is accompanied by bronchiectasis and situs inversus, all secondary to defective ciliary action (Chapter 16).

Necrotizing Lesions of the Nose and Upper Airways (p. 763)

Necrotizing lesions of the nose and upper airways include the following:

■ *Spreading fungal infections*
■ Wegener *granulomatosis* (Chapter 16)
■ *Lethal midline granuloma* or *polymorphic reticulosis*, now thought to represent, in most cases, angiocentric non-Hodgkin lymphoma, a neoplasm of natural killer cells (Chapter 15).

Tumors of the Nose, Sinuses, and Nasopharynx (p. 763)

Tumors of the nose, sinuses, and nasopharynx include the following:

■ *Nasopharyngeal angiofibroma* is a highly vascularized benign tumor that occurs in adolescent boys and may cause serious bleeding during surgery.
■ *Inverted papilloma* is a benign but locally aggressive neoplasm of squamous epithelium.
■ *Isolated plasmacytomas* are made up of mature and immature plasma cells (Chapter 15).
■ *Olfactory neuroblastoma* (esthesioneuroblastoma) is an uncommon, highly malignant tumor composed of small round cells of a neuroendocrine origin.
■ *Nasopharyngeal carcinomas* can be nonkeratinizing squamous cell carcinomas or undifferentiated carcinomas with abundant lymphocytic infiltrate *(lymphoepithelioma)*. These lesions are particularly frequent in parts of Africa and Southern China, where they are common in adults and rare in children. The tumor is closely linked to Epstein-Barr virus infection (Chapter 8). These carcinomas tend to grow silently until they have become unresectable and often spread to cervical or distant nodes. Most are sensitive to radiotherapy, with a 50 to 70% 3-year survival rate.

LARYNX (p. 765)

Inflammations (p. 765)

Laryngitis may occur as a manifestation of allergic, viral, bacterial, or chemical injury but is most commonly the result of nonspecific infection or heavy exposure to tobacco smoke. In heavy smokers, it constitutes an important predisposition to the development of squamous cell cancers. Laryngitis in children caused by *Haemophilus influenzae* may be serious owing to the rapid development of mucosal congestion and edema and airway obstruction. The inspiratory stridor it produces is known as *croup*.

Reactive nodules (vocal cord polyps) occur most often in heavy smokers or singers (singer's nodules). They consist of smooth, rounded excrescences a few millimeters in diameter located on the true vocal cords, consisting of myxoid connective tissue, sometimes quite vascular, covered by squamous epithelium that may be hyperplastic. They virtually never give rise to cancers but change the character of the voice and often cause progressive hoarseness.

Carcinoma of the Larynx (p. 765)

A spectrum of epithelial alterations is seen in the larynx, termed from one end to the other

- *Hyperplasia*
- *Atypical hyperplasia*
- *Dysplasia*
- *Carcinoma* in situ
- *Invasive carcinoma*

The likelihood of development of an overt carcinoma is directly proportional to the level of atypia when the lesion is first seen. The changes are most often related to tobacco smoke, and up to the point of frank cancer, the changes often regress after cessation of smoking. Alcohol is also a risk factor.

About 95% of laryngeal cancers are typical squamous cell lesions, usually developing directly on the vocal cords but also below the cords in the epiglottis or pyriform sinuses. They begin as in-situ lesions but ultimately ulcerate and fungate. They manifest clinically by persistent hoarseness but later may produce pain, dysphagia, and hemoptysis. With surgery, radiation, or both, more than two thirds of patients are cured.

Squamous Papilloma and Papillomatosis
(p. 766)

Squamous papillomas are benign lesions, usually on the true vocal cords. In children, they may be multiple, referred to as *juvenile laryngeal papillomatosis*. Lesions are caused by human papillomavirus types 6 and 11, do not become malignant, but frequently recur. In children, they often regress spontaneously at puberty. Cancerous transformation is rare.

EAR (p. 766)
Inflammations (p. 766)

Otitis media occurs mostly in infants and children and is usually caused by *Streptococcus pneumoniae*, *H. influenzae*, and β-hemolytic streptococci. *Chronic disease* is usually caused by pseudomonas and staphylococcus. *Cholesteatomas* associated with chronic otitis media are cystic lesions 1 to 4 cm in diameter, lined by keratinizing squamous epithelium and filled with amorphous debris, sometimes containing spicules of cholesterol.

Otosclerosis (p. 767)

Otosclerosis refers to *abnormal bone deposition* in the middle ear about the oval window, hampering the mobility of the footplate of the stapes. The basis for the osseous overgrowth is obscure; in most instances, it is familial following autosomal dominant transmission with variable penetrance. The process is slowly progressive and, during the span of decades, leads eventually to marked hearing loss.

NECK (p. 767)
Thyroglossal Duct Cyst (p. 767)

Thyroglossal duct cysts arise from residua of the embryonic origins of the thyroid gland and are discussed in Chapter 24.

Paraganglioma (Carotid Body Tumor)
(p. 768)

Paragangliomas are tumors arising in extra-adrenal paraganglia either in the paravertebral areas or more commonly in the paraganglia around the great vessels of the head and neck, including the *carotid bodies*. They are red, pink, or brown and consist of nests (zellballen) of polygonal chief cells enclosed by trabeculae of fibrous and sustentacular elongated cells. The cells have neuroendocrine granules by electron microscopy and stain positively for neuroendocrine markers (e.g., S-100, chromogranin).

They commonly occur singly and sporadically but may be familial, as part of the multiple endocrine neoplasia II syndrome (Chapter 24) and in this case are usually multiple and bilateral. They may recur after excision in about 50% of cases and ultimately prove fatal largely because of infiltrative growth.

SALIVARY GLANDS (p. 769)
Inflammations (p. 769)

Sialoadenitis may be viral, bacterial, or autoimmune in origin; the last-mentioned usually is associated with the *Sjögren syndrome* (Chapter 7). Bacterial sialoadenitis is usually secondary to ductal obstructions by stones, *sialolithiasis*.

Neoplasms (p. 769)

Salivary glands give rise to a surprising variety of benign and malignant tumors (Table 17–1). About 65 to 80% arise within the parotid, 10% in the submandibular, and the remainder in the minor salivary glands. Fifteen percent to 30% of tumors in the parotids are malignant, in contrast to 40% in the submandibulars and 70 to 90% in the sublingual gland.

PLEOMORPHIC ADENOMA (p. 770)

Pleomorphic adenomas are mixed tumors that are the most common of salivary gland neoplasms. They represent 60% of parotid tumors and show both epithelial and mesenchymal differentiation. They are composed of epithelial nests, cords, or glands dispersed through a matrix showing varying degrees of myxoid, hyaline, chondroid, and even osseous tissue.

The tumors present as painless, slow-growing mobile, discrete masses within the parotid or submandibular areas or in the buccal cavity. They may recur if not well excised, with recurrence ap-

Table 17-1. HISTOLOGIC CLASSIFICATION AND
APPROXIMATE INCIDENCE OF
BENIGN AND MALIGNANT TUMORS
OF THE SALIVARY GLANDS

Benign	Malignant
Pleomorphic adenoma (50%) (mixed tumor)	Mucoepidermoid carcinoma (15%)
Warthin tumor (5–10%)	Adenocarcinoma (NOS) (10%)
Oncocytoma (1%)	Acinic cell carcinoma (5%)
Other adenomas (5–10%)	Adenoid cystic carcinoma (5%)
Basal cell adenoma	Malignant mixed tumor (3–5%)
Canalicular adenoma	Squamous cell carcinoma (1%)
Ductal papillomas	Other carcinomas (2%)

NOS, not otherwise specified.

Data from Ellis GL, Auclair PL: Tumors of the Salivary Glands. Atlas of Tumor Pathology, Third Series. Washington, DC, Armed Forces Institute of Pathology, 1996.

proaching 25% in some series. Malignant transformation occurs in 10% of pleomorphic adenomas of more than 15 years' duration, usually in the form of adenocarcinoma or undifferentiated carcinoma.

WARTHIN TUMOR (PAPILLARY CYSTADENOMA) (p. 771)

Warthin tumor almost always arises in the parotid gland; 10% are multifocal and bilateral. The tumor is most common in smokers. It is well encapsulated and consists of glandular spaces lined by a double layer of epithelial cells resting on a dense lymphoid stroma, sometimes bearing germinal centers. The histogenesis is unknown. The tumors are benign.

MUCOEPIDERMOID CARCINOMA (p. 772)

Mucoepidermoid carcinomas represent about 15% of all salivary gland tumors and are the most common form of malignant tumor primary in the salivary glands. They range in diameter up to 8 cm and lack well-defined capsules. Histologically, they consist of cords, sheets, or cystic configurations of squamous, mucous, or intermediate cells with small-to-large mucus-filled vacuoles highlighted with mucin stains. They can be low-grade, intermediate-grade, or high-grade malignancies. Low-grade tumors may invade locally and recur in 15% of cases, but high-grade tumors recur in about 25% and have only a 50% 5-year survival.

Diseases of the Gastrointestinal Tract

ESOPHAGUS (p. 776)

Key symptoms for esophageal disorders include the following:

- *Dysphagia*: Subjective difficulty in swallowing, encountered with mechanical and functional disorders
- *Heartburn*: Retrosternal burning pain, usually reflecting regurgitation of gastric contents into lower esophagus
- *Hematemesis*: Vomiting of blood, the result of inflammation or ulceration or rupture of blood vessels
- *Pain*: Retrosternal, nonspecific

Anatomic Anomalies (p. 777)
ATRESIA AND FISTULAS (p. 777)

Atresia and fistulas are uncommon, usually discovered soon after birth; many are incompatible with life, often associated with congenital heart disease and other gastrointestinal tract malformations.

- In esophageal *atresia*, a segment of the esophagus is only a thin, noncanalized cord, with blind pouches on either side.
- In 80 to 90% of cases, a *fistula* connects one of the pouches with the trachea or a mainstem bronchus.

STENOSIS, WEBS, AND RINGS (p. 777)

- *Stenosis* may be congenital or acquired in adult life after severe esophageal injury (gastroesophageal reflux, radiation, scleroderma, or caustic injury).
- *Mucosal rings* are smooth ledges of mucosa and a vascularized fibrous core, designated *webs* in upper esophagus and *Schatzki rings* at the gastroesophageal junction. These usually present in adult life.

Features of esophageal narrowing include progressive dysphagia, especially to solid foods.

Lesions Associated With Motor Dysfunction (p. 778)
ACHALASIA (p. 778)

Three features are present in achalasia:

1. Aperistalsis of the esophagus

2. Partial or incomplete relaxation of the lower esophageal sphincter (LES) with swallowing
3. Increased resting tone of the LES

Secondary features are proximal esophageal dilation, dysphagia, and regurgitation. Achalasia presents in young adulthood or earlier and is problematic throughout life. The risk of esophageal carcinoma is 2 to 7%. Other complications include candidal esophagitis, diverticula, and aspiration pneumonia.

Manometry

Manometry shows aperistalsis, impaired relaxation of the LES, and increased LES resting tone.

Morphology

Morphologic features include the following:

- Dilated esophagus above LES
- Thickened (muscular hypertrophy) or thinned (distention) muscular wall
- Diminished myenteric ganglia
- Secondary mucosal damage

SECONDARY ACHALASIA

Secondary achalasia occurs with Chagas disease *(Trypanosoma cruzi)*, disorders of the vagal dorsal motor nuclei (polio, surgical ablation), diabetic autonomic neuropathy, and infiltrative disorders (malignancy, amyloidosis, sarcoidosis).

HIATAL HERNIA (p. 779)

Hiatal hernia refers to a saclike dilation of stomach with protrusion above the diaphragm, with separation of the diaphragmatic crura and widening of the esophageal foramen.

- *Sliding* (axial) *hiatal hernia* (90% of cases): Shortened esophagus, traction of upper stomach into thorax, bell-like dilation of stomach within the thoracic cavity
- *Paraesophageal hiatal hernia* (rolling hernia) (<10% of cases): Cardia of stomach dissects alongside esophagus into thorax, vulnerable to strangulation and infarction

Clinical Findings

Hiatal hernia is reported in up to 1 to 20% of normal adults; it may also affect infants and children. Only 9% have symptoms (retrosternal chest pain, regurgitation of gastric juices). A hiatal hernia may ulcerate or strangulate, causing bleeding or perforation.

DIVERTICULA (p. 779)

A *diverticulum* is an outpouching of the alimentary tract that contains one or more layers of the wall. In the esophagus, they are classified as follows:

- *Pharyngeal (Zenker) diverticulum*: In the upper esophagus, the presumed result of motor dysfunction
- *Traction diverticulum*: More distal location, attributed to fibrosing mediastinal processes or abnormal motility

- *Epiphrenic diverticulum*: Immediately above esophageal sphincter, unclear cause.

LACERATIONS (MALLORY-WEISS SYNDROME)
(p. 779)

Lacerations are longitudinal tears in the esophagus at the esophagogastric junction, attributed to episodes of excessive vomiting in the setting of toxic gastritis, with failure of LES relaxation. Lacerations are most frequently seen in alcoholics. They may lead to potentially massive hematemesis, inflammation, residual ulcer, mediastinitis, or peritonitis.

Morphology

Irregular longitudinal tears span the esophagogastric junction, several millimeters to centimeters in length. Lacerations may involve only mucosa or may penetrate the wall (unusual).

Clinical Findings

Lacerations account for 5 to 10% of upper gastrointestinal bleeding events. Lacerations are not usually fatal, and healing tends to be prompt.

Esophagitis (p. 780)

REFLUX ESOPHAGITIS (p. 780)

Reflux of gastric contents is the foremost cause of esophagitis. Contributing factors include

- Decreased efficacy of esophageal antireflux mechanisms
- The presence of a sliding hiatal hernia
- Delayed gastric emptying and increased gastric volume
- Reduced reparative capability of the esophageal mucosa

Morphology

Morphologic findings (from mild to severe) are as follows:

- Hyperemia and edema
- Thickening of basal zone and thinning of superficial layers of stratified squamous epithelium
- Polymorphonuclear or eosinophilic leukocyte infiltrate
- Superficial necrosis and ulceration with adherent inflammatory exudate

Clinical Findings

Reflux esophagitis occurs usually in adults. Symptoms include dysphagia, heartburn, regurgitation of sour brash, hematemesis, and melena. Stricture or Barrett esophagus can develop as a result of reflux esophagitis.

BARRETT ESOPHAGUS (p. 781)

Barrett esophagus refers to *replacement of the distal esophageal squamous epithelium by a metaplastic columnar epithelium, in response to prolonged injury.* It is most common in adults but may be seen in children and infants.

Pathogenesis (proposed)

Long-standing gastroesophageal reflux leads to inflammation and ulceration of squamous mucosa; healing is by re-epithelialization by pluripotent stem cells, which in the setting of low pH differentiate into more resistant gastric-type or intestinal-type epithelium.

Morphology

Morphologic findings are as follows:

- *Gross*: Red, velvety mucosa existing as an irregular circumferential band at the gastroesophageal junction, linear streaks, or patches in the distal esophagus.
- *Microscopic*: Mixture of gastric-type and intestinal-type columnar epithelial cells (mucin-secreting and absorptive).

Substantial risk of ulceration and stricture exists. Risk of adenocarcinoma is 30 times normal.

INFECTIOUS AND CHEMICAL ESOPHAGITIS
(p. 782)

Unusual causes of esophageal mucosal inflammation include the following:

- Prolonged gastric intubation
- Ingestion of irritants: alcohol, corrosive acids or alkalis, excessively hot fluids, smoking
- Uremia
- Bacteremia or viremia; herpesvirus, cytomegalovirus infection
- Fungal infection: candidiasis, mucormycosis, aspergillosis
- Radiation
- Cytotoxic anticancer therapy
- Systemic desquamative disorders: pemphigoid, epidermolysis bullosa
- Graft-versus-host disease

Varices (p. 783)

Varices occur in 90% of cirrhotic patients, especially alcoholics; hepatic schistosomiasis is a common cause worldwide. Prolonged and severe portal hypertension induces formation of collateral bypass channels: through the coronary veins of the stomach into esophageal subepithelial and submucosal veins *(varices)* and thence to the azygous veins and systemic circulation. Other portosystemic shunts include the rectal canal *(hemorrhoids)* and falciform ligament *(caput medusa).*

MORPHOLOGY

Tortuous dilated veins lying primarily within submucosa of distal esophagus and proximal stomach are seen, with irregular protrusion of overlying mucosa into lumen. Superficial ulceration, inflammation, or adherent blood clot may be apparent.

CLINICAL FINDINGS

Varices are clinically silent until rupture, with catastrophic hematemesis—fatality rate is 40% for each episode of bleeding, with a 90% chance of recurrence within a year in survivors. Massive hematemesis in patients with varices also may be caused by gastritis, esophageal laceration, or peptic ulcer.

Tumors (p. 783)

BENIGN TUMORS (p. 783)

Benign tumors include the following types:

- *Intramural or submucosal*: Leiomyoma, fibroma, lipoma, hemangioma, neurofibroma, lymphangioma
- *Mucosal*: Squamous papilloma, fibrovascular polyp (with overlying epithelium), inflammatory polyp (severely inflamed mesenchyme with overlying epithelium)

They rarely exceed 3 cm in diameter.

MALIGNANT TUMORS (p. 783)

Malignant tumors can be classified as follows:

- Esophageal carcinomas make up 6% of all cancers of the gastrointestinal tract but cause a disproportionately high death rate.
- Malignant stromal tumors (of smooth muscle or fibroblast origin) are rare.

Squamous Cell Carcinoma (p. 783)

Epidemiology. Squamous cell carcinoma occurs in adults older than age 50, more often in men. Incidence varies considerably among geographic areas, with the highest incidence in Northern China, Iran, Russia, and South Africa. Blacks are at greater risk than whites.

Pathogenesis. Pathogenesis is multifactorial, with synergistic interaction of environmental and dietary factors, perhaps modified by genetic factors (Table 18–1).

Morphology. Squamous cell carcinomas begin as in-situ lesions: gray-white, plaquelike thickenings or elevations of mucosa. With progression, the lesions extend longitudinally along axis, circumferentially, and deep (with invasion).

- Distribution (thirds):
  - Upper 20%
  - Middle 50%
  - Lower 30%
- Gross patterns:
  - *Polypoid* (60%)
  - *Necrotizing excavation* (25%)
  - *Diffuse infiltrative* (15%)
- Early, *superficial* carcinoma denotes invasion no deeper than submucosa.
- Usually moderately to well differentiated, with or without keratinization.
- Tend to spread via the rich submucosal lymphatic network to

Table 18-1. FACTORS ASSOCIATED WITH THE DEVELOPMENT OF ESOPHAGEAL SQUAMOUS CELL CARCINOMA

Dietary

Vitamin deficiency (A, C, riboflavin, thiamine, pyridoxine)
Deficiency of trace metals (zinc, molybdenum)
Fungal contamination of foodstuffs
High content of nitrites/nitrosamines
Betel chewing

Lifestyle

Alcohol consumption
Tobacco use
Urban environment

Esophageal Disorders

Long-standing esophagitis
Achalasia
Plummer-Vinson syndrome

Predisposing Influences

Long-standing celiac disease
Ectodermal dysplasia, epidermolysis bullosa
Genetic (racial) predisposition
Tylosis palmaris et plantaris

nearby lymph nodes, and locally by deep extension into adjacent mediastinal structures.

Clinical Findings. Insidious in onset, symptoms develop late in the course: dysphagia, obstruction, weight loss, hemorrhage, sepsis secondary to ulceration, fistula formation into respiratory tree with aspiration.

■ Curative resection possible in 80% of cases.
■ Five-year survival:
  • Superficial, 75%
  • Advanced resectable, 25%
  • All patients with esophageal cancer, 5%

Adenocarcinoma (p. 786)

Adenocarcinoma represents one half of esophageal cancers. Risk factors are as for Barrett mucosa. Adenocarcinoma appears to evolve through dysplastic change in Barrett mucosa.

Pathogenesis. Genetic alterations are well documented: overexpression of *p53* protein, allelic losses at 17p, with abrogation of cell cycle control at the G_1-to-S phase transition.

Morphology. *The vast majority arise from Barrett mucosa in areas of dysplasia*—most are in the distal third of esophagus.

■ *Gross*: May be exophytic nodule or excavated and deeply infiltrative.
■ *Microscopic*: Mucin-producing glandular tumors with intestinal features or diffusely infiltrative signet ring cells; rarely adenosquamous or small cell type.

Clinical Findings. Tumors arise in Barrett mucosa patients older than age 40, more commonly in men than in women, with symptoms as in squamous cell carcinoma. Previous symptoms of gastroesophageal reflux are present in fewer than half of patients.

Overall 5-year survival is less than 30%; screening programs detect disease earlier.

STOMACH (p. 787)
Congenital Anomalies (p. 788)

Uncommon anomalies include *pancreatic heterotopia* in the gastric muscle wall or submucosa or in utero displacement of the stomach cephalad through a *diaphragmatic hernia.* Such hernias are due to a weakness or a defect in the diaphragm (usually on left) and do not involve the hiatal orifice. If herniation of abdominal viscera is substantial, respiratory impairment with pulmonary hypoplasia is life-threatening.

PYLORIC STENOSIS (p. 789)
Congenital Hypertrophic Pyloric Stenosis (p. 789)

Congenital hypertrophic pyloric stenosis refers to hypertrophy and possibly hyperplasia of circular muscle of the muscularis propria of the pyloris. It occurs in 1:300 to 1:900 live births, and the male-female ratio is 4:1. Clinical findings include visible peristalsis and a firm ovoid palpable mass by physical examination. Other characteristics of congenital hypertrophic pyloric stenosis include the following:

- Multifactorial inheritance, high concordance in twins
- Mucosal edema and inflammation, which aggravates narrowing
- Regurgitation and vomiting by third week of life
- Full-thickness, muscle-splitting incision *(pyloromyotomy)* curative

Acquired Pyloric Stenosis (p. 789)

Acquired pyloric stenosis is a long term complication of chronic antral gastritis. Peptic ulcers close to the pylorus and malignancy (carcinoma, lymphoma, pancreatic carcinoma) also are causes.

Gastritis (p. 789)

Gastritis is defined as *inflammation of the gastric mucosa.*

ACUTE GASTRITIS (p. 789)

Acute gastritis is an acute mucosal inflammatory process, usually transient.

Pathogenesis

Etiologic associations are as follows:

- Chronic and heavy use of nonsteroidal anti-inflammatory drugs (NSAIDs), particularly aspirin
- Excessive alcohol consumption
- Heavy smoking
- Cancer chemotherapy
- Uremia
- Systemic infection
- Severe stress (burns, trauma, surgery)
- Ischemia and shock

- Ingestion of acid or alkali
- Gastric irradiation
- Mechanical trauma
- Post–distal gastrectomy

Proposed mechanisms of action include

- Increased acid production with back-diffusion
- Decreased production of surface bicarbonate buffer
- Reduced mucosal blood flow, disruption of mucus layer
- Direct damage to mucosal epithelium

Morphology

Morphologic findings include

- Moderate edema and hyperemia
- Entry of neutrophils into the epithelial layer *(activity)*
- Sloughing of the superficial epithelium *(erosion)*
- Hemorrhage *(acute hemorrhagic erosive gastritis)*

Clinical Findings

Asymptomatic or minor abdominal pain or acute abdominal pain with hematemesis occurs.

CHRONIC GASTRITIS (p. 790)

Chronic gastritis is defined as *the presence of chronic mucosal inflammatory changes leading eventually to mucosal atrophy and epithelial metaplasia.* This condition constitutes a background for dysplasia, hence carcinoma.

Pathogenesis

Etiologic associations are as follows:

- Chronic infection, especially *Helicobacter pylori*, which predisposes to a number of conditions (Table 18–2)
- Immunologic:
  - Antibodies to parietal cells (including the H^+,K^+-ATPase)
  - Gland destruction and atrophy
  - Decreased intrinsic factor secretion by parietal cells, which may lead to pernicious anemia
- Toxic: alcohol and tobacco usage
- Postsurgical: postantrectomy reflux of bile
- Motor/mechanical: obstruction, atony
- Radiation
- Granulomatous conditions: Crohn disease
- Graft-versus-host disease, uremia, amyloidosis

Table 18–2. DISEASES ASSOCIATED WITH *HELICOBACTER PYLORI*

Disease	Association
Chronic gastritis	Strong causal association
Peptic ulcer disease	Strong causal association
Gastric carcinoma	Postulated etiologic role
Gastric lymphoma	Postulated etiologic role

HELICOBACTER PYLORI (p. 790)

H. pylori colonizes more than 50% of Americans older than age 50; it is an S-shaped gram-negative rod and is present in 90% of patients with chronic gastritis of antrum. Specialized traits that allow it to flourish in the stomach include

1. *Motility* via flagella
2. Elaboration of a *urease*, buffering gastric acid
3. Binding to surface epithelial cells via a bacterial *adhesin*

Some strains express the *cagA* and *vacA* cytotoxins, which are proinflammatory peptides.

AUTOIMMUNE GASTRITIS (p. 791)

Autoimmune gastritis accounts for less than 10% of chronic gastritis, owing to autoantibodies to gastric parietal cells and intrinsic factor. It is associated with other autoimmune diseases, including Hashimoto thyroiditis and Addison disease.

Morphology

Reddened, coarse-textured mucosa is seen, which may be boggy or exhibit flattening; distribution is variable.

- *Environmental causes* (including *H. pylori*): variable and patchy distribution of antrum or antrum and corpus
- *Autoimmune*: diffuse damage of body-fundic mucosa

Microscopic findings are as follows:

- Inflammatory infiltrate of lymphocytes and plasma cells in lamina propria, involving either the superficial portion or the entire mucosal thickness
- Activity (intraepithelial neutrophilic infiltrate)
- Regenerative change
- Variable atrophy
- Metaplasia to intestinal-type epithelium
- Dysplasia in some cases of long-standing chronic gastritis

H. pylori, when present, are found nestled in superficial mucous layer.

Clinical Findings

Usually there are few symptoms. Nausea, vomiting, or upper abdominal discomfort may occur; rarely, overt pernicious anemia occurs in autoimmune gastritis. Laboratory findings include gastric hypochlorhydria and serum hypergastrinemia. Long-term risk of cancer is 2 to 4%.

Peptic Ulcer Disease (p. 793)

An ulcer is defined as *a breach in the mucosa of the alimentary tract that extends through the muscularis mucosa into the submucosa or deeper.*

PEPTIC ULCERS (p. 793)

Peptic ulcers are *chronic, most often solitary ulcers in any portion of the alimentary tract arising from exposure to acid-peptic juices.*

Epidemiology

The lifetime likelihood of peptic ulcer is 10% for American men and 4% for women. Most often, middle-aged to older adults are affected. Even with healing, propensity to ulcers remains. There are no genetic tendencies. Duodenal ulcer is more frequent in patients with alcoholic cirrhosis, chronic obstructive pulmonary disease, chronic renal failure, and hyperparathyroidism.

Pathogenesis

Peptic ulcers are *produced by an imbalance between the gastro-duodenal mucosal defense mechanisms and damaging forces of gastric acid and pepsin, combined with superimposed injury from environmental or immunologic agents.* Mucosal defense forces consist of

- Surface mucus secretion
- Bicarbonate secretion into mucus
- Mucosal blood flow
- Apical epithelial cell transport systems
- Epithelial regeneration
- Uncertain role of prostaglandins

Impaired defense occurs in ischemia and shock, with delayed gastric emptying, and with duodenal-gastric reflux. *H. pylori* infection is present in virtually all patients with duodenal ulcers and 70% with gastric ulcers, causing damage by the following:

- *H. pylori* secretes urease, protease, or phospholipases.
- Bacterial lipopolysaccharide attracts inflammatory cells to the mucosa. Neutrophils release myeloperoxidase.
- A bacterial platelet-activating factor promotes thrombotic occlusion of surface capillaries.
- Mucosal damage permits leakage of tissue nutrients into the surface microenvironment, sustaining the bacillus.

Other promoters of gastric mucosal ulceration include the following:

1. Gastric hyperacidity—increased parietal cell mass can arise in the setting of excess gastrin production, as from a gastrinoma causing multiple peptic ulcerations *(Zollinger-Ellison syndrome,* p. 927)
2. Chronic use of NSAIDs, which suppress mucosal prostaglandin synthesis
3. Cigarette smoking, alcoholic cirrhosis, corticosteroids, and hypercalcemia as from chronic renal failure or hyperparathyroidism

Morphology

Ninety-eight percent of ulcers are found in duodenum and stomach, in a ratio of 4:1. Gross findings include a sharply punched-out defect with overhanging mucosal borders and smooth, clean ulcer base. Microscopic findings include four layers:

1. Thin superficial layer of necrotic debris
2. Zone of inflammation
3. Granulation tissue
4. Scar

Surrounding mucosa usually exhibits chronic gastritis; exceptions are acute erosive gastritis and stress ulcers.

Clinical Findings

Epigastric gnawing, burning, or aching pain occurs, which is worse at night and 1 to 3 hours after meals. Nausea, vomiting, bloating, belching, and weight loss occur. Complications include anemia, hemorrhage, perforation, and obstruction. Malignant transformation is rare and related to underlying gastritis.

ACUTE GASTRIC ULCERATION (p. 796)

Acute gastric ulceration refers to focal, acutely developing gastric mucosal defects appearing during severe stress *(stress ulcer)*. This condition is encountered in *shock; extensive burns or severe trauma* (Curling ulcers); and *elevated intracranial pressure*, as in trauma or surgery (Cushing ulcers). Acute gastric ulceration is in a continuum with acute erosive gastritis and so may exhibit only erosions. NSAID use also may cause acute ulceration.

Pathogenesis

Pathogenesis is unclear. It may include

- Impaired oxygenation
- Stimulation of vagal nuclei with hypersecretion of gastric acid
- Systemic acidosis

Morphology

Ulcers are usually less than 1 cm in diameter, multiple, and shallow. Ulcer base is brown (blood); adjacent mucosa is normal (both gross and microscopic).

Clinical Findings

Acute gastric erosions or ulcers occur in 5 to 10% of intensive care unit patients. The single most important determinant of outcome is the *ability to correct the underlying conditions.*

Miscellaneous Conditions (p. 797)

Gastric dilation may arise from gastric outlet obstruction (pyloric stenosis, tumors) or gastric and intestinal atony (ileus). Rarely, gastric rupture may occur. *Bezoars* are luminal concretions of indigestible ingested material: A phytobezoar is derived from plant material; a trichobezoar is a *hairball*.

HYPERTROPHIC GASTROPATHY (p. 797)

Hypertrophic gastropathy refers to uncommon conditions featuring giant cerebriform enlargement of gastric rugal folds, caused by hyperplasia of mucosal epithelial cells.

- *Menetrier disease*: hyperplasia of surface mucosal cells
- *Hypertrophic-hypersecretory gastropathy*: hyperplasia of parietal and chief cells
- *Gastric gland hyperplasia*: secondary to excessive gastrin secretion by a gastrinoma (Zollinger-Ellison syndrome)

Clinical Findings

Conditions may mimic diffuse gastric cancer or lymphoma on radiographic studies; patients are at risk for peptic ulceration. Excess secreted protein may cause hypoalbuminemia and *protein-*

losing gastroenteropathy. The hyperplastic mucosa may become dysplastic, with risk of adenocarcinoma.

GASTRIC VARICES

Gastric varices develop in the setting of portal hypertension, near the gastroesophageal junction. These are less common than esophageal varices.

Tumors (p. 798)
BENIGN TUMORS (p. 798)

In the alimentary tract, polyp *refers to any nodule or mass that projects above the level of the surrounding mucosa* and is generally restricted to *mass lesions arising from the mucosa.*

- The majority of gastric polyps (90%) are *hyperplastic or inflammatory polyps*—smooth surfaced, sessile, or pedunculated, with epithelial tubules and cysts, interspersed with an inflamed stroma. Polyps are often multiple and seen in chronic gastritis. They are regarded as having no malignant potential per se but may be found in stomachs resected for carcinoma.
- *Gastric adenoma* (5 to 10% of gastric polyps) is a true neoplasm with *proliferative dysplastic epithelium;* thereby has malignant potential. Usually single, may be *sessile* (without a stalk) or *pedunculated* (with a stalk). Much more common in colon.

Incidence of gastric adenomas increases with age; up to 40% harbor carcinoma at time of diagnosis. Arise in background of chronic gastritis or genetic polyposis syndromes.

GASTRIC CARCINOMA (p. 798)

Epidemiology

Of gastric malignancies, 90 to 95% are carcinoma (versus lymphomas, carcinoids, spindle cell tumors). Worldwide distribution is widely variable. Incidence has decreased fourfold over the last 60 years, but the prognosis is dismal, and it still represents 2.5% of all cancer deaths in the United States. Five-year survival is 20% overall. There are two types (described later): intestinal and diffuse.

Pathogenesis

Contributing factors for intestinal-type tumors (risk factors for diffuse cancer are poorly defined) are as follows:

- *Environment*:
  1. Diet—lack of refrigeration, use of preservatives, lack of fresh fruit and vegetables
  2. Cigarette smoking increases risk 1.5- to 3.0-fold
- *Host*:
  1. Infection by *H. pylori* leading to chronic gastritis
  2. *Autoimmune gastritis*
  3. *Partial gastrectomy* permitting gastroduodenal reflux

Dysplasia of the gastric mucosa is the final common pathway. Molecular events include genetic instability in DNA repair genes; expression of telomerase; and abnormalities in *c-met*, K-*sam*, and *erb* (growth factor receptor systems).

Morphology

Gross locations of carcinoma are:

- Pylorus and antrum, 50 to 60%
- Cardia, 25%
- Body and fundus, 15 to 25%

Lesser curvature is involved in 40% and greater curvature in 12%. Classification is according to the following:

- *Depth of invasion: Early gastric carcinoma* is confined to the mucosa and submucosa, regardless of presence or absence of lymph node metastases. *Advanced gastric carcinoma* extends beyond the submucosa.
- *Macroscopic growth pattern*: Tumors are exophytic, flat or depressed, or excavated. Uncommonly, diffuse invasion throughout the wall creates a rigid thickened stomach: *linitis plastica.*
- *Histologic subtype* according to *Lauren classification*:
  - *Intestinal*: Gland-forming columnar epithelium; usually mucin producing; usually polypoid expansile growth pattern; almost always associated with mucosal intestinal metaplasia; mean age, 55 years; male-female ratio, 2:1; decreasing incidence
  - *Diffuse*: poorly differentiated, single signet-ring cells; mucin producing; infiltrative growth pattern; mean age, 48 years; male-female ratio, 1:1; no change in incidence
- *Dissemination*: Dissemination to ovaries generates *Krukenberg tumors.*

Clinical Findings

Gastric carcinoma is an insidious disease, initially asymptomatic. Findings include weight loss, abdominal pain, anorexia, vomiting, altered bowel habits, dysphagia, anemia, and hemorrhage. Prognosis depends only on *depth of invasion*:

- Resected early gastric cancer, 90 to 95% 5-year survival
- Advanced disease, less than 15% 5-year survival

LESS COMMON GASTRIC TUMORS (p. 802)

Lymphomas represent 5% of gastric malignancies. Other rare tumors include carcinoid tumors, lipomas, and stromal tumors (featuring smooth muscle, neural, or fibroblastic features). Metastatic tumor may produce a linitis plastica.

SMALL AND LARGE INTESTINES (p. 802)

Congenital Anomalies (p. 804)

Rare anomalies include *duplication* of a portion of small intestine or colon; *malrotation* of the entire bowel during embryologic development; *omphalocele*, in which the abdominal musculature fails to form; and *gastroschisis*, in which a portion of the abdominal wall fails to develop altogether. The first two may be silent for decades, but the latter two are severe to catastrophic in the newborn.

ATRESIA AND STENOSIS (p. 804)

Atresia and stenosis arise from developmental failure (e.g., intrauterine vascular accidents) and intussusception; the duodenum is most commonly affected. Failure of the cloacal diaphragm to rupture leads to *imperforate anus*.

MECKEL DIVERTICULUM (p. 804)

A *diverticulum* is a blind pouch leading off the alimentary tract, lined by mucosa that communicates with the lumen of the gut. Meckel diverticulum is the prototype congenital diverticulum: Persistence of the vitelline duct (connects yolk sac with gut lumen) leaves a solitary diverticulum 30 cm from the ileocecal valve, consisting of a *pouch of mucosa, submucosa, and muscularis propria. Heterotopic gastric (or pancreatic) mucosa may generate symptoms of peptic ulceration or appendicitis.* Diverticula may also intussuscept, incarcerate, or perforate. They present in 2% of the normal population and are usually asymptomatic.

CONGENITAL AGANGLIONIC MEGACOLON—HIRSCHSPRUNG DISEASE
(p. 805)

Arrested migration of neural crest cells into the gut (proximal to distal) *generates an aganglionic segment with functional obstruction and dilation proximal to the affected segment.*

Morphology

Morphologic findings include absence of ganglion cells and ganglia in muscle wall (Auerbach plexus) and submucosa (Meissner plexus) of the affected segment. The rectum is always affected; proximal involvement is more variable. There is progressive dilation and hypertrophy of unaffected proximal colon.

Clinical Findings

Hirschsprung disease occurs in 1:5000 to 1:8000 live births; the male-female ratio is 4:1. There is an association with Down syndrome and neurologic abnormalities. Hirschsprung disease manifests as failure to pass meconium in the neonate or abdominal distention. There is a risk of perforation, sepsis, and enterocolitis with fluid derangement.

Acquired megacolon may occur in Chagas disease, bowel obstruction, inflammatory bowel disease, and psychosomatic disorders.

Enterocolitis (p. 805)
DIARRHEA AND DYSENTERY (p. 805)

Diarrhea is roughly defined as *daily stool production in excess of 250 gm, containing 70 to 95% water,* and is perceived as an *increase in stool volume, fluidity,* or *frequency.* Low-volume, painful diarrhea is known as *dysentery.*

■ *Secretory diarrhea*: Net intestinal fluid secretion greater than 500 ml/day, isotonic with plasma, and persists during fasting.
■ *Osmotic diarrhea*: Osmotic forces exerted by luminal solutes lead to greater than 500 ml stool/day; abates during fasting and exhibits osmotic gap (stool osmolality exceeds electrolyte concentration by >50 mOsm).
■ *Exudative diseases*: Purulent, bloody stools that persist during fasting; frequent but variable volume.

- *Deranged motility*: Variable features, excluding other causes.
- *Malabsorption*: Voluminous, bulky stools with excess fat and osmolarity; abates on fasting.

Major causes are given in Table 18–3; mechanisms may overlap.

INFECTIOUS ENTEROCOLITIS (p. 806)

- More than 12,000 deaths occur *per day* in children in developing countries; one half of all deaths occur before age 5 worldwide.

Table 18–3. MAJOR CAUSES OF DIARRHEAL DISEASES

Secretory Diarrhea

Infectious: viral damage to surface epithelium
    Rotavirus
    Norwalk virus
    Enteric adenoviruses
Infectious: enterotoxin-mediated
    Vibrio cholerae
    Escherichia coli
    Bacillus cereus
    Clostridium perfringens
Neoplastic
    Tumor elaboration of peptides, serotonin, prostaglandins
    Villous adenoma in distal colon (non–hormone mediated)
Excess laxative use

Osmotic Diarrhea

Disaccharidase (lactase) deficiencies
Lactulose therapy (for hepatic encephalopathy, constipation)
Prescribed gut lavage for diagnostic procedures
Antacids ($MgSO_4$ and other magnesium salts)

Exudative Diseases

Infectious: bacterial damage to mucosal epithelium
    Shigella
    Salmonella
    Campylobacter
    Entamoeba histolytica
Idiopathic inflammatory bowel disease
Typhlitis (neutropenic colitis in the immunosuppressed)

Malabsorption

Defective intraluminal digestion
Primary mucosal cell abnormalities
Reduced small intestinal surface area
Lymphatic obstruction
Infectious: impaired mucosal cell absorption
    Giardia lamblia

Deranged Motility

Decreased intestinal transit time
    Surgical reduction of gut length
    Neural dysfunction, including irritable bowel syndrome
    Hyperthyroidism
    Diabetic neuropathy
    Carcinoid syndrome
Decreased motility (increased intestinal transit time)
    Small intestinal diverticula
    Surgical creation of a blind intestinal loop
    Bacterial overgrowth in the small intestine

- Attack rates in industrialized nations are one to two illnesses of either vomiting or diarrhea *per person per year;* 40% of U.S. population is affected per year.
- Parasitic and protozoal disease affect more than *one half of the world's population* on a chronic or recurrent basis.

Viral Gastroenterocolitis (p. 806)

Major viral infections include the following:

- *Rotavirus (group A)*: 70-nm dsDNA virus, person-to-person transmission via food and water, affects 6- to 24-month-old infants. Worldwide, 140 million cases and 1 million deaths occur per year. Minimal infective inoculum is 10 particles. Outbreaks are characteristic.
- *Enteric adenoviruses*: 80-nm dsDNA virus, person-to-person transmission, children younger than 2 years.
- *Astroviruses*: ssRNA viruses affecting children; person-to-person transmission via water, cold foods, and raw shellfish.
- *Small round structured viruses*, of which *Norwalk virus* is the prototype, classified in the family *Caliciviridae*: 27-nm ssRNA viruses; person-to-person transmission via cold food, water, and raw shellfish; affects school-age children to adults. Outbreaks are common after exposure to a common food source.

Morphology. The small intestine exhibits modestly shortened villi, lamina propria inflammation, and damage to surface cells.

Clinical Findings. Incubation periods range from hours to several days; acute illness occurs from 1 to 7 or more days. In addition to diarrhea, anorexia, headache, and fever may develop.

Bacterial Enterocolitis (p. 807)

Mechanisms of bacterial illness are as follows:

- *Ingestion of preformed toxin* in contaminated food (food poisoning): *Staphylococcus aureus, Vibrios, Clostridium perfringens.* Botulism is neurotoxic, not diarrheogenic.
- *Infection by toxigenic organisms*, which proliferate in gut lumen and elaborate an enterotoxin.
- *Infection by enteroinvasive organisms*, which proliferate, invade, and destroy mucosal epithelial cells.

The key bacterial properties by which disease can be produced are:

- *Bacterial adhesion and replication*: To produce disease, ingested organisms must adhere to the mucosal epithelial cells; otherwise, they are swept away. Adherence depends on plasmid-encoded adhesins; proteins are expressed on the bacterial surface.
- *Bacterial enterotoxins*: These are polypeptides that cause diarrhea. Two mechanisms:

  1. *Secretagogues* (e.g., *cholera toxin* from *Vibrio cholerae*), which stimulate fluid secretion by activation of endogenous secretion systems
  2. *Cytotoxins* (e.g., *Shiga Toxin*), which cause direct tissue damage through epithelial cell necrosis
  E. coli produce both forms of toxins.

- *Bacterial invasion*: Microbe-stimulated endocytosis permits intracellular proliferation, cell lysis, cell-to-cell spread, and spread to circulation. This is typical of enteroinvasive *E. coli, Shigella, Salmonella*, and *Yersinia enterocolitica.*

Morphology. Morphologic manifestations are extremely variable. Nonspecific features include damage to surface epithelium, increased mitotic rate, lamina propria hyperemia and edema, and neutrophilic infiltration of lamina propria and epithelium.

- *Salmonella*: Ileum and colon with Peyer patch involvement, *S. typhimurium* causes *typhoid fever* (bacteremia and dissemination to biliary tree, joints, bones, and meninges).
- *Shigella*: Colonic inflammation, erosion, and exudate.
- *Campylobacter jejuni* and other species: Small intestine, appendix, colon, ulcers, inflammation, and exudate.
- *Y. enterocolitica* and *Y. pseudotuberculosis*: Ileum Peyer patches, appendix, colon, and mesenteric lymph nodes with necrotizing granulomas and systemic spread.
- *V. cholerae*: Essentially normal small intestine.
- *Clostridium perfringens*: Usually mild; some strains cause severe necrotizing enterocolitis *(pigbel)*.
- *E. coli*: Enterotoxigenic E. coli* produce cholera-like toxin; *enterohemorrhagic* produce shiga-like toxin; *enteropathogenic* attach and efface epithelium but do not invade; *enteroinvasive* are like shigellosis. All cause traveler's diarrhea.

Clinical Findings. Clinical findings are as follows:

- *Ingestion of preformed toxins*: Explosive diarrhea and abdominal pain within hours.
- *Infection with enteric pathogens*: Incubation period of hours to days, followed by *diarrhea and dehydration or dysentery*, depending on the pathogenic mechanism.
- *Insidious infection*: Yersinial and mycobacterial infection. All enteroinvasive organisms can mimic (or coexist with) acute onset of inflammatory bowel disease.

Necrotizing Enterocolitis (p. 809)

Necrotizing enterocolitis refers to acute, necrotizing inflammation of the small intestine and colon, in low-birth-weight or premature neonates. It is the presumed result of

1. Immaturity of gut immune system
2. Initiation of oral feeding, which initiates release of proinflammatory cytokines by the gut mucosa
3. Gut colonization with bacteria with mucosal exposure to endotoxin
4. Mucosal injury
5. Impaired intestinal blood flow

Rapidly progressive injury results.

Morphology. Mucosal edema, hemorrhage, and necrosis involve the terminal ileum and proximal colon or entire gut.

Clinical Findings. Necrotizing enterocolitis presents as mild gastrointestinal illness or fulminant illness with gangrene, perforation, sepsis, and shock. Massive resection of bowel may be required.

Antibiotic-Associated Colitis—
Pseudomembranous Colitis (p. 809)

Pseudomembranous colitis is an acute colitis characterized by *the formation of an adherent inflammatory membrane (pseudomembrane) overlying sites of mucosal injury*. It is usually caused by toxins of *C. difficile* in the setting of antibiotic therapy.

Morphology. There is plaquelike adhesion of fibrinopurulent-necrotic debris and mucus to damaged colonic mucosa. These pseudomembranes also may form with any severe mucosal injury, such as ischemia, volvulus, or infection.

Clinical Findings. Acute or chronic diarrheal illness occurs with *C. difficile* toxin detectable in stool. Treatment response is prompt.

COLLAGENOUS AND LYMPHOCYTIC COLITIS
(p. 810)

Collagenous and lymphocytic colitis both feature chronic watery diarrhea in middle-aged and older women. *Collagenous colitis* exhibits patches of bandlike collagen under the surface epithelium. *Lymphocytic colitis* exhibits a prominent intraepithelial infiltrate of lymphocytes and is associated with autoimmune diseases and celiac sprue. Both are benign in clinical course.

MISCELLANEOUS INTESTINAL INFLAMMATORY DISORDERS (p. 810)

Parasites and protozoa collectively affect more than one half of the world's population on a chronic or recurrent basis. Key organisms include

1. *Nematodes (roundworms): Strongyloides, Ascaris,* hookworms
2. *Flatworms*: Tapeworms and flukes
3. Protozoa: *Entamoeba histolytica, Giardia lamblia*

In acquired immunodeficiency syndrome (AIDS) patients, microsporidia, cryptosporidia, and *Isospora belli* are frequent causes of diarrheal illness.

- *Transplantation* (bone marrow transplantation especially) may result in graft-versus-host mediated damage to the gut mucosa and may be fatal.
- *Drug-induced intestinal injury* may develop, particularly focal ulceration or mucosal inflammation from NSAID use.
- *Radiation enterocolitis* may be indolent or an inflammatory diarrheal illness.
- *Neutropenic colitis (typhlitis)* arises in neutropenic patients, particularly bone marrow transplant patients.
- *Diversion colitis* is an inflammatory colitis from inadequate nourishment of the colonic mucosa after surgical diversion of the fecal stream (as with an enterostomy).

Malabsorption Syndromes (p. 812)

Malabsorption is characterized by suboptimal absorption of fats, fat-soluble and other vitamins, proteins, carbohydrates, electrolytes, minerals, and water. Malabsorption is the result of disturbed

- *Intraluminal digestion*—secreted enzymes, emulsification
- *Terminal digestion*—enzymes of enterocyte membranes
- *Transepithelial transport* through enterocyte

Table 18–4 classifies malabsorption syndromes. Clinical consequences are as follows:

- *Alimentary tract*: Diarrhea; flatus; pain; weight loss; passage of bulky, frothy, greasy stools. Excessive diarrhea may be life-threatening.

Table 18-4. MAJOR MALABSORPTION SYNDROMES

Defective Intraluminal Digestion

Digestion of fats and proteins
    Pancreatic insufficiency, owing to pancreatitis or cystic fibrosis
    Zollinger-Ellison syndrome, with inactivation of pancreatic enzymes by excess gastric acid secretion
Solubilization of fat, owing to defective bile secretion
    Ileal dysfunction or resection, with decreased bile salt uptake
    Cessation of bile flow from obstruction, hepatic dysfunction
Nutrient preabsorption or modification by bacterial overgrowth

Primary Mucosal Cell Abnormalities

Defective terminal digestion
    Disaccharidase deficiency (lactose intolerance)
    Bacterial overgrowth, with brush border damage
Defective epithelial transport
    Abetalipoproteinemia
    Primary bile acid malabsorption owing to mutations in the ileal bile acid transporter

Reduced Small Intestinal Surface Area

Gluten-sensitive enteropathy (celiac sprue)
Crohn disease

Lymphatic Obstruction

Lymphoma
Tuberculosis and tuberculous lymphadenitis

Infection

Acute infectious enteritis
Parasitic infestation
Tropical sprue
Whipple disease *(Tropheryma whippelii)*

Iatrogenic

Subtotal or total gastrectomy
Short-gut syndrome, after extensive surgical resection
Distal ileal resection or bypass

- *Hematopoietic system*: Anemia, bleeding.
- *Musculoskeletal system*: Osteopenia, tetany.
- *Endocrine system*: Amenorrhea, impotence, infertility, hyperparathyroidism.
- *Skin*: Purpura and petechia, edema, dermatitis.
- *Nervous system*: Peripheral neuropathy.

The most common causes in the United States are celiac sprue, chronic pancreatitis with pancreatic insufficiency, and Crohn disease.

CELIAC SPRUE (p. 813)

Celiac sprue is a chronic disease with a characteristic small intestinal mucosal lesion and impaired nutrient absorption, which improves on withdrawal of wheat gliadins and related grain proteins from the diet. It is also called *gluten-sensitive enteropathy, nontropical sprue,* and *celiac disease*. Celiac sprue is generally a disease of whites, with a prevalence of 1:2000 to 1:3000.

Pathogenesis

A sensitivity to gluten, which contains the gliadin protein component, shared by wheat, oat, barley, and rye, is present.

- *Genetic susceptibility*: Familial clustering; 90 to 95% of patients express the DQw2 (and HLA B8) histocompatibility antigen.
- *Immune-mediated injury*: Serum antibodies to gliadin and potential cross-reactivity to type 12 adenovirus.

Morphology

Diffuse enteritis is present with flattened (atrophic) villi, elongated regenerative crypts, surface epithelial damage with intraepithelial lymphocytes, and robust lamina propria inflammation (lymphocytes, plasma cells, macrophages). Severity decreases in proximal-to-distal intestine and reverts to near-normal upon withdrawal of dietary gluten.

Clinical Findings

- *Symptoms*: Diarrhea, flatulence, weight loss, fatigue. Celiac sprue presents in infants up to mid adult life. Other causes must be excluded; the disease responds to withdrawal of dietary gluten.
- *Complications*: Iron and vitamin deficiencies, 10 to 15% risk of gastrointestinal lymphoma, usually T-cell.

TROPICAL SPRUE (POSTINFECTIOUS SPRUE) (p. 814)

Tropical sprue occurs almost exclusively in people living in or visiting the tropics. The cause is unknown; enterotoxigenic *E. coli* is a possibility. It responds to long-term broad-spectrum antibiotic therapy.

Morphology

Extremely variable intestinal changes are seen, ranging from normal to resembling celiac disease.

- In contrast to celiac disease, the brunt of injury is distal.
- Lamina propria has abundant lymphocytes and more eosinophils than celiac disease.

WHIPPLE DISEASE (p. 814)

Whipple disease is a rare, systemic condition principally involving intestine, central nervous system, and joints. It is attributed to infection by *Tropheryma whippelii*, a gram-positive actinomycete.

Morphology

Small intestinal mucosa is laden with distended macrophages in lamina propria, which contain rod-shaped bacilli by electron microscopy. Similar macrophages are present in lymphatics, lymph nodes, joints, and brain. Inflammation is essentially absent.

Clinical Findings

Clinical findings are as follows:

- Malabsorption occurs with diarrhea, steatorrhea, abdominal cramps, distention, fever, and weight loss; migratory arthritis and heart disease may be presenting problems.

- Usually whites in their thirties to forties are affected; the male-female ratio is 10:1.
- Whipple disease usually responds to antibiotic therapy.

DISACCHARIDASE DEFICIENCY (p. 815)

Disaccharidase deficiency is characterized as follows:

- An apical membrane enzyme of surface absorptive cells.
- With deficiency, lactose remains in lumen and exerts an osmotic pull, leading to diarrhea and malabsorption.
- Rare congenital form: explosive, frothy stools; abdominal distention in infant exposed to milk or milk products.
- Acquired form: common among North American blacks, with milder symptoms. Worsens with enteric infections, owing to superimposed mucosal injury.
- No abnormalities of mucosa or mucosal cells.

ABETALIPOPROTEINEMIA (p. 815)

Abetalipoproteinemia is characterized as follows:

- Familial, autosomal recessive inheritance.
- Inability to synthesize apoproteins required for lipoprotein export from mucosal cells; triglycerides stored in the cells create lipid vacuolation.
- Severe hypolipoproteinemia related to depressed levels of chylomicrons, pre-β-lipoproteins (VLDL), and β-lipoproteins (LDL). Defective lipid membranes of erythrocytes create *burr cell* appearance.
- Presents in infancy, with failure to thrive, diarrhea, and steatorrhea.

Idiopathic Inflammatory Bowel Disease
(p. 815)

Idiopathic inflammatory bowel disease refers to *chronic, relapsing inflammatory disorders of obscure origin*:

- *Crohn disease*: Granulomatous disease affecting any portion of gut, most often small intestine and colon
- *Ulcerative colitis*: Colonic disease, no granulomas

Salient differences are listed in Table 18–5.

CAUSE AND PATHOGENESIS (p. 815)

Both diseases remain unexplained (i.e., are *idiopathic*).

- *Genetic*: Familial aggregations, no particular HLA types.
- *Infectious*: No proven pathogen; many agents mimic inflammatory bowel disease.
- *Mucosal structure*: Possible susceptibility factors—increased intestinal permeability, altered muciproteins
- *Abnormal host immunoreactivity*: Postulated abnormal host response to otherwise innocuous antigenic stimuli
- *Inflammation as final common pathway*: Inflammatory bowel disease ultimately results from *activation of inflammatory cells, whose products cause tissue injury.*

Table 18-5. DISTINCTIVE FEATURES OF CROHN DISEASE AND ULCERATIVE COLITIS

Feature	Crohn Disease—SI*	Crohn Disease—C*	Ulcerative Colitis
Macroscopic			
Bowel region	Ileum ± colon	Colon ± ileum	Colon only
Distribution	Skip lesions	Skip lesions	Diffuse
Stricture	Early	Variable	Late/rare
Wall appearance	Thickened	Thin	Thin
Dilation	No	Yes	Yes
Microscopic			
Pseudopolyps	No to slight	Marked	Marked
Ulcers	Deep, linear	Deep, linear	Superficial
Lymphoid reaction	Marked	Marked	Mild
Fibrosis	Marked	Moderate	Mild
Serositis	Marked	Variable	Mild to none
Granulomas	Yes (50%)	Yes (50%)	No
Fistulas or sinuses	Yes	Yes	No
Clinical			
Fat or vitamin malabsorption	Yes	Yes, if ileum	No
Malignant potential	Yes	Yes	Yes
Response to surgery	Poor	Fair	Good

*SI, Crohn disease of the small intestine; C, Crohn disease of the colon. Features are not all present in a single case.

CROHN DISEASE (p. 816)

Crohn disease is characterized by

1. Sharply delimited and typically transmural involvement of the bowel by inflammatory process with mucosal damage
2. The presence of noncaseating granulomas (but not in all cases)
3. Fissuring and fistula formation
4. Systemic manifestations

Epidemiology

Crohn disease has the following epidemiologic features:

- Annual incidence in United States: 3:100,000
- Presents at any age: young childhood to advanced age
- Peak incidence: teens and twenties
- Females more than males, whites more than nonwhites

Morphology

Distribution is as follows:

- Small intestine alone, 40%
- Small intestine and colon, 30%
- Colon, 39%
- Duodenum, stomach, esophagus, mouth, uncommon

Gross findings include the following:

- Granular serosa with adherent *creeping* mesenteric fat
- Rubbery thick intestinal wall with edema, inflammation, fibrosis, muscular hypertrophy, and often stricture

- Mucosal punched-out *aphthous* ulcers and linear ulcers
- Tendency to fistula and sinus tract formation
- *Sharply demarcated involved bowel segments with intervening normal areas (skip lesions)*

Microscopic findings include the following:

- *Mucosal inflammation* with intraepithelial neutrophils and *crypt abscesses,* lamina propria mononuclear inflammation
- *Ulceration*
- *Chronic mucosal damage*—villus blunting, atrophy, metaplasia, architectural disarray
- *Transmural inflammation* with *lymphoid aggregates*
- *Noncaseating granulomas* in about half of cases–may be present throughout the gut, even in uninvolved segments
- *Fibrosis,* muscle and neural hypertrophy, vasculitis; dysplasia may develop

Clinical Findings

Clinical findings include the following:

- Intermittent attacks of diarrhea, fever, abdominal pain, anorexia, weight loss; intervening asymptomatic periods.
- *Complications* from fibrotic strictures; fistulas to adjacent viscera, abdominal and perineal skin, bladder, vagina; malabsorption and malnutrition; loss of albumin (protein-losing enteropathy).
- With extensive terminal ileal involvement: Vitamin B_{12} deficiency with pernicious anemia and malabsorption of bile salts with steatorrhea.
- Extraintestinal manifestations: Migratory polyarthritis, sacroiliitis, ankylosing spondylitis, erythema nodosum, uveitis, cholangitis, amyloidosis, and risk of bowel cancer.

ULCERATIVE COLITIS (p. 818)

Ulcerative colitis is *an ulceroinflammatory disease limited to the colon, affecting only mucosa and submucosa except in the most severe cases.* In contrast to Crohn disease, *ulcerative colitis extends in a continuous fashion proximally from the rectum, and granulomas are absent.*

Epidemiology

Ulcerative colitis has the following epidemiologic features:

- Annual incidence in United States, 4 to 12 per 100,000.
- Presents in young to older adulthood.
- Peak incidence, 20 to 25 years of age.
- Females more than males, whites more than nonwhites.

Morphology

Gross morphologic findings are as follows:

- Involves rectum and extends proximally in retrograde fashion to involve entire colon (pancolitis).
- Distal ileum may show some inflammation.
- A disease of continuity with no *skip* lesions.
- Mucosa may be reddened, granular, or friable with inflammatory *pseudopolyps,* easy bleeding, and extensive ulceration or may be atrophic and flattened.
- Mural thickening and stricture do not occur.

Microscopically, *mucosal inflammation* is similar to Crohn disease with *crypt abscesses, ulceration, chronic mucosal damage and atrophy*. With treated or inactive disease, regions may appear almost normal microscopically.

Epithelial dysplasia may progress to *carcinoma*. The risk increases with extent of colonic involvement and duration of disease.

Clinical Findings

Clinical findings include the following:

- Intermittent attacks of bloody mucoid diarrhea and abdominal pain; rarely presents as explosive illness with severe electrolyte disturbances and toxic megacolon (a massively dilated, nonfunctional colon).
- *Extraintestinal manifestations*: Migratory polyarthritis, sacroiliitis, ankylosing spondylitis, uveitis, cholangitis and primary sclerosing cholangitis, skin lesions.
- *Risk of carcinoma arising from dysplasia*: Highest risk in patients with pancolitis of greater than 10 years' duration; rate of progression is still low in the ulcerative colitis population.

Vascular Disorders (p. 820)

ISCHEMIC BOWEL DISEASE (p. 820)

Predisposing conditions include the following:

- *Arterial thrombosis*: atherosclerosis, vasculitis, dissecting aneurysm, angiography, surgery, hypercoagulable states
- *Arterial embolism*: Cardiac vegetations, angiography, aortic atheroembolism
- *Venous thrombosis*: Hypercoagulable states, cirrhosis, sepsis, surgery and abdominal trauma, neoplasms
- *Nonocclusive ischemia*: Cardiac failure, shock, dehydration, vasoconstrictive drugs
- *Miscellaneous*: Radiation, volvulus, stricture, herniation

Morphology

Morphologic findings are as follows:

- *Transmural infarction*: Sudden and total occlusion of a major vessel, infarction of all bowel layers. Bowel segment is hemorrhagic as a result of blood reflow into damaged area. Bowel appears rubbery and dusky, bacteria produce gangrene, and perforation develops within days.
- *Mural and mucosal infarction*: Incomplete necrosis or necrosis of mucosa only. Mucosa appears hemorrhagic, but serosa may be normal. Distribution is frequently patchy; inflammation depends on duration of injury. Ischemic changes may be due to any cause (occlusive or nonocclusive).
- *Chronic ischemia*: Causes mucosal inflammation, ulceration, fibrosis, and stricture. Ischemia has a segmental patchy distribution.

Transmural infarction is more common in the small bowel (completely dependent on mesenteric blood supply); large bowel has posterior abdominal wall collaterals.

Clinical Findings

Total infarction imparts 50 to 75% death rate. It usually occurs in severely ill patients and features severe abdominal pain and tenderness, bloody diarrhea or gross melena, nausea, vomiting, bloating, and abdominal wall rigidity. With incomplete infarction, there are nonspecific abdominal complaints, easily confused with acute and chronic inflammatory conditions.

ANGIODYSPLASIA (p. 823)

Angiodysplasia refers to tortuous, abnormal dilations of the submucosal veins that extend into the lamina propria, cecum, and ascending colon and tend to bleed. They range from small, focal ectasias to large, dilated, tortuous venous formations.

Pathogenesis

Acquired ectasias are attributed to partial, intermittent occlusion of submucosal veins in the cecum and ascending colon, the site of maximal wall tension because of its greater diameter (Laplace law).

HEMORRHOIDS (p. 823)

Hemorrhoids refer to variceal dilation of anal and perianal submucosal venous plexuses, affecting 5% of the adult population. Hemorrhoids are associated with constipation (straining at stool), venous stasis of pregnancy, and cirrhosis (portal hypertension).

Morphology

Ectasia of the inferior hemorrhoidal plexus below the anorectal line (external hemorrhoids) is seen as well as in superior hemorrhoidal plexus (internal hemorrhoids). Secondary thrombosis (with recanalization), strangulation, or ulceration with fissure formation may develop.

Diverticular Disease (p. 823)

In contrast to congenital Meckel diverticulum (discussed earlier), *acquired diverticula* may occur in esophagus, stomach, small intestine, and colon. Acquired *colonic diverticula (diverticulosis)* are uncommon in patients younger than age 30 but present in 50% of adults older than age 60 in Western populations.

MORPHOLOGY

Multiple flasklike outpouchings 0.5 to 1 cm in diameter are seen, usually in distal colon. They occur alongside taeniae coli and dissect into appendices epiploicae. The thin wall is lined by mucosa and submucosa and an attenuated-to-absent muscularis propria. Muscularis of intervening bowel wall is hypertrophic. *Diverticulitis*—inflammation of diverticulum after obstruction or perforation—is a complication.

PATHOGENESIS

Pathogenesis includes the following mechanisms:

1. *Focal weakness in bowel wall* at sites of penetrating blood vessels (vasa rectae).
2. *Increased intraluminal pressure* resulting from exaggerated

peristaltic contractions, possibly the result of decreased bulk in diet.

CLINICAL FINDINGS

Diverticular disease is usually asymptomatic; it may be associated with cramping, abdominal discomfort, and constipation. Diverticulitis may lead to pericolic abscesses, sinus tracts, and peritonitis.

Intestinal Obstruction (p. 825)

Table 18–6 lists the major causes of intestinal obstruction.

HERNIAS (p. 826)

Weakness or a defect in the wall of the peritoneal cavity permits protrusion of a peritoneal sac, or *hernial sac.* Segments of viscera may become trapped in them *(external herniation)*; stasis and edema lead to *incarceration*; vascular compromise leads to *strangulation.* Sites include

- Inguinal (internal and external) and femoral canals
- Umbilicus
- Surgical scars
- Retroperitoneal

ADHESIONS (p. 826)

Adhesions refer to localized peritoneal inflammation *(peritonitis)* after surgery, infection, endometriosis, or radiation; healing leads to fibrous bridges between viscera. *Complications* include *internal herniation* (within peritoneal cavity), obstruction, and strangulation of viscera. Adhesions may be congenital.

INTUSSUSCEPTION (p. 826)

Intussusception refers to telescoping of one segment of intestine into the immediately distal segment, usually small bowel. In *in-*

Table 18–6. MAJOR CAUSES OF INTESTINAL OBSTRUCTION

Mechanical Obstruction
Adhesions
Hernias, internal or external
Volvulus
Intussusception
Tumors
Inflammatory strictures
Obstructive gallstones, fecaliths, foreign bodies
Congenital strictures, atresias
Congenital bands
Meconium in cystic fibrosis
Imperforate anus
Pseudo-obstruction
Paralytic ileus (e.g., postoperative)
Vascular—bowel infarction
Myopathies and neuropathies (e.g., Hirschsprung disease)

fants and children, intussusception is spontaneous and reversible. In *adults,* point of traction is usually a tumor.

VOLVULUS (p. 826)

A volvulus is complete twisting of a bowel loop about its mesenteric base. It leads to obstruction and infarction. Volvulus occurs most often in small bowel or redundant loops of sigmoid colon.

Tumors of the Small and Large Intestines
(p. 826)

The colon (including the rectum) is the segment of the gastrointestinal tract most affected by tumors (Table 18–7). Benign tumors, primarily epithelial, are present in 25 to 50% of older adults. Tumors are uncommon in the small intestine.

SMALL INTESTINAL NEOPLASMS (p. 826)

The small intestine represents 75% of the length of the gastrointestinal tract, yet contributes only 3 to 6% of tumors (malignant-benign ratio, 1.5:1). *Benign lesions* include leiomyomas, adenomas, lipomas, neuromas, vascular malformations, and hamartomatous lesions. *Adenomas* frequently occur in the region of the ampulla of Vater, especially in patients with polyposis syndromes (discussed later). *Adenocarcinomas* and *carcinoids* exhibit roughly equal incidence and are discussed later.

Table 18–7. TUMORS OF THE SMALL INTESTINES AND COLON

Non-neoplastic (benign) polyps
  Hyperplastic polyps
  Hamartomatous polyps
    Juvenile polyps
    Peutz-Jeghers polyps
  Inflammatory polyps
  Lymphoid polyps
Neoplastic epithelial lesions
  Benign
    *Adenoma**
  Malignant
    *Adenocarcinoma**
    Carcinoid tumor
    Anal zone carcinoma
Mesenchymal lesions
  Gastrointestinal stromal tumors (gradation
    from benign to malignant)
  Other benign lesions
    Lipoma
    Neuroma
    Angioma
  Kaposi sarcoma
Lymphoma

---

*Denotes the benign and malignant counterparts of the same neoplastic process.

Clinical Findings

Adenomas are silent, unless they obstruct the intestinal lumen or common bile duct. Adenocarcinomas typically present with obstruction (cramping pain, nausea, vomiting), weight loss, and bleeding. Spread to mesentery, regional lymph nodes, and liver is as with colonic adenocarcinoma. Five-year survival is 70% with wide en bloc excision.

TUMORS OF THE COLON AND RECTUM
(p. 827)

DEFINITIONS FOR POLYPS

Polyp   A tumorous mass that protrudes into lumen of the gut.

Pedunculated   With stalk.

Sessile   Without stalk.

Non-neoplastic   Polyps resulting from abnormal mucosal maturation, inflammation, or architecture; no malignant potential.

Neoplastic   Polyps arising from proliferative *dysplasia,* termed *adenomas. Adenomas are precursors to carcinoma.*

Non-Neoplastic Polyps (p. 828)

Non-neoplastic polyps represent 90% of epithelial polyps in the colon.

- *Hyperplastic polyp:* Found in more than one half of persons older than 60 years. Nipple-like hemispheric protrusions are usually less than 5 mm in diameter. Polyps are composed of well-formed mature glands and scant lamina propria. These polyps result from delayed shedding of surface epithelial cells.
- *Juvenile polyp:* Focal hamartomatous malformation of small intestine and colon mucosa, usually sporadic. The vast majority occur in children younger than 5 years old, and most are in the rectum. The rare *juvenile polyposis syndrome* exhibits autosomal dominance, numerous polyps, and increased risk of adenomas and adenocarcinoma. Polyps usually are large (1 to 3 cm), rounded, and pedunculated with cystically dilated glands and abundant lamina propria.
- *Peutz-Jeghers polyp:* Hamartomatous mucosal polyps of small intestine and colon, often sporadic. The rare *Peutz-Jeghers syndrome* exhibits autosomal dominance, melanotic pigmentation of mucosal and skin surfaces, and increased risk of carcinomas (pancreas, breast, lung, ovary, uterus). These are large, pedunculated, lobulated polyps with arborizing smooth muscle surrounding normal abundant glands.
- *Other polyps: Lymphoid aggregates* (normal); *inflammatory polyps* in inflammatory bowel disease; smaller isolated hamartomatous polyps *(retention polyps)* found in colon of adults.

Adenomas (p. 829)

Prevalence of adenomas approaches 50% after age 60 and are frequently multiple. *All adenomas arise as the result of epithelial proliferative dysplasia; adenocarcinoma generally arises from adenomas*. Three histologic appearances are characteristic:

1. *Tubular adenoma*: Tubular glands, smooth surface
2. *Villous adenoma*: Villous frondlike projections
3. *Tubulovillous adenoma*: A mixture of the first two

Most tubular adenomas are small and become pedunculated as they enlarge, whereas most villous adenomas are large and remain sessile during growth. *Risk of coexistent malignancy is correlated with three interdependent features*:

1. *Polyp size*
2. *Histologic architecture*
3. *Severity of dysplasia*

Larger villous adenomas are more likely to harbor severe dysplasia or carcinoma. *Adenomas are slow growing; doubling time is approximately 10 years.*

Morphology. Most (90%) adenomas are in the colon; they may also occur in the stomach and small intestine. Adenomas may be single or multiple. *All adenomas exhibit dysplastic epithelium* (tall, hyperchromatic disorderly cells with increased nuclear-cytoplasmic ratio, cigar-shaped nuclei). Dysplastic cells line the entire colonic crypt and mucosal surface continuously. The degree of dysplasia may be mild (nuclei still basally oriented, mucin production maintained) to severe (stratified nuclei over full thickness of epithelium, no mucin production). All adenomas may harbor *intramucosal carcinoma* (overt malignancy confined to mucosa) or *invasive carcinoma* (invasive into submucosa or deeper), regardless of size or histologic type.

Tubular adenomas begin as smooth contoured bumps in the mucosa involving only a few adjacent crypts; with growth, they become bulky neoplasms (up to 4 cm diameter) and protrude into the lumen—traction creates a submucosal stalk lined by normal mucosa. Branching dysplastic glands are embedded in lamina propria. *Villous adenomas* tend to be larger when discovered and may carpet up to 10 cm of colonic mucosa. Finger-like projections are lined by dysplastic epithelium with a lamina propria core. *Tubulovillous adenomas* are typically intermediate in size, with likelihood of having a stalk, and mixture of architecture.

Clinical Findings. Adenomas may be asymptomatic or cause anemia and occult bleeding. In small intestine, adenomas may cause obstruction and intussusception. Rarely, large villous adenomas may hypersecrete copious amounts of mucus rich in protein and potassium. Clinical impact is as follows:

- *Severe dysplasia (high-grade dysplasia, carcinoma in situ)* cannot yet metastasize and is not yet malignant.
- *Intramucosal carcinoma* is still confined to mucosa, where lymphatic channels are mostly absent (in colon); it has little to no metastatic potential.
- *Invasive adenocarcinoma* is a malignant lesion with metastatic potential because it has crossed into submucosa, which contains lymphatics. Nevertheless, *endoscopic removal of a pedunculated malignant polyp is adequate, provided that*

  1. The invasive adenocarcinoma is superficial and does not approach the margin
  2. There is no vascular or lymphatic invasion
  3. It is not poorly differentiated.

- *Invasive adenocarcinoma arising in a sessile polyp cannot be adequately resected by polypectomy*; further surgery is required.

- *The only adequate treatment for any adenoma is resection,* regardless of whether carcinoma is present. Any residual adenomatous tissue is still a premalignant lesion or may yet harbor invasive adenocarcinoma.

Familial Syndromes (p. 831)

Familial adenomatous polyposis is the archetype of *autosomal dominant* polyposis syndromes:

- Innumerable adenomatous polyps in colon (and elsewhere in the gut); risk of progression to adenocarcinoma is 100%.
- Minimum of 100 colon adenomas required for diagnosis.
- Prophylactic colectomy is curative for colonic risk of cancer; adenomas elsewhere create continued problems.
- Average age of onset is teens to twenties. Progression to cancer occurs in 10 to 15 more years without surgery.

Gardner syndrome is a familial adenomatous polyposis variant that also exhibits multiple osteomas (mandible, skull, long bones), epidermal cysts, fibromatosis (desmoid tumors), abnormal dentition, and higher frequency of duodenal and thyroid cancer. Familial adenomatous polyposis and Gardner syndrome are believed to represent variants of the same genetic condition. *Turcot syndrome* is much rarer with alimentary adenomas and central nervous system tumors (gliomas).

Adenoma-Carcinoma Sequence (p. 831)

Evidence for an adenoma-carcinoma progression includes the following:

- *Epidemiology*: Populations at risk are similar.
- *Topology*: Colorectal distributions are similar.
- *Chronology*: Peak incidence years are offset slightly.
- *Histology*: Adenomas commonly harbor adenocarcinoma.
- *Numerology*: Cancer risk is related to number of polyps.
- *Intervention*: Screening programs for adenomas reduce incidence of colorectal carcinoma.

Genetic alterations in adenomas and colon carcinomas are as follows:

- Familial adenomatous polyposis and Gardner syndrome patients exhibit a somatic mutation in the tumor-suppressor *APC gene* (*a*denomatous *p*olyposis *c*oli). Mutations occur in the tissue of sporadic cancers as well.
- Inherited mutations in *DNA mismatch repair genes* occur in a *hereditary nonpolyposis colorectal cancer syndrome*. This leads to faulty DNA *proofreading,* widespread alterations in the genome, and predisposition to cancer. Sporadic cancers can exhibit the same defect.
- *DNA methylation*: Loss of DNA methyl groups occurs early in colonic adenomas.
- *K-ras gene* and other oncogenes are mutated with increasing frequency as adenoma size increases and in carcinomas.
- Allelic loss on 18q is common in colon cancer at the *DCC locus* (*d*eleted in *c*olon *c*ancer). This is a cell adhesion protein.
- Losses at 17p (site of *p53 gene*) are common in cancers.
- *Telomerase* is an enzyme that maintains chromosome telomere length and cell replicative ability; it is expressed in cancers but not in adenomas.

Cumulative alterations in the genome appear to lead to progressive increases in size, level of dysplasia, and invasive potential of neoplastic lesions. No single event or sequence of events is requisite, but a *multihit* genetic mechanism appears to be operative.

Colorectal Carcinoma (p. 833)

Epidemiology. Colonic carcinoma (55,000 deaths per year) is second only to bronchogenic carcinoma in the United States; 98% are adenocarcinomas. Peak incidence occurs at age 60 to 79 years except in young adults with polyposis syndromes. The male-female ratio is the same except in the rectum, where incidence is slightly more common in men. Worldwide distribution is higher in industrialized countries.

Pathogenesis. Most are thought to arise in polypoid adenomas, but, as noted, a *hereditary nonpolyposis colorectal cancer syndrome* also exists. The genetic syndromes described earlier constitute well-characterized risk groups. For sporadic cancer, *diet* may be important; the risk of cancer is associated with

1. Excess energy intake relative to requirements
2. Low vegetable fiber intake
3. High content of refined carbohydrates
4. High intake of red meat
5. Decreased intake of *protective micronutrients* (vitamins A, C, E)

Such diets may promote increased exposure to bile acids and bacterial degradative byproducts. *Causal relationships are unproven.*

Morphology. Distribution is as follows:

- Cecum/ascending colon, 38%
- Transverse colon, 18%
- Descending colon, 8%
- Rectosigmoid, 35%
- Multiple sites at presentation, 1%

Presentation may be *polypoid, fungating masses* (especially in capacious cecum and right colon) or *annular, encircling masses* with *napkin-ring* obstruction (characteristic of distal colorectum). Both forms penetrate bowel wall over years.

Microscopically, presentation is the same regardless of site: tall, columnar cells resembling neoplastic epithelium of adenomas but now invasive as glands or cell clusters into submucosa and muscularis propria; carcinoma also may be poorly differentiated. Tumors incite a *desmoplastic stromal response*: inflammation and fibrosis of mesenchyme. A minority of tumors produce copious mucin. Less commonly, foci of neuroendocrine differentiation, signet-ring features, or squamous differentiation is apparent.

Clinical Findings. Colorectal carcinoma is asymptomatic for years. Fatigue, weakness, iron deficiency anemia, abdominal discomfort, progressive bowel obstruction, and liver enlargement (metastases) eventually occur. *Prognosis is based on extent of invasion at diagnosis.* Five-year survival depends on the depth of penetration and lymph node involvement, and ranges from 100% for lesions limited to the mucosa to 25% for extensively invasive tumors. Surgery is the only hope for cure.

Carcinoid Tumors (p. 835)

Tumors of gut endocrine cells are termed *carcinoid (cancer-like)*. Most arise in the gut, but also in the pancreas, lungs, biliary tree, and liver. Peak incidence is in the fifties. Carcinoid tumors represent one half of small intestine cancers.

- *Appendiceal, rectal carcinoids infrequently metastasize.*
- *Ileal, gastric, and colonic carcinoids are frequently aggressive.*

Because they arise from gut endocrine cells, many elaborate bioactive products (e.g., amines or peptides).

Morphology. Intramural or submucosal masses are seen—small, firm, and yellow-tan. In the appendix and rectum, masses tend to be solitary; elsewhere, there tend to be multiple nodules. Nodules may cause kinking and obstruction of intestine. Metastases tend to be small and dispersed nodules. *Microscopically,* discrete islands, trabeculae, glands, or sheets of monotonous uniform cells with scant, pink, granular cytoplasm and oval, stippled nuclei are seen, separated by a fibrous stroma.

Clinical Findings. Carcinoid tumors are usually asymptomatic; local symptoms occur from obstruction and bleeding. Inconstant secretory products include

- Gastrin (*Zollinger-Ellison syndrome* with peptic ulceration)
- Adrenocorticotropic hormone (Cushing syndrome)
- Insulin (hyperinsulinism)
- Others

Carcinoid syndrome arises from tumor secretion of seretonin and other bioactive amines; it is seen only with hepatic metastases or with carcinoids outside of the gut:

- *Vasomotor disturbances*: Flushing, cyanosis.
- *Intestinal hypermotility*: Diarrhea, cramps, nausea, vomiting.
- *Asthmatic bronchoconstriction*: Cough, wheezing, dyspnea.
- *Hepatomegaly*: Hepatic metastases—required for intestinal tumors if bioactive amines are to reach the systemic circulation.
- *Systemic fibrosis*: Pulmonic and tricuspid valve thickening and stenosis, endocardial fibrosis, retroperitoneal and pelvic fibrosis, collagenous pleural and intimal aortic plaques.
- Diagnosed by documenting excess 5-hydroxyindoleacetic acid in urine; breakdown product of 5-hydroxytryptamine (serotonin).

Appendiceal and rectal carcinoids are almost always innocuous. Five-year survival rate for other carcinoids is 90%; with hepatic metastases, 5-year survival is 50%.

Gastrointestinal Lymphoma (p. 837)

The gut is the most common location of the 40% of lymphomas arising in sites other than lymph nodes. Although they usually arise as sporadic neoplasms (1 to 3% of gut malignancies), *primary gastrointestinal lymphomas occur more frequently in chronic spruelike malabsorption syndromes, natives of Mediterranean region, congenital immunodeficiency states, human immunodeficiency virus (HIV) infection, and after organ transplantation with immunosuppression.*

- *Sporadic lymphoma*: Most common form in Western hemisphere; B-cell lymphomas also may rise from *mucosa-associated lymphoid tissue (MALT)*. Adults are affected. Distribution is as follows:
  - Stomach, 55 to 60%
  - Small intestine, 25 to 30%
  - Colon, 20 to 25%

Origin may be related to chronic mucosal lymphoid activation, as in chronic inflammation of the stomach in the setting of *H. pylori* infection.

- *Sprue-associated lymphoma*: Younger individuals (30 to 40 years of age), after long duration of malabsorptive disorder; usually T-cell lymphoma. Prognosis is poor.
- *Mediterranean lymphoma*: B-cell lymphoma in children and young adults of Mediterranean ancestry; background of chronic diffuse mucosal plasmacytosis. This is also called *immunoproliferative small intestinal disease*. Prognosis is poor.

Morphology. *Early lesions* are plaquelike expansions of mucosa and submucosa. *Advanced lesions* are full-thickness mural lesions or polypoid, fungating masses protruding into lumen. *Microscopically,* atypical lymphocytes infiltrate mucosa and wall, replacing normal structures. Extreme numbers of lymphocytes may populate the epithelium *(lymphoepithelial lesion).* B-cell lesions (95%) may be low or high grade; T-cell lesions are all high grade.

Clinical Findings. Sporadic lymphomas are amenable to surgical resection and are chemoresponsive. Outcome depends on size, grade, and invasiveness of tumor at time of resection. Lymphomas associated with *H. pylori* infection may be treatable by eradication of *H. pylori*.

Mesenchymal Tumors (p. 838)

Mesenchymal tumors are classified as follows:

- *Lipomas*: Generally submucosal, in small intestine and colon, most common mesenchymal tumor of gut.
- *Gastrointestinal stromal tumors*: Spindle-cell lesions generally of smooth muscle phenotype; may also exhibit neural features. Benign and malignant forms (e.g., leiomyoma, leiomyosarcoma) occur.
- *Kaposi sarcoma*: Visceral involvement common.

Clinical Findings. Most mesenchymal tumors are asymptomatic. Larger lesions may cause mucosal ulceration with bleeding (especially in stomach), obstruction, or intussusception.

APPENDIX (p. 838)
Acute Appendicitis (p. 839)

The most common acute abdominal condition requiring surgery is acute appendicitis. Differential diagnosis includes virtually every acute process that can occur in the abdomen and some of the thorax.

PATHOGENESIS

Obstruction of the lumen (fecalith, calculus, tumor, worms [*Oxyuriasis vermicularis*]) predisposes to buildup of intraluminal pressure, ischemic injury (exacerbated by edema and exudate), and bacterial invasion.

MORPHOLOGY

Morphologic findings are as follows:

- *Early acute appendicitis*: Scant neutrophil exudations throughout the mucosa, submucosa, and muscularis; congestion of subserosal vessels; perivascular neutrophil emigration. Serosa is dull, granular, and red.

■ *Advanced acute appendicitis (acute suppurative appendicitis)*: More severe neutrophilic infiltration; fibrinopurulent serosal exudate; luminal abscess formation with ulceration and suppurative necrosis. Further worsening leads to gangrenous necrosis *(acute gangrenous appendicitis)*, followed by *rupture*.

CLINICAL FINDINGS

Acute appendicitis is mainly a disease of adolescents and young adults but can occur in any age group. *Classic symptoms* are periumbilical pain, then localizing to right lower quadrant; nausea or vomiting; abdominal tenderness; mild fever; and leukocytosis greater than 15,000 cell/mm^3. Symptoms are only variably present or are deceptively absent in very young and elderly patients. Surgically removed appendices may be histologically normal; a false-positive clinical diagnosis rate of 20 to 25% is believed to outweigh the 2% mortality of untreated appendiceal perforation.

■ *Complications*: Perforation, pyelophlebitis and thrombosis of portal venous drainage, liver abscess, bacteremia
■ *Mimics*: Enterocolitis, mesenteric lymphadenitis secondary to enterocolitis, systemic viral infection, acute salpingitis, ectopic pregnancy, mittelschmerz, cystic fibrosis, Meckel diverticulitis

Tumors of the Appendix: Mucocele and Pseudomyxoma Peritonei (p. 840)

Tumors of the appendix are classified as follows:

■ *Mucocele*: Dilation of appendiceal lumen by mucinous secretions. Mucocele is caused by *mucosal hyperplasia*, with non-neoplastic elongated columnar mucous cells producing copious amounts of mucin.
■ *Mucinous cystadenoma*: Neoplastic mucin-producing columnar epithelium. Mechanical distention may lead to appendiceal rupture and spillage of mucin and neoplastic cells into the abdomen; this does not constitute malignant dissemination but rather local rupture.
■ *Mucinous cystadenocarcinoma*: Indistinguishable from cystadenomas except for presence of *invasion of appendiceal wall by now-malignant neoplastic cells and spread beyond appendix as peritoneal implants*. The peritoneal cavity becomes distended with tenacious, semisolid, mucin-containing anaplastic adenocarcinoma cells—*pseudomyxoma peritonei*.

Intraperitoneal dissemination of appendiceal mucinous cystadenocarcinoma progressively fills the abdominal cavity with tumor and mucus and is ultimately fatal.

PERITONEUM (p. 841)
Inflammation (p. 841)

Sterile peritonitis may result from spillage of bile or pancreatic enzymes. *Surgical procedures* may incite foreign body reaction, followed by the development of adhesions. *Endometriosis* (ectopic implants of endometrial tissue) may introduce irritant blood into the peritoneal cavity.

PERITONEAL INFECTION (p. 841)

Bacterial infection may result from appendicitis, ruptured peptic ulcer, cholecystitis, diverticulitis, bowel strangulation, acute salpingitis, abdominal trauma, peritoneal dialysis, or perforated inflammatory conditions of intestines. Spontaneous bacterial peritonitis can develop in the setting of ascites, seen in children with nephrotic syndrome and adult cirrhotic patients.

Morphology

There is dull, gray transformation of normally glistening peritoneal membranes, followed by development of exudate and outright suppuration. Localized abscesses may develop (subhepatic, subdiaphragmatic). Inflammation tends to remain superficial. *Tuberculous peritonitis* produces a plastic exudate with myriad minute granulomas.

Clinical Findings

Infection may heal spontaneously or with therapy. Residual, walled off abscesses may persist, serving as foci for new infection. Exudate may organize, leaving fibrous adhesions.

SCLEROSING RETROPERITONITIS (p. 841)

Sclerosing retroperitonitis refers to dense fibromatous overgrowth of retroperitoneal tissues. Fibrous overgrowth is infiltrative, but accompanying infiltrate of lymphocytes, plasma cells, and neutrophils suggests inflammatory rather than neoplastic disease. Overgrowth may encroach on ureters (leading to hydronephrosis) or bowel segments. Although usually sporadic, sclerosing retroperitonitis is seen in settings of methysergide use (for migraine headaches) and fibrosing disorders (mediastinal fibrosis, sclerosing cholangitis, Riedel fibrosing thyroiditis).

MESENTERIC CYSTS (p. 842)

Mesenteric cysts are cystic masses arising from

- Sequestered lymphatic channels
- Pinched-off enteric diverticula of developing foregut or hindgut
- Cysts of developing urogenital origin
- Cysts from walled-off infections or pancreatic pseudocysts
- Cysts of malignant origin from other sites

TUMORS (p. 842)

Tumors may be primary or secondary.

- *Primary*: Rare mesothelioma (similar to that of pleura and pericardium)
- *Secondary*: Common—any form of advanced cancer extending into peritoneum; tendency to diffuse seeding of peritoneal surfaces.

Diseases of the Liver, Biliary System, and Pancreas

LIVER (p. 846)

General Morphologic and Functional Patterns of Hepatic Injury (p. 847)

The liver is vulnerable to metabolic, toxic, microbial, circulatory, and neoplastic insults. The enormous functional reserve masks the clinical impact of early liver damage. Hepatic injury can take several forms:

- *Inflammation (hepatitis)*: Influx of acute or chronic inflammatory cells. Granulomas may be incited by foreign bodies, organisms, or drugs. Abscesses may occur.
- *Degeneration*: Swelling and edema of hepatocytes. Accumulation of specific material may occur, as with retained bile pigments, iron, copper, or viral particles.
- *Necrosis*: May be caused by virtually any significant insult to the liver: coagulative necrosis (ischemia), *apoptosis* (Councilman bodies) from toxic or immunologic causes, ballooning degeneration (lytic necrosis) from almost any form of injury. Lesions may be focal (scattered through the parenchyma), zonal, submassive, or massive.
- *Regeneration*: Occurs in all but the most fulminant diseases. Hepatocyte proliferation may produce thickened hepatocyte cords or swirls of immature tubular structures.
- *Fibrosis*: Develops in response to inflammation or direct toxic insult. Continuing fibrosis subdivides the liver into nodules of regenerating hepatocytes surrounded by scar tissue, termed *cirrhosis*.

Jaundice and Cholestasis (p. 848)

Yellow discoloration of the skin and sclerae (*jaundice, icterus*) is due to systemic retention of bilirubin. *Cholestasis* is retention of bilirubin and other biliary solutes (e.g., bile salts) and cholesterol.

Jaundice occurs when bilirubin production exceeds hepatic

clearance capacity, via several mechanisms. Unconjugated hyperbilirubinemia occurs from:

- *Bilirubin overproduction*: As from excessive hemolysis of red blood cells, resorption of major hemorrhages, and ineffective erythropoiesis in the bone marrow.
- *Reduced hepatic uptake of bilirubin* formed peripherally: Gilbert syndrome, some drugs (rifampin).
- *Impaired hepatic conjugation of bilirubin*: Transient deficiency of bilirubin uridine diphosphate–glucuronosyltransferase (UGT) in newborns (*neonatal jaundice*) or may be genetic:
  - *Crigler-Najjar syndrome type I* (autosomal recessive): Total absence of bilirubin UGT; fatal.
  - *Crigler-Najjar syndrome type II* (autosomal dominant): Less severe reduction in hepatic bilirubin UGT levels; nonfatal.

Gilbert syndrome is a heterogeneous inherited condition affecting 6% of the population with mild, fluctuating unconjugated hyperbilirubinemia. Mutations in the UGT gene have been reported (missense, or two extra bases—TA—in the 5′ TATAA promoter region of the gene). Gilbert syndrome is usually detected during intercurrent illness or fasting. There are no clinical consequences of this condition.

Conjugated hyperbilirubinemia occurs when greater than 50% of serum bilirubin is conjugated. It is typically associated with cholestasis. Two inherited conditions are as follows:

- *Dubin-Johnson syndrome* (autosomal recessive): Defective canalicular secretion of bilirubin conjugates because the transport protein for bilirubin glucuronides in the canalicular plasma membrane is genetically absent. The liver is brown, with accumulation of pigment granules in hepatocytes (polymers of epinephrine metabolites). Most patients are asymptomatic but jaundiced; life expectancy is normal.
- *Rotor syndrome* (autosomal recessive): Ill-characterized asymptomatic conjugated hyperbilirubinemia.

Cholestasis may result from hepatocellular dysfunction or biliary obstruction. Symptoms include jaundice, *pruritus* from retention of bile acids, or *xanthomas* (skin accumulations of cholesterol). A characteristic laboratory finding is elevated serum alkaline phosphatase because this enzyme is present in bile duct epithelium and in the canalicular membrane of hepatocytes.

MORPHOLOGY

Cholestasis is marked by the following:

- Bile pigment accumulates within the hepatic parenchyma, leading to dilated bile canaliculi and degeneration of hepatocytes.
- With biliary obstruction, portal tracts exhibit distended and proliferating bile ducts, edema, and periductular neutrophils.
- Prolonged obstruction leads to *portal tract fibrosis* and eventually cirrhosis. Necrotic parenchymal foci may coalesce to form *bile lakes*.

CLINICAL FEATURES

- *Cholestasis of intrahepatic origin* (hepatocellular dysfunction or intrahepatic bile duct disease) cannot be benefited by surgery, short of liver transplantation in life-threatening cases.
- *Cholestasis resulting from extrahepatic obstruction* may be

amenable to surgical correction; if uncorrected, the liver becomes cirrhotic.

Hepatic Failure and Cirrhosis (p. 852)

Hepatic failure is a severe clinical consequence of liver disease and develops only with loss of more than 80 to 90% of hepatic function. Clinical features are shown in Table 19–1. Often, patients with marginal hepatic function are tipped toward decompensation by intercurrent disease, which places a greater demand on hepatic function: gastrointestinal hemorrhage, systemic infection, electrolyte disturbances, severe physiologic stress. Few survive with supportive measures; hepatic transplantation may enable survival. Overall mortality is 70 to 95%. Conditions leading to hepatic failure include the following:

- *Massive hepatic necrosis*: As a result of fulminant viral hepatitis or drugs and chemicals (e.g., acetaminophen, halothane, mushroom poisoning).
- *Chronic liver disease*: Relentless chronic hepatitis ending in cirrhosis, including inherited metabolic disorders.
- *Hepatic dysfunction without overt necrosis*: As from tetracycline toxicity or acute fatty liver of pregnancy.

CLINICAL FEATURES

The *clinical signs* include jaundice; hypoalbuminemia; hyperammonemia; fetor hepaticus (a peculiar body odor related to mercaptan formation); and hyperestrogenemia with palmar erythema, spider angiomas of the skin, hypogonadism, and gynecomastia. *Complications* include coagulopathy as a result of inadequate hepatic synthesis of clotting factors, multiple organ failure, hepatic encephalopathy, and hepatorenal syndrome.

HEPATIC ENCEPHALOPATHY (p. 853)

Hepatic encephalopathy is a life-threatening disorder of central nervous system and neuromuscular transmission, accompanied by only minor morphologic changes in brain (e.g., edema, astrocytic

---

Table 19–1.   MAJOR CLINICAL FEATURES OF HEPATIC FAILURE

Jaundice and cholestasis
Hypoalbuminemia
Hypoglycemia
Coagulopathy
Disseminated intravascular coagulation
Hyperammonemia
Fetor hepaticus
Increased serum levels of hepatic enzymes
    Lactate dehydrogenase, alanine, and serine
        aminotransferases
Gynecomastia, testicular atrophy, palmar erythema, spider
    angiomas of skin
Hepatic encephalopathy
Hepatorenal syndrome
Coma

reaction). Pathogenesis is related to severe loss of hepatocellular function and blood shunting around the liver, leading to exposure of the brain to an altered metabolic milieu, of which excess ammonia levels appear to be important. Clinical features include

- Disturbances in consciousness (e.g., behavioral abnormalities, confusion, stupor, coma, death)
- Electroencephalogram changes
- Limb rigidity and hyperreflexia
- Seizures
- Asterixis (a flapping tremor of outstretched hands)

HEPATORENAL SYNDROME (p. 853)

The appearance of renal failure in patients with severe liver disease, in whom there are no intrinsic renal disturbances, also is life-threatening. Kidney function promptly improves if hepatic failure is reversed. Pathophysiology appears to consist of decreased renal perfusion pressure, followed by renal vasoconstriction. Because the renal ability to concentrate urine is retained, oliguria with a hyperosmolar urine devoid of proteins and surprisingly *low in sodium* is characteristic.

CIRRHOSIS (p. 853)

Cirrhosis is among the top 10 leading causes of death in the Western world. It is defined by three characteristics:

1. *Fibrosis*—delicate bands or broad septa
2. *Nodules* created by regeneration of hepatocytes
3. *Disruption of parenchymal architecture of the entire liver*

The fibrosis is generally irreversible and is accompanied by reorganization of the vascular architecture, with formation of abnormal interconnections between inflow and outflow.

Classification is best according to cause. Once cirrhosis has developed, it is often impossible to establish an etiologic diagnosis. The major causes in Western nations are

Alcoholic liver disease	60–70%
Viral hepatitis	10%
Biliary diseases	5–10%
Primary hemochromatosis	5%
Wilson disease	rare
α_1-antitrypsin (α_1-AT) deficiency	rare
Cryptogenic cirrhosis	10–15%

Pathogenesis

The central pathogenetic process is progressive fibrosis. Interstitial collagen (types I and III) is normally in portal tracts and around central veins; occasional bundles are in the space of Disse. A delicate reticulin (collagen type IV) is in the space of Disse. In cirrhosis, types I and III collagen are deposited in all portions of the lobule, and sinusoidal endothelial cells lose fenestrations (*capillarization* of sinusoids). The major source of excess collagen is the perisinusoidal stellate cell (Ito cell). Normally a vitamin A fat-storage cell, Ito cells may become activated and transform into myofibroblast-like cells. Collagen synthesis is stimulated by

- Chronic inflammatory conditions, with cytokine generation
- Release of cytokines by other stimulated cells (Kupffer cells, endothelial cells, hepatocytes, bile duct epithelial cells)

- Disruption of the normal extracellular matrix
- Direct stimulation of stellate cells by toxins

Clinical Features

Cirrhosis may be clinically silent but ultimately leads to anorexia, weight loss, weakness, osteoporosis, and debilitation. Ultimate causes of death are

1. Hepatic failure
2. Complications of portal hypertension
3. Hepatocellular carcinoma

PORTAL HYPERTENSION (p. 855)

Increased resistance to portal blood flow develops from the following conditions:

- *Prehepatic*: Obstructive thrombosis and narrowing of the portal vein or massive splenomegaly with shunting of blood into the splanchnic circulation.
- *Intrahepatic*: Cirrhosis, schistosomiasis, veno-occlusive disease, massive fatty change, diffuse fibrosing granulomatous disease, or nodular regenerative hyperplasia.
- *Posthepatic*: Severe right-sided heart failure, constrictive pericarditis, or hepatic vein outflow obstruction (Budd-Chiari syndrome).

Major clinical consequences of portal hypertension are

- Ascites, especially in cirrhosis
- Formation of portosystemic venous shunts
- Congestive splenomegaly
- Hepatic encephalopathy

Ascites (p. 855)

Ascites is defined as the collection of excess serous fluid in the peritoneal cavity. Pathogenesis involves

- Hepatic sinusoidal hypertension
- Percolation of hepatic lymph into the peritoneal cavity
- Intestinal fluid leakage into the peritoneal cavity
- Renal retention of sodium and water

Portosystemic Shunts (p. 855)

Portosystemic shunts develop because the principal sites for portal-systemic venous bypasses are the following:

- Cardioesophageal junction *(esophagogastric varices)*. These rupture and bleed to cause massive hematemesis and death in one half of cirrhotic patients.
- Rectum (hemorrhoids).
- Retroperitoneum.
- Falciform ligament and umbilicus *(caput medusa)*.

Splenomegaly (p. 856)

Splenomegaly is caused by long-standing congestion and may induce hematologic abnormalities attributable to hypersplenism.

Infectious Disorders (p. 856)

VIRAL HEPATITIS (p. 856)

Any blood-borne infection may involve liver, whether systemic or abdominal in origin, including bacterial, fungal, and parasitic infections, which are discussed elsewhere. Systemic viral infections that may involve the liver include infectious mononucleosis (Epstein-Barr virus); cytomegalovirus; herpesvirus; and, rarely, rubella, adenovirus, enterovirus, and yellow fever. *Unless otherwise specified, viral hepatitis refers to infection of the liver caused by a small group of hepatotropic viruses.* All produce similar patterns of clinical and morphologic acute hepatitis but vary in their potential to induce chronic or fulminant disease or the carrier state.

Hepatitis A Virus (p. 856)

Hepatitis A virus (HAV) was originally called *infectious hepatitis.* HAV causes a benign, self-limited disease, incubation period 2 to 6 weeks. It accounts for 20 to 25% of acute hepatitis in the developing world. Spread is by the fecal-oral route. HAV does not cause chronic disease or the carrier state. Fulminant hepatitis is rare (fatality rate <0.1%). The small, nonenveloped, icosahedral capsid is 27 nm in diameter and a member of the single-stranded RNA picornavirus family. Acute infection is marked by anti-HAV immunoglobulin M (IgM) in serum; IgG appears as IgM declines (within a few months) and can persist for years, conferring immunity.

Hepatitis B Virus (p. 857)

Hepatitis B virus (HBV) was originally called *serum hepatitis;* HBV plays an important role in the development of hepatocellular carcinoma. It affects 300 million people worldwide, with 300,000 new cases in the United States each year. The incubation period is 4 to 26 weeks (typically 6 to 8 weeks). HBV can produce

- An asymptomatic carrier state
- Acute hepatitis with possible complete recovery
- Chronic hepatitis, either indolent or progressive
- Progression to cirrhosis in fewer than 1% of cases
- Fulminant hepatitis with massive liver necrosis

HBV is spread mainly by parenteral routes (transfusion, blood products, needle-stick accidents, shared needles among drug addicts, and during parturition) or via body fluids (saliva, semen, and vaginal fluid), hence the risk of sexual transmission.

Molecular Biology. HBV is a member of the *hepadnavirus* family. It is a DNA virus, spherical, 42-nm diameter (*Dane particle*), 3200-nucleotide double-stranded DNA circle. The viral coat contains surface antigen (HBsAg). Nucleocapsid has HBV DNA, DNA polymerase, hepatitis B core antigen (HBcAg), and X protein (necessary for viral replication and a transcriptional transactivator). HBeAg is elaborated in serum during viral replication and consists of HBcAg plus a *precore* region. HBV mutants may lack the ability to form HBeAg.

Pathogenesis. Pathogenesis involves immunologically mediated hepatocyte necrosis by sensitized cytotoxic CD8+ T cells, attributed to cellular expression of viral antigens during the episomal phase of viral replication (*proliferative phase*). With integration of

HBV DNA into the host genome (*integrative phase*), viral replication ceases, infectivity ends, and active liver damage subsides.

Serum Markers. HBsAg appears before symptoms, peaks during overt disease, and declines over months; it is a marker of active infection. HBeAg, HBV DNA, and DNA polymerase appear soon after HBsAg, before onset of acute disease. HBeAg usually declines within weeks; persistence indicates probable progression to chronic disease. IgM anti-HBc is usually the first antibody to appear, followed shortly by anti-HBe; IgG anti-HBc slowly replaces the IgM. Anti-HBs signifies the end of acute disease and persists for years, conferring immunity. In HBV mutants not expressing serum HBeAg, the inability to form anti-HBeAb carries risk of more fulminant disease.

Hepatitis C Virus (p. 860)

In the United States, 170,000 new cases of hepatitis C virus (HCV) occur per year. Transmission is usually parenteral, causing 90 to 95% of all cases of transfusion-associated hepatitis. Sporadic cases account for 40% of cases. There is a high rate of progression to chronic disease and eventual cirrhosis, exceeding 50%, placing patients at significant risk for developing hepatocellular carcinoma. *Persistent infection and chronic hepatitis are the hallmarks of HCV infection.* Primary risk groups are hemophiliacs, intravenous drug abusers, hemodialysis patients, and homosexuals. Sexual transmission is absent to rare. Incubation period is 2 to 26 weeks (mean, 6 to 12 weeks). Hepatocellular damage is immune mediated.

Molecular Biology. HCV is a small, enveloped single-stranded RNA virus of the Flaviviridae virus family, 30 to 60 nm in diameter. A single, approximately 3010–amino acid polypeptide is processed into nucleocapsid protein, envelope protein, and five nonstructural proteins. Genomic variability constitutes a major obstacle to vaccine development.

Serum Markers. HCV RNA is detectable in blood for 1 to 3 weeks during active infection and persists in many patients despite the presence of neutralizing antibodies. Episodic elevations in serum transaminases are seen in chronic disease states. *Elevated titers of anti-HCV IgG after active infection do not confer effective immunity, either against reactivation of endogenous HCV or by infection with a new HCV strain.*

Hepatitis D Virus (p. 861)

Hepatitis D virus (HDV) is a small, defective RNA virus that can replicate and cause infection only when encapsulated by HBsAg. Hence, *HDV infection can develop only when there is concomitant HBV infection*:

- *Acute coinfection* by HDV and HBV: Mild to fulminant hepatitis; chronicity rarely develops.
- *Superinfection* of chronic HBV by HDV: Eruption of acute hepatitis, conversion of mild chronic disease into fulminant disease or into chronic disease terminating in cirrhosis.

HDV is endemic in Africa, the Middle East, Italy, and elsewhere; in the United States, primarily drug addicts and male homosexuals are infected.

Molecular Biology. HDV is composed of a *Dane particle* with HBV envelope; an internal, 24-kD polypeptide (δ *antigen*, HDV Ag); and a 1689-base circular molecule of genomic single-stranded RNA.

Serum Markers. HDV RNA appears in blood and liver just before and in early acute symptomatic infection. IgM anti-HDV indicates recent HDV exposure. Differentiating acute coinfection from superinfection requires correlation with HBV markers.

Hepatitis E Virus (p. 862)

Hepatitis E virus (HEV) is an enterically transmitted, water-borne infection, with endemics in Asia, Indian subcontinent, and elsewhere; spread is by the fecal-oral route. *There is a high mortality rate in pregnant women (20%)*; otherwise, HEV is a self-limiting disease, with an average incubation period of 6 weeks and no chronic disease tendency.

Molecular Biology. HEV is an unenveloped single-stranded RNA calicivirus, 32 to 34 nm in diameter, with 7.6-kb genome. Antigen (HEV Ag) is found in hepatocytes during active infection.

Other Hepatitis Viruses (p. 862)

The epidemiologic event ascribed to a putative *F* has not been repeated. Hepatitis G virus is a nonpathogenic virus, with serologic evidence of exposure in 1 to 2% of blood donors in the United States.

Clinicopathologic Syndromes (p. 864)

Carrier State. A *carrier* is an individual without manifest symptoms who harbors and therefore can transmit an organism. There are two types: those with little or no adverse effects *(healthy carriers)* and those with chronic disease but few or no symptoms.

- HAV and HEV: Do not produce a carrier state.
- HBV: 90 to 95% of infants infected at birth become carriers; 1 to 10% of individuals infected as adults, especially individuals with impaired immunity.
- HCV: Can clearly induce a carrier state, estimated at 0.2 to 0.6% of the general U.S. population.
- HDV: Low risk of post-transfusion HDV infection.

Acute Viral Hepatitis. Acute viral hepatitis is similar for all hepatitis viruses, with a variable incubation period, asymptomatic preicteric phase, symptomatic icteric phase, and convalescence. It has a fulminant course with high mortality in fewer than 1% of cases.

Chronic Viral Hepatitis. *Chronic viral hepatitis refers to symptomatic, biochemical, or serologic evidence of continuing inflammatory hepatic disease for more than 6 months without steady improvement.* Major causes are viral hepatitis, Wilson disease, α_1-AT deficiency, alcohol, drugs, and autoimmunity. *Cause, rather than histology, is the single most important factor in determining the probability of developing progressive chronic hepatitis.* Likelihood of developing chronic hepatitis is as follows:

- HAV: Extremely rare.
- HBV: Greater than 90% in infected neonates; 5% of adults.
- HCV: *Develops in more than 50% of infected patients, of whom half progress to cirrhosis.*
- HDV: Rare in acute HBV/HDV coinfection but is the most frequent outcome of HDV superinfection.
- HEV: Does not produce chronic hepatitis.

Morphology. The carrier state for HBV may exhibit normal liver architecture and hepatocytes. Isolated cells or clusters show a finely granular, eosinophilic cytoplasm *(ground glass)* and stain positive for HBsAg. Tubules and spheres of HBsAg in the cytoplasm are seen by electron microscopy. HCV carriers exhibit chronic hepatitis.

Acute viral hepatitis can be mimicked by drug reactions. The liver is slightly enlarged and more or less green. Necrosis of scattered hepatocytes, clumps, or an entire lobule occurs; necrotic hepatocytes are eosinophilic and rounded-up *(apoptosis, Councilman bodies)* or swollen *(ballooning degeneration)*. Lymphocytes are present; macrophages engulf necrotic hepatocytes. Lobular architecture is disrupted by necrosis *(lobular disarray)*. Connection of portal-to-central tracts *(bridging necrosis)* is a harbinger of more severe disease. Ancillary features include hypertrophy and hyperplasia of Kupffer cells and sinusoidal lining cells, portal tract inflammation (mainly lymphocytes and macrophages), hepatocellular regeneration, and occasional cholestasis.

Chronic hepatitis ranges from exceedingly mild, to severe, to eventual cirrhosis; it may be mimicked by drug reactions. In mild disease, the chronic inflammatory infiltrate is limited to portal tracts. Progressive disease is marked by extension of chronic inflammation from portal tracts into parenchyma with necrosis of hepatocytes *(interface hepatitis)*; linking of portal-to-portal and portal-to-central tracts constitutes *bridging necrosis. Continued loss of hepatocytes results in fibrous septum formation, which, accompanied by regeneration, results in cirrhosis.*

Clinical Features. Viral hepatitis may be a subclinical event, may run a self-limited course, may persist as indolent disease without progression for many years, or may progress to cirrhosis. Symptoms of acute and chronic hepatitis are similar: fatigue, malaise, anorexia, and bouts of jaundice. With chronic hepatitis, symptoms may persist or be intermittent. Associated findings with chronic liver disease are spider angiomas, palmar erythema, mild hepatosplenomegaly, and hepatic tenderness. Laboratory findings include persistently or intermittently elevated serum liver enzymes, prolonged prothrombin time, hyperglobulinemia, and hyperbilirubinemia. Major causes of death are cirrhosis with liver failure and hepatic encephalopathy, massive hematemesis from esophageal varices, and hepatocellular carcinoma.

Fulminant Hepatitis (p. 867)

Fulminant hepatic failure is hepatic insufficiency progressing from onset to death (or hepatic transplantation) within 2 to 3 weeks. Subfulminant hepatic failure denotes a course of up to 3 months. Causes are listed in Table 19–2; 50 to 65% of cases are viral hepatitis, much of the remainder (25 to 30%) are from drug or chemical toxicity. Fulminant hepatic failure may present with jaundice, encephalopathy, fetor hepaticus, coagulopathy and bleeding, cardiovascular instability, renal failure, adult respiratory distress syndrome, electrolyte and acid-base disturbances, and sepsis. Mortality is 25 to 90% without transplantation.

Morphology. The entire liver, or just portions, may be involved. Affected areas are soft, muddy-red or bile stained; the liver is shrunken. Entire lobules are destroyed, leaving cellular debris and a collapsed reticulin network; inflammation may be minimal. With massive destruction, regeneration is disorderly, and scar may form, producing a coarsely lobulated pattern of cirrhosis.

Table 19-2. CAUSES OF FULMINANT OR SUBFULMINANT HEPATIC FAILURE

Acute viral hepatitis (50–65%)
  Acute hepatitis A
  Acute hepatitis B
  Acute hepatitis C
  Acute hepatitis D (δ)
    Coinfection
    Superinfection
  Acute hepatitis E
  Acute hepatitis due to infection with herpesvirus
      or other viruses
Acute drug-induced hepatitis
Acute hepatitis due to poisoning
  Amanita phalloides (mushroom)
Other causes
  Ischemic liver cell necrosis
  Obstruction of the hepatic veins
    Budd-Chiari syndrome
    Veno-occlusive disease
  Massive malignant infiltration
  Wilson disease
  Microvesicular steatosis
    Acute fatty liver of pregnancy
    Drug-induced microvesicular steatosis
Autoimmune chronic hepatitis
Hyperthermia (heat-stroke)

Liver Abscesses (p. 867)

Liver abscesses are common in developing countries, from parasitic infections (e.g., amebic, echinococcal, other protozoal, or helminthic organisms). Abscesses are uncommon in developed countries, are usually bacterial or candidal, and occur as a complication of infection elsewhere.

- Sources of infection are intra-abdominal via the portal vein, systemic via arterial supply, biliary tree *(ascending cholangitis)*, direct extension, and penetrating injuries.
- Histologic features are nonspecific, although parasitic fragments may be identifiable in tissue sections.

Abscesses are associated with fever, right upper quadrant pain, tender hepatomegaly, and possibly jaundice. Mortality ranges from 30 to 90%; survival is greatly aided by early recognition.

Autoimmune Hepatitis (p. 868)

Autoimmune hepatitis refers to chronic hepatitis in patients with immunologic abnormalities, which responds dramatically to immunosuppressive therapy. It is marked by female predominance, absence of viral serologic markers, elevated serum IgG levels, and high serum titers of autoantibodies in 80% of cases—antinuclear (ANA), anti–smooth muscle (SMA), and antimitochondrial antibodies and increased frequency of HLA B8 or DRw3. A subset exhibit anti–liver and kidney microsome antibodies (LKM). Disease is associated with other autoimmune diseases, such as rheumatoid arthritis, thyroiditis, Sjögren syndrome, and ulcerative colitis. Morphology is similar to chronic viral hepatitis, with robust portal infiltrates of lymphocytes and plasma cells.

Drug-Induced and Toxin-Induced Liver Disease (p. 868)

Exposure to a toxin or therapeutic agent should be included in the differential diagnosis of any form of liver disease. Injury is caused by direct drug toxicity, hepatic conversion of a xenobiotic to an active toxin, or injury via immune mechanisms. Injury may be immediate or develop over weeks to months. Injury may take the form of *hepatocyte necrosis, cholestasis,* or *insidious onset of liver dysfunction. Drug-induced chronic hepatitis is clinically and histologically indistinguishable from chronic viral hepatitis.* Examples are given in Table 19–3.

Alcoholic Liver Disease (p. 869)

Alcohol abuse constitutes the major form of liver disease in most Western countries. More than 10 million Americans are affected, and 200,000 deaths per year in the United States are related to alcohol abuse (including automobile accidents). There

Table 19–3.   DRUG-INDUCED AND TOXIN-INDUCED HEPATIC INJURY

Hepatocellular Damage

Microvesicular fatty change
  Tetracycline, salicylates, yellow phosphorus
Macrovesicular fatty change
  Ethanol, methotrexate, amiodarone
Centrilobular necrosis
  CCl_4, acetaminophen, halothane, rifampin, bromobenzene
Diffuse or massive necrosis
  Halothane, isoniazid, acetaminophen, α-methyldopa, trinitrotoluene, *Amanita phalloides* (mushroom) toxin
Hepatitis, acute and chronic
  α-Methyldopa, isoniazid, nitrofurantoin, phenytoin, oxyphenisatin
Fibrosis-cirrhosis
  Ethanol, methotrexate, amiodarone, most drugs that cause chronic hepatitis
Granuloma formation
  Sulfonamides, α-methyldopa, quinidine, phenylbutazone, hydralazine, allopurinol
Cholestasis (with or without hepatocellular injury)
  Chlorpromazine, anabolic steroids, erythromycin estolate, oral contraceptives, organic arsenicals

Vascular Disorders

Veno-occlusive disease
  Cytotoxic drugs, pyrrolizidine alkaloids (bush tea)
Hepatic or portal vein thrombosis
  Estrogens (and oral contraceptives), cytotoxic drugs
Peliosis hepatis
  Anabolic steroids, oral contraceptives, danazol

Hyperplasia and Neoplasia

Adenoma
  Oral contraceptives
Hepatocellular carcinoma
  Vinyl chloride, aflatoxin, Thorotrast
Cholangiocarcinoma
  Vinyl chloride, inorganic arsenicals, Thorotrast
Angiosarcoma
  Thorotrast

are three distinctive, albeit overlapping, forms of liver disease, characterized by morphology.

HEPATIC STEATOSIS (FATTY LIVER) (p. 869)

In hepatic steatosis, small *(microvesicular)* lipid droplets accumulate in hepatocytes with even moderate intake of alcohol. With chronic alcohol intake, lipid accumulates in *macrovesicular* droplets, displacing the nucleus. At first centrilobular, it may involve the entire lobule over time. The liver becomes enlarged and is soft and yellow. There is little to no fibrosis at the outset and the condition is reversible, but fibrosis may develop.

ALCOHOLIC HEPATITIS (p. 869)

Alcoholic hepatitis is characterized by *liver cell necrosis* (both in the form of ballooning degeneration and apoptosis), particularly in the centrilobular region; *Mallory body* formation (eosinophilic clumps of intermediate filaments); *neutrophilic reaction* to degenerating hepatocytes; inflammation in portal tracts spilling into lobule; and *fibrosis*—sinusoidal, pericentral, and periportal.

ALCOHOLIC CIRRHOSIS (p. 870)

Alcoholic cirrhosis is the final and irreversible outcome of alcoholic liver disease. The liver is transformed from a fatty, enlarged organ to a brown, shrunken, nonfatty organ. Regenerative nodules may be prominent or buried in dense fibrous scar. End-stage alcoholic cirrhosis resembles post–necrotic cirrhosis.

PATHOGENESIS OF ALCOHOLIC LIVER DISEASE (p. 871)

- *Steatosis* results from shunting of substrates toward lipid biosynthesis, impaired lipoprotein assembly and secretion, and increased peripheral catabolism of fat.
- *Cellular injury* results from the following:
  - *Induction of cytochromes P-450* augments biotransformation of other drugs to toxic metabolites.
  - *Free radicals* generated by the microsomal ethanol oxidizing system react with proteins and membranes.
  - *Acetaldehyde* generated from alcohol induces lipid peroxidation and acetaldehyde-protein adduct formation.
- Alcohol induces an *immunologic attack* on hepatic neoantigens, possibly the result of alterations in hepatic proteins.
- Alcohol is a *caloric food source*, displacing nutrients.
- *Fibrosis* is the result of collagen deposition by perisinusoidal stellate cells, eventuating in cirrhosis. Stimuli include
  - *Kupffer cell activation* with proinflammatory cytokine release
  - Amplification of cytokine stimuli by *platelet-activating factor*, a lipid released by endothelial and Kupffer cells
  - *Influx of neutrophils* into the parenchyma, with release of their noxious substances
- *Deranged hepatic blood flow* is the result of progressive fibrosis and alcohol-induced release of vasoconstrictive *endothelins* from sinusoidal endothelial cells.

CLINICAL COURSE (p. 872)

The clinical course for the three forms of alcoholic liver disease is as follows:

- *Hepatic steatosis*: Asymptomatic or mild elevation of serum bilirubin and alkaline phosphatase; reversible.
- *Alcoholic hepatitis*: Acute onset of mild to fulminant hepatic failure; may be transient or fatal.
- *Alcoholic cirrhosis*: Manifests similar to any other form of cirrhosis; irreversible.

Proximate causes of death are hepatic coma, massive gastrointestinal hemorrhage, intercurrent infection, hepatorenal syndrome, and hepatocellular carcinoma.

Inborn Errors of Metabolism and Pediatric Liver Disease (p. 873)

HEMOCHROMATOSIS (p. 873)

Hemochromatosis is defined as *the excessive accumulation of body iron, most of which is deposited in the parenchymal cells of various organs,* particularly liver and pancreas. *Genetic hemochromatosis (hereditary hemochromatosis)* is a homozygous recessive heritable disorder. *Secondary hemochromatosis* denotes disorders with identifiable sources of excess iron (Table 19–4).

Features of fully developed genetic hemochromatosis include micronodular cirrhosis, diabetes mellitus, skin pigmentation, and arthritis. The most common cause of death is hepatocellular carcinoma. Frequency of the genetic hemochromatosis allele is 6% in white populations of Northern European descent; homozygosity in 0.45% and heterozygosity in 11%.

Pathogenesis

The hemochromatosis gene is on the short arm of chromosome 6, close to the HLA locus. The gene is HLA-H, encoding a novel

---

Table 19–4. CLASSIFICATION OF IRON OVERLOAD

Genetic hemochromatosis
Secondary hemochromatosis
   Parenteral iron overload
      Transfusions
         Long-term hemodialysis
         Aplastic anemia
         Sickle cell disease
         Myelodysplastic syndromes
         Leukemias
      Iron-dextran injections
   Ineffective erythropoiesis with increased erythroid activity
      β-Thalassemia
      Sideroblastic anemia
      Pyruvate kinase deficiency
   Increased oral intake of iron
      African iron overload (Bantu siderosis)
   Congenital atransferrinemia
   Chronic liver disease
      Chronic alcoholic liver disease
      Porphyria cutanea tarda

HLA class I–like molecule that interacts with β_2-microglobulin. The most common mutation is cysteine-to-tyrosine substitution at amino acid 282. The fundamental defect appears to be unregulated intestinal absorption of iron; tissue damage is via direct iron toxicity to innocent bystander host tissues. Mechanisms of toxicity include free radical formation with lipid peroxidation, stimulation of collagen formation, and interactions of iron with DNA. Effects are potentially reversible with treatment.

Morphology

Iron accumulates as ferritin and hemosiderin in parenchymal tissues (liver, pancreas, myocardium, endocrine glands) and in synovial joint linings. Prussian blue reaction (potassium ferrocyanide and hydrochloric acid) highlights tissue hemosiderin. *Biochemical determination of hepatic iron content in unfixed tissue is the standard for quantitating liver iron.* Normal is less than 1000 µg/gm dry weight of liver. Adult patients with genetic hemochromatosis exceed 10,000 µg/gm dry weight.

Clinical Features

The male-female ratio is about 6:1, possibly owing to physiologic iron loss in women (e.g., menstruation, pregnancy). Hemochromatosis presents in twenties or thirties with hepatomegaly, abdominal pain, skin pigmentation, diabetes mellitus, cardiac dysfunction, arthritis, and hypogonadism. Potentially fatal complications occur from cirrhosis (including hepatocellular carcinoma) and cardiac disease. Regular phlebotomy is sufficient treatment. Early diagnosis and treatment can enable a normal life expectancy.

WILSON DISEASE (p. 875)

Wilson disease is an autosomal recessive disorder of copper metabolism, marked by the accumulation of toxic levels of copper in liver, brain, and eye (*hepatolenticular degeneration*).

Pathogenesis

A genetic defect is on chromosome 13, in linkage with esterase D locus; gene is ATP7B, encoding a transmembrane copper-transporting adenosine triphosphatase (ATPase), localizing to the hepatocyte canalicular membrane. More than 30 mutations have been identified, and most affected patients are compound heterozygotes with different mutations. Abnormal allele frequency is 1:200; disease incidence is 1:30,000. Disease mechanism is unclear: normal copper absorption and delivery to liver but diminished export from liver into the circulation. The underlying defect may be related to *defective secretion of copper into bile for elimination from the body.* Proposed mechanisms of tissue injury include poisoning of hepatic enzymes, abnormal binding of copper to serum proteins, and formation of free radicals.

Biochemical diagnosis is favored by *a decrease in serum ceruloplasmin* (a copper-binding serum protein), *increase in hepatic copper content, and increased urinary excretion of copper.* Laboratory findings are highly variable.

Morphology

Liver damage may range from minor to severe, in the form of *fatty change*; *acute* and *chronic hepatitis* resembling viral hepatitis but with Mallory bodies, fatty change, and copper accumulation; *cirrhosis* with features of chronic hepatitis; and *massive liver necrosis* (rare).

Clinical Features

Age at onset and clinical presentation are extremely variable—most often acute or chronic liver disease during childhood, adolescence, or early adulthood. Neuropsychiatric disorders also possible, such as mild behavioral changes, frank psychosis, and Parkinson disease–like syndrome. Keyser-Fleischer rings in the eye (copper accumulation in Descemet's membrane) are diagnostic. Copper chelation may ameliorate problems; liver transplantation may be necessary.

α_1-ANTITRYPSIN DEFICIENCY (p. 875)

α_1-AT deficiency is an autosomal recessive disorder with abnormally low serum levels of this major protease inhibitor *(Pi)*; deficiency leads to pulmonary disease (emphysema) and hepatic disease (cholestasis or cirrhosis).

Pathogenesis

α_1-AT is 394–amino acid serum protease inhibitor synthesized primarily in the liver. The gene is on chromosome 14, with more than 75 gene products. Most common allele is PiM, and genotype is PiMM. Homozygotes for the PiZ allele (genotype PiZZ) have circulating α_1-AT levels 10% of normal. Gene frequency of PiZ in the North American white population is 0.0122, with homozygote frequency of 1:7000.

PiZ exhibits a Glu_{342} to Lys_{342} substitution: the nascent polypeptide misfolds and cannot be secreted normally. Impaired hepatic α_1-AT secretion leads to protein accumulation in hepatocytes (within the endoplasmic reticulum); mechanism of liver damage is unclear. Mechanism of lung damage is inadequate levels of this inhibitor of tissue proteases.

Morphology

Lesions include *neonatal hepatitis* (active inflammation with cholestasis) and *childhood* and *adult cirrhosis*. α_1-AT deficiency is diagnosed by periodic acid–Schiff (PAS)–diastase–resistant cytoplasmic globules in hepatocytes.

Clinical Features

Neonatal hepatitis with cholestatic jaundice occurs in 10 to 20% of newborns with α_1-AT deficiency; later presentation may be acute hepatitis or complications of cirrhosis. Hepatocellular carcinoma develops in 2 to 3% of PiZZ adults. Treatment is liver transplantation. Avoidance of smoking is extremely important in patients with pulmonary disease.

NEONATAL HEPATITIS (p. 876)

Neonatal hepatitis is a nonspecific term for hepatic disorders of many possible causes (Table 19–5) in the neonate involving prolonged conjugated hyperbilirubinemia *(neonatal cholestasis)*; hepatomegaly; and variable degrees of hepatic dysfunction, such as hypoprothrombinemia.

Table 19–5. MAJOR CAUSES OF NEONATAL CHOLESTASIS

Bile duct obstruction	
Extrahepatic biliary atresia	
Neonatal infection	
Cytomegalovirus	
Bacterial sepsis	
Urinary tract infection	
Syphilis	
Toxic	
Drugs	
Parenteral nutrition	
Metabolic diseases	
Amino acid	Tyrosinemia
Lipid	Niemann-Pick disease
Carbohydrate	Galactosemia
Bile acid metabolism	D^4-3-oxosteroid 5β-reductase deficiency
Miscellaneous	α_1-Antitrypsin deficiency
Miscellaneous	Cystic fibrosis
Shock/hypoperfusion	
Indian childhood cirrhosis	
Alagille syndrome (paucity of bile ducts)	
Idiopathic neonatal hepatitis	

Morphology

Hepatocytes show necrosis and lobular disarray, panlobular giant cell transformation (multinucleate hepatocytes), prominent cholestasis, inflammation of portal tracts, Kupffer cell reaction, and extramedullary hematopoiesis. Neonatal hepatitis is to be distinguished from the bile duct proliferation seen in obstructive bile duct disease (biliary atresia). No cause is identified in about 50% of cases.

Intrahepatic Biliary Tract Disease (p. 877)

SECONDARY BILIARY CIRRHOSIS (p. 878)

Most common causes of secondary biliary cirrhosis are

- Obstruction from extrahepatic cholelithiasis (stones)
- Biliary atresia
- Malignancies of biliary tree and head of pancreas
- Strictures from previous surgical procedures

Morphology

Cholestasis may be severe but is reversible. *Periportal fibrosis* eventually leads to *cirrhosis*, which is irreversible. End-stage liver is yellow-green and finely divided by fibrous tissue. Small and large bile ducts are distended and contain inspissated bile; ascending bacterial infection incites neutrophilic infiltration of bile ducts and abscess formation.

PRIMARY BILIARY CIRRHOSIS (p. 878)

Primary biliary cirrhosis is a chronic, progressive cholestatic liver disease characterized by destruction of intrahepatic bile ducts, portal inflammation and scarring, and eventual cirrhosis and liver failure. The presymptomatic phase may span two or more decades. It is primarily a disease of middle-aged women. Onset is insidious, with pruritus and hepatomegaly; jaundice and xanthomas (from retained cholesterol) develop later, eventuating in general hepatic failure after a prolonged clinical course. Liver transplantation is required for end-stage disease.

Laboratory findings include elevated serum alkaline phosphatase and cholesterol and serum antimitochondrial antibodies (especially to E-2 subunit of mitochondrial pyruvate dehydrogenase complex) positive in 90% of patients. *Associated conditions* include Sjögren syndrome (dry eyes and mouth), scleroderma, thyroiditis, rheumatoid arthritis, Raynaud phenomenon, membranous glomerulonephritis, and celiac disease. Primary biliary cirrhosis has an autoimmune pathogenesis.

Morphology

Morphologic findings are best described as follows:

1. *Portal tract lesion*: Destruction of interlobular and septal bile ducts by granulomatous inflammation and chronic inflammatory infiltrate of portal tracts
2. *Progressive lesion*: Global involvement of hepatic portal tracts, secondary obstructive changes with eventual cirrhosis
3. *End-stage*: Indistinguishable from other forms of cirrhosis

PRIMARY SCLEROSING CHOLANGITIS
(p. 879)

Primary sclerosing cholangitis is a chronic, progressive cholestatic liver disease characterized by inflammation, obliterative fibrosis, and segmental dilation of the intrahepatic and extrahepatic bile ducts. It is commonly seen in association with inflammatory bowel disease (70% of cases), particularly chronic ulcerative colitis. It is more common in middle-aged men. Pathogenesis is unknown; autoantibodies are usually absent. Primary sclerosing cholangitis runs its course over many years; end-stage disease requires liver transplantation.

Morphology

Morphologic findings include inflammation and concentric fibrosis around bile ducts, progressive atrophy, and obliteration of the bile duct lumen; the ductal obstructions culminate in biliary cirrhosis (and hepatic failure).

ANOMALIES OF THE BILIARY TREE
(p. 880)

Anomalous architecture of the intrahepatic biliary tree includes the following:

- *Von-Meyenberg complexes*: Small clusters of dilated bile ducts or small cysts within a fibrous stroma; incidental portal tract lesion of probable embryologic origin.
- *Polycystic liver disease*: Few to hundreds of biliary epithelium-lined cystic lesions 0.5 to 4 cm in diameter, seen in association with polycystic kidney disease.
- *Congenital hepatic fibrosis*: Incomplete involution of embryonic ductal structures; liver is subdivided by dense fibrous septa with

embedded irregular biliary structures. Portal hypertension, with esophageal varices, may develop.
■ *Caroli disease*: Segmental dilation of larger ducts of intrahepatic biliary tree; complicated by cholelithiasis, hepatic abscesses, and cholangiocarcinoma.

Circulatory Disorders (p. 881)

■ *Obstruction to inflow of blood*:
  • Extrahepatic: Portal vein thrombosis (as from peritoneal sepsis, pancreatitis), postsurgical compromise of hepatic artery
  • Intrahepatic: Thrombosis with infarction (rare), idiopathic fibrosing obliterative portal vein lesions
■ *Compromise to blood flow within the liver*: Cirrhosis is most important cause. Other causes of sinusoidal occlusion leading to parenchymal necrosis include disseminated intravascular coagulation (e.g., eclampsia), sickle cell disease, and sarcoidosis.
■ *Systemic compromise*: As with systemic hypoperfusion (e.g., shock), leads to necrosis of hepatocytes around the terminal hepatic vein (*centrilobular necrosis*). With superimposed passive congestion, as from right-sided heart failure or constrictive pericarditis, there is hemorrhage as well, producing *centrilobular hemorrhagic necrosis*. Protracted right-sided heart failure leads to chronic passive congestion and eventual fibrosis around the terminal hepatic vein (*cardiac sclerosis*)—this may become so severe as to produce essentially a cirrhotic liver.
■ *Peliosis hepatis*: Primary dilation of hepatic sinusoids associated with exposure to anabolic steroids, rarely oral contraceptives and danazol. Liver is mottled and blotchy with irregular blood-filled lakes. Microscopic lesions consist of irregular blood-filled cystic spaces, with or without a lining endothelium.
■ *Hepatic vein outflow obstruction*: Hepatic vein thrombosis (Budd-Chiari syndrome), veno-occlusive disease.

HEPATIC VEIN THROMBOSIS (BUDD-CHIARI SYNDROME) (p. 883)

Budd-Chiari syndrome develops in thrombotic conditions—polycythemia vera, pregnancy and the postpartum state, oral contraceptive use, paroxysmal nocturnal hemoglobinuria, and intra-abdominal cancers (e.g., hepatocellular carcinoma). Membranous webs of inferior vena cava may give rise to obstruction.

Budd-Chiari syndrome is characterized by hepatomegaly, weight gain, ascites, and abdominal pain. This condition may be acute or more chronic. In acute cases, the liver is swollen and red-purple; parenchyma has profound centrilobular congestion and necrosis. Subacute or chronic cases may develop superimposed fibrosis.

VENO-OCCLUSIVE DISEASE (p. 884)

Veno-occlusive disease was originally described in Jamaican drinkers of pyrrolizidine alkaloid–containing bush tea; it now occurs primarily in the bone marrow transplant population as a toxic complication of drug treatment. Clinical features are the same as those of Budd-Chiari syndrome. Veno-occlusive disease is characterized by patchy obliteration of hepatic vein radicles by varying amounts of endothelial swelling and collagen.

Hepatic Disease Associated With Pregnancy (p. 884)

PREECLAMPSIA AND ECLAMPSIA (p. 884)

Preeclampsia affects 7 to 10% of pregnancies and is defined as hypertension, proteinuria, peripheral edema, coagulation abnormalities, and varying degrees of disseminated intravascular coagulation. When hyperreflexia and convulsions occur, the condition is called *eclampsia*. The *HELLP* syndrome (*h*emolysis, *e*levated *l*iver enzymes, and *l*ow *p*latelets) is common in preeclampsia. Definitive treatment is termination of pregnancy.

Morphology

Gross morphologic findings are small red hemorrhagic patches, with occasional yellow or white patches of infarction. Fibrin deposits in periportal sinusoids, periportal necrosis, and hemorrhage occur. Coalescence of hemorrhagic areas leads to hepatic hematomas and potentially fatal intra-abdominal rupture.

ACUTE FATTY LIVER OF PREGNANCY (p. 884)

Incipient hepatic failure in the third trimester of pregnancy leads to bleeding, nausea and vomiting, jaundice, coma, and potentially death. Diagnosis is based on *demonstration of microvesicular fatty transformation of hepatocytes*. Pathogenesis is unknown but may be related to a heterozygous deficiency in long-chain 3-hydroxy-acyl coenzyme A dehydrogenase in the mother and homozygous deficiency in the fetus (with other allele from the father). Definitive treatment is termination of pregnancy.

INTRAHEPATIC CHOLESTASIS OF PREGNANCY (p. 885)

With intrahepatic cholestasis of pregnancy, onset of pruritus and jaundice is in the third trimester of pregnancy; the pathophysiology is related to estrogenic hormones. The liver shows cholestasis. This condition is generally benign, but pruritus may be severe.

Transplantation (p. 885)

DRUG TOXICITY AFTER BONE MARROW TRANSPLANTATION (p. 885)

Administration of cytotoxic drugs before transplantation leads to hepatic dysfunction in up to one half of patients (Table 19–6); dysfunction is heralded by weight gain, tender hepatomegaly, edema, ascites, hyperbilirubinemia, and a fall in urinary sodium excretion. *Clinical features are indistinguishable from veno-occlusive disease.* Morphologic features are nonspecific (hepatocyte necrosis and cholestasis). Outcome depends on severity of hepatic injury.

GRAFT-VERSUS-HOST DISEASE AND LIVER REJECTION (p. 885)

GVHD is characterized by *direct attack of lymphocytes on epithelial cells of the liver*. Acute GVHD generates a picture

Table 19-6. POTENTIAL HEPATIC COMPLICATIONS OF BONE MARROW AND LIVER TRANSPLANTATION

Bone Marrow Transplantation
Conditions present in the liver before transplantation
  Viral hepatitis
  Malignant involvement
  Drug toxicity
  Opportunistic infection
  Biliary tract disease
Posttransplant conditions (listed in approximate order of early to late
   complications)
  Drug toxicity
   Veno-occlusive disease
  Graft-versus-host disease (acute or chronic)
  Opportunistic infection
  Viral hepatitis (hepatotropic)
  Nodular regenerative hyperplasia
  Toxicity from total parenteral nutrition
  Epstein-Barr virus–induced lymphoproliferative disorders
Liver Transplantation
(listed in approximate order of early to late complications)
  Primary graft nonfunction
  Technical problems (e.g., vascular anastomoses)
  Hyperacute rejection
  Acute rejection
  Drug toxicity
  Opportunistic infections
  Technical problems (e.g., biliary anastomosis)
  Nonspecific cholestasis
  Chronic vascular rejection with bile duct damage
  Hepatic artery thrombosis
  Portal vein thrombosis
  Recurrent disease
  Viral hepatitis (hepatotropic)
  Epstein-Barr virus–induced lymphoproliferative disorders

of hepatitis (parenchymal inflammation and hepatocyte necrosis), vascular lymphocytic inflammation and intimal proliferation *(endothelialitis)*, and *destruction of bile ducts. Chronic GVHD* engenders portal tract inflammation, bile duct destruction, and fibrosis.

Acute rejection of liver allografts exhibits portal tract inflammation and vascular changes typical of all solid-organ transplants. *Chronic rejection* may lead to obliteration of arteries, bile ducts, and eventual loss of the graft.

NONIMMUNOLOGIC DAMAGE TO LIVER GRAFTS (p. 886)

- Hyperacute rejection is rare.
- Preservation injury occurs from oxygen radical damage to a hypoxic organ that has insufficient reserve of oxygen scavengers.
- Technical complications include hepatic artery or portal vein occlusion and bile duct obstruction as from stricture.

Tumors and Tumorous Conditions (p. 886)

Hemangiomas and biliary cysts are common benign lesions.

NODULAR HYPERPLASIAS (p. 886)

Nodular hyperplasias are solitary or multiple benign hepatocellular nodules in the absence of cirrhosis; the putative cause is focal obliteration of the hepatic vasculature, with compensatory hypertrophy of well-vascularized lobules. *Focal nodular hyperplasia* occurs in young to middle-aged adults and is an irregular, unencapsulated tumor containing a central stellate fibrous scar. *Nodular regenerative hyperplasia* is a diffuse nodular transformation of the liver *without fibrosis*, occurring in association with virtually any systemic inflammatory condition; it may pose problems in distinguishing from portal hypertension.

ADENOMAS (p. 887)

Liver cell adenomas are benign neoplasms of hepatocytes up to 30 cm in diameter occurring in younger women, typically taking oral contraceptives. Adenomas may be confused with malignancy, may rupture with massive hemorrhage, and rarely may harbor hepatocellular carcinoma. Adenomas are composed of sheets and cords of hepatocytes, with arteries and veins; *portal tracts with bile ducts are absent*.

MALIGNANT TUMORS (p. 888)

Most tumors involving the liver are metastatic. Most primary liver cancers are hepatocellular carcinomas. Rare variants are the following:

- *Hepatoblastoma*: A tumor of young childhood, exhibiting *epithelial* features of the fetal liver or *mixed* features of epithelial and mesenchymal differentiation
- *Angiosarcoma*: Similar to those occurring elsewhere, associated with exposure to vinyl chloride, arsenic, and Thorotrast (a thyroid contrast agent of the 1950s)

PRIMARY CARCINOMA OF THE LIVER
(p. 888)

Hepatocellular Carcinoma (p. 888)

Hepatocellular carcinoma, constituting 90% of primary liver cancers, arises in the middle to late decades of life; the male-female ratio is 3 to 4:1. A strong causal relationship has been established between hepatotropic viral infection (especially HBV and HCV) and hepatocellular carcinoma.

Epidemiology. Global distribution is closely linked to distribution of HBV infection, with higher incidence in men and black populations in any geographic area. Hepatocellular carcinoma represents 40% of all cancers in high-incidence locales (Africa, Southeast Asia); 2 to 3% of cancers in the United States and Western Europe are hepatocellular carcinoma. Hepatocellular carcinoma is strongly associated with protracted HBV infection, particularly when acquired early in life, presumably after integration of HBV into the hepatocellular genome. Chronic HCV infection is also strongly implicated. Other associated environmental influences are cirrhosis (alcoholism, primary hemochromatosis, tyrosinemia) and environmental and iatrogenic carcinogens (aflatoxin B_1 from *Aspergillus*, Thorotrast). Individuals infected with HBV from birth may develop hepatocellular carcinoma at age 20 to 40; other risk populations develop hepatocellular carcinoma later in life.

Pathogenesis. For HBV-related malignancy, key events appear to be

1. Integration of HBV DNA into host genome at random sites, which induces genomic host instability
2. Possible oncogenic transformation events

The role of HBV X protein as a transactivator is unclear. Fungal *aflatoxins* in contaminated grains act as carcinogens by intercollating into host DNA. Exposure of HBV-infected individuals to aflatoxins in endemic areas of the world appears to be synergistic in promoting hepatocellular carcinoma development. *Universal vaccination against HBV of children in endemic areas may dramatically decrease the incidence of hepatocellular carcinoma.*

Morphology. Gross findings are a unifocal mass, multifocal nodules, or a diffusely infiltrative cancer with massive liver enlargement. Hepatocellular carcinoma more often occurs in cirrhotic livers. Malignant foci are pale pink-yellow or bile-stained; intrahepatic spread and vascular invasion are common.

Lesions may range from well differentiated to highly anaplastic and undifferentiated.

- *Well differentiated*: Hepatocytes arranged in trabecular (sinusoidal) or acinar (tubular) pseudoglandular patterns
- *Poorly differentiated*: Markedly pleomorphic giant cells; small, completely undifferentiated cells; spindle cells; or completely anaplastic cells

Hepatocellular features include formation of bile (by light microscopy) or bile canaliculi (by electron microscopy); cytoplasmic inclusions resembling Mallory bodies; positive staining for α-fetoprotein and α_1-antitrypsin.

Clinical Features. Features include hepatomegaly, right upper quadrant pain, weight loss, or elevated serum levels of α-fetoprotein. Prognosis depends on the resectability of the tumor. In Western countries, survival is dismal; death occurs within 6 months of diagnosis.

Fibrolamellar Variant of Hepatocellular Carcinoma (p. 890)

The fibrolamellar variant of hepatocellular carcinoma arises in the absence of identifiable risk factors or underlying liver disease in children, adolescents, and young adults. This variant is more often resectable; at 5 years, survival is 60%. Usually a single, sometimes encapsulated multinodular mass is present. The mass contains prominent fibrous bands separating trabeculae of large, eosinophilic polygonal hepatocytes. Cytoplasmic hyalin globules and PAS-positive inclusions may be present.

Cholangiocarcinoma (p. 890)

Cholangiocarcinoma arises from elements of the intrahepatic biliary tree. Causal associations include prior treatment with Thorotrast, protracted parasitic infection of the biliary tree with Clonorchis *(Opisthorchis sinensis)* and its close relatives, and Caroli disease; most cases arise without antecedent risk conditions.

As with hepatocellular carcinoma, cholangiocarcinoma may appear as a unifocal large mass, multifocal, or diffusely infiltrative. In contrast to hepatocellular carcinoma, tumor is typically pale (because biliary epithelium does not secrete bilirubin pigment) and firm and is composed of bile ductular elements that may be well or more poorly differentiated, resembling adenocarcinomas elsewhere in the alimentary tract. Mixed variants of *hepatocellular-cholangiocarcinoma* may rarely occur. Clinical outlook is dismal because they are rarely resectable.

METASTATIC TUMORS (p. 891)

The liver and lung are the visceral organs most often involved in the metastatic spread of cancers. Thus, the overwhelming majority of hepatic malignancy is metastatic in origin, most commonly from carcinomas of the breast, lung, and colon. Any cancer in any site of the body may spread to the liver, including those of the blood-forming elements. Typically, multiple implants are present, with massive enlargement of the liver. Metastases that outgrow their blood supply become centrally necrotic. Massive involvement of the liver may be present before hepatic failure develops.

BILIARY SYSTEM (p. 891)

Congenital Anomalies (p. 893)

In the normal anatomy of the biliary tree, the pancreatic duct and common bile duct join to form a common intrapancreatic channel, or the ducts enter the duodenum separately. Abnormal variants of gallbladder are folded fundus *(phrygian cap)*, congenitally *absent*, *duplicated*, *bilobed*, or *aberrant location*.

Disorders of the Gallbladder (p. 893)

CHOLELITHIASIS (GALLSTONES) (p. 893)

Bile enables the hepatic elimination of cholesterol (as free cholesterol and as bile salts), bilirubin, and xenobiotics from the body. Detergent bile salts are necessary for dispersion and hydrolysis of dietary lipid, facilitating intestinal lipid absorption. Cholesterol is solubilized by bile salts and cosecreted lecithin; supersaturation of bile with cholesterol or bilirubin salts predisposes to stone formation. There are two kinds of stones:

1. *Cholesterol* (>50% crystalline cholesterol monohydrate)
2. *Pigmented* (predominantly bilirubin calcium salts)

Prevalence and Risk Factors

Gallstones afflict 10 to 20% of adult populations in developed countries. Patients with cholesterol gallstones exhibit the following risk factors:

- Native Americans, adults in industrialized countries
- Increasing age, with a male-female ratio of 1:2
- Estrogenic influences, clofibrate, obesity, or rapid weight loss
- Gallbladder stasis, as in spinal cord injury or pregnancy
- Hypercholesterolemic syndromes

Patients with pigmented gallstones exhibit the following risk factors:

- Asian more than Western, rural more than urban

- Chronic hemolytic syndromes or biliary tract infection (as with bacteria or parasites)
- Ileal disease (resection or bypass) or cystic fibrosis with pancreatic insufficiency

Pathogenesis

Four conditions are necessary for formation of cholesterol stones:

1. *Bile must be supersaturated with cholesterol.*
2. *Gallbladder hypomotility promotes crystal nucleation.*
3. *Cholesterol nucleation in bile is accelerated.*
4. *Mucus hypersecretion in the gallbladder traps the crystals, permitting their agglomeration into stones.*

Nucleation is promoted by microprecipitates of calcium salts (inorganic or bilirubin salts).

The pathogenesis of pigmented stones is based on the presence in the biliary tree of unconjugated bilirubin and precipitation of calcium bilirubin salts. Infection of the biliary tract with *Escherichia coli, Ascaris lumbricoides,* or the liver fluke *Opisthorchis sinensis* promotes deconjugation of bilirubin glucuronides secreted by the liver. Chronic hemolytic conditions promote formation of unconjugated bilirubin in the biliary tree.

Morphology

Cholesterol stones arise exclusively in the gallbladder and are pale yellow and hard. Single stones are ovoid; multiple stones tend to be faceted. Bilirubin salts may impart black color. *Pigmented stones* are classified as *black* and *brown.* Black pigment stones are found in sterile gallbladders, and brown stones are found in infected intrahepatic or extrahepatic bile ducts. Both are soft and usually multiple; brown stones are greasy. Based on calcium content, cholesterol stones are more often radiolucent, and pigment stones are more often radiopaque.

Clinical Features

Seventy percent to 80% of gallstone patients remain asymptomatic throughout life. *Asymptomatic patients become symptomatic at the rate of 1 to 3% per year, and risk diminishes with time. Symptoms* include spasmodic, *colicky* pain, owing to obstruction of bile ducts by passing stones. Gallbladder obstruction per se generates right upper abdominal pain. *Complications* are gallbladder inflammation *(cholecystitis),* empyema, perforation, fistulas, biliary tree inflammation *(cholangitis),* obstructive cholestasis or pancreatitis, and erosion of a gallstone into adjacent bowel *(gallstone ileus).* Clear mucinous secretions in an obstructed gallbladder distend the gallbladder *(mucocele).*

CHOLECYSTITIS (p. 895)

Acute Cholecystitis (p. 895)

Acute cholecystitis is an acute inflammation of the gallbladder, precipitated 90% of the time by gallstone obstruction of the neck or cystic duct. Cases without gallstone obstruction usually occur in the severely ill patient, in the following conditions: postoperative state, severe trauma, severe burns, multisystem organ failure, sepsis, prolonged hyperalimentation, or postpartum state. For both cases with obstruction and cases without obstruction, *symptoms* are an attack of right upper quadrant or epigastric pain, mild fever, anorexia, tachycardia, diaphoresis, and nausea and vomiting. Jaundice suggests common bile duct obstruction.

Pathogenesis. Acute inflammation in the setting of gallstone obstruction is initiated by chemical irritation of the gallbladder by bile acids, with release of inflammatory mediators (lysolecithin, prostaglandins), gallbladder dysmotility, distention, and ischemia. Bacterial contamination is a later complication. In the severely ill patient, cholecystitis is thought to be the direct result of ischemic compromise of the gallbladder.

Morphology. An enlarged, tense gallbladder is observed, bright red to blotchy green-black with a serosal covering of fibrin. Luminal contents may be turbid or outright purulent.

Clinical Features. Acute cholecystitis may be mild and intermittent or may be a surgical emergency. Self-limited attacks subside over several days; overall mortality is less than 1%. In the severely ill patient, the symptoms may not be evident, and mortality is higher. Complications include

- Bacterial superinfection with cholangitis and sepsis
- Gallbladder perforation or rupture
- Enteric fistula formation
- Aggravation of preexisting illness

Chronic Cholecystitis (p. 897)

Chronic cholecystitis may arise from repeated bouts of symptomatic acute cholecystitis or in the absence of antecedent attacks. Although gallstones are usually present, they may not play a direct role in the initiation of inflammation. Rather, chronic supersaturation of bile with cholesterol permits cholesterol suffusion of the gallbladder wall and initiation of inflammation and gallbladder dysmotility. Patient populations and symptoms are the same as for the acute form.

Morphology. Gallbladder may be contracted (from fibrosis), normal in size, or enlarged (from obstruction). The wall is variably thickened and gray-white. Mucosa is generally preserved but may be atrophied. Cholesterol-laden macrophages in the lamina propria are frequently seen *(cholesterolosis)*. Gallstones are frequent. Inflammation in the mucosa and wall is variable; mucosal outpouchings through the wall *(Rokitansky-Aschoff sinuses)* may be present. Rare findings are mural dystrophic calcification *(porcelain gallbladder)* and a fibrosed, nodular gallbladder with marked histiocytic inflammation *(xanthogranulomatous cholecystitis)*.

Clinical Features. Recurrent attacks of steady or colicky epigastric or right upper quadrant pain occur. Complications include

- Bacterial superinfection
- Gallbladder perforation with peritonitis
- Biliary-enteric fistula
- Aggravation of coexisting medical illnesses

Disorders of the Extrahepatic Bile Ducts
(p. 898)

CHOLEDOCHOLITHIASIS AND ASCENDING CHOLANGITIS (p. 898)

Choledocholithiasis is the presence of stones within the biliary tree, occurring in about 10% of patients with cholelithiasis. In

Western nations, almost all stones are derived from the gallbladder and are cholesterol stones. In Asia, stones are usually primary and pigmented. *Symptoms* include those from obstruction, pancreatitis, cholangitis, hepatic abscess, secondary biliary cirrhosis, and acute calculous cholecystitis.

Ascending cholangitis refers to bacterial infection of the bile ducts; it usually arises in the setting of choledocholithiasis. Uncommon causes include indwelling stents or catheters, tumors, acute pancreatitis, and benign strictures. Infections are usually ascending bacteria (e.g., *E. coli*, *Klebsiella*, other enteroforms), entering the biliary tract through the sphincter of Oddi.

BILIARY ATRESIA (p. 898)

Extrahepatic biliary atresia is complete obstruction of bile flow owing to destruction or absence of all or part of the extrahepatic bile ducts; it occurs in 1:10,000 live births.

Pathogenesis. Biliary tree is intact at birth, with progressive inflammatory destruction after birth. The cause is unknown.

Morphology. Inflammation and fibrosing stricture of both extrahepatic and, with progression of disease, intrahepatic biliary tree are seen. The liver shows florid features of bile duct obstruction:

- Marked bile ductular proliferation
- Portal tract edema
- Fibrosis progressing to cirrhosis within 3 to 6 months

Clinical Features. Clinical features include neonatal cholestasis in an infant of normal birth weight and postnatal weight gain. If untreated, death occurs within 2 years of birth; liver transplantation is curative.

CHOLEDOCHAL CYSTS (p. 899)

Choledochal cysts are congenital dilations of the common bile duct, presenting most often in children before age 10 with nonspecific symptoms of jaundice, recurrent abdominal pain, or both. The cysts predispose to stone formation, stenosis and stricture, pancreatitis, obstructive biliary complications, and bile duct carcinoma in the adult.

Tumors (p. 899)

The primary neoplasms of the gallbladder are epithelial. Adenomas are described in Chapter 18.

CARCINOMA OF THE GALLBLADDER
(p. 899)

Carcinoma of the gallbladder is the fifth most common cancer of the digestive tract, slightly more common in women, most often presenting in patients in their sixties. Gallstones coexist in 60 to 90% of patients in Western nations, but it is unclear whether there is a causal relationship. Chronic gallbladder inflammation (with or without stones) may be a more critical risk factor. Gallstones are less common in Asian populations, where pyogenic and parasitic disease dominate.

Morphology

There are two patterns of growth:

1. *Infiltrating* (diffuse thickening and induration of gallbladder)

2. *Exophytic* (growth into the lumen as an irregular, cauliflower-like mass)

Most are adenocarcinomas, with histologic patterns of papillary; infiltrating; moderate to poorly differentiated to undifferentiated; and, rarely, squamous or adenosquamous, carcinoid, or mesenchymal. *Patterns of spread* include local invasion of liver; extension to cystic duct and portohepatic lymph nodes; and seeding of peritoneum, viscera, and lungs. Tumors are usually unresectable when discovered.

Clinical Features

Symptoms are insidious and indistinguishable from those caused by cholelithiasis. Preoperative diagnosis at a resectable stage is rare. Prognosis rarely is good.

CARCINOMA OF THE EXTRAHEPATIC BILE DUCTS (p. 899)

Carcinoma of the extrahepatic bile ducts refers to distinctly uncommon malignancies of the extrahepatic biliary tree down to the ampulla of Vater. There is an apparent increased risk in patients with choledochal cysts, ulcerative colitis, and chronic biliary infection with *C. sinensis* and *Giardia lamblia*.

Morphology

Most are adenocarcinomas; uncommonly, squamous metaplasia gives rise to squamous cell carcinomas or adenosquamous carcinomas. Carcinoma may take the form of papillary exophytic masses, intraductal nodules, or diffuse infiltrative lesions of the duct walls. Tumors arising at the confluence of the right and left hepatic bile ducts are called *Klatskin tumors*, notable for slow growth, sclerosing behavior, and infrequency of distant metastasis.

Clinical Features

Symptoms are similar to those of cholelithiasis. There is progressive obstruction, which may wax and wane as necrosis of tumor reestablishes ductal lumen. Most have invaded adjacent structures at the time of diagnosis, and the prognosis is only fair.

PANCREAS (p. 902)

Exocrine Pancreas (p. 902)

CONGENITAL ANOMALIES (p. 904)

Congenital anomalies include the following:

- *Agenesis*: Associated with other severe congenital malformations, usually incompatible with life.
- *Hypoplasia; pancreas divisum*: Persistence as dorsal and ventral pancreas.
- *Annular pancreas*: Pancreatic head encircles the duodenum with risk of obstruction; persistence of two separate pancreatic ducts from dorsal and ventral pancreas—predisposes to recurrent pancreatitis.
- *Aberrant (or ectopic) pancreas*: Found in 2% of all routine postmortem examinations. Located in stomach, duodenum, jejunum, Meckel diverticulum, and ileum. Single or multiple firm,

yellow-gray nests measuring several millimeters to 3 to 4 cm in diameter in wall of gut, typically submucosal.

PANCREATITIS (p. 904)

Acute Pancreatitis (p. 904)

Acute pancreatitis is an acute condition typically presenting with abdominal pain, associated with raised levels of pancreatic enzymes (amylase and lipase) in blood or urine. The mild form features interstitial edema and inflammation of the pancreas *(acute interstitial pancreatitis)*. With more severe pancreatitis, tissue necrosis develops *(acute necrotizing pancreatitis)*. The most severe form, *acute hemorrhagic pancreatitis*, exhibits extensive hemorrhage into the parenchyma of the pancreas.

Associated Conditions. About 80% of cases are associated with cholelithiasis and alcoholism (Table 19–7).

Pathogenesis. The pancreas secretes 22 enzymes. Proteases, elastases, and phospholipase are secreted as proenzymes and normally require activation by trypsin in the duodenum. Trypsin itself is activated by duodenal enteropeptidase. Amylases and lipase are secreted in their active form. Features of pancreatitis include *tissue proteolysis, lipolysis, and hemorrhage*, resulting from the destructive effect of pancreatic enzymes released from acinar cells. Locally activated trypsin converts other proenzymes to active enzymes and converts prekallikrein to kallikrein, activating the kinin system and clotting, leading to local inflammation and thrombosis.

Proposed mechanisms for activation of pancreatic enzymes are as follows:

- *Pancreatic duct obstruction*: By gallstones, with impaction in the ampulla of Vater and pancreatic duct obstruction. An en-

Table 19–7.   ETIOLOGIC FACTORS IN ACUTE PANCREATITIS

Metabolic
Alcoholism*
Hyperlipoproteinemia
Hypercalcemia
Drugs (e.g., thiazide diuretics)
Genetic
Mechanical
Gallstones*
Traumatic injury
Iatrogenic injury
Perioperative injury
Endoscopic procedures with dye injection
Vascular
Shock
Atheroembolism
Polyarteritis nodosa
Infectious
Mumps
Coxsackievirus
Mycoplasma pneumoniae

*Most common conditions associated with acute (and chronic) pancreatitis.

zyme-rich interstitial fluid accumulates, and resident tissue leukocytes release proinflammatory cytokines, promoting local inflammation and edema.

- *Primary acinar cell injury*: Damage by viruses (mumps), drugs, trauma, and the ischemia of shock.
- *Defective intracellular transport of proenzymes*: Acinar cell digestive enzymes are misdirected toward lysosomes rather than toward secretion; lysosomal hydrolysis of the proenzymes promotes local release of activated enzymes.

Alcohol is proposed to promote acinar cell injury (possibly by misdirected intracellular transport of proenzymes) and promotes the deposition of inspissated protein plugs within pancreatic ducts, leading to local obstruction and inflammation.

Morphology. The basic pancreatic alterations are as follows:

1. Leakage of the vasculature to cause edema
2. Necrosis of regional fat by lipolytic enzymes
3. An acute inflammatory reaction
4. Proteolytic destruction of the pancreatic substance
5. Destruction of blood vessels with subsequent interstitial hemorrhage

Mild pancreatitis (acute interstitial pancreatitis) features only the first three alterations listed. Acute necrotizing pancreatitis generates gray-white necrosis of the parenchyma and chalky white fat necrosis. Peritoneal fluid is serous, slightly turbid, and brown-tinged with globules of oil. With acute hemorrhagic pancreatitis, the pancreas exhibits a variegated pattern of blue-black hemorrhages and gray-white necrotic softening alternating with sprinkled foci of yellow-white, chalky fat necrosis. Resolution leaves diffuse or focal parenchymal fibrosis, calcification, and irregular ductal dilation.

Clinical Features. Full-blown, acute pancreatitis is a medical emergency with acute abdomen, constant and intense abdominal pain with upper back radiation, peripheral vascular collapse, and shock from explosive activation of the systemic inflammatory response. Death occurs from shock, acute respiratory distress syndrome, or acute renal failure. Laboratory findings include marked elevation of the serum amylase during the first 24 hours, followed within 72 to 96 hours by a rising serum lipase. Glycosuria occurs in 10% of cases. Hypocalcemia may result from precipitation of calcium soaps in the fat necrosis; if persistent, it is a poor prognostic sign. In less severe cases, common sequelae are a sterile *pancreatic abscess* from liquefaction of the tissue and *pancreatic pseudocyst* from aberrant drainage of pancreatic secretions.

Chronic Pancreatitis (p. 907)

Chronic pancreatitis is characterized by repeated bouts of mild to moderate pancreatic inflammation, with continued loss of pancreatic parenchyma and replacement by fibrous tissue. This disease is more debilitating than life-threatening because of progressive loss of pancreatic function. Associated conditions are alcoholism and biliary tract disease. Less commonly, hypercalcemia, hyperlipidemia, pancreas divisum, familial hereditary pancreatitis (autosomal recessive condition featuring an arginine-to-histidine substitution at residue 117 of trypsinogen), and protein-deficient malnutrition occur. Postulated inciting events are as follows:

1. *Ductal obstruction by concretions* (as with alcohol)
2. *Abnormal secretion of proteins*, including decreased acinar

secretion of *lithostatine*, a protein proposed to inhibit intraluminal precipitation of calcium carbonates

3. *Oxidative stress* from alcohol-induced oxygen radical generation

4. *Interstitial fibrosis* initiated by acute pancreatitis.

Morphology. Morphologic findings include irregularly distributed fibrosis, reduced number and size of acini with relative sparing of the islets of Langerhans, and variable obstruction of pancreatic ducts. The pancreas is hard with foci of calcification; fully developed calculi may be present (*chronic calcifying pancreatitis*) in alcoholics. *Chronic obstructive pancreatitis* with impacted ampullary stones is centered around ducts and irregular in its glandular distribution. Pseudocyst formation is common, especially in alcoholics.

Clinical Features. Chronic pancreatitis can be silent, or recurrent attacks of pain may occur at scattered intervals. Attacks are precipitated by alcohol abuse, overeating, and drug use. Late complications include

- Diarrhea (malabsorption)
- Steatorrhea
- Diabetes
- Pseudocyst

TUMORS (p. 909)

Non-Neoplastic Cysts (p. 909)

Congenital Cysts. Congenital cysts are defined as anomalous development of the pancreatic ducts. Cysts frequently coexist with kidney and liver cysts in *congenital polycystic disease*. In *von Hippel–Lindau disease*, pancreatic cysts and angiomas of the central nervous system occur.

Pseudocysts. Pseudocysts are localized collections of fluid representing sequestered pancreatic secretions, almost always arising after bouts of acute or chronic pancreatitis. They do not possess an epithelial lining but instead are lined by fibrosed inflammatory tissue. They are usually unilocular. *Symptoms* include abdominal pain. They may become infected or hemorrhagic.

Neoplasms (p. 909)

Cystic Tumors. Cystic tumors constitute fewer than 5% of pancreatic neoplasms. Tumors are usually located in the body or tail and present as painless, slow-growing masses.

- *Serous microcystic adenoma*: Predominantly in women older than age 65. Tumors are usually solitary, 6 to 10 cm in diameter, well circumscribed, and round. Tumors are made up of numerous tiny cysts; a few larger ones are filled with serous, clear, watery fluid and lined with a bland serous epithelium; sometimes there is a central fibrous core. Prognosis is excellent, with little risk of malignant transformation.
- *Mucinous cystic tumor*: Unilocular or multiloculated cystic neoplasms up to 10 cm in diameter filled with mucinous material and lined by mucin-producing tall columnar cells (except when compressed into a flattened epithelium). Tumors usually in women and may vary from benign (cystadenoma) to borderline to malignant (cystadenocarcinoma), on the basis of epithelial pleomorphism and evidence of invasion and metastasis. Prognosis depends on adequacy of surgical resection.

■ *Solid-cystic papillary cystic tumor*: A round, well-circumscribed tumor with solid and cystic regions; the latter are primarily due to hemorrhage and cystic degeneration. Tumor cells are small and uniform, growing in solid sheets or papillary projections. Tumors are seen in adolescent girls and women younger than age 35; prognosis is usually excellent, although metastases can occur.

Carcinoma of the Pancreas. Carcinoma of the pancreas refers to carcinomas of the exocrine pancreas, almost always arising from ductal epithelial cells.

Epidemiology. Carcinoma of the pancreas accounts for 5% of all cancer deaths in the United States. Incidence rates are higher in smokers than nonsmokers; alcohol consumption imposes a modestly increased risk. Peak incidence is between 60 and 80 years of age, with 28,000 new patients identified each year in the United States. Five-year survival is less than 4%.

Pathogenesis. Although pancreatic cancer may arise in patients with chronic pancreatitis, this is most likely the result of the common risk factors of smoking and alcohol consumption. K-*ras* mutations are observed in greater than 90% of pancreatic cancers, and 60 to 80% exhibit mutations in *p53*. The reasons for this striking pattern of genetic alterations are not yet known.

Morphology. Distribution is as follows:

■ Head, 60%
■ Body, 15%
■ Tail, 5%
■ Diffuse or widely spread, 20%

Tumors may be small and ill defined or large (8 to 10 cm), with extensive local invasion and regional metastasis. *Microscopically*, more or less differentiated glandular patterns (*adenocarcinoma*) arise from ductal epithelium, mucus or non–mucus secreting. Rare histologic variants include

■ *Adenosquamous carcinoma*
■ *Anaplastic carcinoma* with giant cell formation
■ *Acinar cell carcinoma* (arising from acinar cells with abundant eosinophilic cytoplasm)

Periampullary carcinomas refer to pancreatic carcinomas in the immediate vicinity of the ampulla of Vater as well as tumors of the most distal common bile duct and ampulla itself.

Clinical Features. Insidious growth occurs over years; 85% are unresectable at presentation, with a dismal outlook: First-year mortality exceeds 80%. Weight loss and pain are typical presenting symptoms; obstructive jaundice develops with tumors in the head or periampullary region. Massive metastasis to the liver occurs via splenic vein invasion. Migratory thrombophlebitis (*Trousseau sign*) may occur with pancreatic and pulmonary neoplasms or other visceral cancers.

Endocrine Pancreas (p. 911)

DIABETES MELLITUS (p. 913)

Diabetes mellitus refers to a group of disorders exhibiting a defective or deficient insulin secretory response, glucose underutilization, and hyperglycemia. The net effect is a chronic disorder of carbohydrate, fat, and protein metabolism with long-term complications affecting the *blood vessels*, *kidneys*, *eyes*, and *nerves*.

Classification and Incidence

Table 19–8 compares types I and II diabetes.

- ■ *Primary diabetes*
  - *Type I diabetes mellitus* (formerly called *insulin-dependent diabetes mellitus*) occurs in 10 to 20% of cases.
  - *Type II diabetes mellitus* (formerly called *non–insulin-dependent diabetes mellitus*) occurs in most of the remainder of cases.
  - *Genetic defects* are involved in several rare autosomal dominant forms of diabetes mellitus, including defects in β cell function (formerly called *maturity-onset diabetes of the young*) and insulin action.
  - About 3% of the world population, or about 100 million people, suffer from diabetes. In the United States, 13 million people are affected, with an annual mortality rate of about 54,000.
- ■ *Secondary diabetes*
  - Hyperglycemia is associated with identifiable causes of islet destruction or insulin dysfunction.
  - *Diseases of the exocrine pancreas* include inflammatory pancreatic disease (pancreatitis), surgery (pancreatectomy), pancreatic cancer, cystic fibrosis, hemochromatosis.
  - *Endocrine disorders causing insulin resistance* include acromegaly, Cushing syndrome, tumors (pheochromocytoma, pituitary tumors, glucagonoma, somatostatinoma, aldosteronoma), hyperthyroidism.
  - *Drug-induced or chemical-induced disorders* occur from glucocorticoids, thyroid hormone, Vancor (rat poison that destroys β cells), and others.

Table 19–8.   COMPARISON OF TYPE I AND TYPE II DIABETES

	Type I (IDDM)*	Type II (NIDDM)*
Clinical	Onset <20 y	Onset >30 y
	Normal weight	Obese
	Decreased blood insulin	Normal or increased blood insulin
	Anti-islet cell antibodies	No islet cell antibodies
	Ketoacidosis common	Ketoacidosis rare
Genetics	50% concordance in twins	90–100% concordance in twins
	HLA-D linked	No HLA association
Pathogenesis	Genetic susceptibility, autoimmunity, environmental triggering	Deranged insulin secretion with some insulin deficiency, insulin resistance
Insulin Status	Severe insulin deficiency	Relative insulin deficiency
Islet Cells	Insulitis early	No insulitis
	Marked atrophy and fibrosis	Focal atrophy and amyloid
	Severe β-cell depletion	Mild β-cell depletion

*Former terminology: IDDM, insulin-dependent diabetes mellitus; NIDDM, non–insulin-dependent diabetes mellitus.

- *Infections that destroy* β *cells* include congenital rubella, cytomegalovirus.
- *Gestational diabetes mellitus* occurs during pregnancy.
- Other genetic disorders are sometimes associated with diabetes, especially Down syndrome.

Pathogenesis

Normal Insulin Physiology. Glucose homeostasis is regulated by

1. Glucose production in the liver
2. Uptake and utilization of glucose by peripheral tissues
3. Insulin secretion by β cells in the pancreatic islets of Langerhans

Glucose is the most important stimulus for insulin synthesis and release; neural costimulation is necessary for insulin synthesis. Insulin is an anabolic hormone, necessary for uptake of glucose and amino acids by peripheral tissues (especially skeletal and heart muscle, fibroblasts, and adipose tissue), glycogen formation in the liver and skeletal muscles, glucose conversion to triglycerides, nucleic acid synthesis, and protein synthesis. Impaired peripheral tissue utilization of glucose can arise from an absolute lack of insulin or insulin resistance. The result is a rise in circulating levels of glucose to abnormally high levels.

Type I Diabetes. In type I diabetes, a severe, absolute lack of insulin is caused by a reduction in the pancreatic β cell mass. Interlocking mechanisms are as follows:

- *Genetic susceptibility* to altered immune regulation: About 20 chromosomal susceptibility regions have been identified. The strongest association is related to HLA class II inheritance; about 95% of white patients with type I diabetes have either HLA-DR3 or HLA-DR4 alleles or both versus 45% in the general population. It is proposed that particular HLA genes affect the potential immune responsiveness to a pancreatic β cell antigen.
- *Autoimmunity* to islet β cells, with lymphocytic inflammation of islets *(insulitis)*: About 70 to 80% of patients have islet cell autoantibodies, including antibodies to glutamic acid decarboxylase, *islet autoantigen 2* (a tyrosine phosphatase), and insulin. β cells are selectively destroyed. There is a 10% coincidence of Graves disease, Addison disease, thyroiditis, and pernicious anemia.
- Triggering of autoimmunity by an *environmental insult*: There is marked variability between world populations in the incidence of type I diabetes, and seasonal trends are observed. *Viruses* are suspected as initiators.

Postulated Scenario. Mild environmental β cell injury is induced by a viral infection, followed by an autoimmune reaction against altered β cells in persons with HLA-linked susceptibility. Possible mechanisms for triggering the autoimmune reaction include

1. Cross-reaction between a viral and host protein (e.g., a six–amino acid sequence shared by host glutamic acid decarboxylase and the P2-C replicative complex of coxsackie B4 virus), termed *molecular mimicry*
2. *Exposure of previously sequestered antigens when the* β *cell is damaged*

Chemical toxins (e.g., streptozotocin, alloxan, pentamidine) may act directly on islet cells or may trigger autoimmunity. *Molecular mimicry* after development of antibodies to the bovine serum albumin found in *cow's milk* also may trigger autoimmunity.

Type II Diabetes Mellitus. Type II diabetes mellitus is by far the more common type, with an even greater role for genetic susceptibility. This disease appears to result from a collection of multiple genetic defects, each contributing its own predisposing risk and modified by environmental factors. Key physiologic events are as follows:

- *Deranged β cell secretion of insulin*: Early in the disease, the normal pulsatile, oscillating pattern of insulin secretion is lost, and the insulin response to glucose is obtunded. Later, a mild to moderate absolute deficiency in insulin secretion develops. Loss of β cell mass is only a late event.
- *Insulin resistance*: Insulin resistance refers to reduced responsiveness of peripheral tissues to the actions of insulin. The number of insulin receptors decrease, and intracellular receptor signaling is impaired.
- *Obesity* is an extremely important environmental influence because it appears to increase insulin resistance (a similar phenomenon is observed during pregnancy). About 80% of type II diabetics are obese, and weight loss can improve the diabetic condition.

Several autosomal dominant genetic deficiencies of β cell function cause severe impairment of insulin regulation:

- *Chromosome 12, mutation in the hepatic nuclear factor-1α gene (HNF-1α)*: HNF-1α is a transcription factor that functions as a weak transactivator of the insulin-I gene. This was formerly called *MODY3*, for maturity-onset diabetes of the young type 3.
- *Chromosome 7, mutation in the glucokinase gene*: This reduces the ability of the β cell to *sense* glucose. This was formerly called *MODY2*.
- *Chromosome 20, mutation in the hepatic nuclear factor 4α gene (HNF-4α)*: HNF-4α is a member of the steroid/thyroid hormone receptor superfamily and an upstream regulator of HNF-1α expression. This was formerly called *MODY1*.

Pathogenesis of the Complications of Diabetes

Metabolic Complications. Insulin is a major anabolic hormone; deranged insulin function affects glucose, fat, and protein metabolism. Counterregulatory hormones (e.g., growth hormone, epinephrine) are secreted unopposed; peripheral tissues cannot accumulate glucose. Excess glycosuria induces osmotic diuresis and *polyuria*, with profound loss of water and electrolytes. Intense thirst *(polydipsia)* develops, with increased appetite *(polyphagia)*, completing the classic diabetic triad.

- *Diabetic ketoacidosis*: Occurs exclusively in type II diabetes as a result of severe insulin deficiency and absolute or relative increases in glucagon: excessive release of free fatty acids from adipose tissue and hepatic oxidation, which generates ketone bodies (butyric acid and acetoacetic acid). Ketonemia and ketonuria, with dehydration, generate life-threatening *systemic metabolic ketoacidosis*.
- *Nonketotic hyperosmolar coma*: Can develop in type II diabetics in the setting of severe dehydration (from sustained hyperglycemic diuresis) and an inability to drink water.

Long-Term Complications. Long-term complications are dominated by

- *Microangiopathy*
- *Retinopathy*
- *Nephropathy*
- *Neuropathy*

Late systemic complications are the major causes of morbidity and mortality of diabetes; onset and severity are extremely variable. The key metabolic causes appear to be as follows:

- *Nonenzymatic glycosylation*: Glucose chemically attaches to amino groups of proteins, reflected in *glycosylated hemoglobin* (HbA$_{1c}$) blood levels. With glycosylation of collagens and other long-lived proteins, *irreversible advanced glycosylation end products (AGE)* accumulate over the lifetime of blood vessel walls. AGE formation of proteins, lipids, and nucleic acids leads to
  - Protein cross-linking (trapping (among others) plasma lipoproteins in vessel walls
  - Reduction in normal proteolysis
  - AGE binding to cell receptors, inducing a variety of (undesired) biologic activities
- *Intracellular hyperglycemia with disturbances in polyol pathways*: Some tissues (nerve, lens, kidney, blood vessels) that do not require insulin develop increased intracellular glucose, which is metabolized to *sorbitol* and then *fructose*. The osmotic load leads to influx of water and osmotic cell injury. Sorbitol decreases phosphoinositide metabolism and signal transduction.

Morphology of Diabetes and Its Late Complications

Pancreas (Variable). There is a reduction in size of the pancreas and number of islets (especially type I diabetes mellitus), an increase in islets in infants of diabetic mothers, β cell degranulation, and fibrosis of islets. Other findings include amyloid (amylin) replacement of islets and leukocytic infiltrations, especially *insulitis* (a heavy lymphocytic infiltrate within and about islets) in newly symptomatic type I diabetics.

Vascular System. Accelerated *atherosclerosis* in the aorta and large-sized and medium-sized arteries increases the risk for myocardial infarction, cerebral stroke, aortic aneurysms, and gangrene of the lower extremities. *Hyaline arteriolosclerosis*, the vascular lesion associated with hypertension, is more prevalent and more severe in diabetics. Contributing influences to the vascular lesions include the following:

- *Hyperlipidemia* with *reduction in high-density lipoprotein levels* in type II diabetics
- *Nonenzymatic glycosylation* of low-density lipoprotein (LDL), rendering it more recognizable by the LDL receptor
- *LDL cross-linking to collagen*, retarding efflux of cholesterol from vascular wall
- *Increased platelet adhesiveness*
- Obesity
- Hypertension

Diabetic Microangiopathy. Diffuse thickening of basement membranes of small arteries and capillaries occurs in all patients and is related to hyperglycemia and AGEs. It is most evident in capillaries of the skin, skeletal muscles, retina, renal glomeruli, and renal medulla. It may affect nonvascular structures, such as renal tubules, Bowman capsule, peripheral nerves, and placenta. This basement membrane change is seen in all patients and is related to hyperglycemia and AGEs. Capillaries are actually more leaky than normal to plasma proteins.

Diabetic Nephropathy. The kidneys are the most severely damaged organ in diabetics, and renal failure is a major cause of mortality.

- *Glomerular involvement*: Diffuse glomerulosclerosis, nodular glomerulosclerosis, or exudative lesions, resulting in progressive proteinuria and chronic renal failure
- *Vascular*: Arteriosclerosis, including benign nephrosclerosis with hypertension
- *Infection*: Bacterial urinary tract infection, with *pyelonephritis* and sometimes *necrotizing papillitis*

Diabetic Ocular Complications. Visual impairment resulting from *diabetic retinopathy, cataract formation*, or *glaucoma* affects virtually all diabetics. *Nonproliferative retinopathy* consists of intraretinal and preretinal hemorrhages, exudates, edema, thickening of retinal capillaries, and microaneurysms. *Proliferative retinopathy* is the process of neovascularization and fibrosis of the retina, which can especially lead to blindness.

Diabetic Neuropathy. A *symmetric peripheral neuropathy* affecting motor and sensory nerves of the lower extremities is attributable to Schwann cell injury, myelin degeneration, and axonal damage. *Autonomic neuropathy* may lead to sexual impotence and bowel and bladder dysfunction. Focal neurologic impairment (*diabetic mononeuropathy*) is most likely due to microangiopathy.

Clinical Features

Type I Diabetes Mellitus. Type I diabetes mellitus begins by age 20 and is dominated by *signs of altered metabolism*: polyuria, polydipsia, and polyphagia. *Chemical indices* include ketoacidosis, low or absent plasma insulin, and elevated plasma glucose. There is an absolute need for insulin replacement. Metabolic derangement and insulin need are directly related to physiologic stress, including deviations from normal dietary intake, increased physical activity, infections, and surgery.

Type II Diabetes Mellitus. Type II diabetes mellitus patients are usually older than age 40, with polydipsia and polyuria and, often (but not necessarily), obesity. Metabolic derangements are usually mild and controllable with dietary restriction or insulin.

Complications of Both Types. Complications of both types of diabetes mellitus include the following:

- Atherosclerotic events: myocardial infarction, cerebrovascular accidents, gangrene of the lower extremity, renal insufficiency
- Diabetic microangiopathy: blindness, peripheral neuropathy
- Increased susceptibility to infection

ISLET CELL TUMORS (p. 926)

Islet cell tumors are rare compared with tumors of the exocrine pancreas. Tumors are

- Hormonally functional or nonfunctional
- Single or multiple
- Benign or malignant

β *Cell Tumors (Insulinoma)* (p. 926)

β cell tumors are the most common islet cell tumor. Tumors may elaborate sufficient insulin to cause hypoglycemia; symptomatic attacks occur with serum glucose less than 50 mg/dl. *Symptoms* include confusion, stupor, and loss of consciousness. Attacks are promptly relieved by glucose feeding or infusion.

Morphology. Of tumors, 70% are solitary adenomas, 10% are multiple adenomas, 10% are metastasizing carcinomas, and the remainder are diffuse islet hyperplasia and adenomas in ectopic pancreatic tissue. They may be minute (<0.5 cm) to greater than 2 cm diameter lesions, usually encapsulated, firm, yellow-brown nodules composed of cords and nests of well-differentiated β cells, with typical β cell granules by electron microscopy. Diffuse hyperplasia is characteristic of infants born to diabetic mothers, subjected to sustained hyperglycemia in utero.

Zollinger-Ellison Syndrome (Gastrinoma) (p. 927)

Zollinger-Ellison syndrome comprises a triad of recalcitrant peptic ulcer disease, gastric hypersecretion, and an endocrine cell tumor elaborating gastrin.

Morphology. Sixty percent of gastrinomas are malignant, with spread to lymph nodes and metastasis; 40% are benign. Gastrinomas are most common in the pancreas, but 10 to 15% arise in the duodenum. The histologic and ultrastructural features are similar to normal intestinal and gastric G cells. Peptic ulcers are in the usual sites in the stomach or duodenum in 75% of cases; abnormally located ulcers in the stomach or first and second portion of duodenum occur in 25%. The stomach shows hyperplasia of parietal cells.

Clinical Features. Features include striking gastric hypersecretion with intractable ulcers and severe diarrhea, with fluid and electrolyte imbalance and malabsorption. Surgical removal is extraordinarily difficult, with recurrence of symptoms postsurgically common.

Other Rare Islet Cell Tumors (p. 927)

Elaboration of multiple hormones is occasionally seen in *multihormonal tumors*: insulin, glucagon, gastrin, adrenocorticotropic hormone (ACTH), melanocyte-stimulating hormone, vasopressin, norepinephrine, and serotonin.

- α *Cell tumors (glucagonomas)*: Associated with extremely high plasma glucagon levels, mild features of diabetes mellitus, migratory necrotizing skin erythema, and anemia. These tumors are seen in perimenopausal and postmenopausal women.
- δ *Cell tumors (somatostatinomas)*: Associated with high plasma somatostatin levels. These tumors have features of diabetes mellitus, cholelithiasis, steatorrhea, and hypochlorhydria.
- *VIPoma (diarrheogenic islet cell tumor)*: Watery diarrhea, hypokalemia, achlorhydria; associated with neural crest tumors.
- *Pancreatic carcinoid tumors*: Serotonin-producing; rare.
- *Pancreatic polypeptide-secreting islet cell tumors*: Rare, asymptomatic.

The Kidney and Lower Urinary Tract

KIDNEY (p. 935)

Renal diseases are traditionally divided into four categories, based on the four basic anatomic compartments:

1. Glomeruli
2. Tubules
3. Interstitium
4. Blood vessels

Many disorders affect more than one structure, however, and the anatomic interdependence of these compartments means that damage to one secondarily affects the others. In particular, there is a tendency for all forms of *chronic* renal disease ultimately to destroy all four components of the kidney, culminating in end-stage kidneys and chronic renal failure.

Clinical Manifestations of Renal Diseases
(p. 935)

Clinical manifestations of renal diseases are grouped into reasonably well-defined syndromes.

- *Acute nephritic syndrome:* Seen with certain glomerular diseases (e.g., poststreptococcal glomerulonephritis). It is characterized by the acute onset of usually grossly visible hematuria, mild to moderate proteinuria, and hypertension.
- *Nephrotic syndrome:* Characterized by heavy proteinuria (>3.5 gm/day), hypoalbuminemia, severe edema, hyperlipidemia, and lipiduria (oval fat bodies in urine).
- *Asymptomatic hematuria or proteinuria:* Usually a manifestation of subtle or mild glomerular abnormalities.
- *Acute renal failure:* Dominated by the recent onset of azotemia with oliguria or anuria resulting from severe injury to glomeruli, tubules, interstitium, or blood vessels.
- *Chronic renal failure:* Characterized by prolonged uremia. It is the end result of all chronic renal diseases.
- *Renal tubular defects:* Dominated by polyuria, nocturia, and electrolyte disorders (e.g., metabolic acidosis). These are seen in acquired or genetic diseases affecting the tubules, interstitium, or both.
- *Urinary tract infections:* Affecting the kidney (pyelonephritis) or bladder (cystitis), leading to bacteriuria, pyuria, or both.

■ *Nephrolithiasis:* Manifested by renal colic, hematuria, and recurrent stone formation.

Renal Failure (p. 936)

Renal failure is characterized as follows:

■ *Azotemia* refers to an elevation of the blood urea nitrogen (BUN) and creatinine levels and is largely related to decreased glomerular filtration rate (GFR).

■ *Prerenal azotemia* occurs with hypoperfusion of the kidneys, as occurs with congestive heart failure, shock, volume depletion, and hemorrhage.

■ *Postrenal azotemia* occurs with urinary outflow obstruction below the level of the kidney.

■ *Uremia* is characterized by azotemia associated with a constellation of clinical signs and symptoms (Table 20–1) and is the *sine qua non* of chronic renal failure.

Stages of progression in renal disease are as follows:

1. Diminished renal reserve (approximately 50% of normal GFR)
2. Renal insufficiency (20 to 50% of normal GFR)
3. Renal failure (<20 to 25% of normal GFR)
4. End-stage renal disease (<5% of normal GFR)

Table 20–1.   PRINCIPAL SYSTEMIC MANIFESTATIONS OF CHRONIC RENAL FAILURE AND UREMIA

Fluid and Electrolytes
Dehydration
Edema
Metabolic acidosis

Calcium Phosphate and Bone
Hyperphosphatemia
Hypocalcemia
Secondary hyperparathyroidism
Renal osteodystrophy

Hematologic
Anemia
Bleeding diathesis

Cardiopulmonary
Hypertension
Congestive heart failure
Pulmonary edema
Uremic pericarditis

Gastrointestinal
Nausea and vomiting
Bleeding
Esophagitis, gastritis, colitis

Neuromuscular
Myopathy
Peripheral neuropathy
Encephalopathy

Dermatologic
Sallow color
Pruritus
Dermatitis

Congenital Anomalies (p. 936)

About 10% of newborns have potentially significant malformations of the urinary system. Renal dysplasias and hypoplasias account for 20% of chronic renal failure in children. Most arise from developmental defects rather than inherited genes.

- *Renal agenesis:*
  - *Bilateral* absence of renal development is incompatible with life.
  - *Unilateral* agenesis is associated with compensatory hypertrophy of the remaining kidney, which in later life may develop progressive glomerulosclerosis and renal failure.
- *Hypoplasia:* Failure of kidneys to develop to normal size, usually unilateral. A truly hypoplastic kidney shows no scars and possesses a reduced number of renal lobes and pyramids (six or fewer).
- *Ectopic kidneys:* Lie either just above the pelvic brim or sometimes within the pelvis. Kinking or tortuosity of the ureters may cause urinary obstruction, predisposing to bacterial infection.
- *Horseshoe kidney:* Fusion of the upper (10%) or lower (90%) poles produces a horseshoe-shaped structure continuous across the midline anterior to the great vessels.

Cystic Diseases of the Kidney (p. 937)

CYSTIC RENAL DYSPLASIA (p. 937)

Cystic renal dysplasia refers to sporadic, nonfamilial disease resulting from abnormal metanephric differentiation. It is frequently associated with obstructive abnormalities of the ureter and lower urinary tract. Dysplasia may be unilateral or bilateral. Affected kidneys are enlarged and multicystic and histologically show immature ducts surrounded by undifferentiated mesenchyme, often with focal cartilage formation.

AUTOSOMAL DOMINANT (ADULT) POLYCYSTIC KIDNEY DISEASE (p. 937)

Autosomal dominant polycystic kidney disease affects 1:400 to 1:1000 persons and accounts for about 10% of cases of chronic renal failure. The genetic defect has high penetrance, about 75% of affected individuals developing overt disease by age 75.

Genetics and Pathogenesis

The disease is genetically heterogeneous, caused by mutations of three separate genes:

- The *PKD1* gene, located on chromosome 16p13.3, accounts for about 85% of cases and encodes a large (460 kD) protein named *polycystin 1*. Although its precise function is unknown, it has homologies to proteins involved in cell-cell and cell-matrix interactions as well as specific repeated so-called PKD domains.
- The *PKD2* gene is on chromosome 4q13-23, and its mutations are present in about 10% of families. Its product, *polycystin 2*, is an integral membrane protein with homologies to certain calcium and sodium channel proteins as well as to a portion of polycystin 1.

- A *PKD3* gene, responsible for a minority of cases, has yet to be mapped.

How do defects in these proteins cause cyst formation? The answer is unclear, but it is thought that the mutations result in *altered cell-cell matrix interactions important in tubular epithelial cell growth and differentiation.*

Clinical and Morphologic Features

Polycystic changes are always bilateral and present from early childhood to as late as 80 years of age. Patients have flank pain from hemorrhage into cysts, hematuria, hypertension, proteinuria, progressive renal failure, and bilateral abdominal masses inducing a dragging sensation. Progression is accentuated in the presence of hypertension.

- The kidneys are enlarged, achieving massive size, and are composed of a mass of cysts up to 3 to 4 cm in diameter. Cysts arise anywhere along the nephron and compress adjacent parenchyma. In late disease, there is interstitial inflammation and fibrosis.
- Of patients, 40% have scattered *liver cysts* (polycystic liver disease), and 10 to 30% have *cerebral berry aneurysms,* which cause death from subarachnoid hemorrhage in 5 to 10% of patients. Mitral valve prolapse occurs in 20 to 25%.
- About 40% die of hypertensive or coronary heart disease, 25% of infection, 15% from ruptured berry aneurysm or hypertensive brain hemorrhage, and the rest of other causes.

AUTOSOMAL RECESSIVE (CHILDHOOD) POLYCYSTIC KIDNEY DISEASE (p. 940)

Autosomal recessive polycystic kidney disease is a rare bilateral anomaly presenting at perinatal, neonatal, infantile, and juvenile periods. Infants usually succumb rapidly to renal failure. Kidneys are enlarged by multiple, cylindrically dilated collecting ducts, which are oriented at right angles to the cortex and fill both the cortex and the medulla. The liver almost always has cysts and proliferating bile ducts, which in the infantile and juvenile forms give rise to *congenital hepatic fibrosis.*

MEDULLARY SPONGE KIDNEY (p. 940)

The term *medullary sponge kidney* should be restricted to lesions consisting of multiple cystic dilations in the collecting ducts of the medulla, usually presenting in adults. Most frequently an innocuous lesion discovered radiographically, it may predispose to renal calculi.

NEPHRONOPHTHISIS—UREMIC MEDULLARY CYSTIC DISEASE COMPLEX (p. 940)

Uremic medullary cystic disease complex is a family of progressive renal disorders, usually beginning in childhood, characterized by small cysts in the medulla (especially the corticomedullary area) associated with cortical tubular atrophy and interstitial fibrosis. There are four variants:

1. Sporadic, nonfamilial (20%)
2. Familial juvenile nephronophthisis (50%) inherited as an autosomal recessive disease

3. Renal-retinal (recessive) dysplasia (15%)
4. Adult-onset (dominant) medullary cystic disease (15%)

Children present with polyuria, sodium wasting, and tubular acidosis, followed by progression to renal failure. The gene, in some families with familial juvenile nephronophthisis, on chromosome 2q13, encodes a protein with an SH3 domain. These disorders should be strongly considered in children or adolescents with otherwise unexplained chronic renal failure, a positive family history, and chronic tubulointerstitial nephritis on biopsy.

ACQUIRED (DIALYSIS-ASSOCIATED) CYSTIC DISEASE (p. 941)

The end-stage kidneys of patients undergoing prolonged renal dialysis may develop multiple cortical and medullary cysts. The cysts are often lined by atypical, hyperplastic epithelium that can undergo malignant transformation to renal cell carcinoma.

SIMPLE CYSTS (p. 942)

Commonly encountered, single or multiple cysts of the cortex (rarely medulla) are lined by low cuboidal epithelium and usually are 2 to 5 cm in diameter but can measure up to 10 cm. They show smooth walls and are filled with clear serous fluid, but on occasion hemorrhage and stromal reaction may cause flank pain and irregular contours, thus mimicking renal carcinoma.

Glomerular Diseases (p. 942)

Glomerular injury is a major cause of renal disease.

- In *primary glomerulonephritis* (GN), the kidney is the principal organ involved.
- In *secondary glomerular disease,* the kidney is one of many organ systems damaged by a systemic disease (Table 20–2).
- *Chronic GN* is one of the most common causes of chronic renal failure in humans.

Some glomerular diseases cause mainly the nephritic syndrome, others cause mainly a nephrotic syndrome, and some may cause mixtures of both.

PATHOGENESIS OF GLOMERULAR INJURY (p. 943)

Immune mechanisms predominate in glomerular injury, but a variety of nonimmune factors may also initiate GN or cause its progression.

Immune Mechanisms

The deposition of antigen-antibody complexes in glomeruli is a major mechanism of glomerular injury, whether they are formed in situ with glomerular antigens or are trapped circulating complexes (Table 20–3). With in situ *immune mechanisms,* antibodies can be directed against the following:

- *Fixed intrinsic antigens:* Examples include:
  1. *Anti–glomerular basement membrane (GBM) nephritis,* an autoimmune disease in which antibodies bind to the noncol-

Table 20–2. GLOMERULAR DISEASES

Primary Glomerulopathies
Acute diffuse proliferative glomerulonephritis
Poststreptococcal
Nonpoststreptococcal
Rapidly progressive (crescentic) glomerulonephritis
Membranous glomerulopathy
Lipoid nephrosis (minimal change disease)
Focal segmental glomerulosclerosis
Membranoproliferative glomerulonephritis
IgA nephropathy
Focal proliferative glomerulonephritis
Chronic glomerulonephritis

Systemic Diseases
Systemic lupus erythematosus
Diabetes mellitus
Amyloidosis
Goodpasture syndrome
Polyarteritis nodosa
Wegener granulomatosis
Henoch-Schönlein purpura
Bacterial endocarditis

Hereditary Disorders
Alport syndrome
Thin membrane disease
Fabry disease

lagenous domain of the α3 chain of collagen type IV in the GBM, inducing a *linear* pattern of staining by immunofluorescence microscopy. Anti-GBM GN accounts for 5% of primary GN in humans.

2. *Heymann nephritis,* in which antibodies react with an antigen on visceral epithelial cells consisting of a large 330-kD protein called *megalin,* complexed to a smaller 44-kD protein called *receptor-associated protein* (RAP). The resultant le-

Table 20–3. IMMUNE MECHANISMS OF GLOMERULAR INJURY

Antibody-mediated injury
  In situ immune complex deposition
    Fixed intrinsic tissue antigens
      Goodpasture antigen (anti-GBM nephritis)
      Heymann antigen (membranous glomerulonephritis)
      Mesangial antigens
      Others
    Planted antigens
      Exogenous (infectious agents, drugs)
      Endogenous (DNA, immunoglobulins, immune complexes, IgA)
  Circulating immune complex deposition
    Endogenous antigens (e.g., DNA, tumor antigens)
    Exogenous antigens (e.g., infectious products)
  Cytotoxic antibodies
Cell-mediated immune injury
Activation of alternative complement pathway

GBM, glomerular basement membrane.

sions are characterized by *subepithelial deposits* of antigen-antibody complexes resembling those in human *membranous GN.* The deposits give a *granular* pattern of staining for immunoglobulin G (IgG) and complement by immunofluorescence microscopy.

- *Planted circulating exogenous* (e.g., infectious agents) or *endogenous* (e.g., DNA) *antigens.*

With *circulating immune complexes,* the antigens may be endogenous (e.g., thyroglobulin) or exogenous (e.g., infectious agents), but in human GN they are frequently unknown. The complexes are deposited usually subendothelially or in the mesangium and give a granular pattern of immunofluorescence. Once immune complexes are deposited in glomeruli, injury is induced by both cellular and soluble mediators, including

- *Neutrophils,* which release proteases, oxygen free radicals, and arachidonic acid metabolites, often in response to complement activation
- *Monocytes, macrophages, lymphocytes, and natural killer (NK) cells,* which release cytokines, cytotoxic cell mediators, growth factors, and other biologically active molecules (Chapter 3)
- *Platelets,* which aggregate and release eicosanoids and growth factors
- *Resident glomerular cells, particularly mesangial cells,* which can initiate inflammatory responses by releasing cytokines, oxygen free radicals, eicosanoids, and endothelin
- *C5b-C9,* the terminal membrane attack complex of complement, which causes cell lysis
- *Coagulation proteins,* especially fibrin, which may stimulate crescent formation in crescentic GN
- *Hemodynamic regulators* (e.g., eicosanoids, nitric oxide, endothelin)
- *Cytokines* (e.g., interleukin-1, tumor necrosis factor) and *chemokines* (e.g. MCP-1).
- *Growth factors* (e.g., platelet-derived growth factor, transforming growth factor-β [the latter being important for extracellular matrix deposition in glomerulosclerosis].)

Nonimmune Mechanisms of Progression in Glomerular Diseases

Once any renal disease, glomerular or otherwise, destroys functioning nephrons and reduces the GFR to about 30 to 50% of normal, progression to end-stage renal failure can proceed at a relatively constant rate, independent of the original stimulus or activity of the underlying disease. The two major histologic characteristics of such progressive renal damage are *focal segmental glomerulosclerosis* and *tubulointerstitial inflammation and fibrosis.*

The *glomerulosclerosis* appears to be initiated by the *adaptive change* that occurs in the relatively unaffected glomeruli of diseased kidneys. Similar changes occur in rats subjected to ablation of renal mass by subtotal nephrectomy. *Compensatory hypertrophy* of the remaining glomeruli maintains renal function in these animals, but proteinuria and glomerulosclerosis soon develop, leading eventually to total glomerular sclerosis and uremia. The glomerular hypertrophy is associated with *hemodynamic changes,* including increases in single-nephron GFR, blood flow, and transcapillary pressure (capillary hypertension), and often with systemic hypertension.

The *tubulointerstitial injury* is a component of many acute and chronic glomerulonephritides. *There is often a much better correlation of decline in renal function with the extent of tubulo-interstitial damage than with the severity of glomerular injury.* Many factors may lead to tubulointerstitial injury, including ischemia distal to sclerotic glomeruli, concomitant immune reactions to shared tubular and glomerular antigens, phosphate or ammonia retention leading to interstitial fibrosis, and the effects of *proteinuria* on tubular cell structure and function. Proteinuria is thought to cause *direct injury to and activation of tubular cells.* Activated tubular cells, in turn, elaborate proinflammatory cytokines and growth factors that contribute to interstitial fibrosis.

TYPES OF GLOMERULAR DISEASE (p. 949)

Acute Proliferative, Poststreptococcal, Postinfectious Glomerulonephritis (p. 949)

Acute proliferative, poststreptococcal, postinfectious GN is characterized by the *acute nephritic syndrome (hematuria, red cell casts, and usually moderate proteinuria and edema),* which presents 1 to 4 weeks after a streptococcal infection of the throat or, less commonly in the United States, the skin. Other bacterial, viral, and parasitic infections can produce the same disease picture. Poststreptococcal GN is an antibody-mediated disease in its acute form, but the precise streptococcal antigen involved is still unclear. Only certain strains (types 12, 4, 1) of group A β-hemolytic streptococci are nephritogenic.

- Biopsy specimens show *diffuse* GN (all glomeruli involved and *global* hypercellularity) resulting from proliferation of endothelial, mesangial, and epithelial cells and from infiltration by neutrophils and monocytes.
- Immunofluorescence shows a granular pattern of IgG, IgM, and C3 deposition, and electron microscopy shows subepithelial, *humplike* deposits, supporting the belief that the mechanism is immune complex deposition.
- There are elevated levels of serum antistreptococcal antibody, decreased serum complement C3 concentrations, and commonly cryoglobulins in the serum.
- Clinically, more than 95% of children recover. A few develop a rapidly progressive form of the disease, and the remainder progress to chronic renal failure. In adults, the epidemic form has a good prognosis, but only 60% recover after the sporadic form; the remainder develop rapidly progressive disease, chronic renal failure, or delayed but eventual resolution.

Rapidly Progressive (Crescentic) Glomerulonephritis (p. 951)

Rapidly progressive GN (RPGN) is a *clinicopathologic syndrome characterized by the accumulation of cells in Bowman space in the form of crescents accompanied by a rapid, progressive decline in renal function.* RPGN is divided into three broad groups. In each group, the disease may be associated with another systemic disorder, or it may be idiopathic (Table 20–4).

- *Type I RPGN* is an anti-glomerular basement membrane (GBM) disease characterized by linear deposits of IgG and, in many

Table 20–4. RAPIDLY PROGRESSIVE
GLOMERULONEPHRITIS (RPGN)

Type 1 RPGN (Anti-GBM)
Idiopathic
Goodpasture syndrome
Type II RPGN (Immune Complex)
Idiopathic
Postinfectious
Systemic lupus erythematosus
Henoch-Schönlein purpura (IgA)
Others
Type III RPGN (Pauci-immune)
(ANCA associated)
Idiopathic
Wegener granulomatosis
Microscopic polyarteritis nodosa

GBM, glomerular basement membrane; ANCA, antineutrophil cytoplasmic autoantibodies.

cases, C3 in the GBM. In some of these patients, the anti-GBM antibodies cross-react with pulmonary alveolar basement membranes to produce pulmonary hemorrhages (*Goodpasture syndrome*). What triggers these antibodies is unclear in most patients. There is a high prevalence of certain HLA subtypes and haplotypes, a finding consistent with genetic predisposition to autoimmunity.

■ *Type II RPGN* is an *immune complex–mediated disease.* It can be a complication of any of the immune complex nephritides, including postinfectious GN, but in some cases, the underlying cause is undetermined. In all of these cases, immunofluorescence studies reveal the characteristic (*lumpy bumpy*) granular pattern of staining.

■ *Type III RPGN,* also called *pauci-immune type,* is defined by the lack of either anti-GBM antibodies or immune complexes. Most of these patients have *antineutrophil cytoplasmic antibody* (ANCA) in the serum, which plays a role in some vasculitides. In some cases, type III RPGN is a component of a systemic vasculitis, such as Wegener granulomatosis or microscopic polyarteritis. In many cases, however, pauci-immune crescentic glomerulonephritis is isolated and hence *idiopathic.* More than 90% of such idiopathic cases have C-ANCA or P-ANCA in the sera, as described in Chapter 12.

Idiopathic cases are distributed as follows:

1. One fourth have anti-GBM disease (RPGN type I) without lung involvement.
2. One fourth have type II RPGN.
3. One half are pauci-immune or have type III RPGN.

The common denominator in all types of RPGN is severe glomerular injury.

■ The *histologic picture* of RPGN is dominated by the distinctive *crescents* formed by proliferation of parietal cells and by migration of monocytes and macrophages into Bowman space. Neutrophils and lymphocytes may also be present. Electron microscopy may, as expected, disclose subepithelial deposits in some cases but in all cases shows distinct *ruptures in the GBM*. In time, most crescents undergo sclerosis.

■ The *clinical manifestations* of all forms include hematuria with red cell casts in the urine, moderate proteinuria, and variable hypertension and edema. In Goodpasture syndrome, the course may be dominated by recurrent hemoptysis. Serum analyses for anti-GBM, antinuclear antibodies, and ANCA are helpful in the diagnosis of specific subtypes. The renal involvement is usually progressive during a matter of weeks, culminating in severe oliguria. Recovery of function may follow early intensive plasmapheresis (plasma exchange) combined with steroids and cytotoxic agents in Goodpasture syndrome.

NEPHROTIC SYNDROME (p. 952)

Nephrotic syndrome results from excessive permeability of the glomerular capillary wall to plasma proteins with proteinuria greater than 3.5 gm per day. Depending on the lesions, the proteinuria may be highly selective, mostly of low-molecular-weight proteins (albumin and transferrin); with more severe injury, poorly selective proteinuria appears of higher-molecular-weight proteins as well as albumin. The heavy proteinuria leads to hypoalbuminemia, decreased colloid osmotic pressure, and edema. There are also *sodium and water retention, hyperlipidemia, lipiduria, vulnerability to infection, and thrombotic complications*. The diseases causing the nephrotic syndrome in children and adults are listed in Table 20–5.

Membranous Glomerulonephritis (p. 953)

Membranous GN is a major cause of nephrotic syndrome in adults and is manifested by diffuse thickening of the glomerular

Table 20–5. CAUSES OF NEPHROTIC SYNDROME

	Prevalence (%)*	
	Children	*Adults*
Primary Glomerular Disease		
Membranous glomerulonephritis	5	40
Lipoid nephrosis	65	15
Focal segmental glomerulosclerosis	10	15
Membranoproliferative glomerulonephritis	10	7
Other proliferative glomerulonephritis (focal, *pure mesangial,* IgA nephropathy)	10	23
Systemic Diseases		
Diabetes mellitus		
Amyloidosis		
Systemic lupus erythematosus		
Drugs (gold, penicillamine, street heroin)		
Infections (malaria, syphilis, hepatitis B, acquired immunodeficiency syndrome)		
Malignant disease (carcinoma, melanoma)		
Miscellaneous (bee-sting allergy, hereditary nephritis)		

*Approximate prevalence of primary disease = 95% in children and 60% in adults.
Approximate prevalence of systemic disease = 5% in children and 40% in adults.

capillary wall owing to immunoglobulin-containing, electron-dense deposits along the *subepithelial* side of the GBM. The disease is idiopathic in 85% of patients; the remainder have secondary disease associated with underlying malignant tumors (lung, colon, melanoma), systemic lupus erythematosus, exposure to gold or mercury, drugs (penicillamine, captopril), infections (hepatitis B, syphilis, schistosomiasis, malaria), and metabolic disorders (thyroiditis). It is now thought that idiopathic membranous GN is caused by autoantibodies to visceral epithelial antigens, such as the megalin complex.

- By light microscopy, there is diffuse thickening of the capillary wall, hence the term membranous. Immunofluorescence studies show immunoglobulins and complement in a *diffuse granular pattern* along the GBM. By electron microscopy, there are subepithelial deposits along the GBM.
- The condition usually starts with the insidious onset of nephrotic syndrome or subnephrotic-range proteinuria. Up to 40% of cases progress to renal insufficiency over an unpredictable time span of 2 to 20 years. It is necessary in any patient with membranous GN first to rule out the secondary causes cited previously.

Minimal Change Disease (Lipoid Nephrosis) (p. 954)

Lipoid nephrosis is the major cause of nephrotic syndrome in children. *It is characterized by normal glomeruli on light microscopy but uniform and diffuse effacement of the foot processes of visceral epithelial cells on electron microscopy.* Immunofluorescence shows no immune deposits. The most characteristic feature of this condition is the dramatic response to corticosteroid therapy.

The cause and pathogenesis are unknown, but several features suggest an immune defect of T cells resulting in the elaboration of a cytokine-like circulating substance that affects visceral epithelial cells and increases glomerular permeability. Certain rare congenital forms of lipoid nephrosis are caused by mutations in an adhesive protein *(nephrin)* present in visceral epithelial slits. Despite the heavy proteinuria, the long-term prognosis is excellent for children and adults.

Focal Segmental Glomerulosclerosis (p. 956)

A cause of nephrotic syndrome or heavy proteinuria, focal segmental glomerulosclerosis (FSG) is characterized by *sclerosis of some, but not all, glomeruli (thus, it is focal), and in the affected glomeruli, only a portion of the capillary tuft is involved (segmental).* FSG can be

- Idiopathic
- Superimposed on another primary glomerular disease (e.g., IgA nephropathy)
- Associated with loss of renal mass (renal ablation FSG) as the result of chronic reflux, analgesic abuse, or unilateral renal agenesis
- Secondary to other known disorders (e.g., heroin abuse, human immunodeficiency virus [HIV] infection)
- In certain forms, inherited

Whether idiopathic FSG is a subform of severe lipoid nephrosis is controversial. The primary lesion in glomeruli is *visceral epithelial damage* (detachment) in affected glomerular segments. In contrast to minimal change disease, the proteinuria is relatively nonselective, and there is progressive segmental sclerosis (with associated IgM and C3 deposition). In addition, patients with FSG are more likely to suffer hematuria, reduced GFR, and hypertension. Idiopathic FSG responds poorly to steroids, and progression to chronic renal failure is common. Recurrences are seen in 25 to 50% of patients receiving allografts, with proteinuria occurring rapidly after transplantation. A circulating factor, perhaps a cytokine, is now suspected as the initiator of the lesions, but certain cases are familial, and mutations in visceral epithelial cell proteins are suspected.

In the FSG associated with HIV infection, there is more frequent *collapse* and *sclerosis* of the entire glomerular tuft (collapsing variant of FSG) as well as the presence of *endothelial tubuloreticular inclusions* by electron microscopy.

Membranoproliferative Glomerular Nephritis (p. 958)

The name membranoproliferative GN implies both thickened capillary loops and proliferation of glomerular cells. It accounts for 5 to 10% of nephrotic syndrome in children and adults, but some patients have hematuria or proteinuria, and others demonstrate a combined *nephritic-nephrotic* picture. Glomeruli have a *lobular* appearance because of mesangial proliferation, and the capillary wall has a *double-contour* or *tram-track* appearance. The latter is caused by extension of the mesangium around the inside of the capillary loop, so-called *mesangial interposition,* accounting for the alternative name *mesangiocapillary* GN.

There are two major types of membranoproliferative GN:

- *Type I* shows subendothelial electron-dense deposits and occasional subepithelial and mesangial deposits of C3, early complement components (C1q and C4), and immunoglobulins in a granular manner. Type I changes can occur in patients with systemic lupus erythematosus, hepatitis B, hepatitis C with cryoglobulinemia, infected ventriculoatrial shunts, schistosomiasis, α_1-antitrypsin deficiency, chronic liver disease, and certain malignancies.
- *Type II (dense-deposit disease)* shows the GBM to contain electron-dense material in a ribbon-like fashion. Subepithelial *humplike* deposits are also found occasionally. C3 is present, but there are no early complement components.

Type I disease appears related to immune complexes, whereas type II exhibits evidence of alternate complement pathway activation (decreased serum C3, properdin, and factor B). Most type II patients have *C3 nephritic factor* in the serum, an autoantibody against C3 convertase that stabilizes the C3 convertase activity.

Although steroids may slow the progression of membranoproliferative GN, about 50% of patients develop chronic renal failure within 10 years. There is a high recurrence rate in transplant recipients, particularly those with type II disease.

IgA Nephropathy (Berger Disease) (p. 961)

Berger disease is one of the most common glomerular diseases and is a major cause of recurrent glomerular hematuria. It is characterized by mesangial proliferation and *IgA deposition* by immunofluorescence microscopy. By light microscopy, the glomeruli may appear nearly normal, showing only mesangial hypercellularity, or reveal focal proliferative sclerotic lesions.

The pathogenesis is unclear. The data suggest a genetic or

acquired defect in immune regulation leading to increased mucosal IgA secretion in response to ingested or inhaled antigens with deposition of IgA aggregates or complexes in the mesangium. How these cause disease is unknown. Decreased clearance of IgA complexes by the liver is also associated with IgA deposition. Similar IgA deposits are seen in *Henoch-Schönlein purpura* in children.

The hematuria typically lasts for several days then subsides, only to recur every few months. Although most patients have an initial benign course, chronic renal failure develops in up to 50% over a period of 20 years. Recurrence occurs in 20 to 60% of grafts. Onset in old age, heavy proteinuria, hypertension, crescents, and vascular sclerosis portend a poorer prognosis.

FOCAL PROLIFERATIVE GLOMERULONEPHRITIS (p. 962)

Focal GN is a histologic entity marked by glomerular proliferation or damage restricted to segments of individual glomeruli (segmental) and involving only some glomeruli (focal). There are three circumstances in which this picture may be observed; in each case, the histology may change with the extent and progression of the underlying disease:

1. An early or mild manifestation of a systemic disease that might otherwise involve all segments (global) of all glomeruli (diffuse), such as systemic lupus erythematosus, polyarteritis nodosa, Henoch-Schönlein purpura, Goodpasture disease, subacute bacterial endocarditis, and Wegener granulomatosis
2. A component of a known glomerular disease (e.g., IgA nephropathy)
3. A form of primary idiopathic focal GN, a diagnosis made by excluding other potential causes

CHRONIC GLOMERULONEPHRITIS (p. 963)

Chronic GN refers to an end-stage pool of glomerular diseases fed by a number of different glomerulonephritides. Some contributors and the percentage of cases progressing to chronic GN are as follows:

- Poststreptococcal GN (1 to 2%)
- RPGN (90%)
- Membranous GN (40%)
- Focal glomerulosclerosis (50 to 80%)
- Membranoproliferative GN (50%)
- IgA nephropathy (30 to 50%)

Some cases arise mysteriously with no history of any well-recognized form of early GN. Glomeruli in chronic GN are totally replaced by hyalinized connective tissue, making it difficult to know the nature of the antecedent lesion. An overview of the various forms of primary GN is presented in Table 20–6.

Glomerular Lesions Associated With Systemic Disease (p. 964)

The following systemic diseases have glomerular associations:

- *Systemic lupus erythematosus* (p. 965): Covered in detail in Chapter 7.

- *Henoch-Schönlein purpura* (p. 965): Purpuric skin lesions (leukocytoclastic vasculitis), abdominal symptoms (pain, vomiting, bleeding), arthralgia, and GN. GN lesions vary from focal mesangial proliferation to crescentic GN but are always associated with *mesangial IgA deposition*. This condition usually occurs in children, and the course is variable. For most children, resolution of the lesions is the rule. Chronic renal failure may ensue, however, especially in those with diffuse lesions or the nephrotic syndrome. There is progressive renal failure in those with crescents.

- *Bacterial endocarditis* (p. 966): Variably severe, immune complex–mediated GN showing a morphologic continuum from focal necrotizing GN to diffuse GN, sometimes with crescents.

- *Diabetic glomerulosclerosis* (p. 966): Produces proteinuria (sometimes in the nephrotic range) in about 50% of type I and type II diabetics. It is usually discovered 12 to 22 years after diabetes appears (in type I) and heralds the onset of end-stage renal disease 4 to 5 years later in about 30% of juvenile diabetics. Morphologic changes in glomeruli include
  1. Capillary basement membrane thickening
  2. Diffuse diabetic glomerulosclerosis
  3. Nodular glomerulosclerosis (the latter also known as *Kimmelstiel-Wilson disease*)

Diabetics also develop hyaline arteriosclerosis and pyelonephritis, sometimes associated with papillary necrosis. Diabetes and renal changes are further discussed in Chapter 19.

- *Amyloidosis* (p. 968): Amyloid deposited in glomeruli and in vessel walls in either primary or secondary forms, producing heavy proteinuria. Eventually end-stage renal disease occurs, but the kidneys tend to be of normal size or slightly enlarged.

- *Miscellaneous:* Goodpasture syndrome, polyarteritis nodosa, allergic vasculitis, and Wegener granulomatosis all produce a similar form of GN ranging from focal segmental necrotizing GN to crescentic GN. Essential mixed cryoglobulinemia can induce cutaneous vasculitis, synovitis, and GN. Plasma cell dyscrasias can be associated with amyloidosis, monoclonal cryoglobulinemia, and a peculiar nodular GN (granular dense deposits) ascribed to the deposition of nonfibrillar light chains usually of the κ type, known as *light-chain glomerulopathy* (p. 968).

Hereditary Nephritis (p. 962)

Hereditary nephritis comprises a heterogeneous group of hereditary renal diseases manifesting primarily as GN, usually presenting with hematuria, and sometimes progressing to renal failure. *The best characterized—Alport syndrome—has GN associated with nerve deafness, lens dislocation, cataracts, and corneal dystrophy.* In most patients, electron microscopy demonstrates irregular thickening of the GBM, with pronounced splitting of the lamina densa. The X-linked form of the disease, in which males are most severely affected, is due to mutations in the gene encoding the $\alpha 5$ chain of collagen type IV, a component of the GBM. As a result of this defect, there is decreased synthesis of the $\alpha 3$ chain; thus kidneys from these patients do not recognize the Goodpasture antigen.

Thin membrane disease (p. 963) is associated with the fairly common entity of benign (asymptomatic) familial hematuria. Re-

Table 20–6. SUMMARY OF MAJOR PRIMARY GLOMERULONEPHRITIDES

Disease	Most Frequent Clinical Presentation	Pathogenesis	Glomerular Pathology Light Microscopy	Glomerular Pathology Fluorescence Microscopy	Glomerular Pathology Electron Microscopy
Poststreptococcal glomerulonephritis	Acute nephritis	Antibody mediated; circulating or planted antigen	Diffuse proliferation; leukocytic infiltration	Granular IgG and C3 in GBM and mesangium	Subepithelial humps
Goodpasture syndrome	Rapidly progressive glomerulonephritis	Anti-GBM COL4-A3 antigen	Proliferation; crescents	Linear IgG and C3; fibrin in crescents	No deposits; GBM disruptions; fibrin
Idiopathic RPGN	Rapidly progressive glomerulonephritis	Anti-GBM Immune complex ANCA-associated	Proliferation; focal necrosis; crescents	Linear IgG and C3 Granular Negative or equivocal	No deposits Deposits may be present No deposits
Membranous glomerulonephritis	Nephrotic syndrome	In situ antibody-mediated antigen: megalin complex	Diffuse capillary wall thickening	Granular IgG and C3; diffuse	Subepithelial deposits

484

	Clinical presentation	Pathogenesis	Light microscopy	Immunofluorescence	Electron microscopy
Lipoid nephrosis	Nephrotic syndrome	Unknown, loss of glomerular polyanions	Normal; lipid in tubules	Negative	Loss of foot processes; no deposits
Focal segmental glomerulosclerosis	Nephrotic syndrome; non-nephrotic proteinuria	Unknown Ablation nephropathy ?Plasma factor	Focal and segmental sclerosis and hyalinosis	Focal; IgM and C3	Loss of foot processes; epithelial denudation
Membranoproliferative glomerulonephritis type I	Nephrotic syndrome	(I) Immune complex	Mesangial proliferation; basement membrane thickening; splitting	(I) IgG + C3; C1 + C4	(I) Subendothelial deposits
Type II	Hematuria Chronic renal failure	(II) Autoantibody: alternative complement pathway		(II) C3 ± IgG; no C1 or C4	(II) Dense-deposit disease
IgA nephropathy	Recurrent hematuria or proteinuria	Unknown; see text	Focal proliferative glomerulonephritis; mesangial widening	IgA + IgG, IgM, and C3 in mesangium	Mesangial and paramesangial dense deposits
Chronic glomerulonephritis	Chronic renal failure	Variable	Hyalinized glomeruli	Granular or negative	

GBM, glomerular basement membrane; RPGN, rapidly progressive glomerulonephritis; ANCA, antineutrophil cytoplasmic antibody.

nal function is normal, and the prognosis is excellent. The GBM is 150 to 225 nm in thickness by electron microscopy (normal, 300 to 400 nm). The genetic basis is still unclear.

Acute Renal Failure (p. 969)

Acute renal failure signifies acute suppression of renal function in 24 hours, often with a fall in urine output to less than 400 ml. Acute renal failure is caused by

- Organic vascular obstruction
- Severe glomerular disease
- Acute tubulointerstitial nephritis
- Massive infection, especially with papillary necrosis
- Disseminated intravascular coagulation
- Acute tubular necrosis (ATN) (the most common cause)

ACUTE TUBULAR NECROSIS (p. 969)

ATN is characterized by destruction of renal tubular epithelial cells either from *ischemia* or *nephrotoxins.*

- *Ischemic ATN* occurs after shock produced by sepsis, burns, crush injury, or circulatory collapse (ATN is uncommon after hemorrhagic shock).
- *Nephrotoxic ATN* is caused by a wide variety of drugs (e.g., gentamicin, cephalosporin, methoxyflurane, cyclosporine, contrast media) and toxins (e.g., mercury; lead; arsenic; methyl alcohol; ethylene glycol; and certain mushrooms, insecticides, and herbicides). ATN may also follow massive hemoglobinuria or myoglobinuria (from rhabdomyolysis), usually associated with dehydration and hypoxia.

Although the morphologic abnormalities may be subtle by microscopy, careful studies reveal the following:

- *Ischemic ATN* shows patchy tubular necrosis mostly in the straight segments of the proximal tubules and ascending limbs of Henle loops.
- *Nephrotoxic ATN* shows variable degrees of tubular necrosis mostly in proximal tubules, although other tubular segments can be affected.
- In both types, the distal tubules and collecting ducts contain casts. The recovery phase shows epithelial regeneration (i.e., flattened tubular cells and mitotic figures).

Although the exact pathogenesis of acute renal failure in ATN is debated, it is thought that reversible and irreversible tubular damage are primary events leading to (Fig. 20–1):

- Arteriolar vasoconstriction, associated with tubuloglomerular feedback and involving the renin-angiotensin mechanism or with endothelial dysfunction resulting in increased endothelin and decreased nitric oxide and prostaglandin I_2
- Tubular obstruction by casts derived from necrotic and apoptotic epithelial cells
- Back-leak of tubular fluids
- Altered glomerular ultrafiltration

The clinical course of ATN proceeds through

1. *An initiating stage* (dominated by the inciting event)

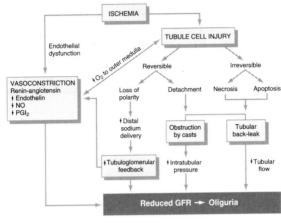

Figure 20–1 ■

Possible pathogenetic mechanisms in ischemic acute renal failure.

2. *A maintenance stage* (dominated by persistent renal failure and hyperkalemia)

3. *A recovery stage* (dominated by polyuria and perhaps hypokalemia).

The prognosis depends on the cause:

■ Good for nephrotoxic ATN
■ Poor for ATN when secondary to overwhelming sepsis

Pyelonephritis and Urinary Tract Infection
(p. 972)

Urinary tract infection (UTI) denotes infection of the bladder (cystitis), the kidneys (pyelonephritis), or both. UTI may be clinically silent (asymptomatic bacteriuria) but more often causes dysuria and frequency and (in pyelonephritis) flank pain and fever. UTI is much more common in women, perhaps because of a shorter urethra and hormonal changes affecting mucosal adherence of bacteria. Other risk factors for UTI include long-term catheterization; pregnancy; diabetes mellitus; immunosuppression; and lower urinary tract obstruction resulting from congenital defects, benign prostatic hypertrophy, tumors, or calculi.

PATHOGENESIS

Pyelonephritis is most commonly the result of *ascending infection,* the consequence of

1. *Bacterial colonization* of the distal urethra and introitus in women, followed by

2. *Multiplication of bacteria in the bladder (cystitis),* followed by

3. *Vesicoureteral reflux* through an incompetent vesicoureteral orifice, and

4. *Intrarenal reflux through open papillae to renal tissue*

- Vesicoureteral reflux is most often due to congenital defects in the intravesicular portion of the ureter and may be accentuated by cystitis, allowing retrograde seeding of the renal pelvis and renal papillae. *Escherichia coli, Proteus,* and *Enterobacter* are the most frequent culprits.
- *Hematogenous seeding of kidneys* occurs most often in the setting of septicemia or infective endocarditis, is frequently due to *Staphylococcus* or *E. coli,* and is enhanced by urinary obstruction.

ACUTE PYELONEPHRITIS (p. 974)

Acute infection of the kidney is marked by patchy, suppurative inflammation; tubular necrosis; and neutrophilic casts. More advanced changes include *abscesses, necrotizing papillitis* (especially in diabetics and in those with obstruction), *pyonephrosis* (pelvis filled with pus), *perinephric abscesses,* and eventually renal scars with fibrotic deformation of the cortex and underlying calyx and pelvis (see chronic pyelonephritis, next).

Clinically, acute pyelonephritis is associated with flank pain, fever, dysuria, pyuria (with pus casts in the urine), and bacteriuria. Uncomplicated acute pyelonephritis follows a benign course with antibiotic therapy but may recur or progress in the presence of vesicoureteral reflux, obstruction, immunocompromise, diabetes, and other conditions.

CHRONIC PYELONEPHRITIS AND REFLUX NEPHROPATHY (p. 975)

Chronic pyelonephritis (CPN) is a disorder in which *tubulointerstitial inflammation causes discrete, corticomedullary scars overlying dilated, blunted, and deformed calyces.* CPN is the cause of 10 to 20% of cases of chronic renal failure. It can be divided into two forms: *obstructive CPN* and *reflux nephropathy–associated CPN.*

- In *obstructive CPN,* chronic obstruction predisposes the kidney to infections, and multiple recurrences over time produce CPN. It is usually caused by enteric bacteria.
- *Reflux nephropathy–associated CPN* is the most common cause of CPN. It begins in childhood, as a result of infection superimposed on congenital vesicoureteral reflux and intrarenal reflux. Reflux nephropathy may have a silent, insidious onset, sometimes presenting with hypertension or evidence of renal dysfunction in the absence of persisting infection.
- *Morphologically,* both types of CPN are associated with broad scars, deformed calyces, and significant tubulointerstitial inflammation and fibrosis. Secondary FGS and hypertensive changes can also be present.
- *Xanthogranulomatous pyelonephritis* is an uncommon form of CPN associated with gram-negative infections, in which a mixed inflammatory infiltrate with abundant foamy macrophages produces large, yellow-orange nodules that can clinically and radiologically mimic renal cell carcinoma.

Acute Drug-Induced Interstitial Nephritis (p. 977)

Acute drug-induced interstitial nephritis is an adverse hypersensitivity reaction to a variety of drugs. It begins 2 to 40 days after exposure to drugs (e.g., methicillin, ampicillin, rifampicin, thiazides, various nonsteroidal anti-inflammatory drugs, phenindione). The disorder is immunologically mediated, with drugs acting usually as haptens. During secretion by tubules, they covalently bind to cytoplasmic or extracellular matrix components, become immunogenic, and induce antibody (IgE) and T cell–mediated immune reactions.

The clinical features are variably characterized by fever, eosinophilia, skin rash, hematuria, mild proteinuria, sterile pyuria, azotemia, and in some patients acute renal failure. Withdrawal of drug is followed by recovery in most patients. Biopsy specimen shows edema, patchy tubular necrosis, and tubulointerstitial infiltrates, with variable combinations of lymphocytes, histiocytes, eosinophils, neutrophils, plasma cells, and occasionally well-formed granulomas.

Analgesic Abuse Nephropathy (p. 978)

Analgesic abuse nephropathy is caused by excessive intake of analgesic mixtures. It is characterized by *chronic tubulointerstitial nephritis with papillary necrosis. Most affected patients consume phenacetin-containing mixtures, and cases ascribed to aspirin, phenacetin, or acetaminophen alone are uncommon.* The drugs act synergistically to cause papillary necrosis first; the tubulointerstitial nephritis is secondary.

Patients may have polyuria, headaches, anemia, gastrointestinal symptoms, pyuria, UTIs, and hypertension. Chronic renal failure may result, but drug withdrawal often stabilizes renal function. Renal papillary necrosis can be diagnosed by radiographic means. Papillary necrosis is not specific for analgesic nephropathy, being also seen in diabetes mellitus, sickle cell disease, and urinary tract obstruction. These patients have an increased incidence of transitional cell carcinoma of the renal pelvis.

Other Tubulointerstitial Diseases (p. 979)

Other tubulointerstitial diseases are as follows:

■ *Urate nephropathy:* This can cause acute renal failure or chronic renal failure, depending on the time course of uric acid crystal deposition. The former is particularly apt to occur in patients with hematolymphoid malignancies who are undergoing chemotherapy; the latter is likely to occur in patients with gout. Patients with increased exposure to lead may develop gout and a chronic interstitial disease.
■ *Hypercalcemia:* From whatever cause, hypercalcemia can cause stones (nephrolithiasis) or deposition within the kidney (nephrocalcinosis). Both may lead to renal insufficiency.
■ *Multiple myeloma:* Proteinuria and acute or chronic renal failure is seen. Renal insufficiency occurs in half the patients with this disease. Several factors contribute to renal damage:

 1. *Bence Jones proteinuria and cast nephropathy:* Two mechanisms account for the renal toxicity of Bence Jones proteins. First, some light chains are directly toxic to epithelial cells. Second, Bence Jones proteins combine with the urinary glycoprotein (Tamm-Horsfall protein) under acidic conditions to form large, histologically distinct tubular casts that obstruct the tubular lumens and induce a peritubular inflammatory reaction (cast nephropathy).

2. *Amyloidosis:* This occurs in 6 to 24% of patients with myeloma.
3. *Light-chain nephropathy:* In some patients, light chains deposit in glomeruli in nonfibrillar forms, causing a glomerulopathy, or around tubules, causing a tubulointerstitial nephritis.
4. *Hypercalcemia and hyperuricemia:* These conditions are often present in these patients.
5. *Vascular disease:* Vascular disease occurs in the usually elderly population affected with myeloma.
6. *Urinary tract obstruction:* This may lead to secondary pyelonephritis.

Diseases of Blood Vessels (p. 981)

Nearly all diseases of the kidney and many systemic diseases secondarily affect the blood vessels of the kidney. In particular, hypertension has marked effects on the renal vessels, and, conversely, the vascular changes augment the hypertension.

BENIGN NEPHROSCLEROSIS (p. 981)

Benign nephrosclerosis is the term used for changes in the kidney associated with sclerosis of renal arterioles and small arteries. The vascular lesions are characterized by narrowing of the lumens of the arterioles, caused by thickening and hyalinization of the walls. Larger muscular arteries show *fibroelastic hyperplasia,* with medial and intimal thickening. The changes are more severe in patients with essential hypertension, diabetes mellitus, or both. *The vascular lesions cause diffuse ischemic atrophy of nephrons, hence the relatively small kidneys and diffuse granular surfaces seen grossly in this condition.* Benign nephrosclerosis rarely causes renal failure, but mild proteinuria can occur. Three groups of patients are at risk of developing renal failure: blacks; those with more severe blood pressure elevations; those with second underlying diseases, particularly diabetes.

MALIGNANT NEPHROSCLEROSIS AND ACCELERATED HYPERTENSION (p. 982)

Malignant nephrosclerosis is the kidney disease associated with an accelerated phase of hypertension. Although occasionally developing in previously normotensive people, most cases are superimposed on preexisting benign essential hypertension, chronic renal disease (particularly GN or reflux nephropathy), or scleroderma.

The condition occurs in 1 to 5% of patients with hypertension and in pure form is most frequent in black men. Its pathogenesis involves injury and fibrinoid necrosis of the vessel walls caused by severe hypertension, intravascular thrombosis, and arteriolar wall thickening, all leading to renal ischemia and stimulation of the renin-angiotensin and other vasoconstrictive systems leading to a perpetuating cycle of increased blood pressure.

Pathologic changes include *fibrinoid necrosis of arterioles (necrotizing arteriolitis); hyperplastic arteriolosclerosis (onion-skinning); and necrotizing glomerulitis, often associated with a thrombotic microangiopathy.* Onset of diffuse intravascular coagulation may trigger malignant hypertension. Patients have a diastolic pressure greater than 130 mm Hg, marked proteinuria, hematuria, papilledema, encephalopathy, cardiovascular abnormalities, and eventually renal failure. There are marked increases in plasma renin, angiotensin, and aldosterone.

RENAL ARTERY STENOSIS (p. 984)

Unilateral renal artery stenosis accounts for 2 to 5% of cases of renal hypertension, resulting from excessive renin secretion by the involved kidney. Of stenoses, 70% are caused by obstructive *atheromatous plaque* at the origin of the renal artery and the remainder by *fibromuscular dysplasia.* The latter is a heterogeneous group of disorders, usually occurring at a younger age (twenties to thirties), characterized by nonarteriosclerotic *intimal, medial, or adventitial* thickening. Before arteriosclerosis develops in the opposite kidney, surgery cures about 80% with fibromuscular dysplasia and 60% with atherosclerotic stenosis.

THROMBOTIC MICROANGIOPATHIES (p. 985)

A group of diseases with overlapping clinical manifestations (e.g., microangiopathic hemolytic anemia, thrombocytopenia, renal failure, and manifestations of intravascular coagulation) are all characterized morphologically by thromboses in the interlobular arteries, afferent arterioles, and glomeruli, together with necrosis and thickening of the vessel walls. The morphologic changes are similar to those in malignant hypertension, but in this group the changes may precede the development of hypertension or be seen in its absence. The diseases include

- Classic (childhood) hemolytic-uremic syndrome (HUS)
- Adult HUS associated with infection, antiphospholipid antibodies, contraceptives, complications of pregnancy, certain drugs, and *scleroderma*
- Idiopathic HUS thrombotic thrombocytopenic purpura (TTP)

Although these diseases may have diverse causes, endothelial injury and intravascular platelet aggregation and coagulation appear to be shared pathogenetic mechanisms.

Classic (Childhood) Hemolytic-Uremic Syndrome
(p. 985)

Classic HUS usually occurs after a gastrointestinal or flulike prodrome and is manifested by acute renal failure with oliguria, hematuria, microangiopathic hemolytic anemia, hypertension, and (in some patients) neurologic signs. Up to 75% of patients are infected with *verocytotoxin-producing E. coli.*

Pathogenesis is related to the endothelial effects of the Shiga-like verotoxin:

- Increased leukocyte adhesion
- Increased endothelin and decreased nitric oxide production (both favoring vasoconstriction)
- Endothelial lysis

Kidneys show patchy renal cortical necrosis, glomerular capillary wall thickening (owing to deposits of fibrin-related materials), and arteriolar changes (fibrinoid necrosis, intimal hyperplasia, and thrombi).

Adult Hemolytic-Uremic Syndrome/Thrombotic Thrombocytopenic Purpura (p. 986)

HUS/TTP occurs in adults in a variety of settings:

1. *In association with infection,* such as typhoid fever, *E. coli* septicemia, viral infections, and shigellosis—postinfectious HUS.

2. In the *antiphospholipid syndrome,* either primary or secondary to systemic lupus erythematosis (lupus anticoagulant) (Chapter 5).

3. In women in relation to complications of pregnancy (placental hemorrhage) or the postpartum period. So-called *postpartum renal failure* usually occurs after an uneventful pregnancy, 1 day to several months after delivery, and is characterized by microangiopathic hemolytic anemia, oliguria, anuria, and initially mild hypertension.

4. Associated with *vascular renal diseases,* such as scleroderma, and malignant hypertension.

5. In patients treated with chemotherapeutic and immunosuppressive drugs, such as mitomycin and bleomycin.

Idiopathic TTP and various forms of HUS overlap considerably both clinically and morphologically. *Classic idiopathic TTP* is manifested by fever, neurologic symptoms, hemolytic anemia, thrombocytopenic purpura, and thrombi in glomerular capillaries and afferent arterioles. The disease is more common in women, mostly younger than 40 years. The thrombi are composed largely of platelets and are found in arterioles of many organs throughout the body. Untreated, the disease was once highly fatal, but exchange transfusions and corticosteroid therapy have reduced mortality to less than 50%.

ATHEROEMBOLIC RENAL DISEASE (p. 986)

Cholesterol crystals and debris embolize from atheromatous plaques after manipulation of severely diseased aortas, usually for repair of aortic aneurysms or during intra-aortic cannulation. They lodge in intrarenal vessels, causing arterial narrowing and focal ischemic injury. Rarely, renal function becomes compromised.

RENAL INFARCTS (p. 987)

Kidneys are favored sites of infarction because they receive 25% of cardiac output. Infarcts usually develop in a clinical setting of atrial fibrillation or myocardial infarction complicated by mural thrombosis. Most renal infarcts are asymptomatic but may cause pain and hematuria. Large infarcts of one kidney can cause hypertension.

Urinary Tract Obstruction (Obstructive Uropathy) (p. 988)

Obstruction increases susceptibility to infection and to stone formation. Unrelieved obstruction almost always leads to permanent renal atrophy. *Hydronephrosis is the term used to describe dilation of the renal pelvis and calyces associated with progressive atrophy of the kidney owing to obstruction of the outflow of urine.* Causes of urinary tract obstruction include

- Congenital anomalies (urethral valves, urethral strictures, meatal stenosis, bladder neck obstruction, ureteropelvic junction narrowing or obstruction, severe vesicoureteral reflux)

- Urinary calculi
- Prostatic hypertrophy or carcinoma
- Tumors
- Inflammation (prostatitis, ureteritis, urethritis, retroperitoneal fibrosis)
- Sloughed papillae or blood clots
- Normal pregnancy
- Functional disorders (neurogenic bladder)

When obstruction is sudden and complete, the reduction of GFR usually leads to only mild dilation of the pelvis and calyces but sometimes to atrophy of the renal parenchyma. When the obstruction is subtotal or intermittent, GFR is not suppressed, and progressive dilation ensues. Unilateral (complete or partial) obstruction may remain silent for long periods because the unaffected kidney can maintain adequate renal function. In bilateral partial obstruction, the earliest manifestations are inability to concentrate the urine, reflected by polyuria and sometimes acquired distal tubular acidosis, salt wasting, renal calculi, tubulointerstitial nephritis, atrophy, and hypertension.

UROLITHIASIS (RENAL CALCULI, STONES)
(p. 989)

Renal stones can arise at any level in the urinary tract, frequently causing clinical symptoms, such as obstruction, ulceration, bleeding, and pain (known as *renal colic*). They also predispose to renal infection. There are four types of calculi (Table 20–7):

1. About 75% of stones are *calcium containing,* composed of calcium oxalate or calcium oxalate mixed with calcium phosphate.

2. About 15% are so-called *triple stones* or struvite stones composed of magnesium ammonium phosphate.

3. Six percent are uric acid stones.

4. One percent to 2% are made up of cystine.

Table 20-7.   PREVALENCE OF VARIOUS TYPES OF RENAL STONES

	Percentage of All Stones
Calcium oxalate (phosphate)	75
Idiopathic hypercalciuria (50%)	
Hypercalciuria and hypercalcemia (10%)	
Hyperoxaluria (5%)	
Enteric (4.5%)	
Primary (0.5%)	
Hyperuricosuria (20%)	
Hypocitraturia	
No known metabolic abnormality (15–20%)	
Struvite (magnesium ammonium phosphate)	10–15
Uric acid	6
Associated with hyperuricemia	
Associated with hyperuricosuria	
Idiopathic (50% of uric stones)	
Cystine	1–2
Others or unknown	± 10

An organic matrix of mucoprotein, making up 1 to 5% of the stone by weight, is present in all calculi.

- *Calcium-containing stones* are usually associated with hypercalcemia and hypercalciuria (about 60%); hyperoxaluria and hyperuricosuria are associated in others. In about 25%, there is no demonstrable metabolic abnormality.
- *Struvite stones* are associated with infection by urea-splitting bacteria that convert urea to ammonia. So-called *staghorn* calculi are almost always associated with infection.
- *Uric acid stones* may or may not form in the presence of hyperuricemia or hyperuricosuria.

Increased concentrations of stone constituents, changes in urinary pH, decreased urine volume, and bacteria all play a role in stone formation, but many calculi occur in the absence of these factors. Thus, loss of *inhibitors* of crystal formation is postulated to play a role in the pathogenesis of some stones. These include citrate, pyrophosphate, glycosaminoglycans, and glycoproteins (nephrocalcin).

Tumors of the Kidney
(p. 990)

BENIGN TUMORS (p. 991)

Benign tumors include the following:

- *Renal papillary adenoma:* Small, discrete (usually yellow) tumors occur in 7 to 22% of autopsies. Histologically, most consist of vacuolated epithelial cells forming tubules and complex branching papillary structures. The cells may be histologically indistinguishable from those of low-grade papillary renal cell carcinoma, and they share some of their cytogenetic features. Most are small (0.5 mm in diameter). Tumors greater than 3 cm in diameter are considered early cancers.
- *Renal fibroma or hamartoma:* Small (<1 cm) nodules of fibroblast-like cells and collagen are found in the medulla; these are completely benign.
- *Angiomyolipoma:* Angiomyolipoma is often associated with tuberous sclerosis (25 to 50% of patients) and is considered a hamartomatous malformation.
- *Oncocytomas:* These are epithelial tumors composed of eosinophilic epithelial cells, arising from the intercalated cells of collecting ducts. On electron microscopy, the cells are packed with mitochondria. They may be large (up to 12 cm) but almost never metastasize.

MALIGNANT TUMORS (p. 991)

Renal Cell Carcinoma (Hypernephroma or Adenocarcinoma of Kidney) (p. 991)

Renal cell carcinomas represent about 1 to 3% of all visceral cancers and 85% of renal cancers in adults. They occur usually in patients in their fifties and sixties and show a male preponderance. Tobacco is the most prominent risk factor. Most renal cancer is sporadic, but unusual forms of autosomal dominant familial cancers account for 4%.

- *von Hippel–Lindau (VHL) syndrome:* Of patients with VHL, 50 to 70% develop renal cysts and bilateral, often multiple renal cell carcinomas. The VHL gene is implicated in carcinogenesis of both familial and sporadic clear cell tumors.

- *Hereditary (familial) clear cell carcinoma:* This occurs without the other manifestations of VHL.
- *Hereditary papillary carcinoma:* This autosomal dominant form is manifested by multiple bilateral tumors with papillary histology and ascribed to mutations in the *MET* protooncogene.

The major types of tumor are as follows:

- *Clear cell (nonpapillary) carcinoma* is the most common type, accounting for 70 to 80% of renal cell carcinoma. Tumors are made up of cells with clear or granular cytoplasm and are *nonpapillary.* In 98% of these tumors, *whether familial, sporadic, or associated with VHL,* there is a deletion or unbalanced chromosomal translocation involving 3p14 to 3p26, a locus that harbors the *VHL,* a tumor-suppressor gene.
- *Papillary carcinoma* accounts for 10 to 15% of renal cell cancers. It occurs in both familial and sporadic forms. The gene for the familial form, on chromosome 7, encompasses the locus for *MET,* a protooncogene that exhibits both germ line and somatic mutations. A second gene called *PRCC* (for papillary renal cell carcinoma) on chromosome 1 is implicated in sporadic tumors, largely in children.
- *Chromophobe renal carcinoma* represents 5% of renal cell cancers and is manifested by cells with prominent cell membranes and pale eosinophilic cytoplasm, usually with a halo around the nucleus. These tumors exhibit multiple chromosome losses and extreme hypodiploidy. They are thought to grow from intercalated cells of collecting ducts and have an excellent prognosis.

Morphologically, renal clear cell carcinomas appear as spherical masses, 3 to 15 cm in diameter, composed of bright yellow-gray-white tissue that distorts the renal outline. There are commonly large areas of ischemic opaque, gray-white necrosis; foci of hemorrhagic discoloration; and areas of softening. Tumors may bulge into the calyces and pelvis and invade the renal vein and grow as a solid column of cells within this vessel. *Clinically,* patients may show hematuria (90%), fever, constitutional symptoms, or a paraneoplastic syndrome (polycythemia, hypercalcemia, hypertension, feminization or masculinization, Cushing syndrome, eosinophilia, leukemoid reaction, and amyloidosis).

Prognosis depends on tumor size and the extent of spread (either local or distant) at diagnosis. Renal cell carcinoma has a tendency to metastasize widely before giving rise to any local symptoms; in 25% of new patients, there is radiographic evidence of metastases at presentation. Time course of disease is variable, but on average 45% survive 5 years and up to 70% in the absence of distant metastasis at diagnosis.

Urothelial Carcinomas of Renal Pelvis (p. 994)

About 5 to 10% of renal tumors occur in the pelvis, where they present early because of obstruction. Their histology exactly mimics urothelial tumors in the bladder, ranging from well-differentiated papillary lesions to anaplastic, invasive carcinomas. They are often multifocal, and in 50% of cases there is a synchronous or metachronous bladder tumor. Despite these observations, evidence suggests they are clonal in origin. Five-year survival varies from 70% for low-grade superficial tumors to 10% for high-grade infiltrating tumors.

LOWER URINARY TRACT (p. 998)

Ureters (p. 999)

Congenital anomalies occur in 2 to 3% of autopsies and for the most part are of only incidental interest without clinical relevance. *Ureteropelvic junction narrowing or obstruction* can cause hydronephrosis, however. They may be congenital or acquired; the latter are ascribed to disorganized smooth muscle at the junction, excess stromal deposition of collagen, or rarely extrinsic compression by aberrant polar renal vessels. Tumors (p. 999) can be urothelial or connective tissue in origin and reflect features analogous to tumors in the renal pelvis and bladder.

OBSTRUCTIVE LESIONS (p. 999)

The major causes of ureteral obstruction are listed in Table 20–8.

Sclerosing Retroperitonitis (Retroperitoneal Fibromatosis) (p. 1000)

Sclerosing retroperitonitis is a rare cause of obstruction and hydronephrosis. It is characterized by ill-defined fibrous masses that begin over the sacral promontory, encircle the lower abdominal aorta, and extend laterally through the retroperitoneum to enclose and encroach on the ureters. Microscopically the fibrosis is marked by a prominent inflammatory infiltrate of lymphocytes,

Table 20–8. MAJOR CAUSES OF URETERAL OBSTRUCTION

Intrinsic	
Calculi	Of renal origin, rarely >5 mm in diameter
	Larger renal stones cannot enter ureters
	Impact at loci of ureteral narrowing—ureteropelvic junction, where ureters cross iliac vessels and where they enter bladder—and cause excruciating *renal colic*
Strictures	Congenital or acquired (inflammations, sclerosing retroperitoneal fibrosis)
Tumorous masses	Transitional cell carcinomas arising in ureters
	Rarely, benign tumors or fibroepithelial polyps
Blood clots	Massive hematuria from renal calculi, tumors, or papillary necrosis
Neurogenic causes	Interruption of the neural pathways to the bladder
Extrinsic	
Pregnancy	Physiologic relaxation of smooth muscle or pressure on ureters at pelvic brim from enlarging fundus
Periureteral inflammation	Salpingitis, diverticulitis, peritonitis, sclerosing retroperitoneal fibrosis
Endometriosis	With pelvic lesions, followed by scarring
Tumors	Cancers of the rectum, bladder, prostate, ovaries, uterus, cervix, lymphomas, sarcomas
	Ureteral obstruction is one of the major causes of death from cervical carcinoma

often with germinal centers, plasma cells, and eosinophils. Sometimes, foci of fat necrosis and granulomatous inflammation are present. The cause is unclear.

Urinary Bladder (p. 1000)

CONGENITAL ANOMALIES (p. 1000)

Diverticula, outpouchings of the bladder wall between the crisscrossing muscle bundles, may arise as congenital defects but more commonly are acquired lesions from persistent urethral obstruction. They are the sites of urinary stasis and predispose to infection and the formation of bladder calculi. They also predispose to vesicoureteric reflux, and rarely carcinomas may arise within them.

Exstrophy of the bladder is due to a defect in the anterior abdominal wall, wherein the bladder communicates directly through a large defect with the body surface or lies as an exposed sac. Chronic infections supervene, and there is an increased incidence of carcinoma, mostly adenocarcinoma.

INFLAMMATIONS (p. 1001)

Acute and Chronic Cystitis (p. 1001)

Lower UTIs have already been discussed, but in addition to the common causal agents of infectious cystitis (*E. coli, Proteus, Klebsiella,* and *Enterobacter*), *tuberculous cystitis* can be a sequel to renal tuberculosis. *Candida* and *Cryptococcus* can cause cystitis in immunosuppressed patients or those receiving long-term antibiotics. *Schistosomiasis* predisposing to bladder cancer is common in Middle Eastern countries, notably Egypt. *Adenovirus, Chlamydia, Mycoplasma,* and *radiation* can cause cystitis. The *antitumor agents* cyclophosphamide and busulfan have produced hemorrhagic cystitis. Often the cystitis associated with long-term indwelling catheters results in mucosal bulges into the lumen, forming polyps (polypoid cystitis), a lesion that should not be mistaken for papillary carcinoma. The symptoms caused by cystitis include urinary frequency, lower abdominal pain, and pain or burning on urination (dysuria).

Interstitial Cystitis (Hunner Ulcer). Interstitial cystitis is a form of chronic cystitis, occurring usually in women, causing pain and dysuria. Histologically, there is localized ulceration with inflammation and fibrosis of all layers of the bladder wall. Mast cells may be prominent.

Malakoplakia. Malakoplakia is a type of chronic bacterial cystitis characterized by soft, yellow, slightly raised mucosal plaques, 3 to 4 cm in diameter. The plaques consist of lymphocytes and foamy histiocytes, the latter containing periodic acid–Schiff–positive granules and *targetoid* intracellular structures called *Michaelis-Gutmann bodies.* The intracellular material represents incompletely digested bacteria. Identical lesions occur in the colon, lungs, bones, kidney, prostate, and epididymis and are sometimes associated with immunosuppression. *E. coli* is the most common causative organism.

Cystitis Glandularis and Cystitis Cystica. These are common lesions in which nests of transitional epithelium (Brunn nests) grow downward into the lamina propria and undergo transformation of their central epithelial cells into cuboidal or columnar epithelium lining slitlike *(cystitis glandularis)* or cystic spaces *(cystitis cystica).* Typical goblet cells are sometimes present, and the epithelium resembles intestinal mucosa *(intestinal metaplasia).* Both variants are common microscopic incidental findings in relatively normal bladders but are more prominent in inflamed and chronically irritated bladders. *Lesions exhibiting extensive intestinal metaplasia are at increased risk for the development of adenocarcinoma.*

NEOPLASMS (p. 1003)

About 95% of bladder tumors are of epithelial—urothelial (transitional)—origin, the remainder being mesenchymal.

Urothelial (Transitional Cell) Tumors (p. 1003)

Urothelial tumors represent about 95% of all bladder tumors and run the gamut from small benign lesions that may never recur, to tumors of low or indeterminate malignant potential, to lesions that invade the bladder wall and frequently metastasize. Many are multifocal at presentation. Histologic grading of these tumors, to predict behavior, has been a subject of great debate. Table 20–9 lists two of many systems of grading these tumors. The older (1972) and commonly used World Health Organization (WHO) classification grades tumors into a rare totally benign papilloma and three grades of transitional cell carcinoma (grades I, II, and III). A more recent classification recognizes a rare benign papilloma, a group of papillary urothelial neoplasms of low malignant potential, and two grades of carcinoma (low and high grade).

Grossly, tumors vary from purely papillary to nodular or flat to mixed papillary and nodular. The tumors may also be invasive or noninvasive. Multicentric origins may produce separate tumors. The histologic changes encompass a spectrum from benign papillomas, which resemble normal transitional epithelium, to highly aggressive anaplastic cancers. Overall, about half of bladder cancers are high-grade lesions. Most arise from the lateral or posterior walls at the bladder base.

Papillomas and low-grade lesions are almost always papillary. Higher grades may be flat or papillary. Many grade III lesions may be fungating, necrotic, sometimes ulcerative tumors that have unmistakably invaded deeply. Less than 10% of low-grade cancers invade, but as many as 80% of high-grade transitional cell carcinomas are invasive. In advanced stages, there is invasion of the adjacent prostate, seminal vesicles, ureters, and retroperitoneum

---

Table 20–9. GRADING OF UROTHELIAL (TRANSITIONAL CELL) TUMORS

WHO Grading	ISUP Consensus*
Papilloma	Urothelial papilloma
TCC grade I	Urothelial neoplasm of low malignant potential
TCC grade II	Urothelial carcinoma, low grade
TCC grade III	Urothelial carcinoma, high grade

WHO, World Health Organizations; ISUP, International Society of Urological Pathology; TCC, transitional cell carcinoma.

*Tentative (*Grades in WHO classification do not strictly correspond to ISUP terminology*).

and metastases to regional lymph nodes. Hematogenous dissemination, principally to the liver, lungs, and bone marrow, occurs late, with highly anaplastic tumors.

Carcinoma in situ is a high-grade flat lesion confined to the bladder mucosa. It appears as an area of mucosal reddening, granularity, or thickening without producing an evident intraluminal mass. It is commonly multifocal and may involve most of the bladder surface and extend into the ureters and urethra. Although carcinoma in situ is most often found in bladders harboring well-defined transitional cell carcinoma, about 1 to 5% of cases occur in the absence of such tumors. In time, some of these lesions become invasive.

The extent of spread at the time of initial diagnosis is the most important factor in determining the outlook for a patient. Thus, staging, in addition to grade, is critical in the assessment of bladder neoplasms. *Squamous cell carcinomas* represent about 3 to 7% of bladder cancers in the United States, but in countries endemic for urinary schistosomiasis, they occur much more frequently.

Epidemiology and Pathogenesis. The incidence of carcinoma of the bladder resembles that of bronchogenic carcinoma, being more common in men than in women, in industrialized than in developing nations, and in urban than in rural dwellers. About 80% of patients are between the ages of 50 and 80 years. Factors implicated in the causation of transitional cell carcinoma include

- *Cigarette smoking*
- *Industrial exposure to arylamines,* particularly 2-naphthylamine
- *Schistosoma haematobium* infections in areas where these are endemic (Egypt, Sudan)
- *Heavy long-term exposure to cyclophosphamide,* an immuno-suppressive agent

The cytogenetic and molecular alterations are heterogeneous, but most tumors, even when multicentric, are clonal. Particularly common (occurring in 30 to 60% of tumors studied) are chromosome 9 monosomy or deletions of 9p and 9q. The 9p deletions involve the tumor-suppressor gene *p16* (*MTS1,* INK4a), which encodes an inhibitor of a cyclin-dependent kinase, and also the related *p15.* Additionally, many invasive transitional cell carcinomas show *deletions of 17p,* including the region of the *p53* gene as well as mutations in the *p53* gene, suggesting that alterations in *p53* contribute to the progression of transitional cell carcinoma. The *13q* deletion is that of the *retinoblastoma gene* and is also present in invasive tumors. Deletions of *14q* are seen exclusively in flat lesions or invasive tumors.

Clinical Course. Bladder tumors produce painless hematuria, sometimes with frequency and urgency. About 60% of neoplasms, when first discovered, are single, and 70% are localized to the bladder. Patients with urothelial tumors, whatever their grade, have a tendency to develop new tumors after excision, and recurrences may exhibit a higher grade. Overall, about 50% of papillomas and low-grade carcinomas recur, in contrast to 80 to 90% of high-grade tumors.

The prognosis depends on the histologic grade of the tumor and on the stage when it is first diagnosed. Papillomas and grade I cancers (those of low malignant potential) yield a 98% 10-year survival rate regardless of the number of recurrences. In contrast, only about 40% of individuals with a grade III cancer survive 10 years; the tumor is progressive in 65%.

Urethra (p. 1009)

Urethritis can be caused by gonococci and nongonococci. The nongonococcal forms can be caused by *E. coli,* other enteric organisms, *Chlamydia,* and *Mycoplasma.* The *caruncle* is a red, polypoid inflammatory tumor, 1 to 1.5 cm in diameter, of the external urethral meatus in women; excision is curative. Malignant tumors are rare, usually squamous cell carcinoma.

Diseases of the Male Genital Tract

PENIS (p. 1011)

Congenital Anomalies (p. 1011)

Congenital anomalies include the following conditions:

- A variety of abnormalities occur in size and form, including aplasia or hypoplasia; hypertrophy; duplication; and, more commonly, *hypospadias*, *epispadias*, and *phimosis*.
- Malformations of the urethral groove and canal may produce abnormal urethral orifices involving the *ventral* or *dorsal* aspects of the penis, designated *hypospadias* or *epispadias*. These may be associated with other urogenital malformations, including *undescended testes*, and may produce lower urinary tract *obstruction* and *sterility*.
- *Phimosis* designates an abnormally small orifice in the prepuce; it may arise as a primary developmental defect but is more frequently secondary to inflammation. Phimosis predisposes to secondary *infections* and *carcinoma*, owing to chronic accumulation of secretions and other debris under the foreskin. *Paraphimosis* refers to abnormal, painful swelling of the glans penis after forceful retraction of a phimotic prepuce; it may cause urethral obstruction.

Inflammations (p. 1012)

Inflammations characteristically involve both the glans penis and the prepuce.

- *Nonspecific* inflammatory processes and specific *sexually transmitted diseases* (e.g., syphilis, gonorrhea, chancroid, lymphopathia venereum, genital herpes, granuloma inguinale) occur.
- *Balanoposthitis* refers to nonspecific infection of the glans penis and prepuce, generally associated with *phimosis* or a *redundant prepuce*, and resultant chronic accumulation of smegma; it may be caused by a wide variety of bacteria, fungi, mycoplasmas, and chlamydiae.

Tumors (p. 1012)

Tumors of the penis include *benign tumors*, *carcinoma* in situ, and *malignant tumors*.

BENIGN TUMORS (p. 1012)

Condyloma Acuminatum (p. 1012)

- Condyloma acuminatum is a benign epithelial proliferation caused by *human papilloma virus* (HPV), especially types 6 and 11.
- Condyloma acuminatum may involve mucocutaneous genital surfaces of either sex; *sexual contact* is the most likely mode of transmission. It is most common after puberty; its presence in a prepubertal child should arouse suspicion of sexual abuse.
- Gross morphology is that of a sessile or pedunculated papillary excrescence, often involving the coronal sulcus or inner surface of the prepuce.
- Histologic characteristics include branching stromal papillae covered by hyperplastic stratified squamous epithelium, often associated with prominent hyperkeratosis. Vacuolation of superficial epithelial cells *(koilocytosis)* is common. Maturation of epithelial cells is orderly, in contrast to carcinoma in situ.
- Most lesions remain benign; they may recur owing to persistence of HPV infection.

CARCINOMA IN SITU (p. 1013)

Carcinoma in situ indicates cytologic evidence of malignancy (e.g., marked dysplasia, hyperchromasia, pleomorphism) confined to epithelium (i.e., no invasion of underlying connective tissue). Variants include Bowen disease, erythroplasia of Queyrat, and bowenoid papulosis.

Bowen Disease (p. 1013)

Bowen disease may occur in the genital region in both men and women, generally those older than age 35. In men, the disease presents most commonly as a thickened, gray-white plaque over the shaft of the penis. Microscopic features include marked epithelial atypia with complete loss of normal surface maturation but *no invasion* of underlying stroma. Transition to invasive squamous cell carcinoma is estimated to occur in approximately 10% of cases; there is a possible association with *visceral malignancies*.

Erythroplasia of Queyrat (p. 1013)

Erythroplasia of Queyrat presents as a single or multiple, shiny red, sometimes velvety plaque on the glans and prepuce. Histologic features and evolution are comparable to those of Bowen disease. There is no association with visceral malignancy.

Bowenoid Papulosis (p. 1014)

Bowenoid papulosis presents as multiple, pigmented papular lesions on external genitalia; it may mimic condyloma acuminatum grossly. Patients are generally younger than those with Bowen disease. Bowenoid papulosis is histologically indistinguishable from Bowen disease, but, in contrast to Bowen disease, evolution into invasive carcinoma is rare.

MALIGNANT TUMORS (p. 1014)

Squamous Cell Carcinoma (p. 1014)

- Squamous cell carcinoma accounts for 1% of cancers in men in the United States; prevalence is higher in regions where circumcision is not routinely practiced. Most cases are seen between ages 40 and 70 years.

- Potential causes include *carcinogens* within smegma accumulating under the foreskin and *HPV* types 16 and 18.
- Squamous cell carcinoma typically presents as epithelial thickening on the glans or inner surface of the prepuce, progressing to ulceroinfiltrative or exophytic growth eroding the penile tip, shaft, or both.
- Histologic appearance is identical to squamous cell carcinomas involving other cutaneous sites.
- Clinical course is characterized by slow growth, with metastases to regional (inguinal and iliac) lymph nodes; distant metastases are uncommon. The 5-year survival rate is 66% for lesions confined to the penis and 27% with regional node involvement.
- Verrucous carcinoma, also called *giant condyloma* or *Buschke-Löwenstein tumor*, is an uncommon well-differentiated form of squamous cell carcinoma with low malignant potential.

TESTIS AND EPIDIDYMIS (p. 1014)
Congenital Anomalies (p. 1015)

Anomalies include cryptorchidism, aplasia, fusion (synorchism), and a variety of developmental cysts.

CRYPTORCHIDISM (p. 1015)

- Cryptorchidism affects 1% of 1-year-old boys.
- Cryptorchidism represents *failure of descent*; testes may be found anywhere along the normal path of descent, from the abdominal cavity to the inguinal canal.
- Most cases are idiopathic; other causes include
  1. Genetic abnormalities (e.g., trisomy 13)
  2. Hormonal abnormalities
- Most cases are unilateral; 25% are bilateral.
- Histologic changes may be apparent as early as 2 years of age, including *decreased germ cell development*, *thickening* and *hyalinization* of seminiferous tubular basement membrane, interstitial *fibrosis*, and relative sparing of Leydig cells. Regressive changes may also occur in the contralateral descended testis.
- Clinical significance is related to high prevalence of *inguinal hernias*, *sterility*, and a 5- to 10-fold increased incidence of *testicular neoplasms*; surgical correction (orchiopexy) decreases the likelihood of sterility if performed early but does *not* decrease the risk of neoplasia, which may occur in either testis.

Atrophy (p. 1016)

Atrophy is characterized as follows:

- May be secondary to cryptorchidism, vascular disease, inflammatory disorders, hypopituitarism, malnutrition, obstruction of outflow of semen, elevated levels of female sex hormones (endogenous or exogenous), persistently elevated levels of follicle-stimulating hormone, radiation, and chemotherapy.
- May also be encountered as a *primary developmental abnormality* in patients with Klinefelter syndrome.
- Morphologic alterations identical to those in cryptorchidism.

Inflammations (p. 1016)

Inflammatory conditions are generally more common in the epididymis than in the testis; however, some infections, notably syphilis, may begin in the testis with secondary involvement of the epididymis. Inflammatory diseases include *nonspecific* epididymitis and orchitis, *granulomatous (autoimmune)* orchitis, and several *specific* infectious diseases (e.g., gonorrhea, mumps, tuberculosis, syphilis).

NONSPECIFIC EPIDIDYMITIS AND ORCHITIS (p. 1016)

- Nonspecific epididymitis and orchitis are often associated with infection of the *urinary tract*, with secondary infection of the epididymis via the vas deferens or lymphatics of the spermatic cord.
- Causes vary with the age of the patient and include
  - Gram-negative rods associated with genitourinary malformations in pediatric patients
  - *Chlamydia trachomatis* and *Neisseria gonorrhoeae* in sexually active men younger than age 35
  - *Escherichia coli* and *Pseudomonas* species in older men
- Nonspecific interstitial congestion, edema, and neutrophilic infiltrates occur in the early stages, with subsequent involvement of tubules; severe cases may progress to generalized suppuration of the entire epididymis. Inflammation may extend to the testis via efferent ductules or local lymphatic channels. Scarring of the testis and epididymis may occur with resultant *infertility*. Leydig cells are less severely affected, and sexual activity generally is not disturbed.

GRANULOMATOUS (AUTOIMMUNE) ORCHITIS (p. 1017)

- Granulomatous orchitis is an uncommon cause of *unilateral testicular enlargement* in middle-aged men. It has a possible *autoimmune* origin.
- Most cases present with sudden onset of a tender testicular mass, sometimes associated with fever; it may be painless in some patients and difficult to distinguish from testicular neoplasia.
- *Granulomas* occur within testicular tubules and adjacent connective tissue, accompanied by occasional plasma cells and neutrophils. Lesions must be differentiated from granulomas of tuberculosis.

SPECIFIC INFLAMMATIONS (p. 1017)

Gonorrhea (p. 1017)

- Most cases of gonorrhea represent *retrograde extension* of infection from the posterior urethra to the prostate, seminal vesicles, and epididymis.
- The inflammatory pattern is identical to that seen in nonspecific epididymitis and orchitis (discussed previously); infection may extend to the testis and produce suppurative orchitis in untreated cases.

Mumps (p. 1017)

- Orchitis is uncommon in children; it develops in 20 to 30% of postpubertal males with mumps.
- Orchitis typically develops about 1 week after onset of parotid inflammation; it may precede parotitis or occur in the absence of parotitis in a minority of patients.
- Orchitis is not usually associated with sterility, owing to unilateral testicular involvement and the patchy, predominantly interstitial pattern of inflammation.

Tuberculosis (p. 1017)

- Inflammation almost always begins in the *epididymis*, with secondary involvement of the testis.
- There is granulomatous inflammation associated with caseous necrosis, identical to active tuberculosis in other sites.

Syphilis (p. 1017)

- Inflammation virtually always begins as *orchitis*, with secondary involvement of the epididymis; it may present as isolated orchitis, without involvement of adnexal structures. Orchitis may occur in both congenital and acquired syphilis.
- May produce nodular *gummas* or *diffuse interstitial inflammation*. Interstitial changes include edema, lymphoplasmacytic inflammatory cells, and typical obliterative endarteritis.

Vascular Disturbances (Torsion) (p. 1017)

Vascular disturbances, referred to as *torsion*, are characterized as follows:

- Torsion occurs secondary to twisting of the spermatic cord, with resultant *venous obstruction*; arteries may also be occluded but often remain patent because of thicker walls.
- Torsion typically occurs in patients with preexisting structural lesions, such as incompletely descended testicles, absence of scrotal ligaments, or testicular atrophy. Torsion is generally precipitated by trauma or other violent movement.
- Changes range from congestion and interstitial hemorrhage to extensive hemorrhagic necrosis, depending on the duration and severity of the process.

Testicular Tumors (p. 1017)

A wide range of histologic types of testicular tumors are recognized, giving rise to many different classification schemes. Tumors can be divided into two major groups:

1. *Germ cell tumors* (accounting for approximately 95% of cases)
2. *Nongerminal tumors* (stromal or sex cord tumors)

Most germ cell tumors are aggressive lesions, although outlook has improved considerably with current therapy.

GERM CELL TUMORS (p. 1018)

Incidence of germ cell tumors is approximately 6:100,000 men annually, with peak incidence between ages 15 and 34 years. Germ cell tumors account for 10% of cancer deaths in this age group.

Classification and Histogenesis

Diverse classification schemes are based on a wide spectrum of morphologic patterns and variable concepts of histogenesis. Testicular germ cell neoplasms may contain a *single* histologic pattern (40% of cases) or a *mixture* of patterns (60% of cases). Most tumors arise from a focus of intratubular carcinoma in situ. The neoplastic germ cells may give rise to *seminoma* or transform into a *totipotential* neoplastic cell (embryonal carcinoma) capable of further differentiation. Germ cell neoplasms accordingly may be divided broadly into *seminomas* and *nonseminomatous tumors*. The *World Health Organization classification* of testicular neoplasms (Table 21–1) is the most widely used scheme in the United States.

Pathogenesis

Important risk factors include the following:

1. *Cryptorchidism*: Associated with 10% of testicular tumors.
2. *Genetic factors*: Higher risk of testicular neoplasia among siblings of patients with testicular tumors; some familial clustering reported. Significant racial differences also exist (rare in African blacks).
3. *Testicular dysgenesis*: Includes testicular feminization and Klinefelter syndrome.

Cytogenetic abnormalities involving *chromosome 12* are common; *i(12p)* is present in 90% of testicular germ cell tumors. In the remaining cases, extra genetic material derived from 12p is found in other chromosomes, thus implicating genes located on the short arm of chromosome 12.

Table 21-1. WORLD HEALTH ORGANIZATION PATHOLOGIC CLASSIFICATION OF TESTICULAR TUMORS

Germ Cell Tumors

Tumors of one histologic pattern
  Seminoma
  Spermatocytic seminoma
  Embryonal carcinoma
  Yolk sac tumor (embryonal carcinoma, infantile type)
  Polyembryoma choriocarcinoma
  Teratomas
    Mature
    Immature
    With malignant transformation
Tumors showing more than one histologic pattern
  Embryonal carcinoma plus teratoma (teratocarcinoma)
  Choriocarcinoma and any other types (specify types)
  Other combinations (specify)
Sex Cord–Stromal Tumors

Well-differentiated forms
  Leydig cell tumor
  Sertoli cell tumor
  Granulosa cell tumor
Mixed forms (specify)
Incompletely differentiated forms

Seminoma (p. 1019)

- Seminoma accounts for 50% of all testicular germ cell tumors; it is the most likely germ cell neoplasm to present with a single histologic pattern.
- Peak incidence is in the thirties.
- Variants include
  - Classic seminoma (85% of seminomas)
  - Anaplastic seminoma (5 to 10%)
  - Spermatocytic seminoma (4 to 6%) (discussed later)
- Seminoma presents as a homogeneous, lobulated, gray-white mass, generally devoid of hemorrhage or necrosis; the tunica albuginea usually remains intact. Microscopically, the mass is composed of large polyhedral *seminoma cells* containing abundant clear cytoplasm, large nuclei, and prominent nucleoli; cytoplasmic glycogen is typically present. A fibrous stroma of variable density divides the neoplastic cells into irregular *lobules*; an accompanying *lymphocytic infiltrate* (usually T cell) is present in most cases; granulomas may also be present. Neoplastic giant cells and syncytial cells resembling placental syncytiotrophoblast may be seen in some cases; human chorionic gonadotropin (HCG) is present in such cells and presumably accounts for the elevated serum HCG levels demonstrable in some patients with pure seminoma. The tumor cells contain placental alkaline phosphatase. Classic seminoma cells do not contain α-fetoprotein (AFP). *Anaplastic seminomas* are distinguished from classic seminomas by greater nuclear atypia and a higher mitotic rate.
- Histologically identical tumors may occur in the ovary (dysgerminomas) and central nervous system (germinomas).

Spermatocytic Seminoma (p. 1020)

- Spermatocytic seminomas are uncommon neoplasms, occurring in *patients older* than those with classic seminoma.
- These are *indolent* growths, with virtually no tendency to metastasize.
- Lesions tend to be larger than those of classic seminoma. Lesions are composed of a *mixed* population of cells, including smaller (6 to 8 mm) cells resembling secondary spermatocytes (hence the *spermatocytic* designation), medium-sized (15 to 18 mm) cells, and scattered giant cells.

Embryonal Carcinoma (p. 1020)

- Peak incidence is in the 20- to 30-year age group. Embryonal carcinoma is more *aggressive* than seminoma, although developments in chemotherapy have improved the prognosis considerably.
- Lesions may be small and confined to the testis; most examples are poorly demarcated, gray-white masses punctuated by foci of hemorrhage, necrosis, or both. They may extend through the tunica albuginea into the epididymis or spermatic cord. Microscopically, they are composed of primitive epithelial cells with indistinct cell borders, forming irregular sheets, tubules, alveoli, and papillary structures. Mitotic figures and neoplastic giant cells are common; syncytial cells positive for HCG and AFP may be detected and, when present, indicate a *mixed germ cell tumor* with concomitant trophoblastic or yolk sac differentiation.

Yolk Sac Tumor (p. 1021)

- Yolk sac tumor is the most common testicular neoplasm in infants and young children; synonyms include *infantile embryonal carcinoma* and *endodermal sinus tumor*. Prognosis is good in children up to 3 years of age.
- Most adult cases occur as a component of a *mixed* germ cell neoplasm.
- Pure forms present as infiltrative, homogeneous, yellow-white mucinous lesions. Microscopically, they are composed of cuboidal neoplastic cells arrayed in a lacelike (reticular) network; solid areas and papillae may also be seen. Structures resembling primitive glomeruli, so-called *endodermal sinuses*, are seen in 50% of cases. Eosinophilic, hyalin globules containing immunoreactive *AFP* and α_1-*antitrypsin* are present within and around the neoplastic cells.

Choriocarcinoma (p. 1021)

- Choriocarcinoma is a highly malignant neoplasm composed of both cytotrophoblastic and syncytiotrophoblastic elements.
- Similar neoplasms may occur in the ovary, placenta, or ectopic pluripotential germ cell rests in other sites (e.g., mediastinum, abdomen). This neoplasm is rare in pure form within the testis; it is more often encountered as a component of a *mixed germ cell neoplasm*.
- The primary testicular neoplasm is often quite small, even in the presence of widespread systemic metastases. The gross appearance ranges from a bulky, hemorrhagic mass to an inconspicuous lesion replaced by a fibrous scar. Histologically, it is composed of polygonal, comparatively uniform cytotrophoblastic cells growing in sheets and cords, admixed with multinucleated syncytiotrophoblastic cells; well-developed villi are not seen. HCG is readily demonstrable within the cytoplasm of the syncytiotrophoblastic elements.

Teratoma (p.1021)

- Teratomas are a group of neoplasms exhibiting evidence of simultaneous differentiation along endodermal, mesodermal, and ectodermal lines. They may occur at any age.
- Variants include the following:
  1. *Mature teratomas* are composed of a haphazard array of *differentiated* mesodermal (e.g., muscle, cartilage, adipose tissue), ectodermal (e.g., neural tissue, skin), and endodermal (e.g., gut, bronchial epithelium) elements. Mature teratomas are more common in infants and children; diagnosis of pure testicular teratoma should be made with extreme caution in adults, owing to the likelihood of concomitant malignant germ cell elements elsewhere in the neoplasm.
  2. *Immature teratomas* contain elements of three germ layers in incomplete stages of differentiation. They should be regarded as malignant, even though cytologic features of malignancy may be inconspicuous.
  3. *Teratoma with malignant transformation* is characterized by malignancy, generally in the form of a carcinoma (e.g., squamous cell carcinoma or adenocarcinoma) developing within a mature teratoma.

Mixed Tumors (p. 1022)

- Mixed tumors account in aggregate for approximately 50% of germ cell neoplasms.

- Histologic patterns are variable; the most common includes a mixture of teratoma, embryonal carcinoma, yolk sac tumor, and HCG-containing giant cells. *Teratocarcinoma* designates neoplasms containing both teratoma and embryonal carcinoma. Metastases from such lesions may contain virtually any germ cell element, including elements not present in the primary tumor.

Clinical Features of Germ Cell Neoplasms

- Most cases present with *painless enlargement of the testis*; neoplasia should be considered in the differential diagnosis of *all* testicular masses, even those that are painful. Clinical evaluation, however, does not reliably distinguish between the various types of germ cell tumors.
- *Lymphatic* metastases are most common in *retroperitoneal para-aortic* nodes but may occur in more distant sites (e.g., mediastinal and supraclavicular nodes); the *lungs* are the most common site for *hematogenous* metastases, followed by liver, brain, and bone. The histologic appearance of metastases may be identical to that of primary tumor or may contain other germ cell elements (e.g., teratomatous metastases in a patient with a primary embryonal carcinoma).
- The biologic behavior of nonseminomatous germ cell tumors (NSGCTs) is, in general, more aggressive than that of seminomas. Roughly 70% of seminomas present with localized (clinical stage I) disease; in contrast, 60% of NSGCTs present with advanced (stage II or III) disease. Extensive metastases may be present even with small primary lesions, particularly in the case of choriocarcinoma.
- *Clinical staging* is accomplished via physical examination, radiographic imaging of the retroperitoneum and chest, and assay of various tumor markers (see later). Clinical stages are as follows:
  - Stage I: Tumor confined to the testis
  - Stage II: Metastases limited to retroperitoneal nodes below the diaphragm
  - Stage III: Metastases outside the retroperitoneal nodes or above the diaphragm
- Several peptides may be produced by germ cell neoplasms and can be detected in body fluids by sensitive assays; AFP and HCG are the most commonly assayed. Lactate dehydrogenase, although not specific for testicular tumors, is produced by the tumor cells, and the degree of elevation provides a rough measure of tumor burden. Serum markers are of value to
  - *Evaluate* testicular masses
  - *Stage* germ cell tumors
  - Assess tumor burden
  - Monitor the response of a germ cell tumor to therapy
- Treatment includes radiation and chemotherapy, depending on the histologic type of the neoplasm (seminoma versus NSGCT) and the stage of disease; chemotherapy, in particular, has dramatically improved the prognosis of patients with NSGCT.

TUMORS OF SEX CORD—GONADAL STROMA (p. 1024)

Classification of sex cord tumors is based on differentiation into Leydig or Sertoli cells.

Leydig (Interstitial) Cell Tumors (p. 1024)

- Leydig cell tumors are relatively uncommon neoplasms, accounting for 2% of all testicular tumors; most occur between the ages of 20 and 60 years, but they may be found at any age.
- Tumors may elaborate androgens or mixtures of androgens and other steroids (estrogens, corticosteroids).
- Clinical manifestations include a *testicular mass* and changes referable to *hormonal abnormalities* (e.g., gynecomastia, sexual precocity in prepubertal boys).
- Tumors are grossly circumscribed nodules with a homogeneous, golden brown cut surface. Microscopically, they are composed of polygonal cells with abundant granular, eosinophilic cytoplasm and indistinct cell borders. Lipochrome pigment, lipid droplets, and eosinophilic Reinke crystalloids are commonly present. Ten percent of tumors invade, metastasize, or both invade and metastasize.

Sertoli Cell Tumors (Androblastoma) (p. 1024)

- These are uncommon neoplasms, composed of Sertoli cells or a mixture of Sertoli and granulosa cells.
- Tumors may elaborate androgens or estrogens but rarely in sufficient quantity to produce precocious masculinization or feminization.
- Tumors present as homogeneous gray-white–to–yellow masses of variable size. The microscopic picture is dominated by cells with tall, columnar cytoplasm, often forming cords reminiscent of immature seminiferous tubules. Most are benign; 10% demonstrate invasion, metastases, or both.

TESTICULAR LYMPHOMAS (p. 1024)

Testicular lymphomas are characterized as follows:

- They account for 5% of all testicular neoplasms; they are the most common testicular neoplasm in patients older than age 60.
- Most are diffuse, large cell, non-Hodgkin lymphomas and disseminate widely; the prognosis is accordingly poor.

MISCELLANEOUS LESIONS OF TUNICA VAGINALIS (p. 1025)

Conditions include the following:

1. *Hydrocele*: Accumulation of serous fluid within the tunica vaginalis, either secondary to generalized edema or due to incomplete closure of the processus vaginalis. A hydrocele may become secondarily infected.

2. *Hematocele*: Accumulation of blood within the tunica vaginalis secondary to trauma, torsion, or hemorrhage; a generalized bleeding diathesis; or, rarely, invasion of the tunica by neoplasms.

3. *Chylocele*: Accumulation of lymphatic fluid within the tunica vaginalis, secondary to lymphatic obstruction (e.g., in patients with elephantiasis).

4. *Spermatocele*: Local accumulation of semen in the spermatic cord, generally within a dilated duct in the head of the epididymis.

5. *Varicocele*: Local accumulation of blood within a dilated vein in the spermatic cord; more appropriately designated *cystic venous varix*.

PROSTATE (p. 1025)

Major disorders of the prostate include inflammations (prostatitis), nodular hyperplasia, and carcinoma.

Inflammations (p. 1025)

Conditions include *acute bacterial prostatitis*, *chronic bacterial prostatitis*, and *chronic abacterial prostatitis*. Diagnosis is based on microscopic examination and culture of fractionated urine specimens and prostatic secretions expressed by prostatic massage. Diagnosis of prostatitis is based on the presence of more than 15 leukocytes per high-power field in a urine fraction containing expressed prostatic secretions. In *bacterial* prostatitis, cultures of prostatic secretions are positive, and bacterial counts are significantly higher (>1 log) than in cultures of urethral and bladder urine.

ACUTE BACTERIAL PROSTATITIS (p. 1026)

- Most cases are caused by organisms associated with urinary tract infections (e.g., *E.coli* and other gram-negative rods), *Enterococcus*, or *Staphylococcus aureus*.
- Organisms reach the prostate via *direct extension* from the urethra or urinary bladder or by *lymphatic* or *hematogenous seeding* from more distant sites. This may follow *catheterization or surgical manipulation* of the urethra or prostate.
- Acute bacterial prostatitis presents with fever; chills; dysuria; and a boggy, markedly tender prostate. Diagnosis is based on clinical features and urine culture.

CHRONIC BACTERIAL PROSTATITIS (p. 1026)

- Chronic bacterial prostatitis may be asymptomatic or associated with low back pain, suprapubic and perineal discomfort, and dysuria; it is frequently associated with a history of *recurrent urinary tract infections* caused by the same organism.
- *Diagnosis* is established by demonstration of leukocytes in expressed prostatic secretions (discussed previously) and positive bacterial cultures in prostatic secretions and urine; most cases are caused by organisms similar to those responsible for acute prostatitis.
- Most cases appear *insidiously*, without a history of acute prostatitis.

CHRONIC ABACTERIAL PROSTATITIS (p. 1026)

- This is the most common form of prostatitis; it typically affects sexually active men.
- Manifestations are similar to those of chronic bacterial prostatitis but *without* a history of recurrent urinary tract infections.
- Expressed prostatic secretions contain more than 15 leukocytes per high-power field; cultures are uniformly *negative*.
- The cause is uncertain; potential pathogens include *Ureaplasma urealyticum* and *Chlamydia trachomatis*.

MORPHOLOGY

- *Acute* cases are associated with variable degrees of edema, congestion, and neutrophilic infiltration of parenchyma; neutrophils may also be present in glandular lumens. Severe cases are associated with a variable degree of parenchymal necrosis and abscess formation.

- *Chronic* cases are manifested histologically by aggregates of macrophages, lymphocytes, plasma cells, and neutrophils within prostatic parenchyma. Diagnosis should *not* be based solely on the presence of lymphocytes within the prostatic stroma because isolated lymphoid aggregates may be encountered in otherwise normal glands in elderly patients.

Nodular Hyperplasia (Benign Prostatic Hyperplasia) (p. 1027)

Nodular hyperplasia, *benign prostatic hyperplasia*, is characterized as follows:

- Benign prostatic hyperplasia is present in approximately 20% of men at age 40 years, increasing to 70% by age 60 years and to 90% by age 70 years.
- This condition is asymptomatic in most patients; a minority require surgical intervention.
- The cause is uncertain but likely related to effects of *androgens*; dihydrotestosterone, derived from testosterone via 5α-reductase activity, probably mediates prostatic growth. Estrogen (estradiol) may further sensitize the prostate to the effects of dihydrotestosterone.

MORPHOLOGY

- The gland is enlarged by nodules of variable size arising in the *inner* (periurethral) portion. Nodules arising lateral to the urethra may compress the urethral lumen to a slitlike orifice; those arising more medially may project directly into the floor of the proximal urethra, contributing to obstruction. In other cases, nodules project into the lumen of the bladder and produce a ball-valve obstruction at the mouth of the urethra. Cut surface demonstrates well-demarcated nodules involving the inner portion of the prostate.
- Microscopically, nodules are composed of variable mixtures of proliferating *glands* and *fibromuscular stroma*; cystic dilation of glandular elements is common and contributes further to nodularity. Hyperplastic glandular epithelium may form irregular papillae but retains two cell layers characteristic of normal prostatic glands. Other changes include areas of *squamous metaplasia* and *infarcts*.

CLINICAL FEATURES

- Manifestations related to *urinary tract obstruction* include
  - Urinary frequency, nocturia, and difficulty starting and stopping the stream of urine
  - Acute urinary retention
  - Chronic urinary stasis with resultant bacterial overgrowth and urinary tract infection
- Chronic obstruction may result in a variety of secondary structural alterations, including
  - Hypertrophy of the urinary bladder
  - Urinary bladder diverticula
  - Hydronephrosis

- *No relationship* has been established between nodular hyperplasia of the prostate and prostatic carcinoma.

Carcinoma of Prostate (p. 1029)

Prostatic carcinoma is characterized as follows:

- Prostatic carcinoma is the *most common* form of cancer in men; currently, it is the second leading cause of cancer death among men. Approximately 300,000 new cases are detected annually. Postmortem and surgical biopsy material indicate an even larger number of *incidental* (occult) prostatic carcinomas.
- Prostatic carcinoma occurs predominantly in men older than age 50.
- This disease is rare in Asians; it is more common in blacks than in whites.
- The *etiology* remains unknown; clinical and epidemiologic data suggest that advancing age, race, *hormonal influences*, genetic factors, and environmental factors (e.g., diet) all play a role in its development.
  - A role for *hormonal influences*, in particular, is suggested by the retardation of the growth of some prostatic carcinomas by castration or estrogen administration and by the presence of androgen receptors on both normal and neoplastic prostatic epithelium.
  - In approximately 10% of white American men, prostate cancer occurs in a familial form, and in a third of these cases, a cancer susceptibility gene has been mapped to 1q24-25.

MORPHOLOGY

- Most cases (70%) arise in the *peripheral* part of the prostate, particularly in the *posterior* region, facilitating palpation during rectal examination.
- Primary lesions characteristically are poorly demarcated, firm, gritty foci, often somewhat yellower than the adjacent nonneoplastic parenchyma. Locally advanced cases may infiltrate the seminal vesicles and urinary bladder; invasion of the rectum may occur but is uncommon. *Lymphatic metastases* occur initially in obturator nodes, followed by spread to perivesical, hypogastric, iliac, presacral, and para-aortic nodes. *Hematogenous dissemination* occurs primarily to bone, most often in the form of *osteoblastic* metastases.
- Microscopically the vast majority of prostatic carcinomas are *adenocarcinomas*, ranging from well-differentiated lesions to poorly differentiated neoplastic cells forming sheets and cords. Well-differentiated lesions may be difficult to distinguish from nodular hyperplasia in some cases but contain acini that are smaller and more *closely spaced (back to back)* than those encountered in hyperplasia and lined by a *single layer* of epithelial cells. Invasion of vascular channels and perineural spaces aids in the diagnosis of malignancy.
- Dysplastic change (prostatic intraepithelial neoplasia) is common in the epithelium of adjacent ducts and presumably represents the precursor of invasive carcinoma.

GRADING AND STAGING

- *Grading* systems attempt to define histologic criteria (degree of differentiation, nuclear atypia, growth pattern) that predict the biologic behavior of a carcinoma. Several available systems (e.g., the Gleason system) provide a good correlation between the histologic appearance of a carcinoma and the clinical stage and prognosis of the neoplasm.

- Staging of disease is also important in the selection of therapy and determination of prognosis (Fig. 21–1).
- DNA ploidy of tumor cells provides additional prognostic information (prognosis is worse for aneuploid and tetraploid tumors than for diploid tumors).

CLINICAL FEATURES

- A minority of cases are diagnosed in *asymptomatic* patients (stage A); the prognosis is generally favorable for stage A_1 cases (carcinoma identified in <5% of tissue resected) and more ominous for A_2 lesions.
- Approximately 60% of patients present with *clinically* localized disease (i.e., stage A or B), but a third of these have micrometastases and hence truly belong to stage D. Most of these do not have urinary symptoms and are detected by digital rectal examination and elevation of serum prostate-specific antigen (PSA) levels.
- Greater than 50% present with stage C or D (as assessed by clinical and pathologic staging); they usually have signs and symptoms of *urinary obstruction, local pain,* or *bone pain.* Urinary obstruction does not occur in the early stages of the disease, owing to the origin of most carcinomas in the periphery of the prostate. *Osteoblastic metastases* in elderly men are virtually diagnostic of metastatic prostatic carcinoma.

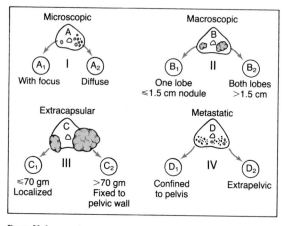

Figure 21–1

Staging of prostate cancer. *Stage A:* Microscopic, not clinically palpable tumor (A_1, with focus in <5% of tissue examined, low grade; A_2, with multiple areas, >5%, or Gleason grade higher than 4). *Stage B:* Palpable, macroscopic tumor. *Stage C:* Tumor with extracapsular extension but still clinically localized. *Stage D:* Demonstrated metastatic tumor. The tumor, node, and metastasis (TNM) staging for local tumors is indicated by Roman numerals I through IV. (Redrawn and adapted from Gittes RF: Carcinoma of the prostate. N Engl J Med 324:240, 1991. Copyright 1991, Massachusetts Medical Society. All rights reserved.)

- Rectal digital examination, supplemented by transrectal sonography or transperineal needle biopsy, is a useful method of diagnosing early prostatic carcinoma. *Lymphatic metastases* may be diagnosed by a variety of methods, including lymphangiography, computed tomography scan, and histologic examination of lymphadenectomy specimens during staging procedures. Skeletal surveys and bone scans are useful in the diagnosis of *skeletal metastases.*

- Serum *prostatic acid phosphatase* measurements are useful in the diagnosis and staging of patients with prostatic carcinoma; however, PSA measurements have largely replaced acid phosphatase levels in the management of prostate cancer. Increasing levels indicate the progression of the carcinoma.

- Serum PSA levels are elevated in patients with both localized and advanced carcinoma; lesser elevations may be seen in prostatic hyperplasia. In most laboratories, 4 ng/ml is used as a cut-off point between normal and abnormal; however, values between 4 and 10 ng/ml can occur in non-neoplastic conditions, such as nodular hyperplasia. Within this range, the ratio of free PSA to that bound to α_1-antichymotrypsin is considered useful in distinguishing prostatic cancer from benign prostatic diseases; the percentage of free PSA is lower (when compared to other prostate diseases) in prostate cancer. Monitoring PSA levels is also particularly useful in assessing response to therapy or progression of disease.

- The treatment and prognosis of prostatic carcinoma are influenced primarily by the stage of the disease. Localized (stage A or B) disease is treated primarily with *surgery, radiotherapy,* or a combination of the two, with a 15-year survival rate of 90%. *Hormonal* treatment includes orchiectomy or the administration of estrogens or synthetic analogs of luteinizing hormone–releasing hormone; it is used primarily in patients with advanced disease.

Diseases of the Female Genital Tract

VULVA (p. 1040)

Bartholin Cyst (p. 1040)

Bartholin cyst results from inflammatory occlusion of the main ducts of Bartholin vulvovaginal glands. Gonorrheal and other infections may have caused the inflammatory obstruction, which also occasionally produces abscesses that must be drained. Uninflamed cysts are lined by transitional or flattened epithelium.

Vestibular Adenitis (p. 1040)

Vestibular adenitis is a poorly understood inflammatory condition of the minor vestibular glands that results in exquisitely painful ulcerative lesions.

Non-Neoplastic Epithelial Disorders (p. 1040)

Non-neoplastic epithelial disorders refers to benign mucosal alterations of the vulva, which should be differentiated from the more ominous dysplasias and cancer (p. 1042). There are two main varieties:

1. *Lichen sclerosus* consists of yellowish blue papules or macules that eventually coalesce into thin, gray, parchment-like areas. Microscopically, there is epithelial thinning and subepithelial fibrosis (occasionally marked hyperkeratosis) and mononuclear perivascular reaction. The cause is unknown.
2. *Squamous hyperplasia* is characterized by thickened hyperplastic epithelium, hyperkeratosis, and leukocytic dermal inflammation. The lesions appear as white plaques, clinically called *leukoplakia.*

Clinically, leukoplakia can denote a benign condition (e.g., vitiligo, chronic dermatitis) or an atypical and malignant lesion. Biopsy is therefore indicated in all such lesions. Neither lichen sclerosus nor hyperplasia is considered premalignant per se. Both, however, are often found in association with vulvar carcinoma. The reason for this is unknown.

Benign Neoplasms (p. 1042)

PAPILLARY HIDRADENOMA (p. 1042)

Papillary hidradenoma is a benign tumor arising from modified apocrine sweat glands, presenting as a sharply circumscribed nodule that consists of tubular ducts lined by nonciliated columnar cells underlain by a layer of flattened myoepithelial cells.

CONDYLOMA ACUMINATUM (p. 1043)

Condyloma acuminatum is a wartlike, verrucous lesion that occurs on the vulva, perineum, vagina, and (rarely) cervix. The lesions are sexually transmitted and induced by human papillomavirus (HPV), mostly types 6 and 11.

Histologically, the lesions consist of a treelike proliferation of stratified squamous epithelium with a peculiar perinuclear vacuolization of squamous cells called *koilocytosis* attributed to a viral effect. The lesions are benign but are often multiple.

Premalignant and Malignant Neoplasms
(p. 1043)

Vulvar dysplasia, or vulvar intraepithelial neoplasia (VIN), presents as multicentric mucosal, sometimes raised, lesions characterized histologically by nuclear and epithelial atypia, increased mitoses, and lack of surface differentiation. The degree of epithelial atypia may vary and in its most severe form is called *carcinoma in situ* (VIN III, Bowen disease). HPV, mostly type 16, is present in 80 to 90% of cases of VIN and may play some causal role. Untreated, the lesions may progress to invasive carcinoma, particularly in older (>40 years) or immunosuppressed patients.

Invasive vulvar carcinomas usually occur in women older than age 60 and may arise from HPV-associated VIN lesions (one third) or as HPV-negative, well-differentiated carcinomas, the latter in association with hyperplasia, lichen sclerosus, or normal mucosa. Tumors metastasizing to regional lymph nodes indicate a poor prognosis.

EXTRAMAMMARY PAGET DISEASE (p. 1044)

Extramammary Paget disease appears as a red, crusted, sharply demarcated, maplike area, mostly on the labia majora. It is characterized histologically by large, anaplastic, sometimes vacuolated tumor cells lying singly or in small clusters *within the epidermis and its appendages.* The tumor cells are mucin positive. Most lesions are confined to the epidermis.

- *In contrast to Paget disease of the nipple (p. 1107), in which 100% of cases have an underlying ductal breast carcinoma, an underlying or adjacent sweat gland adenocarcinoma in the vulva is uncommon in vulvar Paget disease.*
- *Other vulvar carcinomas* include basal cell carcinoma, adenocarcinoma arising in Bartholin glands or sweat glands, and malignant melanoma; the last-mentioned has a poor prognosis.

VAGINA (p. 1045)

Carcinoma (p. 1045)

Primary carcinoma of the vagina is rare. The most common type is *squamous cell carcinoma*, accounting for 95% of cases. The peak incidence is between 60 and 70 years of age. From 1 to 2% of women with cervical carcinoma develop a vaginal carcinoma.

Grossly the lesions are either plaquelike or occasionally fungating. They invade the cervix and perivaginal structures, such as the urethra, urinary bladder, and rectum.

Vaginal adenocarcinomas are rare but important because of the *increased frequency of clear cell adenocarcinoma in young women whose mothers were treated with diethylstilbestrol (DES) during pregnancy (for a threatened abortion).* Only 0.14% of DES-exposed young women develop adenocarcinoma. The tumors are discovered in patients between the ages of 15 and 20 years and are composed of glands lined by vacuolated, glycogen-containing clear cells. Early detection through careful follow-up of daughters of DES-exposed women is mandatory.

Embryonal Rhabdomyosarcoma (p. 1046)

Embryonal rhabdomyosarcoma is an uncommon, highly malignant vaginal tumor consisting of embryonal rhabdomyoblasts in infants and children. The tumors are polypoid, bulky masses with grapelike clusters that may protrude from the vagina. The tumor cells are small, have oval nuclei, and have small protrusions of cytoplasm from one end (*tennis-racket* cells).

Pelvic Inflammatory Disease (p. 1039)

A variety of organisms may infect the lower and upper genital tract. *Pelvic inflammatory disease* (PID) refers to an ascending infection that begins in the vulva or vaginal glands but usually spreads upward through the entire genital tract, potentially involving all the structures of the female genital system.

There are at least three known causes of PID:

1. The *gonococcus*, the most common, as part of a gonorrheal infection
2. Postabortal and postpartum PID, usually caused by staphylococci, streptococci, coliform bacteria, or *Clostridium perfringens*
3. Chlamydial infection

Gonococcal inflammation begins in Bartholin glands, in Skene ducts and periurethral glands, or sometimes in the endocervical glands. The organisms then spread upward over the mucosal surfaces, eventually to involve fallopian tubes and tubo-ovarian regions. Gonococcal disease is characterized by an acute suppurative reaction, largely confined to the superficial mucosa and underlying submucosa.

Acute suppurative salpingitis is the most significant pathologic lesion. This may lead to salpingo-oophoritis, pyosalpinx (pus in the distended tubes), and tubo-ovarian abscesses. Untreated or poorly treated infection results in chronic salpingitis, with tubo-ovarian adhesions and fibrosis of the fallopian tube, occlusion of its lumen, and resultant infertility.

In *postabortal* and *postpartum PID*, caused by a variety of organisms, infection spreads through the uterine wall to involve the serosa and peritoneum. Bacteremia is a frequent complication of this type of PID. Other complications of PID include

1. Peritonitis
2. Intestinal obstruction
3. Infertility
4. Ectopic tubal pregnancy

CERVIX (p. 1047)

Inflammations (p. 1047)

ACUTE AND CHRONIC CERVICITIS (p. 1047)

Cervicitis can be caused either by specific infections, such as gonococci, chlamydia, *Trichomonas vaginalis*, *Candida*, and *Mycoplasma*, or by endogenous vaginal aerobes and anaerobes, including streptococci, enterococci, *Escherichia coli*, and staphylococci (nonspecific cervicitis).

- *Acute cervicitis* is most commonly encountered postpartally and is characterized by acute infiltration of neutrophils beneath the lining mucosa.
- *Chronic cervicitis* is far more common and, although it may be caused by one of the pathogens previously mentioned, is often of unknown etiology. Inflammation may lead to stenosis of cervical gland ducts and the formation of *nabothian cysts* lined by columnar epithelium. There may also be squamous metaplasia of endocervical glands.
- Chronic cervicitis is benign and is present to some degree in every cervix during the reproductive years. If the epithelial response to inflammation is exuberant *(reactive atypia)*, cervical intraepithelial neoplasia (CIN) must be excluded.

ENDOCERVICAL POLYPS (p. 1048)

Endocervical polyps are benign tumors made up of connective tissue stroma harboring dilated glands and covered by endocervical epithelium.

INTRAEPITHELIAL AND INVASIVE SQUAMOUS CELL NEOPLASIA (p. 1048)

Intraepithelial and invasive squamous cell neoplasia is one of the most common tumors in women. Its peak incidence is at 40 to 45 years old for invasive cancer. Cervical carcinoma is usually preceded by *cervical dysplasia* (CIN). The peak incidence of CIN III (carcinoma in situ) is 30 years.

The *epidemiology* of increased risk for cervical cancer and precancerous dysplasia is first intercourse at an early age, multiple sex partners, and high-risk male sex partners; the high incidence in married women and rarity in virgins and nuns suggests sexual transmission of an oncogenic agent from male to female at an early age.

Currently, HPV is being implicated as a *promoter* of cervical carcinoma. HPV infection with types 6 and 11 and other low-risk HPV predominate in condylomas and very low-grade dysplasias (CIN I). Higher-grade dysplasias (CIN II and III) predominately contain high-risk HPV types (16, 18, 31, 33, 35, 39). Cofactors could be other viruses, such as herpes type II, bacteria, tobacco, other environmental agents, or host factors.

Morphology

These cancers arise from precursor lesions. Precancerous lesions are classified according to the degree of epithelial maturation and the distribution of cytologic atypia:

- *CIN I* (including condyloma), in which the atypia is predominately in the superficial cell layers (koilocytosis), with preservation of epithelial maturation
- *CIN II*, in which the atypia is conspicuous in both the superficial and the basal cell layers, but with decreasing maturation
- *CIN III*, in which the atypia is in all cell layers but with minimal or no maturation (carcinoma in situ)

Risk of progression to malignancy is proportional to the grade of CIN, but the rates of progression are not uniform. Carcinoma in situ is clearly a precursor of invasive carcinoma, the latter developing in up to 70% of women followed without treatment after a diagnosis of carcinoma in situ.

Invasive cervical carcinoma manifests itself in three gross morphologic patterns: exophytic or fungating, ulcerating, and infiltrative. Histologically, 65% of tumors are large cell, nonkeratinizing, and moderately well differentiated. Some 25% are large and keratinizing, and the rest are composed of small, undifferentiated squamous cells.

Stages of cervical cancer are as follows:

- 0: Carcinoma in situ
- I: Carcinoma confined to the cervix
  - IA: Preclinical carcinoma diagnosed only by microscopy
  - IB: Histologically invasive carcinoma greater than 5 mm in depth
- II: Carcinoma extends beyond the cervix but not into the pelvic wall; into the vagina but not the lower third
- III: Carcinoma extends to the pelvic wall or lower third of the vagina
- IV: Carcinoma has extended beyond the pelvis

The survival of squamous cell carcinoma depends on the stage:

- 0: 100% cure
- I: 80 to 90%
- II: 75%
- III: 35%
- IV: 10 to 15%

Of cervical carcinomas, 25% consist of adenocarcinomas, adenosquamous carcinomas, and undifferentiated carcinomas.

BODY OF UTERUS AND ENDOMETRIUM
(p. 1054)

Functional Menstrual Disorders (Dysfunctional Uterine Bleeding) (p. 1055)

The most common gynecologic problem in women, during active reproductive life, is excessive bleeding during or between menstrual periods. The causes of abnormal bleeding are many and vary among women of different age groups (Table 22–1). In some instances, bleeding is a result of a well-defined organic lesion, such as a leiomyoma, carcinoma, or polyp, but the largest single group is so-called *dysfunctional uterine bleeding*, defined as abnormal bleeding in the absence of an organic lesion.

An important cause of dysfunctional uterine bleeding is lack of ovulation, called *anovulatory cycle*, which occurs as a result of

- An endocrine disorder, such as thyroid or adrenal disease or pituitary tumors

Table 22-1. CAUSES OF ABNORMAL UTERINE
BLEEDING BY AGE GROUP

Age	Cause(s)
Prepuberty	Precocious puberty (hypothalamic, pituitary, or ovarian origin)
Adolescence	Anovulatory cycle
Reproductive age	Complications of pregnancy (abortion, trophoblastic disease, ectopic pregnancy)
	Organic lesions (leiomyomas, adenomyosis, polyps, endometrial hyperplasia, carcinoma)
	Anovulatory cycle
	Ovulatory dysfunctional bleeding (e.g., inadequate luteal phase)
Perimenopause	Anovulatory cycle
	Irregular shedding
	Organic lesions (carcinoma, hyperplasia, polyps)
Postmenopause	Organic lesions (carcinoma, hyperplasia, polyps)
	Endometrial atrophy

- A primary lesion of the ovary, such as a functioning estrogenic ovarian tumor or polycystic ovaries
- A generalized metabolic disturbance, such as obesity or malnutrition
- Unexplained causes

Morphologically, in all these circumstances, the endometrium reveals a persistent proliferative pattern with possibly mild hyperplasia.

Inflammations (p. 1057)

Chronic endometritis occurs in

- Patients suffering from chronic PID
- Tuberculosis of the female genital tract
- Postabortal or postpartal endometrial cavities, usually as a result of retained gestational tissue
- Patients with intrauterine contraceptive devices

In about 15% of patients, there is no predisposing condition, and the cause is unknown. Chronic endometritis is associated clinically with abnormal endometrial bleeding and histologically with infiltration of plasma cells and macrophages into the endometrium.

Adenomyosis (p. 1057)

Adenomyosis refers to nests of endometrium in the myometrium of the uterine wall. The condition causes uterine enlargement and irregular thickening of the uterine wall and is diagnosed histologically by the finding of endometrial stroma and glands in the myometrium.

Endometriosis (p. 1057)

Endometriosis describes the presence of endometrial glands or stroma in abnormal locations *outside* the uterus. This condition involves the ovaries, uterine ligaments, rectovaginal septum, pelvic peritoneum, and laparotomy scars and, rarely, the umbilicus, vagina, vulva, or appendix.

- Endometriosis presents clinically as severe dysmenorrhea and pelvic pain and *is a common cause of female infertility.*
- Endometrial foci are under the influence of ovarian hormones and therefore undergo cyclic menstrual changes with periodic bleeding.
- A definite histologic diagnosis requires two of the three following features:
  1. Endometrial glands in the ectopic lesions
  2. Stroma in the ectopic lesions
  3. Hemosiderin pigment in the ectopic lesions

Endometrial Polyps (p. 1058)

Endometrial polyps are sessile tumors composed of endometrial glands and stroma. They may be associated with hyperestrogenism or tamoxifen therapy. These polyps are usually benign but occasionally may harbor endometrial hyperplasia or cancer.

Endometrial Hyperplasia (p. 1059)

Endometrial hyperplasia is an important cause of abnormal uterine bleeding, a result of a variety of disordered glandular and stromal growth patterns. *Although endometrial hyperplasia per se is benign, hyperplasias in which there are atypical changes in cells (cellular atypia) are precancerous lesions. Similar to endometrial adenocarcinoma* (p. 1061), hyperplasia is associated with hyperestrogenism.

Histologically, there are two general categories of hyperplasia:

1. Low-grade hyperplasias include
   - ❏ *Simple hyperplasia without atypia* (also known as *cystic* or *mild hyperplasia*), in which benign hyperplastic glands become cystically dilated
   - ❏ *Complex hyperplasia*, in which glands of varying size are crowded together into clusters *(back to back)*, but there is no cellular atypia
2. High-grade hyperplasias include *atypical hyperplasia*, in which the glandular complexity is accompanied by *cellular atypia* of the hyperplastic epithelium.

All these types produce abnormal uterine bleeding, but *only atypical hyperplasia is associated with a significant frequency of progression to carcinoma.*

Malignant Tumors of the Endometrium (p. 1061)

CARCINOMA OF ENDOMETRIUM (p. 1061)

Endometrial carcinoma accounts for 7% of all invasive cancers in women. The peak age incidence is 55 to 65 years. An increased incidence is associated with

- Obesity
- Diabetes
- Hypertension
- Infertility

There is compelling evidence that prolonged estrogen stimulation plays some causal role.

Morphology

Grossly, endometrial carcinoma presents either as a localized polypoid tumor or as a diffuse spreading lesion involving the entire endometrial surface. *Histologically*, most endometrial carcinomas are adenocarcinomas. Biologically the less aggressive tumors include well-differentiated carcinomas closely resembling normal endometrial glands (endometrioid), with *squamous*, *secretory*, or *mucinous* differentiation. More aggressive neoplasms are poorly differentiated carcinomas, including *clear cell carcinomas* and *papillary serous carcinomas*.

The patient usually presents with abnormal bleeding. The prognosis depends on the state of the disease and is excellent in patients in whom the carcinoma is confined to the corpus uteri itself.

MESENCHYMAL TUMORS (p. 1062)

Malignant mixed mesodermal (mixed müllerian) tumors are relatively rare tumors derived from primitive stromal cells, originally derived from müllerian mesoderm. They consist of malignant glandular and stromal elements; the stromal sarcomatous elements may show muscle, cartilage, and osteoid differentiation. Grossly the tumors protrude into the endometrial cavity and vagina and are bulky and polypoid.

Clinically the tumors occur in postmenopausal women and are associated with postmenopausal bleeding. They are highly malignant and have a 5-year survival rate of 25%.

Endometrial stromal tumors are varied and include the following types:

- *Benign stromal nodules*: Nodules of stromal cells within the myometrium.
- *Low-grade stromal sarcoma or endolymphatic stromal myosis*: Masses of well-differentiated endometrial stroma that penetrate lymphatic channels.
- *Endometrial stromal sarcoma*: An overtly cancerous counterpart in which the cells display atypia and mitoses. These tumors are capable of widespread metastases.

Tumors of the Myometrium (p. 1063)

LEIOMYOMA (p. 1063)

Leiomyomas are the most common tumors in women, composed of benign masses of smooth muscle cells. They are most common in women in active reproductive life and are related to estrogenic stimulation.

Morphology

Lesions are sharply circumscribed, discrete, round, firm, gray-white nodules that occur within the myometrium (intramural), beneath the serosa (subserosal), or immediately beneath the endometrium (submucosal). They may undergo cystic degeneration and calcification. Leiomyomas may be asymptomatic or may be associated with abnormal uterine bleeding, pain, urinary bladder disorders, and impaired fertility. Malignant transformation is extremely rare.

LEIOMYOSARCOMAS (p. 1064)

Leiomyosarcomas are uncommon malignancies that form bulky, fleshy masses in the uterine wall. They are differentiated from benign leiomyomas by the presence of

1. More than 10 mitoses per 10 high-power fields, with or without cellular atypia
2. Five to 10 mitoses per 10 high-power fields with cellular atypism

These tumors disseminate throughout the abdominal cavity and metastasize. The 5-year survival rate is 40%.

FALLOPIAN TUBES (p. 1065)

Inflammations (p. 1065)

Suppurative salpingitis is due to infection with pyogenic organisms, including streptococci, staphylococci, and gonococci, and is a part of PID. *Tuberculous salpingitis* is due to hematogenous spread of tuberculosis into the tubes and is sometimes associated with tuberculosis of the endometrium and peritoneum. Both forms of salpingitis are associated with infertility.

Tumors (p. 1065)

Tumors of the fallopian tubes are rare. The most common is an *adenocarcinoma*, which resembles serous adenocarcinoma of the ovary.

OVARIES (p. 1066)

Non-Neoplastic Cysts (p. 1066)

Follicular and *luteal cysts* are common, measure 1 to 8 cm in diameter, and are lined by follicular or luteinized cells. They may be asymptomatic or may rupture, causing a peritoneal reaction and pain.

Polycystic ovarian syndrome (Stein-Leventhal syndrome) is a disorder of young women and is associated with oligomenorrhea, infertility, hirsutism, sometimes obesity, persistent anovulation, and fibrotic cystic ovaries. Patients exhibit excessive production of androgens, increased conversion of androgen to estrogen, and inappropriate gonadotropin production by the pituitary. The ovaries are large; white; studded with subcortical cysts 0.5 to 1 cm in diameter; and covered by a thickened, fibrosed outer tunica. The pathogenesis is unknown, but this is an important cause of infertility.

Tumors (p. 1067)

Ovarian tumors are common forms of neoplasia in women and arise from the surface epithelium, germ cells, or sex cord–stroma (Tables 22–2 and 22–3). The malignant tumors collectively account for about 6% of all cancers in women. Risk factors include nulliparity and family history.

Table 22-2. OVARIAN NEOPLASMS (1993 WORLD HEALTH ORGANIZATION CLASSIFICATION)*

Surface epithelial-stromal tumors
 Serous tumors
  Benign (cystadenoma)
  Of borderline malignancy
  Malignant (serous cystadenocarcinoma)
 Mucinous tumors, endocervical-like and intestinal-type
  Benign
  Of borderline malignancy
  Malignant
 Endometrioid tumors
  Benign
  Of borderline malignancy
  Malignant
  Epithelial–stromal
   Adenosarcoma
   Mesodermal (müllerian) mixed tumor
  Clear cell tumors
   Benign
   Of borderline malignancy
   Malignant
  Transitional cell tumors
   Brenner tumor
   Brenner tumor of borderline malignancy
   Malignant Brenner tumor
   Transitional cell carcinoma (non-Brenner type)
Sex cord–stromal tumors
 Granulosa–stromal cell tumors
  Granulosa cell tumors
  Tumors of the thecoma-fibroma group
 Sertoli–stromal cell tumors; androblastomas
 Sex cord tumor with annular tubules
 Gynandroblastoma
 Steroid (lipid) cell tumors
Germ cell tumors
 Teratoma
  Immature
  Mature (adult)
   Solid
   Cystic (dermoid cyst)
  Monodermal (e.g., struma ovarii, carcinoid)
 Dysgerminoma
 Yolk sac tumor (endodermal sinus tumor)
 Mixed germ cell tumors
Malignant, NOS
Metastatic nonovarian cancer (from nonovarian primary)

*Modified.
NOS, not otherwise specified.

TUMORS OF SURFACE EPITHELIUM (p. 1068)

Serous Tumors (p. 1069)

Serous tumors are the most common cystic neoplasms. Cysts are lined by tall, columnar, ciliated epithelial cells and filled with serous fluid. *Serous tumors can be*

- *Benign (60%)*
- *Frankly malignant (25%)*
- *Of low malignant potential (also called borderline) (15%)*

Table 22-3. CERTAIN FREQUENCY DATA FOR
MAJOR OVARIAN TUMORS

Type	Percentage of Malignant Ovarian Tumors	Percentage That Are Bilateral
Serous	40	
Benign (60%)		25
Borderline (15%)		30
Malignant (25%)		65
Mucinous	10	
Benign (80%)		5
Borderline (10%)		10
Malignant (10%)		20
Endometrioid carcinoma	20	40
Undifferentiated carcinoma	10	—
Clear cell carcinoma	6	40
Granuloma cell tumor	5	5
Teratoma		
Benign (96%)	1	15
Malignant (4%)		Rare
Metastatic	5	>50
Others	3	—

They present grossly as large (up to 40 cm in diameter), spherical or ovoid masses. The benign cystadenomas have a smooth and glistening inner lining. The *cystadenocarcinomas* often have small, mural, solid nodularities; papillary projections; and capillary invasion.

- Twenty percent of benign tumors, 30% of borderline tumors, and approximately 66% of malignant forms are bilateral.
- In benign tumors, the lining epithelium is composed of a single layer of tall, columnar, ciliated epithelial cells with small, microscopic papillae.
- Frankly malignant cystadenocarcinomas have multilayered epithelium with many papillary areas and the formation of large, solid epithelial masses with atypical cells in places invading the stroma.
- Tumors of low malignant potential show epithelial atypia and solid areas but no obvious invasion of the stroma.

Mucinous Tumors (p. 1070)

In contrast to serous neoplasms, 80% of mucinous tumors are benign, and only 5 to 10% are malignant.

- *Grossly* the tumors tend to produce large cystic masses (exceeding the size of serous tumors), often multiloculated and filled with sticky, gelatinous fluid. Five percent of benign tumors and 20% of carcinomas are bilateral.
- *Histologically* the tumors are lined by tall, columnar epithelium showing apical mucinous vacuolation. In cystadenocarcinomas, the papillary projections are more numerous, mural nodules are present, and epithelial cells show atypia and invade the capsule.
- Borderline tumors have similar atypia but are noninvasive.
- Mucinous tumors can seed the peritoneal cavity with multiple implants, filling it with mucinous secretions to produce *pseudomyxoma peritonei*. This disorder is strongly associated with

an appendiceal primary mucinous tumor, with secondary spread to the ovaries and peritoneum.

Endometrioid Tumors (p. 1071)

Endometrioid tumors account for 20% of all ovarian cancers and are distinguished from serous and mucinous tumors by the close resemblance of tubular glands to benign or malignant endometrium. In 15 to 30% of endometrioid carcinomas, independent endometrial carcinomas appear.

Grossly the ovarian lesions are a combination of solid and cystic masses. Of these carcinomas, 40% are bilateral, and histologically the glandular patterns bear a strong resemblance to endometrial adenocarcinoma.

Brenner Tumor (p. 1072)

Brenner tumors are usually small, solid tumors that are characterized by dense fibrous stroma and nests of transitional cells resembling urinary transitional or rarely columnar epithelium. They are occasionally encountered in the wall of mucinous cystadenomas and are usually unilateral; the vast majority are benign.

Clinical Course of Surface Epithelial Tumors (p. 1073)

All large epithelial tumors cause similar symptoms, including lower abdominal pain, abdominal enlargement, and gastrointestinal and urinary complaints. Benign tumors are resected with cure. Carcinomas in time extend through the capsule and seed the peritoneal cavity, occasionally causing massive ascites.

Carcinomas grow slowly and usually are first seen when the lesions are no longer confined to the ovary. They thus have a relatively poor prognosis. Metastases occur to the other ovary, to lymph nodes, and eventually to distant organs.

GERM CELL TUMORS (p. 1073)

Germ cell tumors represent 15 to 20% of all ovarian tumors. They are similar to germ cell tumors in men and are presumed to arise from totipotential germ cells capable of differentiating into the three germ cell layers.

Teratomas (p. 1073)

Teratomas are divided into mature and monodermal (specialized) teratomas.

Mature (Benign) Teratomas. Most mature teratomas are cystic, relatively small, and known as *dermoid cysts*. They are lined by skin with adnexal structures and filled with hair-bearing sebaceous secretion. The tumors are bilateral in 10 to 15% of cases and histologically reveal epidermis, hair follicles and other skin adnexae, and tooth structures. Cartilage, bone, thyroid tissue, and other organ formations can also be found.

Dermoid cysts are clinically benign and are cured by resection. About 1% undergo malignant transformation of any of the component elements but most commonly develop into squamous cell carcinoma.

Monodermal or Specialized Teratomas. Monodermal teratomas differentiate along the line of a single abnormal tissue. The most common is struma ovarii, composed entirely of mature thyroid tissue. Another example is the ovarian carcinoid, similar to carcinoids elsewhere.

Malignant Germ Cell Tumors (p. 1075)

Malignant germ cell tumors include immature teratomas, dysgerminomas, endodermal sinus tumor, and choriocarcinomas.

Immature (Malignant) Teratomas. These rare tumors differ from benign teratomas in that embryonic (rather than adult) elements derived from more than one of the three germ layers are usually present. These tumors are most common in adolescents and young women.

- *Grossly* the tumors are bulky and predominantly solid with areas of necrosis and hemorrhage.
- *Microscopically* there are varied amounts of immature tissue differentiating toward cartilage, glands, bone, muscle, nerve, and others. Extraovarian spread of immature teratomas depends primarily on the degree of immaturity of the tissues. Most are malignant, grow rapidly, and metastasize widely. They can be cured with chemotherapy if treated early.

Dysgerminoma. Dysgerminoma is the ovarian counterpart of testicular seminoma. The tumors are uncommon and may occur in childhood or in the teens and twenties. Most are nonfunctional.

Of lesions, 80 to 90% are unilateral. The tumors are solid, yellowish white to gray-pink, and fleshy. Histologically, they consist of sheets and cords of large vesicular cells separated by scant fibrous stroma.

All dysgerminomas are malignant, but only about one third are highly aggressive. They are also radiosensitive and chemosensitive and thus have a relatively good prognosis if treated early.

Endodermal Sinus Tumor. This rare tumor is thought to be derived from multipotential embryonal carcinoma cells differentiating toward yolk sac structures. The tumor consists histologically of cystic spaces into which protrude papillary projections with central blood vessels enveloped by immature epithelium (glomeruloid). Intracellular and extracellular hyalin droplets are characteristic, some of which can be shown to be α-fetoprotein. The tumors occur in children and young women and grow rapidly and aggressively.

Choriocarcinoma. Choriocarcinoma arises in the ovary from the teratogenous development of germ cells. Most such tumors exist in combination with other germ cell tumors. *Histologically*, they are identical to the more common placental lesions and, similar to gestational choriocarcinoma, elaborate chorionic gonadotropins (p. 1076). Ovarian choriocarcinomas are highly malignant, metastasize widely, and are much more resistant to chemotherapy than their placental counterparts.

SEX CORD–STROMAL TUMORS (p. 1076)

Sex cord–stromal tumors originate either from the sex cords of the embryonic gonad or from the stroma of the ovary. The tumors are frequently functional and mostly have feminizing effects.

Granulosa–Theca Cell Tumors (p. 1076)

Granulosa–theca cell tumors are composed of various combinations of granulosa and theca cells. Two thirds occur in postmenopausal women.

- The tumors are usually unilateral and solid and have a white-yellow coloration. The granulosa cell component consists of small cuboidal-to-polygonal cells growing in cords, sheets, or strands; the thecal cell components are composed of sheets of plump spindle cells closely resembling those of a fibroma. Thecal cells contain lipid droplets.

■ Granulosa–theca cell tumors have the potential of elaborating large amounts of estrogen and thus of producing precocious sexual development and endometrial hyperplasia and predispose to endometrial carcinoma.

■ All granulosa cell tumors are potentially malignant, with clinical malignancy occurring in 5 to 25%. They are slow growing, however, and the 10-year survival rate is almost 85%. Pure thecomas are benign.

Fibromas (p. 1077)

Fibromas are common forms of ovarian neoplasms. They are usually unilateral, solid, hard, gray-white masses made up histologically of well-differentiated fibroblasts. Of fibromas, 40% are associated with hydrothorax (usually right-sided) and ascites (Meigs syndrome).

Sertoli–Leydig Cell Tumors (p. 1078)

Sertoli–Leydig cell tumors recapitulate the cells of the testes and commonly produce masculinization or defeminization. They are usually unilateral and consist histologically of tubules composed of tubular Sertoli cells or Leydig cells interspersed with stroma.

METASTATIC TUMORS (p. 1079)

Metastases of abdominal and breast tumors to the ovary are common. *Krukenberg tumor* refers to metastatic ovarian cancer (usually bilateral) composed of mucin-producing signet cells that metastasize from the gastrointestinal tract, mostly the stomach.

GESTATIONAL AND PLACENTAL DISORDERS (p. 1079)

Gestational and placental disorders can be divided into disorders of early and late pregnancy.

Ectopic Pregnancy (p. 1079)

Ectopic pregnancy denotes implantation of the embryo in any site other than the uterus—most commonly the fallopian tubes (90%) but also rarely in the ovary or abdominal cavity. Predisposing factors include PID with chronic salpingitis and peritubular adhesions, but 50% occur in apparently normal tubes.

Tubal pregnancy has one of four outcomes:

1. Intratubal hemorrhage with the formation of hematosalpinx
2. Tubal rupture with intraperitoneal hemorrhage
3. Spontaneous regression with resorption of the products of conception
4. Extrusion into the abdominal cavity (tubal abortion)

Tubal rupture is a medical emergency characterized by an acute abdomen and shock. Early diagnosis is critical and can be suggested by high human chorionic gonadotropin (HCG) levels, ultrasonographic findings, and an endometrial biopsy specimen showing decidual changes and absent chorionic villi.

Placental Inflammations and Infections
(p. 1082)

Placental infection occurs by two pathways:

1. Ascending through the birth canal
2. Hematogenous (transplacental infection)

Ascending infections are the most common. They are most often bacterial and associated with premature rupture of membranes. Bacterial infection results in chorioamnionitis characterized by a neutrophilic infiltration of the chorion and amnion and acute vasculitis in the umbilical cord.

Toxemia of Pregnancy (p. 1082)

Toxemia of pregnancy refers to a symptom complex characterized by hypertension, proteinuria, and edema (preeclampsia). Eclampsia is the severe form associated with convulsions and coma. Toxemia occurs in 6% of pregnancies, usually in the last trimester, and is most common in primiparas.

PATHOGENESIS

The pathogenesis is unclear. It is thought, however, that primary causes, such as immune or genetic factors, result in mechanical or functional obstruction of uterine spiral arterioles. One theory proposes that inadequate implantation results in decreased uteroplacental perfusion and placental ischemia. This situation results in increased production of vasoconstrictors (e.g., thromboxane, angiotensin) and decreased vasodilators (e.g., prostaglandin I_2, prostaglandin E_2), leading to arterial vasoconstriction and systemic hypertension.

- Placental ischemia also results in endothelial injury and activation of disseminated intravascular coagulation, which accounts for the decreased glomerular filtration rate and proteinuria, central nervous system disturbances, abnormal liver function tests, and fibrin thrombi and ischemia in most other organs.
- *Clinically* preeclampsia usually occurs after the 32nd week of pregnancy and is characterized by hypertension, edema, proteinuria, headaches, and visual disturbances. Mild toxemia can be controlled by bed rest, diet, and antihypertensive agents, but induction of delivery is the only definitive treatment for established preeclampsia and eclampsia.

Gestational Trophoblastic Disease (p. 1084)

Gestational trophoblastic disease is a spectrum of tumors and tumor-like conditions of progressive malignant potential, characterized by proliferation of trophoblastic tissue. The lesions include hydatidiform mole (complete and partial), invasive mole, and choriocarcinoma.

HYDATIDIFORM MOLE (p. 1085)

Hydatidiform mole is characterized by cystic swelling of the chorionic villi, accompanied by variable trophoblastic prolifera-

Table 22–4. FEATURES OF COMPLETE VERSUS PARTIAL HYDATIDIFORM MOLE

Feature	Complete Mole	Partial Mole
Karyotype	46, XX(46,XY)	Triploid
Villous edema	All villi	Some villi
Trophoblast proliferation	Diffuse; circumferential	Focal; slight
Atypia	Often present	Absent
Serum HCG	Elevated	Less elevated
HCG in tissue	+ + + +	+
Behavior	2% choriocarcinoma	Rare choriocarcinoma

HCG, Human chorionic gonadotropin.

tion; this is a common precursor of choriocarcinoma. Moles present in the fourth or fifth month of pregnancy with vaginal bleeding. There are two types of benign noninvasive moles, *complete* and *partial*, that can be differentiated by histologic, cytogenetic, and flow cytometric studies (Table 22–4).

- *Grossly*, moles consist of masses of thin-walled, translucent, cystic, grapelike structures. Fetal parts are rarely seen in complete moles and are more common in partial moles.
- *Microscopically*, complete moles show hydropic swelling of villi, inadequate vascularization of villi, and significant trophoblastic proliferation. Partial moles show only focal edema and focal and slight trophoblastic proliferation. Most complete moles have diploid karyotypes, whereas partial moles are usually triploid.
- Moles can be diagnosed by ultrasound examination and by quantitative analysis of serum HCG, revealing levels exceeding those produced by a normal pregnancy of similar age. Once complete moles are curetted, 80 to 90% give no further difficulty, 10% develop into invasive moles, and 2.5% develop into choriocarcinoma. Follow-up with periodic determination of HCG is essential in these patients.

INVASIVE MOLE (p. 1087)

An invasive mole penetrates and may even perforate the uterine wall, marked by active proliferation of both cytotrophoblasts and syncytiotrophoblasts. It does not metastasize. It is associated with a persistent elevated HCG level and varying degrees of luteinization of the ovaries. The tumor responds well to chemotherapy.

CHORIOCARCINOMA (p. 1087)

Choriocarcinoma is a malignant tumor arising in 1:20,000 to 1:30,000 pregnancies in the United States, but it is much more common in some Asian and African countries. *Of lesions, 50% arise in hydatidiform mole, 25% in previous abortions, 22% in normal pregnancies, and the rest in ectopic pregnancies.*

- *Grossly* the tumor is large, soft, yellowish white, and fleshy with areas of necrosis and hemorrhage.
- *Histologically,* it consists of abnormal proliferations of both cytotrophoblasts and syncytiotrophoblasts. The tumor invades

the underlying endometrium; penetrates blood vessels and lymphatics; and metastasizes to the lungs, bone marrow, liver, and other organs.

■ Clinically, choriocarcinomas are manifested by vaginal bleeding and discharge that may appear in the course of an apparently normal pregnancy, after a miscarriage, or after a curettage. HCG titers are elevated to levels above those seen in hydatidiform mole. When the condition is first discovered, widespread metastases may have already occurred.

■ *Gestational choriocarcinomas are highly sensitive to chemotherapy,* and cures can be achieved even in patients with metastatic disease.

PLACENTAL SITE TROPHOBLASTIC TUMOR
(p. 1089)

Placental site trophoblastic tumor is a rare tumor composed of proliferating *intermediate trophoblasts* that are larger than cytotrophoblasts but mononuclear rather than syncytial. The lesion differs from that of choriocarcinoma by the absence of cytotrophoblastic elements and low levels of HCG production. Most are locally invasive only. Malignant variants are distinguished by a high mitotic index, extensive necrosis, and local spread. About 10% result in metastases and death.

Diseases of the Breast

The preponderance of breast lesions occur in women. In men, the rudimentary breast appears to be resistant to pathogenetic stimuli, although breast lesions, including carcinoma, can occur. Breast lesions present most commonly as palpable masses or mammographic abnormalities and less commonly as inflammatory lesions or nipple secretions.

DISORDERS OF DEVELOPMENT (p. 1096)

Disorders of development are as follows:

- Supernumerary nipples or breast tissue occurs along the milk line in some women and undergo hyperplasia during pregnancy. They are rarely the site of breast cancers.
- Congenital inversion of the nipple may mimic inversion owing to retraction by an invasive carcinoma.
- Accessory axillary breast tissue is uncommon but may be the site of origin of tumors or with lactation and enlargement be confused with a lymphoid malignancy or metastasis from a breast cancer.

INFLAMMATIONS (p. 1096)

Inflammatory conditions include the following:

- *Acute mastitis and breast abscess* are common complications of breast-feeding after the development of cracks or fissures of the nipple and infection by skin bacteria.
- *Periductal mastitis* (recurrent subareolar abscess, squamous metaplasia of lactiferous ducts) presents as a painful subareolar mass secondary to an inflammatory response to keratin debris from ruptured ducts. It is often complicated by formation of a periareolar fistulous tract. Appropriate treatment includes surgical excision of the involved ducts. Almost all patients have a history of smoking.
- *Mammary duct ectasia* usually presents as a poorly defined periareolar mass with thick nipple secretion, which can mimic carcinoma. It is characterized by inspissation of secretions, duct dilation, and periductal inflammation and is most common in women in their forties to fifties. It is not associated with tobacco use.
- *Fat necrosis*, after trauma, surgery, or radiation therapy, is followed by inflammation and fibrosis and can present as a hard

mass grossly resembling cancer or as mammographic calcifications.

- *Granulomatous mastitis* can be associated with systemic diseases (sarcoid, Wegener granulomatosis) or be primary in the breast (granulomatous lobular mastitis).
- *Silicone breast implants* may incite a chronic inflammatory and fibrotic response, particularly if there is seepage or rupture. A definite association with systemic rheumatic diseases has not yet been established.
- *Inflammatory carcinoma* mimics inflammation by obstruction of dermal lymphatics by tumor emboli. It should always be suspected when mastitis appears in nonlactating women.

FIBROCYSTIC CHANGES (p. 1098)

Fibrocystic change refers to a heterogeneous group of morphologic patterns within the breast showing various combinations of cyst formation, apocrine metaplasia, adenosis, and fibrosis after cyst rupture. These alterations may produce palpable lumps but are more commonly so mild as to be clinically silent.

In unselected autopsies, grossly apparent changes were present in 20% of individuals, but microscopic changes were visible in 59%. These changes are unusual before adolescence, are most common between the ages of 20 and 40 years, peak in perimenopausal years, and rarely develop after menopause.

The pathogenesis remains obscure. Relative or absolute estrogen excess and progesterone deficiency appear important, but abnormal end-organ responses to hormones may also be contributory. There are three dominant morphologic patterns:

1. The cysts are usually multifocal and bilateral and may yield a shotty texture.
2. Fibrosis occurs when cysts rupture, releasing secretory debris into the stroma resulting in inflammation and fibrosis. This change contributes to the palpable firmness of the breast.
3. Adenosis is an increase in the number of acini per lobule. The acini often become dilated and may contain calcifications.

In the absence of proliferative breast disease (see later), the above-mentioned fibrocystic changes do not increase the risk of developing cancer. These changes come to clinical attention when they mimic cancer by producing palpable lumps, mammographic densities or calcifications, or nipple discharge. About half of all surgical operations on the breast are due to fibrocystic changes.

PROLIFERATIVE BREAST DISEASE (p. 1100)

The changes discussed here under *proliferative breast disease* are sometimes included within the spectrum of fibrocystic change. Proliferative changes in the breast, however, are associated with an increased risk of cancer and have been identified by examining benign breast biopsy specimens of women who later developed cancer. These changes fall into three groups:

1. Moderate to florid *epithelial cell hyperplasia* is defined by an increase in the number of cells above the basement membrane ranging from two to at least four cells deep. It may be due to increased proliferation or, more likely, failure of cells to undergo apoptosis. *Atypical ductal hyperplasia* refers to lesions that closely resemble ductal carcinoma in situ (DCIS). Such changes are worri-

some particularly because about 40% are clonal, and sometimes multiple clones are present. *Atypical lobular rather than ductal hyperplasia* refers to lesions within acini that resemble lobular carcinoma in situ (LCIS) but are less extensive. Extension of the hyperplasia into the ducts is associated with an increased risk of invasive cancer.

2. *Sclerosing adenosis* is characterized by an increase in acini to at least twofold over a normal lobule with compression and distortion of the acini by the surrounding stroma.

3. *Small duct papillomas* occur deep within the breast and are characterized by cells covering fibrovascular cores extending into duct lumens.

Proliferative breast disease increases the risk for the subsequent development of cancer:

- *No increased risk of carcinoma*: Cysts, apocrine metaplasia, adenosis, mild epithelial hyperplasia
- *Slightly increased risk, 1.5-fold to 2-fold*: Epithelial hyperplasia (moderate to florid), sclerosing adenosis, papillomas
- *Moderately increased risk, 4-fold to 5-fold*: Atypical ductal hyperplasia, atypical lobular hyperplasia

The vast majority of women with these changes never develop breast cancer. When carcinoma does develop, both breasts are at equal risk.

TUMORS (p. 1102)

Stromal Tumors (p. 1102)

FIBROADENOMA (p. 1102)

Fibroadenoma is the most common benign tumor of the female breast, occurring most often during the reproductive period. Some appear after cyclosporine therapy. Fibroadenomas present clinically as well-circumscribed palpable masses or ovoid mammographic densities. During pregnancy, fibroadenomas may grow in size and sometimes infarct. In older women, fibroadenomas may calcify and present as a cluster of mammographic calcifications. Although benign, they may be associated with proliferative changes and incur a slightly increased risk of cancer.

Grossly, these lesions appear as solitary white, rubbery nodules from 1 to 10 cm in diameter. *Histologically*, these are biphasic lesions consisting of stroma and epithelium lining cystic spaces sometimes compressed by the stroma. They are thought to arise from breast-specific lobular stroma and thus are found only in the breast. The stroma is often clonal and may have cytogenetic aberrations, whereas the epithelial component is polyclonal. Other benign, circumscribed mass-forming lesions include *tubular adenoma, lactating adenoma,* pseudoangiomatous stromal hyperplasia, and fibrous tumors.

Phyllodes Tumor (p. 1103)

Phyllodes tumors, similar to fibroadenomas, arise from specialized breast stroma and are biphasic. They usually present as palpable masses in women in their fifties to sixties, 10 to 20 years older than women with fibroadenomas. The stroma frequently overgrows the epithelial component forming clefts and slits creating leaflike fronds of tumor (*phyllodes* means leaflike). Phyllodes tumors can be large, causing breast distortion and pressure necrosis of overlying skin. Their cellularity, mitotic activity, stromal overgrowth, and invasiveness differentiate them from fibroadenomas.

Most phyllodes tumors behave in a benign fashion and can be cured by local excision. A few may recur locally after excision, and rare tumors are highly malignant and can metastasize hematogenously, usually to the lungs. Only the stromal component metastasizes. Changes suggesting malignant potential include cytologic pleomorphism, high mitotic activity, overgrowth of the stromal component, invasion into adjacent breast tissue, and sarcomatous differentiation.

Sarcomas (p. 1104)

All types of connective tissue sarcomas (e.g., leiomyosarcoma, chondrosarcoma, osteosarcoma) can occur rarely in the breast. Sarcomatous differentiation can also occur in phyllodes tumors and carcinomas (*metaplastic carcinomas*). Angiosarcomas may arise spontaneously, after radiation therapy for breast cancer, or in the skin of a chronically edematous arm after mastectomy (Stewart-Treves syndrome).

Epithelial Tumors (p. 1104)

LARGE DUCT PAPILLOMA (p. 1104)

Papillary growths within a lactiferous duct are usually solitary, rarely can be palpated as a mass, and usually present as unilateral serous or bloody nipple discharge. When solitary, they are benign, albeit clonal. When multiple papillomas are present, they impose an increased risk of cancer. Although nipple discharge is most commonly associated with benign papillomas, it can be associated with carcinoma in 7% of women younger than 60 years of age and in 30% of older women.

CARCINOMA OF BREAST (p. 1104)

Carcinomas of the breast arise from epithelial cells. Currently, about one in nine women develops breast cancer during her lifetime, and about one third succumb to the disease.

Incidence and Epidemiology

Breast cancer is found more commonly in the following groups:

- Women with a strong family history of breast carcinoma in premenopausal women: The risk increases in proportion to the number of first-degree relatives with cancer. Specific genes linked to genetic inheritance are *BRCA1*, *BRCA2*, p53 (Li-Fraumeni syndrome), ATM (ataxia-telangiectasia), and the gene causing Cowden disease. *BRCA1* and *BRCA2* account for the majority of hereditary cancers. Genetic inheritance is associated with fewer than 10% of all breast cancer cases, however.
- Older women: Risk continues to increase with age. Carcinoma rarely develops before the age of 25 years except in some familial cases. The average age at diagnosis is 64 years.
- Women with proliferative breast disease, particularly when changes are atypical.
- Women with carcinoma of the contralateral breast or endometrium.

- Women with radiation exposure at a young age (e.g., in the treatment of Hodgkin disease).
- Women in United States and Northern Europe as compared to women in Asia and other countries.
- Women who have an early menarche and late menopause (long reproductive life).
- Nulliparous women as compared to multiparous women (unremitting exposure to ovarian cycles).
- Women having their first child after the age of 30.
- Obese postmenopausal women: Attributed to synthesis of estrogens in fat depots. Obesity in younger women *decreases* the risk because of an association with anovulatory cycles.

The risk of breast cancer from exogenous estrogens for menopausal symptoms or oral contraception remains controversial. Any associated risk is likely to be small.

Etiology and Pathogenesis

Although the cause remains unknown, the following influences appear important:

- *Genetic factors*: Their role is supported by the higher incidence in first-degree relatives of carcinoma patients. The majority of women in families with *BRCA1* and *BRCA2* mutations associated with breast cancer develop the disease.
- *Hormone imbalances*: Many well-established risk factors (e.g., long duration of reproductive life, nulliparity, obesity, late age at first child) are associated with increased exposure to endogenous estrogens. Some carcinomas secrete autocrine growth factors, such as epidermal growth factor, transforming growth factor, and others, in response to estrogen, which may lead to tumor progression.
- *Environmental influences*: Large differences in the incidence of breast cancer in different countries and the increase in breast cancer incidence in immigrants to high-risk countries suggest that environmental influences play a role and that some of these influences may be modifiable. Dietary fat has been implicated, but specific foods that can modify risk have not been identified. Mouse mammary tumor virus can cause breast cancer in suckling mice, but a similar oncogenic virus in humans has not been demonstrated. Environmental pollutants that may have estrogenic effects in humans are under intense scrutiny but have not yet been proven to be risk factors.

Cellular Changes in Breast Cancer Progression

Numerous cellular changes are found in breast carcinomas, including increased expression of oncogenes (e.g., c-*erb*-B2 [Her2/neu], INT2, c-*ras*, c-*myc*); decreased expression or function of tumor-suppressor genes (e.g., NM23, p53, RB); alterations in cell structure (e.g., increased expression of vimentin, decreased expression of fodrin); loss of cell adhesion (e.g., E-cadherin, integrins); increased expression of cell cycle proteins (e.g., cyclins, Ki-67, proliferating cell nuclear antigen); increased expression of angiogenic factors (e.g., vascular endothelial growth factor, fibroblast growth factor); and increased expression of proteases (e.g., cathepsin D, stromelysins). All of these changes occur in some, but not all, carcinomas, suggesting that the malignant phenotype is due to an accumulation of a variety of changes and not an orderly progression.

Distribution and Classification

Distribution of breast carcinomas is as follows:

- About 50% in the upper outer quadrant
- 10% in each of the remaining quadrants
- 20% in the central or subareolar region

The current classification of the major types of breast carcinoma is as follows:

- In situ (noninvasive): 15 to 30% of all cancers
  - DCIS (intraductal carcinoma)
  - LCIS (lobular carcinoma)
- Invasive (infiltrating): 70 to 85% of all cancers
  - Invasive ductal carcinoma (no special type [NST]): 79%
  - Invasive lobular carcinoma: 10%
  - Medullary carcinoma: 2%
  - Colloid carcinoma (mucinous carcinoma): 2%
  - Tubular or cribriform carcinoma: 6%
  - Papillary carcinoma: 1%

Before mammographic screening, fewer than 5% of carcinomas were detected while in situ. In screened populations, almost half of all carcinomas are detected before invasion has occurred. Because not all women undergo screening and some carcinomas occur in young women before screening, however, the majority of cancers are invasive at the time of detection.

In Situ (Noninvasive) Carcinoma

Ductal Carcinoma in Situ. DCIS is characterized by proliferations of tumor cells within ducts and lobules that are confined by the basement membrane. DCIS has been traditionally classified by morphologic patterns into solid, cribriform, papillary, micropapillary, and comedo types. New classification systems are being developed that use nuclear grade and the presence or absence of necrosis.

- DCIS can spread from lactiferous ducts into the contiguous skin of the nipple without violating the basement membrane barrier. This is termed *Paget disease of the nipple*. The nipple appears eczematous or ulcerated.
- DCIS is most commonly detected as mammographic calcifications. It rarely presents as a palpable mass, a mammographic density, or nipple secretion.
- The natural history of DCIS is known only from the study of small cohorts of women with missed diagnoses of DCIS who were treated with biopsy alone. Of these women, with small noncomedo DCIS, about one third develop invasive carcinoma when followed for 30 years. The carcinomas arise in the same breast and the same quadrant as the DCIS. It is likely that cases of higher-grade or more extensive DCIS become invasive at a higher rate. The current treatment of DCIS is aimed at eradicating the lesion by surgery (mastectomy) or surgery and radiation (breast conservation).

Lobular Carcinoma in Situ. LCIS is characterized by a proliferation of small, uniform cells within ducts and lobules that fill, distend, or distort at least 50% of the acinar units of a single lobule and are confined by the basement membrane.

- LCIS is always an incidental finding because it never forms a mass and is rarely associated with calcifications.
- Invasive carcinoma develops in 25 to 30% of women with LCIS if followed for 20 years. In contrast to DCIS, both breasts are at equal risk. Thus, surgical treatment requires bilateral mastectomy. In most cases, women can be followed with mammography and without surgery.

Invasive (Infiltrating) Carcinoma

Invasive Ductal Carcinoma. This type includes the majority of carcinomas that cannot be classified as any other subtype and so are called no special type (NST). *Histologically* the tumor is composed of malignant cells disposed in cords, often single-file, solid cell nests, tubules, anastomosing sheets, and various mixtures of all these. These cells are dispersed in a dense stromal reaction responsible for the hard consistency of the tumor (scirrhous carcinoma).

Invasive Lobular Carcinoma. This type accounts for 5 to 10% of invasive carcinomas. It tends to be more frequently multifocal and bilateral than other breast carcinomas.

Tumors can be scirrhous or can have a diffusely invasive pattern that is difficult to detect clinically and mammographically. Histologically the tumor is composed of small, uniform cells forming strands of infiltrating tumor cells, sometimes arranged concentrically about ducts *(bull's eye lesions).*

Lobular carcinomas more frequently metastasize to cerebrospinal fluid (carcinomatous meningitis), serosal surfaces, ovary and uterus, and bone marrow than other subtypes.

Medullary Carcinoma. This type accounts for 1 to 5% of breast carcinomas and occurs in a younger group than women with other forms of breast cancer. This type is found disproportionately in women carrying *BRCA1* mutations and accounts for 13% of carcinomas in this cohort.

Medullary carcinoma presents as a relatively large, soft, well-circumscribed tumor averaging 2 to 3 cm in diameter. Histologically, medullary carcinoma shows

1. Absence of desmoplasia
2. A moderately dense lymphoplasmacytic infiltrate
3. Large, pleomorphic tumor cells growing in solid, syncytium-like, anastomosing masses

Colloid or Mucinous Carcinoma. This type accounts for about 1 to 6% of breast carcinomas, is slow growing, and occurs most commonly in older women. Morphologically, it appears as soft, gelatinous masses composed of lakes of lightly staining mucin, within which are floating small islands of well-differentiated tumor cells.

Tubular or Cribriform Carcinoma. Tubular carcinomas account for up to 10% of carcinomas less than 1 cm in size. They are usually detected as mammographic spiculated masses. The entire tumor comprises well-formed tubules with low-grade nuclei. This histologic type has the best prognosis.

Papillary Carcinoma. This is a rare type of carcinoma representing fewer than 1% overall. Papillary architecture is much more common in in situ lesions.

Mammographic Appearance of Breast Carcinoma

The principal radiologic signs of breast carcinoma are the following:

- *Densities*: Most neoplasms grow as solid masses and are radiologically more dense than the intermingled connective and adipose tissue of the normal breast. Invasive carcinomas most commonly present as a spiculated density with irregular borders. Postinflammatory changes or complex sclerosing lesions can rarely also have this appearance. Well-circumscribed densities with smooth borders are most often benign lesions, such as cysts or fibroadenomas. Invasive carcinomas (most commonly medullary or colloid carcinoma) can also be well-circumscribed.
- *Architectural distortion*: The normal parenchymal pattern is altered when compared with the remainder of the breast, the opposite breast, or prior mammograms. This change may be due to a diffusely invasive carcinoma that infiltrates in and around adipose tissue without replacing it. This appearance is most commonly seen with lobular carcinomas.
- *Calcifications*: Calcium deposits form on either secretory material or necrotic debris. Calcifications associated with malignancy are more commonly small, irregular, numerous, and clustered or linear and branching. DCIS is the most common malignancy associated with calcifications.
- *Changes over time*: The inexorable growth of malignancies may be seen by comparison of sequential mammograms for developing densities, architectural distortion, or increases in the number of calcifications.

Some carcinomas, even if palpable, may not be detectable by mammography. The principal reasons are

- Surrounding dense stroma (especially in younger women)
- Absence of calcifications
- Small size
- Location close to the chest wall or in the periphery of the breast

Thus, failure to image a palpable mass by mammography is not a useful sign of benignancy.

Features Common to All Invasive Carcinomas

Local invasion into adjacent structures produces tumor fixation, retraction of the nipple, and dimpling of the skin. Extensive lymphatic blockage by tumor can result in lymphedema, causing the breast skin to resemble an orange peel *(peau d'orange)*. Inflammatory carcinomas present as a markedly enlarged erythematous and swollen breast. Although inflammation is absent, these diffusely infiltrating carcinomas mimic inflammatory changes by involving numerous dermal lymphatics and rarely form a palpable mass.

About one third of breast carcinomas present with lymph node metastases. Although any breast cancer can metastasize to axillary, supraclavicular, or internal mammary nodes, tumors in the outer quadrant tend to metastasize to axillary nodes, whereas tumors in the inner quadrants and center of the breast tend to metastasize to internal mammary nodes. Other favored sites of spread are skin, bones, lung, liver, and adrenals.

Clinical Course

Although the course of any specific breast cancer patient cannot be predicted with certainty, there are a number of prognostic factors that are closely associated with outcome. The most important of these (tumor size, locally advanced disease, lymph node metastases, and distant metastases) are used for clinical staging. On average, cancers are 2- to 3-cm palpable masses when first diagnosed, and about one third have already metastasized to axillary or other nodes.

- Lymph node metastases are the most important prognostic factor. Prognosis worsens as the number of involved nodes increases:
  - With no involvement, the 10-year survival is 70 to 80%.
  - If 10 or more nodes are involved, the 10-year survival is 10 to 15%.
- Locally advanced disease (invasion into skin or chest wall) confers a poor prognosis.
- Tumor size affects prognosis: The larger the tumor, the worse the prognosis.
- Histologic subtypes: All special subtypes have a better prognosis when compared with NST cancers, with tubular and colloid carcinomas having the best prognosis.
- Tumor grade: Poorly differentiated carcinomas have a worse prognosis.
- Estrogen/progesterone receptor status: Carcinomas with hormone receptors have a slightly better prognosis and can often be treated with less toxic hormonal therapies.
- Lymphovascular invasion can be seen around carcinomas within the breast and is a poor prognostic factor in women without lymph node metastases. Involvement of dermal lymphatics is associated with the clinical appearance of inflammatory carcinoma and bodes a poor prognosis with 3-year survival only 3 to 10%.
- Proliferation, measured by a variety of different methods, is a poor prognostic factor if higher than average.
- DNA content, if abnormal (i.e., increased over that found in normal diploid cells) is a poor prognostic factor.
- Expression of oncogenes (e.g., c-*erb*-B2) and loss of expression of tumor-suppressor genes are associated with poor prognosis and are often found in carcinomas with other poor prognostic factors.
- Angiogenesis is increased around and within carcinomas and is a poor prognostic factor if the number of vessels is above average.
- Proteases may be involved in invasion by degrading extracellular matrix and may be a poor prognostic factor.

Current therapeutic approaches include local and regional control, using combinations of surgery (mastectomy or breast conservation—*lumpectomy*) and postoperative radiation, and systemic control, using hormonal treatment, chemotherapy, or both. Newer therapeutic strategies include inhibition (by pharmacologic agents or specific antibodies) of membrane-bound growth factor receptors (e.g., c-*erb*-B2), stromal proteases, and inhibition of angiogenesis.

MALE BREAST (p. 1117)

Gynecomastia, or enlargement of the male breast, is of chief importance as an indicator of an imbalance between estrogens and androgens. It may be found during puberty, in Klinefelter syndrome, as a manifestation of hormone-producing tumors (e.g., Leydig cell or Sertoli cell tumors), in men with cirrhosis, or as a side effect of drugs (e.g., marijuana, anabolic steroids, some psychoactive agents). Histologically, there is proliferation of both epithelial and stromal components.

Carcinoma of the male breast is rare. Risk factors and prognostic factors are similar to those of women. Male breast cancer is strongly associated with *BRCA2* in some families but has not been associated with *BRCA1*.

The same histologic types of breast cancer are found in men and women. Because of the scant amount of surrounding breast tissue in men, carcinomas tend to invade skin and chest wall earlier and present at higher stages. Matched by stage, prognosis is similar in men and women.

Diseases of the Endocrine System

The endocrine system orchestrates a state of metabolic equilibrium, or *homeostasis*, between the various organs of the body. Signaling by extracellular secreted molecules can be classified into several types: autocrine, paracrine, or endocrine, based on the distance over which the signal acts. In *endocrine* signaling, the secreted molecules, or hormones, act on target cells distant from their site of synthesis. An endocrine hormone is frequently carried by the blood from its site of release to its target. Increased activity of the target tissue, in turn, can down-regulate the activity of the gland secreting the stimulating hormone, a process known as *feedback inhibition*. Hormones can be classified into several broad categories, which act on different types of receptors:

- *Signaling molecules which interact with cell-surface receptors.* This large class of compounds is composed of two groups:
  1. Peptide hormones, such as growth hormone and insulin
  2. Small molecules, such as epinephrine and histamine, that are derived from amino acids and function as hormones
- *Steroid hormones that diffuse across the plasma membrane and interact with intracellular receptors*, which, in turn, activate expression of specific genes.

Endocrine diseases can be generally classified as

- Diseases of *underproduction* or *overproduction* of hormones and their resulting metabolic and clinical consequences.
- Diseases associated with the development of *mass lesions*. The mass lesions may be nonfunctional, or they may be associated with overproduction or underproduction of hormones.

PITUITARY GLAND (p. 1122)

The pituitary gland is located at the base of the brain, where it lies nestled within the confines of the sella turcica. Along with the hypothalamus, the pituitary gland plays a critical role in the regulation of most of the other endocrine glands. It is composed of two morphologically and functionally distinct components:

1. Anterior lobe *(adenohypophysis)*
2. Posterior lobe *(neurohypophysis)*

Diseases of the pituitary can be divided into those that primarily affect the anterior lobe and those that predominantly affect the posterior lobe.

- Diseases of the *anterior pituitary* may come to clinical attention because of *endocrine effects*, such as increased or decreased secretion of hormones, designated *hyperpituitarism* or *hypopituitarism*. This secretory activity is normally regulated by hypothalamic-releasing factors or an inhibitor factor controlling release of prolactin. In most cases, *hyperpituitarism* is intrinsic to the pituitary and caused by a functional adenoma within the anterior lobe. *Hypopituitarism* may be caused by a variety of destructive processes, including ischemic injury, radiation, inflammatory reactions, and nonfunctioning neoplasms. In addition to endocrine abnormalities, diseases of the anterior pituitary may also be manifested by *local mass effects*, including radiographic enlargement of the sella turcica, visual field abnormalities resulting from encroachment of mass lesions on the visual pathways, and evidence of increased intracranial pressure.

■ Diseases of the *posterior pituitary* may come to clinical attention because of increased or decreased secretion of one of its products (e.g., *antidiuretic hormone* [ADH]).

Hyperpituitarism and Pituitary Adenomas
(p. 1123)

Excess production of anterior pituitary hormones is most often caused by an adenoma in the anterior lobe. Less commonly, excess production is due to primary hypothalamic disorders and *rarely* by carcinomas of the anterior pituitary. Hormones most commonly produced by functional adenomas include *prolactin (Prl), growth hormone (GH), and adrenocorticotropic hormone (ACTH)*. *Thyroid-stimulating hormone (TSH)*–secreting and *gonadotropin (follicle-stimulating hormone [FSH] or luteinizing hormone [LH])*–secreting adenomas are *rare*. Functional pituitary adenomas are usually composed of a single cell type and produce a single predominant hormone, although some adenomas generate more than one hormone, most commonly *GH* and *Prl*. Pituitary adenomas may be nonfunctional and cause hypopituitarism by destroying adjacent native anterior pituitary parenchyma.

Pituitary adenomas are responsible for about 10% of intracranial neoplasms and microadenomas are discovered in up to 25% of routine autopsies. They are usually found in adults with a peak incidence from the thirties to fifties.

Most pituitary adenomas are monoclonal in origin, even those that are plurihormonal, suggesting that most arise from a single somatic cell. Molecular studies demonstrate mutations constitutively activating guanosine triphosphate (GTP)–binding proteins in subsets of pituitary adenomas.

MORPHOLOGY

Pituitary adenomas can be divided into *microadenomas* (<10 mm in diameter) and *macroadenomas* (>10 mm in diameter). They are usually solitary and, in early stages, form discrete soft masses within the sella. Larger adenomas may compress or even infiltrate adjacent structures (e.g., cavernous sinus, base of brain, sphenoid bone).

Microscopically, adenomas are generally composed of uniform or *monomorphous* cells, in contrast to the normal pluricellular anterior pituitary. The neoplastic cells may be arrayed in sheets, cords, nests, or papillae and have only a scanty reticulin network. Nuclear atypia may be present but does not imply malignancy as well as necrosis and hemorrhage. Ultrastructurally, variable numbers of membrane-bound *secretory granules* are present in the cytoplasm of most cells.

PROLACTINOMAS (p. 1125)

Prolactinomas are the *most common* functional pituitary tumor, accounting for about 30% of all adenomas. Most are *macroadenomas*, composed of *sparsely granulated* acidophilic or chromophobic cells. Immunostaining for Prl is required to demonstrate the secretory product in histologic sections. Prl secretion by these adenomas is characterized by its *efficiency*—even microadenomas secrete sufficient Prl to cause hyperprolactinemia—and by its *proportionality*—serum Prl concentrations tend to correlate with the size of the adenoma.

Clinical manifestations of increased serum levels of Prl, or *prolactinoma*, are amenorrhea, galactorrhea, loss of libido, and infertility. The diagnosis of a pituitary adenoma is made more readily in women than in men because of the sensitivity of menses to disruption by hyperprolactinemia. This tumor underlies almost a quarter of cases of amenorrhea. In contrast, in men and older women, the hormonal manifestations may be subtle, allowing the tumors to reach considerable size before being detected clinically.

Hyperprolactinemia may result from causes other than Prl-secreting pituitary adenomas. Physiologic hyperprolactinemia occurs in pregnancy, in which serum Prl levels increase throughout pregnancy, reaching a peak at delivery. Pathologic hyperprolactinemia can also result from *lactotroph hyperplasia*, such as when there is interference with normal dopamine inhibition of Prl secretion. This inhibition may occur as a result of damage to the dopaminergic neurons of the hypothalamus, pituitary stalk section (e.g., owing to head trauma), or drugs that block dopamine receptors on lactotroph cells. Any mass in the suprasellar compartment may disturb the normal inhibitory influence of the hypothalamus on Prl secretion, resulting in hyperprolactinoma—a phenomenon called the *stalk effect*. *A mild elevation in serum Prl in a patient with a pituitary adenoma, therefore, does not necessarily indicate a Prl-secreting tumor.*

GROWTH HORMONE (SOMATOTROPH CELL) ADENOMAS (p. 1126)

GH-secreting tumors are the second most common type of functioning adenoma and are responsible for the vast majority of examples of *excess GH*, with associated acromegaly or gigantism. Microscopically, GH-containing adenomas are composed of granulated cells, which appear acidophilic or chromophobic in routine sections. Immunocytochemical stains demonstrate GH within the cytoplasm of the neoplastic cells. In addition, small amounts of immunoreactive Prl are often present.

Persistent hypersecretion of GH stimulates the hepatic secretion of insulin-like growth factor-I (IGF-I), which causes many of the clinical manifestations. If somatotropic adenomas appear in children before the epiphyses have closed, the elevated levels of GH result in *gigantism*. This condition is characterized by a generalized increase in body size, with disproportionately long arms and legs. If the increased levels of GH first appear after closure of the epiphyses, patients develop *acromegaly*. Features include enlargement of head, hands, feet, jaw, tongue, and soft tissues.

The goals of treatment are to restore GH levels to normal and to decrease symptoms referable to a pituitary mass lesion, while not causing hypopituitarism. The tumor can be surgically removed by a transsphenoidal approach or destroyed by radiation therapy, or the GH secretion can be reduced by drug therapy.

CORTICOTROPH TUMORS (p. 1126)

Corticotroph adenomas are usually small microadenomas at the time of diagnosis. These tumors are basophilic or chromophobic. Immunostaining for ACTH yields a strong reaction in basophilic adenomas. Chromophobic tumors are often larger and produce symptoms from local mass effects. *Crooke basophilic hyaline change* may be seen in the cytoplasm of corticotroph cells, including those in the non-neoplastic surrounding gland.

Excess production of ACTH by the corticotroph adenoma leads to adrenal hypersecretion of cortisol and the production of *hypercortisolism* (also known as *Cushing syndrome*). This syndrome is discussed in more detail later with the diseases of the adrenal gland. It can be caused by a wide variety of conditions in addition to ACTH-producing pituitary tumors.

OTHER FUNCTIONING ADENOMAS (p. 1127)

Pituitary adenomas may elaborate more than one hormone. As described earlier, somatotroph adenomas commonly contain immunoreactive Prl. In some tumors, designated *mixed adenomas*, more than one cell population is present. In other cases, a single cell type is apparently capable of synthesizing more than one hormone. A few comments are made about several of the less frequent functioning tumors:

- *Gonadotroph (LH and FSH producing) adenomas*: These adenomas comprise 10 to 15% of pituitary adenomas. Gonadotroph adenomas are most frequently found in middle-aged men and women when they become large enough to cause neurologic symptoms, such as impaired vision, headaches, diplopia, or pituitary apoplexy. Pituitary hormone deficiencies can also be found, most commonly impaired secretion of LH. The result in men is low serum testosterone, which results in decreased energy and libido. The result in premenopausal women is amenorrhea.
- *Thyrotroph (TSH producing) adenomas*: These are rare, accounting for approximately 1% of all pituitary adenomas, and are a rare cause of hyperthyroidism.
- *Nonsecretory pituitary adenomas*: A substantial number of pituitary adenomas generate no detectable hormonal product and are designated *null cell adenomas*. These nonfunctional tumors account for approximately 20% of all pituitary adenomas. Patients with null cell adenomas typically present with mass effects.
- *Pituitary carcinomas*: Pituitary carcinomas are quite rare, and most are not functional. The diagnosis of carcinoma requires the demonstration of metastases.

Hypopituitarism (p. 1127)

Hypopituitarism refers to decreased secretion of pituitary hormones, which can result from diseases of the hypothalamus or of the pituitary, requiring that approximately 75% of the parenchyma be destroyed or absent.

- *Tumors and other mass lesions*: Pituitary adenomas as well as metastatic malignancies and cysts can induce hypopituitarism. Any mass lesion in the sellae can cause damage by exerting pressure on adjacent pituitary cells.
- *Pituitary surgery or radiation*: Surgical excision of a pituitary adenoma may inadvertently remove sufficient normal tissue to result in hypopituitarism. Radiation of the pituitary, used to prevent regrowth of residual tumor after surgery, exposes the nonadenomatous pituitary to the same radiation.
- *Rathke cleft cyst*: These cysts can accumulate proteinaceous fluid and expand causing symptoms.
- *Pituitary apoplexy*: This is a sudden hemorrhage into the pituitary gland, often occurring into a pituitary adenoma. In its most dramatic presentation, apoplexy causes a rapid increase in the size of the tumor and the sudden onset of excruciating headache, diplopia resulting from pressure on the oculomotor nerves, and hypopituitarism.
- *Ischemic necrosis of the pituitary and Sheehan syndrome*: The anterior pituitary can tolerate ischemia reasonably well, although damage from 75% causes hypopituitarism. *Sheehan syndrome*, or postpartum necrosis of the anterior pituitary, is the most common form of clinically significant ischemic necrosis of the anterior pituitary. This syndrome results from sudden infarction of the anterior lobe precipitated by obstetric hemorrhage or shock. Pituitary necrosis may also be encountered in other conditions, such as disseminated intravascular coagulation or (more rarely) sickle cell anemia, elevated intracranial pressure, traumatic injury, and shock of any origin. The infarcted adenohypophysis at the outset appears soft, pale, and ischemic or hemorrhagic. Over time, the ischemic area is resorbed and replaced by fibrous tissue.
- *Empty sella syndrome*: Any condition that destroys part or all of the pituitary gland, such as ablation of the pituitary by surgery or radiation, can result in an *empty sella*. *Empty sella syndrome* refers to the presence of an enlarged, empty sella turcica that is not filled with pituitary tissue. There are two types:
  1. In a *primary* empty sella, there is a defect in the diaphragma sellae that allows the arachnoid mater and cerebrospinal fluid to herniate into the sella, resulting in expansion of the sella and compression of the pituitary.
  2. In *secondary* empty sella, a mass, such as a pituitary adenoma, enlarges the sella but then is removed by surgery or radiation. Hypopituitarism can result from the treatment or spontaneous infarction.

Posterior Pituitary Syndromes (p. 1129)

The posterior pituitary is composed of modified glial cells and axonal processes extending from nerve cell bodies in the supraoptic and paraventricular nuclei of the hypothalamus. These neurons produce two peptides: *ADH* and *oxytocin*. Oxytocin stimulates contraction of the uterine smooth muscle cells in the gravid uterus and those that surround the lactiferous ducts of the mammary glands. Inappropriate oxytocin secretion has not been associated with clinical abnormalities. ADH is a nonapeptide hormone synthesized predominantly in the supraoptic nucleus and is involved in the control of water conservation. The clinically relevant posterior pituitary syndromes involve ADH and include *diabetes insipidus* and *secretion of inappropriately high levels of ADH*.

- *ADH deficiency (diabetes insipidus)*: ADH deficiency causes diabetes insipidus, a condition characterized by excessive urination (polyuria) as a result of an inability of the kidney to resorb water properly from the urine, excessive thirst (polydipsia), and *hypernatremia*. It can result from a variety of processes, including head trauma, tumors, and inflammatory disorders of the hypothalamus and pituitary, as well as surgical procedures involving these organs.
- *Syndrome of inappropriate ADH secretion (SIADH)*: ADH excess causes resorption of excessive amounts of free water, resulting in *hyponatremia*. The most frequent causes of SIADH include the secretion of ectopic ADH by *malignant neoplasms* (particularly small cell carcinomas of the lung); non-neoplastic diseases of the lung (e.g., pulmonary tuberculosis, pneumonia); and local injury to the hypothalamus, posterior pituitary, or both. The clinical manifestations of SIADH are dominated by hyponatremia, cerebral edema, and resultant neurologic dysfunction.

Hypothalamic Suprasellar Neoplasms
(p. 1129)

Hypothalamic suprasellar neoplasms may induce hypofunction or hyperfunction of the anterior pituitary, diabetes insipidus, or combinations of these manifestations. The most commonly implicated lesions are *gliomas* (sometimes arising in the chiasm; Chapter 30) and *craniopharyngiomas*.

CRANIOPHARYNGIOMA (p. 1129)

The craniopharyngioma is thought to be derived from vestigial remnants of Rathke pouch. These slow-growing tumors account for about 5% of intracranial tumors. Most of these tumors are suprasellar, and they may encroach on the hypothalamus, third ventricle, or optic chiasm. Although they occur most commonly during childhood and adolescence, about 50% present clinically after age 20. Children usually come to clinical attention because of endocrine deficiencies, such as growth retardation; adults present with visual disturbances.

Morphology

These tumors are characteristically cystic, and calcification is present in 75%. They are composed of a mixture of squamous epithelial elements and delicate reticular stroma, recapitulating the appearance of the enamel organ of a developing tooth; gliosis is common at the periphery. Rupture of cyst contents may provoke a vigorous inflammatory reaction. Malignancy is *rare*.

THYROID GLAND (p. 1130)

Diseases of the thyroid are of great importance because they are relatively common in the general population, and most are amenable to medical or surgical management. They include conditions associated with excessive release of thyroid hormone (hyperthyroidism), those associated with thyroid hormone deficiency (hypothyroidism), and focal or diffuse mass lesions of the thyroid.

Thyrotoxicosis (Hyperthyroidism) (p. 1131)

Thyrotoxicosis is a *hypermetabolic state* caused by increased levels of circulating triiodothyronine (T_3) and thyroxine (T_4). It can be caused by a variety of disorders:

- *Diffuse hyperplasia* of the thyroid associated with Graves disease (accounts for 85% of cases)
- Ingestion of *exogenous thyroid hormone* (administered for hypothyroidism)
- Hyperfunctional *multinodular goiter*
- Hyperfunctional *adenoma* of the thyroid
- Thyroiditis

CLINICAL COURSE

The clinical manifestations of hyperthyroidism include changes referable to the *hypermetabolic state* induced by excess thyroid hormone as well as those related to overactivity of the *sympathetic nervous system*.

- *Cardiac manifestations are among the earliest and most consistent features of hyperthyroidism.* Patients with hyperthyroidism can have an increase in cardiac output, as a result of both increased cardiac contractility and increased peripheral oxygen requirements. Tachycardia, palpitations, and cardiomegaly are common. Arrhythmias, particularly atrial fibrillation, occur frequently and are more common in older patients. The origin of thyrotoxic cardiomyopathy is uncertain.
- *Ocular changes* often call attention to hyperthyroidism. A wide, staring gaze and lid lag are present owing to sympathetic overstimulation of the levator palpebrae superioris. Only patients with Graves disease have ophthalmopathy (see later).
- In the *neuromuscular system*, overactivity of the sympathetic nervous system produces tremor, hyperactivity, emotional lability, anxiety, inability to concentrate, and insomnia.
- The *skin* of thyrotoxic patients tends to be warm, moist, and flushed because of increased blood flow and peripheral vasodilation to increase heat loss. Infiltrative dermopathy is seen only in Graves hyperthyroidism and is discussed later.
- In the *gastrointestinal system*, weight loss is due primarily to increased calorigenesis and secondarily to increased gut motility resulting from increased sympathetic activity. The weight loss occurs despite an increased appetite and hyperphagia.

Determining the decreased serum TSH concentration (feedback inhibition of the pituitary), in conjunction with a measurement of unbound *(free)* T_4, provides the best initial screen for cases of suspected hyperthyroidism.

Hypothyroidism (p. 1132)

Hypothyroidism is caused by any structural or functional derangement that interferes with the production of adequate levels of thyroid hormone. As in the case of hyperthyroidism, this disorder is divided into primary and secondary categories, depending on whether the hypothyroidism arises from an intrinsic abnormality in the thyroid or occurs as a result of hypothalamic or pituitary disease.

- *Primary hypothyroidism* accounts for the majority of cases of hypothyroidism. The most common cause of hypothyroidism in iodine-sufficient areas of the world is *chronic autoimmune thyroiditis*, or Hashimoto thyroiditis. This condition is variously reported to cause 15 to 60% of cases of hypothyroidism. *Hypothyroidism can follow thyroid surgery, follow radiation, be drug induced, or occur as a result of an infiltrative disorder.*

- *Secondary hypothyroidism is caused by TSH deficiency, and tertiary (central) hypothyroidism is caused by thyrotropin-releasing hormone deficiency.* Secondary hypothyroidism can result from any of the causes of hypopituitarism, frequently a pituitary tumor, although other causes include postpartum pituitary necrosis, trauma, and nonpituitary tumors.

Clinical manifestations of hypothyroidism include *cretinism* if thyroid deficiency develops during the perinatal period or infancy and *myxedema* in older children and adults.

- *Cretinism* may occur in both the *endemic* form, associated with dietary iodine deficiency and endemic goiter, and the *sporadic* form, often associated with a biosynthetic defect in hormone synthesis. Manifestations include impaired development of the skeletal system and central nervous system, with severe mental retardation, short stature, coarse facial features with wide-set eyes, an enlarged and protruding tongue, and umbilical hernia.
- *Myxedema* refers to hypothyroidism developing in the older child or adult. The older child shows signs and symptoms intermediate between those of the cretin and those of the adult with hypothyroidism, which is manifested by an insidious slowing of physical and mental activity, associated with fatigue, cold intolerance, and apathy. *Signs* include periorbital edema, coarsening of skin and facial features, cardiomegaly, pericardial effusion, hair loss, and accumulation of mucopolysaccharide-rich ground substance within the dermis *(myxedema)* and other tissues.

Thyroiditis (p. 1133)

Inflammation of the thyroid gland, or thyroiditis, encompasses a diverse group of disorders characterized by some form of thyroid inflammation. These diseases include conditions that result in acute illness with severe thyroid pain (e.g., infectious thyroiditis, subacute granulomatous thyroiditis) and disorders in which there is relatively little inflammation and the illness is manifested primarily by thyroid dysfunction (subacute lymphocytic [painless] thyroiditis and fibrous [Reidel] thyroiditis).

Acute infections may reach the thyroid gland via hematogenous spread or through direct seeding of the gland, such as via a fistula from the piriform sinus. Other infections of the thyroid are more chronic and include mycobacterial, fungal, and *Pneumocystis* infections, which occur in immunocompromised patients. The inflammatory involvement may cause sudden onset of neck pain and tenderness in the area of the gland and is accompanied by fever, chills, and other signs of infection.

Hashimoto Thyroiditis (p. 1134)

Hashimoto thyroiditis, an insidiously developing condition, is the most common cause of hypothyroidism in areas of the world where iodine levels are sufficient. It is characterized by gradual thyroid failure because of an autoimmune-mediated destruction of the thyroid gland. Hashimoto thyroiditis is most prevalent between

45 and 65 years of age, with a female predominance of 10:1 to 20:1. It is a major cause of nonendemic goiter in children.

PATHOGENESIS

Although both cellular and humoral factors contribute to thyroid injury and hypothyroidism in Hashimoto thyroiditis, this disease is believed to be caused primarily by a defect in the function of thyroid-specific suppressor T cells. This defect results in the emergence of CD4 + *helper T cells* directed at the thyroid and the production of *autoantibodies* to various components of the thyroid follicle (thyroglobulin, thyroid peroxidase, TSH receptor, and others). It is uncertain whether humoral mechanisms, cell-mediated injury, or both cause the damage to the thyroid gland. Although the cause is uncertain, there may be a *genetic* component because some cases are associated with HLA-DR5, and others with severe thyroid atrophy are linked to HLA-DR3. Hashimoto thyroiditis is associated with *other autoimmune diseases*, including systemic lupus erythematosus, Sjögren syndrome, rheumatoid arthritis, pernicious anemia, type II diabetes, and Graves disease.

MORPHOLOGY

The thyroid is a diffusely enlarged, often asymmetric, gland with an intact capsule. The parenchyma is generally paler than normal. Microscopic changes include an exuberant infiltrate of lymphocytes, plasma cells, and macrophages, often associated with germinal centers; abundant eosinophilic granular cytoplasm in residual follicular cells (*Hürthle* cells or *oncocytes*); and delicate fibrosis. An *atrophic variant* is associated with more extensive fibrosis and less inflammation; the gland is often reduced in size.

CLINICAL COURSE

Hashimoto thyroiditis comes to clinical attention as painless enlargement of the thyroid, *usually associated with some degree of hypothyroidism* in a middle-aged woman. *Hyperthyroidism (hashitoxicosis)* may be seen early in the course of the disease, associated with the presence of anti-TSH receptor antibodies, but it is transient. There is a small risk of subsequent lymphoma.

Subacute (Granulomatous) Thyroiditis
(p. 1135)

Subacute thyroiditis, which is also referred to as *granulomatous thyroiditis* or *de Quervain thyroiditis*, occurs much less frequently than Hashimoto disease. This disorder is most common between the ages of 30 and 50 and affects women considerably more often than men (3:1 to 5:1).

PATHOGENESIS

Subacute thyroiditis is believed to be caused by a *viral infection* or a postviral inflammatory process. The majority of patients have a history of an upper respiratory infection just before the onset of thyroiditis. Cases have been reported in association with coxsackievirus, mumps, measles, adenovirus, and other viral illnesses. There is a fairly strong association with HLA-B35.

MORPHOLOGY

Subacute thyroiditis is characterized by variable enlargement of the gland, which may be symmetric or irregular. Histologically the changes are patchy and depend on the stage of the disease. Early lesions include *disruption of thyroid follicles* with a *neutrophilic* infiltrate. Later the more characteristic features appear in the form of aggregations of lymphocytes, histiocytes, and plasma cells about collapsed and damaged thyroid follicles. *Multinucleate giant cells* enclose naked pools or fragments of colloid.

CLINICAL COURSE

The presentation of subacute thyroiditis may be sudden or gradual. It is characterized by pain in the neck, which may radiate to the jaw, throat, or ears, particularly when swallowing. Fever, fatigue, malaise, anorexia, and myalgia accompany the variable enlargement of the thyroid. The thyroid inflammation and the resultant hyperthyroidism are transient, usually diminishing in 2 to 6 weeks, even if the patient is not treated. It may be followed by a period of transient, usually asymptomatic hypothyroidism lasting from 2 to 8 weeks, but recovery is virtually always complete.

Subacute Lymphocytic (Painless) Thyroiditis (p. 1136)

Subacute thyroiditis is an uncommon cause of hyperthyroidism or painless enlargement of the gland. It is most common in women in the postpartum period. Self-limited, it may be followed by *hypo*thyroidism. It is an inflammatory disorder of unknown etiology defined histologically by *nonspecific lymphoid infiltration* of the thyroid parenchyma; there is no germinal center formation or significant plasma cell infiltrate. *No* clear association with viral infection, subacute granulomatous thyroiditis, or Hashimoto disease has been described.

The principal clinical manifestation of painless thyroiditis is hyperthyroidism. Symptoms usually develop over 1 to 2 weeks and last from 2 to 8 weeks before subsiding. The patient may have any of the common findings in hyperthyroidism (e.g., palpitations, tachycardia, tremor, weakness, and fatigue).

Riedel Thyroiditis (p. 1136)

Riedel fibrosing thyroiditis is an uncommon *fibrosing* process of unknown etiology associated with replacement of thyroid parenchyma by dense fibrous tissue penetrating the capsule and extending into *contiguous neck structures*. Manifestations include glandular atrophy and hypothyroidism. The disorder may be mistaken for an infiltrating neoplasm. It may be associated with idiopathic fibrosis in other sites.

Graves Disease (p. 1136)

Graves disease, the most common cause of endogenous hyperthyroidism, is characterized by

■ *Hyperthyroidism* resulting from hyperfunctional, diffuse enlargement of the thyroid, which is always present

- Infiltrative ophthalmopathy with resultant exophthalmos, in most, but not all, cases
- Localized, infiltrative *dermopathy* sometimes called *pretibial myxedema*, which is present in a minority of patients.

Graves disease has a peak incidence between the ages of 20 and 40, with *women being affected up to seven times more often than men*. Graves disease is a common disorder that is said to be present in 1.5 to 2.0% of women in the United States. Genetic factors are important in the onset of Graves disease. It is associated with HLA-B8 and DR3 and with *other autoimmune disorders*, including Hashimoto disease, pernicious anemia, and rheumatoid arthritis.

PATHOGENESIS

Evidence points to an autoimmune disorder produced by autoantibodies to the TSH receptor, thyroglobulin, and thyroid hormones (T_3 and T_4).

- *Autoantibodies to the TSH receptor* or thyroid-stimulating immunoglobulin are found in patients with Graves disease. The antibody is relatively specific for Graves disease, in contrast to thyroglobulin and thyroid peroxidase antibodies.
- *Thyroid growth-stimulating immunoglobulins* are also directed against the TSH receptor and have been implicated in the proliferation of thyroid follicular epithelium.
- *TSH-binding inhibitor immunoglobulins* prevent TSH from binding normally to its receptor on thyroid epithelial cells. In so doing, these antibodies mimic the action of TSH, resulting in the stimulation of thyroid epithelial cell activity, whereas other forms may actually *inhibit* thyroid cell function.

The trigger for the initiation of the autoimmune reaction in Graves disease remains uncertain but may involve the following:

- *Molecular mimicry*: This implies structural similarity between some infectious or other exogenous agent and human cell proteins, such that antibodies formed in response to the exogenous agent react with one or more of the thyroid proteins.
- *Primary T-cell autoimmunity*: Thyroid epithelial cells can express specific types of major histocompatibility complex proteins that are recognized by T cells in association with processed peptides derived from thyroid antigens. These activated T cells then cooperate with B cells, enhancing formation of a range of thyroid-specific autoantibodies from the B cells, including antibodies against the TSH receptor.

MORPHOLOGY

The gland is mildly and *symmetrically enlarged*, with an intact capsule and soft parenchyma. Microscopic changes include widespread *hypertrophy* and *hyperplasia* of follicular epithelium, manifested by crowding of the columnar cells into irregular papillary folds. Colloid is substantially decreased. Interfollicular parenchyma contains *hyperplastic lymphoid tissue* and increased numbers of blood vessels.

Preoperative therapy influences the histologic appearance:

- *Thiouracil* exaggerates hyperplasia.
- *Iodine* promotes devascularization, colloid accumulation, and follicular involution.

Changes in extrathyroidal tissue include generalized lymphoid hyperplasia. In patients with ophthalmopathy, the tissues of the orbit are edematous because of the presence of hydrophilic muco-polysaccharides. In addition, there is infiltration by lymphocytes and fibrosis late in the course of the disease.

CLINICAL FEATURES

The clinical findings in Graves disease include changes referable to *thyrotoxicosis* as well as those associated uniquely with Graves disease—*diffuse hyperplasia of the thyroid, ophthalmopathy,* and *dermopathy.* Ophthalmopathy may be self-limited or may progress to severe proptosis despite control of the thyrotoxicosis. Laboratory values include *elevated free T_4 and T_3 levels* and depressed TSH levels. Because of ongoing stimulation of the thyroid follicles, *iodine uptake is elevated,* and *radioiodine scans show a diffuse uptake of iodine.*

Diffuse and Multinodular Goiter (p. 1138)

Enlargement of the thyroid, or *goiter,* is the most common manifestation of thyroid disease. *The presence of goiter reflects impaired synthesis of thyroid hormone,* most often due to dietary iodine deficiency.

Diffuse Nontoxic (Simple) Goiter (p. 1138)

Diffuse nontoxic (simple) goiter specifies a form that diffusely involves the entire gland without producing nodularity. Because the enlarged follicles are filled with colloid, the term *colloid goiter* has been applied to this condition. It occurs in both an endemic and a sporadic distribution.

- *Endemic goiter* occurs in geographical areas where the soil, water, and food supply contain only low levels of iodine. Such conditions are particularly common in mountainous areas of the world, including the Alps, Andes, and Himalayas. The lack of iodine leads to decreased synthesis of thyroid hormone and a *compensatory increase in TSH,* leading to follicular cell hypertrophy and hyperplasia and goitrous enlargement. With increasing dietary iodine supplementation, the frequency and severity of endemic goiter have declined significantly.
- *Sporadic goiter* occurs less frequently than does endemic goiter. There is a striking female preponderance and a peak incidence in young adult life. Sporadic goiter can be caused by a number of conditions, including the ingestion of substances that interfere with thyroid hormone synthesis (goitrogens, found in a variety of vegetables and plants). In other instances, goiter may result from hereditary enzymatic defects that interfere with thyroid hormone synthesis, all transmitted as autosomal recessive conditions. These defects in thyroid hormone synthesis include defects in iodine transport, organification, dehalogenation, and iodotyrosine coupling.

MORPHOLOGY

Two stages can be identified in the evolution of diffuse nontoxic goiter: the *hyperplastic stage* and *colloid involution.* In the hyperplastic stage, the thyroid gland is diffuse and symmetrically enlarged. Initial histologic changes include *hypertrophy* and *hyperplasia* of follicular epithelium with *scant colloid.* Later changes as the demand for thyroid hormone is met include accumulation of colloid and variable atrophy of follicular epithelium. If the demand for thyroid hormone decreases, the stimulated follicular epithelium involutes to form an enlarged, colloid-rich gland *(colloid goiter)*.

CLINICAL FEATURES

The clinical significance of nontoxic diffuse goiter in adults depends largely on its ability to achieve a state of euthyroidism, which is generally the rule, and the manifestations related to enlargement of the gland. Hypothyroidism is more common in children with underlying biosynthetic defects.

Multinodular Goiter (p. 1139)

Recurrent episodes of stimulation and involution of a diffuse goiter generate a more irregular enlargement of the thyroid, termed *multinodular goiter*. Most long-standing simple goiters convert into multinodular goiters. They may be nontoxic or may induce thyrotoxicosis (toxic multinodular goiter or Plummer disease). *Multinodular goiters produce the most extreme thyroid enlargements and are more frequently mistaken for neoplastic involvement than any other form of thyroid disease.*

MORPHOLOGY

Multinodular goiters are multilobulated, asymmetrically enlarged glands. Glands may become massively enlarged (>2000 gm). The pattern of enlargement is quite irregular and can produce lateral pressure on the trachea and esophagus. In other instances, the goiter grows behind the sternum, trachea, and clavicles to produce the so-called *intrathoracic* or *plunging goiter*. The irregular *nodularity* of the gland is associated with focal hemorrhage, fibrosis, calcification, and cystic change. Histologic changes include a variable degree of *colloid* accumulation, follicular *epithelial hyperplasia*, and follicular *involution* with focal intervening areas of scarring and hemorrhage.

CLINICAL FEATURES

Clinical features include

1. Signs and symptoms referable to *mass effect*
2. Occasionally, abnormal thyroid function as a result of hyperactivity of a focal nodule with resultant *thyrotoxicosis* (rarely associated with hypothyroidism)

Problems related to *mass effect* include cosmetic deformity, esophageal compression with dysphagia, tracheal compression, and, occasionally, obstruction of the superior vena cava. Hemorrhage into goiter may cause pain and contribute to mass effect. Most patients are euthyroid, but *thyrotoxicosis* occurs in a substantial minority of patients. Infiltrative ophthalmopathy and dermopathy are *not* seen in the absence of concomitant Graves disease. *Cardiovascular manifestations* (tachycardia, atrial fibrillation, congestive heart failure) may be prominent. Laboratory findings include variable elevations in T_3, T_4, and radioactive iodine uptake; scintiscans reveal irregular functional activity with patchy or focal accumulations of radioiodine. Distinction between multinodular goiter and neoplasm may be difficult, especially in patients with a dominant mass.

Neoplasms (p. 1140)

Solitary thyroid nodules are present in 2 to 4% of the U.S. population, although the estimated incidence is significantly higher in endemic goitrous regions. Single nodules are about four times more common in women than in men, and the incidence of thyroid nodules increases throughout life. Most solitary nodules of the thyroid prove to be benign lesions, either follicular adenomas or localized, non-neoplastic conditions (e.g., nodular hyperplasia, simple cysts, or foci of thyroiditis).

Among thyroid neoplasms, greater than 90% prove to be *adenomas*. Several clinical criteria may provide a clue as to the nature of the thyroid nodule:

- *Solitary nodules* are more likely to be neoplastic than are multiple nodules.
- *Nodules in younger patients* (<40 years old) are more likely to be neoplastic than are those in older patients.
- *Nodules in men* are more likely to be neoplastic than are those in women.
- A history of *radiation treatment* to the head and neck region is associated with an increased incidence of thyroid malignancy.
- Nodules that take up radioactive iodine in imaging studies (*hot* or functioning nodules) are more likely to be benign than malignant.
- *Fine-needle aspiration* biopsy is often useful in the evaluation of thyroid nodules.

ADENOMAS (p. 1140)

Adenomas of the thyroid are discrete, solitary masses. There are multiple histologic variants, all representing *follicular neoplasms*. Adenomas are rarely the precursors of cancer.

Pathogenesis

Somatic mutations in some of the components of thyrotropin (TSH) receptor signaling system cause chronic stimulation of the cyclic adenosine monophosphate (cAMP) pathway, generating cells that acquire a growth advantage. This results in clonal expansion of specific epithelial cells, leading to the formation of autonomous monoclonal thyroid adenomas. For example, somatic mutations have been identified in Gsα in 12 to 38% of thyroid adenomas. Overall, mutations leading to constitutive activation of the cAMP cascade appear to cause a large proportion (50 to 75%) of autonomously functioning thyroid adenomas.

Morphology

The typical thyroid adenoma is a well-demarcated, solitary lesion, occasionally accompanied by fibrosis, hemorrhage, or calcification. It is sharply demarcated from the adjacent parenchyma by a well-defined fibrous capsule. The tumor compresses the surrounding gland, which is notable for the absence of multinodularity. Histologic patterns range from closely apposed nests and trabeculae reminiscent of developing (embryonal) thyroid to well-developed follicles containing abundant colloid (follicular adenomas). *Hürthle cell* adenomas feature granular, eosinophilic cells containing abundant mitochondria.

Clinical Features

A thyroid adenoma typically presents as a painless mass that must be differentiated from a carcinoma. Most adenomas take up less radioactive iodine than does normal thyroid parenchyma and are *cold* (nonfunctioning) on scans, but some are *hot*, helping to distinguish them from nonfunctioning cancers. About 10% of *cold* nodules eventually prove to be malignant. Fine-needle aspiration biopsy is frequently used to evaluate suspected adenomas before surgical excision.

CARCINOMAS (p. 1142)

Carcinomas of the thyroid are relatively uncommon in the United States, accounting for about 1.5% of all cancers. Most cases occur in adults, with a female predominance. Most (90 to 95%) are *well-differentiated lesions* and are therefore relatively not aggressive. The major subtypes of thyroid carcinoma and their relative frequencies include

- Papillary carcinoma: 75 to 85% of cases
- Follicular carcinoma: 10 to 20% of cases
- Medullary carcinoma: 5% of cases
- Anaplastic carcinomas: less than 5% of cases

Pathogenesis

The major risk factor predisposing to thyroid cancer is exposure to *ionizing radiation*, particularly during the first two decades of life. Certain thyroid diseases, such as nodular goiter and autoimmune thyroid disease (Hashimoto thyroiditis), have also been implicated as predisposing factors.

The activation or mutation of certain *oncogenes* is important in the development of some thyroid carcinomas. Perhaps the most notable is the *RET protooncogene, a tyrosine kinase that plays a role in both papillary and medullary thyroid carcinomas.* The RET gene is mutated in most families with *multiple endocrine neoplasia type II (MEN II)*, a heritable disorder that involves the triad of medullary thyroid carcinoma, pheochromocytoma, and hyperparathyroidism (see later).

Papillary Carcinoma (p. 1143)

Papillary carcinomas are the most common form of thyroid cancer. They occur at any age but occur most often in women in their twenties to forties and account for the vast majority of thyroid carcinomas associated with previous exposure to ionizing radiation. They often appear as *multifocal tumors* because of their propensity for lymphatic invasion.

Morphology

The tumors are solitary or multifocal lesions that may infiltrate the adjacent parenchyma and are sometimes associated with calcification or cystic change. The microscopic appearance ranges from lesions that are predominantly *papillary* in architecture to those with mostly *follicular* elements (follicular variant of papillary carcinoma).

Other features include

- Hypochromatic empty nuclei devoid of nucleoli *(Orphan Annie eyes)* and nuclear grooves (the diagnostic features of papillary carcinomas)

- Eosinophilic intranuclear inclusions (cytoplasmic invaginations)
- Psammoma bodies

Histologic variants of papillary carcinoma include
- *Encapsulated variant* (previously designated *papillary adenoma*)
- *Follicular variant* (distinguished by the nuclei from true follicular carcinoma, which carries a worse prognosis)
- *Tall cell variant* (occurs in older individuals; associated with poorer prognosis than other papillary carcinomas)

Clinical Course. Most papillary carcinomas present as asymptomatic thyroid nodules, but the first manifestation may be a mass in a cervical lymph node. The tumor involves *regional nodes* in 50% of cases at time of diagnosis, although distant metastases are uncommon at presentation (5%). The carcinoma, which is usually a single nodule, moves freely during swallowing and is not distinguishable from a benign nodule. Hoarseness, dysphagia, cough, or dyspnea suggests advanced disease. Prognosis is generally excellent (90% survival at 20 years); favorable factors include confinement of the lesion to the thyroid and well-differentiated histology.

Follicular Carcinoma (p. 1144)

Follicular carcinomas account for *10 to 20%* of thyroid cancers. These tumors have a peak incidence in the forties to fifties and a female predominance (3:1). There is an increased prevalence in areas of dietary *iodine deficiency*, suggesting that multinodular goiter may predispose to follicular carcinoma.

Morphology

Follicular carcinomas are single nodules that may be well circumscribed or infiltrative. Sharply demarcated lesions may be exceedingly difficult to distinguish from follicular adenomas. Microscopically, architecture of the tumors may vary considerably; the nuclear features noted in papillary carcinomas (described earlier) are absent. Most have a microfollicular pattern, with relatively uniform, colloid-filled follicles reminiscent of normal thyroid. Other patterns include a trabecular and sheetlike architecture. Some variants contain large numbers of eosinophilic cells resembling Hürthle cells. The presence of capsular and vascular invasion increases the likelihood of metastases; the majority of metastases are *hematogenous* (bone, lungs, liver).

Clinical Course

Prognosis is influenced by the size of the lesion, presence or absence of capsular or vascular invasion, presence of metastases, and degree of histologic anaplasia. Better-differentiated lesions may take up *radioactive iodine*, which may be used to identify and palliate metastatic lesions. Follicular carcinomas are treated with lobectomy or subtotal thyroidectomy.

Medullary Thyroid Carcinoma (p. 1145)

Medullary carcinomas of the thyroid are *neuroendocrine* neoplasms originating from the parafollicular cells, or C-cells, of the thyroid. The cells of medullary carcinomas, similar to normal C-cells, secrete *calcitonin* and possibly other secretory products as well. The tumors arise sporadically in about 80% of cases. The remainder occur in the setting of MEN syndrome IIa or IIb. Peak incidence is in the forties to fifties for sporadic cases and the twenties to thirties for MEN-associated cases. Germ line mutations in the *RET proto-oncogene* play an important role in the development of medullary carcinomas associated with the MEN IIa syndrome.

Morphology

Medullary carcinomas can arise as a solitary nodule or may present as multiple lesions involving both lobes of the thyroid. Sporadic cases tend to originate in one lobe, whereas familial cases are usually bilateral and multicentric. Microscopic features include polygonal to spindle-shaped cells arrayed in nests, trabeculae, and, occasionally, follicles. *Amyloid deposits*, derived from altered calcitonin molecules, are present in the adjacent stroma in many cases. Foci of *C-cell hyperplasia* are often present in familial cases but are typically absent in sporadic cases.

Clinical Course

Clinical features vary, depending on whether the case is sporadic or familial.

■ *Sporadic cases* usually present as a thyroid mass, sometimes associated with dysphagia, hoarseness, or cough; occasional cases may present with manifestations related to the secretion of a peptide product (e.g., diarrhea resulting from calcitonin or vasoactive intestinal polypeptide).
■ *Familial cases* are usually detected through screening of asymptomatic relatives of affected patients for abnormal serum calcitonin levels.

The prognosis is variable; sporadic lesions and those associated with MEN IIb are often aggressive. Lesions arising in patients with isolated familial medullary carcinoma syndrome are more often indolent.

Anaplastic Carcinoma (p. 1147)

Anaplastic carcinomas of the thyroid are aggressive undifferentiated tumors of the thyroid follicular epithelium. They account for less than 5% of thyroid carcinomas and are most common in elderly patients, particularly in areas of endemic goiter. Microscopically, these neoplasms are composed of highly anaplastic cells, which may take one of three histologic patterns:

1. Large, pleomorphic giant cells
2. Spindle cells with a sarcomatous appearance
3. Small anaplastic cells resembling those seen in small cell carcinomas arising in other sites

The tumors have a dismal prognosis. Dissemination is common, but death is usually attributable to aggressive local growth.

Congenital Anomalies (p. 1147)

Thyroglossal duct (cyst) is the most common clinically significant congenital anomaly arising as a remnant of the tubular development of the thyroid gland. It may present at any age, as a midline cyst or mass anterior to the trachea. Histologic features include squamous epithelium in segments occurring high in the neck and thyroidal acinar epithelium in lesions arising more inferiorly. Lymphocytic infiltrates are often conspicuous. They may become infected and form abscess cavities; rarely, they may give rise to carcinoma.

PARATHYROID GLANDS (p. 1147)

The activity of the parathyroids is controlled by the level of free (ionized) calcium in the bloodstream. Decreased levels of free calcium stimulate the synthesis and secretion of *parathyroid hormone (PTH)*. The metabolic functions of PTH in supporting serum calcium level can be summarized as follows:

- PTH activates osteoclasts, thereby mobilizing calcium from bone.
- PTH increases the renal tubular reabsorption of calcium, thereby conserving free calcium.
- PTH increases the conversion of vitamin D to its active 1,25-$(OH)_2D_3$ form in the kidneys.
- PTH increases urinary phosphate excretion, thereby lowering the serum phosphate level.
- PTH augments gastrointestinal calcium absorption.

The net result of these activities is an increase in the serum level of free calcium that inhibits further PTH secretion in a classic feedback loop.

Hypercalcemia is one of a number of changes induced by elevated levels of PTH and is a relatively common complication of malignancy. Hypercalcium of malignancy is due to increased bone resorption and subsequent release of calcium, which can occur by two mechanisms:

- Osteolytic metastases and local release of cytokines
- Release of parathyroid hormone–related protein

Hyperparathyroidism occurs in two major forms, *primary* and *secondary*. The first condition represents an autonomous overproduction of PTH, whereas the latter conditions typically occur as a secondary phenomenon in patients with chronic renal insufficiency.

Primary Hyperparathyroidism (p. 1148)

Primary hyperparathyroidism is one of the most common endocrine disorders; it is an important cause of *hypercalcemia*, or an increase in the level of serum ionized calcium. The frequency of the various parathyroid lesions underlying the hyperfunction is as follows:

- Adenoma: 75 to 80%
- Primary hyperplasia (diffuse or nodular): 10 to 15%
- Parathyroid carcinoma: less than 5%

The annual incidence of primary hyperparathyroidism is roughly 25 cases per 100,000 in United States and Europe; most cases occur in patients in their fifties and older, with a female predominance (3:1). Most cases occur sporadically, although some are caused by inherited syndromes, such as MEN I.

In more than 95% of cases, the disorder is caused by sporadic parathyroid adenomas or sporadic hyperplasia. Among the *sporadic adenomas*, there are two notable tumor-specific (i.e., not germ line) chromosome defects in genes that appear related to the clonal origin of some of these tumors:

- *Parathyroid adenoma 1 (PRAD 1)*: PRAD 1 encodes cyclin D1, a major regulator of the cell cycle.
- *MEN I*: Homozygous loss of the MEN I gene, a putative suppressor gene on chromosome 11q13, is demonstrated in familial MEN I cases of parathyroid adenoma and in some sporadic parathyroid tumors.

MORPHOLOGY

The morphologic changes seen in primary hyperparathyroidism include those in the parathyroid glands as well as those in other organs affected by elevated levels of calcium.

- *Parathyroid adenomas* are usually *solitary*, averaging 0.5 to 5.0 gm, and are surrounded by a delicate capsule. In contrast to primary hyperplasia, the remaining glands are usually normal in size as a result of feedback inhibition by the elevations in serum calcium. Microscopically, parathyroid adenomas are composed of predominantly *chief cells* arrayed in uniform sheets, trabeculae, or follicles; foci of oxyphil cells may be present.
- *Primary hyperplasia* may occur sporadically, or in association with MEN syndromes I and IIa. It usually involves *all glands* histologically, although *asymmetric* involvement may be seen, particularly in cases of nodular hyperplasia. The combined weight of the affected glands rarely exceeds 1.0 gm. Microscopically the most common pattern seen is that of chief cell hyperplasia, which may involve the glands in a diffuse or multinodular pattern. Cells may form solid sheets, trabeculae, nests, or follicles; fat cells are usually interspersed.
- *Parathyroid carcinoma* may be fairly circumscribed lesions that are difficult to distinguish from adenomas, both grossly and microscopically. These tumors enlarge one parathyroid gland and consist of gray-white, irregular masses that sometimes exceed 10 gm in weight. The cells of parathyroid carcinomas are usually uniform and not too dissimilar from normal parathyroid cells. Diagnosis of malignancy is based on the presence of *local invasion*, *metastases*, or both.
- *Other organs*:
  - Skeletal changes include osteoclast activation, which causes bone resorption. In severe cases, the marrow of affected bones contains increased amounts of fibrous tissue accompanied by foci of hemorrhage and cyst formation *(osteitis fibrosa cystica)*
  - Hypercalcemia favors formation of urinary tract stones *(nephrolithiasis)*, calcification of the renal interstitium and tubules *(nephrocalcinosis)*, and metastatic calcifications in other tissues.

CLINICAL FEATURES

Primary hyperparathyroidism usually presents in two general ways:

- *Asymptomatic hyperparathyroidism*: *Routine serum calcium determinations* in medical evaluations have resulted in the diagnosis of most cases of primary hyperparathyroidism at an earlier stage. In patients with primary hyperparathyroidism, serum PTH levels are inappropriately elevated for the level of serum calcium, whereas PTH levels are low to undetectable in the hypercalcemia resulting from nonparathyroid diseases.

- *Symptomatic primary hyperparathyroidism*: The signs and symptoms of hyperparathyroidism reflect the combined effects of increased PTH secretion and hypercalcemia. Primary hyperparathyroidism has been traditionally associated with a constellation of symptoms that have included *painful bones, renal stones, abdominal groans, and psychic moans*. The clinical manifestations affect multiple systems and include:
  - *Bone disease*: Bone pain, secondary to fractures of bones weakened by osteoporosis
  - *Renal disease*: Nephrolithiasis (renal stones) with attendant pain and obstructive uropathy
  - *Gastrointestinal disturbances*: Constipation, nausea, peptic ulcers, pancreatitis, and gallstones
  - *Central nervous system alterations*: Depression, lethargy, and eventually seizures
  - *Neuromuscular abnormalities*: Complaints of weakness, fatigue
  - *Cardiac manifestations*: Aortic and mitral valve calcifications

Secondary Hyperparathyroidism (p. 1150)

Secondary hyperparathyroidism is caused by any condition associated with a chronic depression in the serum calcium level because low serum calcium leads to compensatory overactivity of the parathyroids. *Renal failure is, by far, the most common cause of secondary hyperparathyroidism.* The pathogenesis in renal failure is related to phosphate retention and hypocalcemia, with compensatory hypersecretion of PTH. Impaired gastrointestinal calcium absorption because of reduced 1,25-$(OH)_2D_3$ synthesis and skeletal resistance to the effects of PTH and vitamin D may also contribute. *Morphology* of parathyroid glands is identical to that of primary hyperplasia. Skeletal changes, including osteitis fibrosa cystica (usually not as severe as that in primary disease) and osteomalacia, are present, and *metastatic calcifications* may be seen in many tissues. The condition may remit with correction of underlying renal failure; occasionally an *autonomous adenoma* may develop (*tertiary* hyperparathyroidism).

Hypoparathyroidism (p. 1151)

There are multiple causes of hypoparathyroidism:

- *Surgically induced*
- *Congenital absence* of all glands (e.g., DiGeorge syndrome)
- *Autoimmune destruction of the gland*
- *Familial hypoparathyroidism*

The major clinical manifestations of hypoparathyroidism include

- *Neuromuscular manifestations*, such as tetany, muscle cramps, carpopedal spasms, laryngeal stridor, and convulsions
- *Mental status changes*, such as irritability or psychosis
- *Intracranial manifestations*, such as parkinsonian-like movement disorders and elevated intracranial pressure with papilledema
- *Ocular* changes with calcification of the lens leading to cataract formation

■ *Cardiac* conduction defects, which produce a characteristic prolongation of the QT interval in the electrocardiogram

Pseudohypoparathyroidism (p. 1151)

The pathogenesis of pseudohypoparathyroidism is related to *abnormalities in the PTH receptor complex* and loss of responsiveness to PTH. This situation results in hypocalcemia, compensatory parathyroid hyperfunction, and a variety of skeletal and developmental abnormalities. Patients with this disorder may have short stature, round face, short neck, and short metacarpals and metatarsals.

ADRENAL CORTEX (p. 1152)

Adrenocortical Hyperfunction (Hyperadrenalism) (p. 1152)

There are three basic types of corticosteroids elaborated by the adrenal cortex (glucocorticoids, mineralocorticoids, and sex steroids) and three distinctive hyperadrenal clinical syndromes:

1. Cushing syndrome (excess cortisol)
2. Hyperaldosteronism
3. Adrenogenital syndromes (excess androgens)

Hypercortisolism (Cushing Syndrome) (p. 1152)

Cushing syndrome is caused by an elevation in glucocorticoid levels. There are *multiple etiologies*:

■ Administration of exogenous glucocorticoids, the most common cause
■ Primary hypothalamic—pituitary diseases associated with hypersecretion of ACTH
■ Hypersecretion of cortisol by an adrenal adenoma, carcinoma, or nodular hyperplasia
■ The secretion of ectopic ACTH by a nonendocrine neoplasm

Pituitary hypersecretion of ACTH (also called Cushing *disease*) is encountered most commonly in young adult life with a female predominance (5:1). It accounts for more than half of the cases of *endogenous* hypercortisolism. Most cases are associated with an ACTH-producing *pituitary adenoma* (may be basophilic or sparsely granulated *chromophobic neoplasm*); *corticotroph hyperplasia* accounts for 15% of cases. The adrenals are bilaterally hyperplastic, and elevated serum ACTH is usually readily detectable.

Primary *adrenal neoplasms*, such as adrenal adenoma, carcinoma, and primary cortical hyperplasia, account, in aggregate, for 20 to 25% of cases of endogenous Cushing syndrome. These lesions are independent of ACTH because the adrenals function autonomously. Adenomas and carcinomas are equally common in adults; carcinomas predominate in children. Hypercortisolism is usually more marked with carcinomas than with adenomas or hyperplasia. In patients with a unilateral neoplasm, native adrenal cortex is usually atrophic because of *ACTH suppression* and low levels of ACTH.

Ectopic ACTH secretion by nonpituitary tumors accounts for 15 to 30% of cases of endogenous Cushing syndrome and is seen most commonly in men in their forties and fifties. It is most commonly associated with *small cell carcinoma of lung*, carcinoid tumors of the bronchus or pancreas, medullary carcinoma of the thyroid, and islet cell tumors of the pancreas (e.g., gastrinomas). It may rarely be associated with *ectopic secretion of corticotropin-releasing factor*, with resultant overproduction of ACTH and hypercortisolism. The adrenals are bilaterally hyperplastic.

MORPHOLOGY

The pituitary shows *Crooke hyaline change* within basophils (described earlier), caused by elevated glucocorticoid levels. The morphology of the adrenal glands depends on the cause of the hypercortisolism. *Diffuse adrenal cortical hyperplasia* is present in 60 to 70% of cases of Cushing syndrome; the glands are enlarged and affected bilaterally. *Nodular adrenal cortical hyperplasia* is present in 15 to 20% of cases; the appearance of the cortex between nodules is identical to that in diffuse hyperplasia, suggesting that nodular hyperplasia probably evolves from the latter. *ACTH levels are elevated* in most cases of hyperplasia. *Adrenal cortical adenomas and carcinomas* resemble nonfunctional cortical neoplasms (described later). Lesions occur most commonly in the thirties to fifties, with a female predominance. Adenomas are generally small and well circumscribed; carcinomas tend to be larger and unencapsulated. The zona reticularis and fasciculata of the adjacent residual cortex and the contralateral gland are *atrophic*; the zona glomerulosa is intact.

CLINICAL COURSE

The clinical features of Cushing syndrome include

- Central obesity (85 to 90%)
- Moon facies (85%)
- Weakness and fatigability (85%)
- Hirsutism (75%)
- Hypertension (75%)
- Plethora (75%)
- Glucose intolerance/diabetes (75%/20%)
- Osteoporosis (75%)
- Neuropsychiatric abnormalities (75 to 80%)
- Menstrual abnormalities (70%)
- Cutaneous striae (50%)
- Delayed wound healing/bruisability

Determining the cause of Cushing syndrome depends on measuring the level of serum ACTH and determination of urinary steroid excretion after administration of dexamethasone to suppress ACTH levels. These results coupled with imaging of pituitary and adrenals are necessary to characterize Cushing syndrome fully.

Primary Hyperaldosteronism (p. 1155)

Primary hyperaldosteronism is characterized by chronic excess aldosterone secretion. *Excessive levels of aldosterone cause sodium retention and potassium excretion, with resultant hypertension and hypokalemia.*

Primary hyperaldosteronism indicates an autonomous overproduction of aldosterone, with resultant suppression of the renin angiotensin system and decreased levels of plasma renin activity. Primary hyperaldosteronism is caused either by an aldosterone-producing adrenocortical neoplasm, usually an adenoma, or by primary adrenocortical hyperplasia. A solitary aldosterone-secreting adenoma accounts for about 65% of cases (Conn syndrome).

In *secondary hyperaldosteronism*, aldosterone release occurs in response to activation of the renin-angiotensin system and is encountered in conditions such as congestive heart failure, decreased renal perfusion, and pregnancy.

MORPHOLOGY

Aldosterone-producing adenomas are usually *solitary, small, encapsulated lesions*; they occur more commonly on the left side. *Peak incidence* is in the thirties to forties, usually in women. They may be buried within the adrenal and not apparent externally; cut surface is usually bright yellow, reflecting high lipid content. Constituent lipid-laden cells more often resemble cells of zona fasciculata than zona glomerulosa. *Bilateral idiopathic hyperplasia* is characterized by hyperplasia of cells resembling normal zona glomerulosa, interspersed with nodules resembling zona fasciculata.

CLINICAL COURSE

The clinical manifestations of primary hyperaldosteronism are those of hypertension and hypokalemia. Hypokalemia results from renal potassium wasting and can cause a variety of neuromuscular manifestations, including weakness, paresthesias, visual disturbances, and occasionally frank tetany. Sodium retention increases the total body sodium and expands the extracellular fluid volume. The hypertension is, in some part, a result of the sodium retention.

Adrenogenital Syndromes (p. 1157)

Disorders of sexual differentiation, such as virilization in the female and precocious puberty in the male, may be caused by primary gonadal or adrenal disorders:

- Androgen-secreting adrenal cortical *neoplasms.*
- *Congenital metabolic defects* in corticosteroid biosynthesis, leading to decreased glucocorticoid production, a compensatory increase in ACTH secretion, adrenal hyperplasia, and increased production of other cortical steroids, including androgens. Certain enzymatic defects may also be associated with *salt wasting* resulting from impaired aldosterone production.

21-HYDROXYLASE DEFICIENCY (p. 1157)

Defective conversion of progesterone to 11-deoxycorticosterone by 21-hydroxylase accounts for 85 to 90% of cases of congenital adrenal hyperplasia. All adrenogenital syndromes are autosomal recessive disorders. Three distinctive syndromes have been segregated:

1. Salt-wasting adrenogenitalism is associated with a complete absence of hydroxylase activity and resultant mineralocorticoid and cortisol deficiency syndrome usually recognized after birth, with virilization in females, salt wasting, hyponatremia, hyperkalemia, and cardiovascular collapse.

2. Simple virilizing adrenogenitalism without salt wasting is associated with incomplete loss of hydroxylase activity.

3. Nonclassic adrenogenitalism implies mild disease that may be entirely asymptomatic or associated only with symptoms of androgen excess during childhood or puberty.

Morphologic changes include substantial, bilateral adrenal enlargement; cortex is widened and nodular and appears brown because of lipid depletion. The clinical features of this disorder are determined by the specific enzyme deficiency and include abnormalities related to androgen excess; sodium deficiency; and, in severe cases, glucocorticoid deficiency. Patients with congenital adrenal hyperplasia are treated with exogenous glucocorticoids.

Adrenal Insufficiency (p. 1159)

PRIMARY ACUTE ADRENOCORTICAL INSUFFICIENCY (p. 1159)

Primary acute adrenocortical insufficiency may be caused by any lesion of the adrenal cortex that impairs corticosteroid production or may be secondary to ACTH deficiency. Patterns include

- Primary acute adrenocortical insufficiency (adrenal crisis)
- Primary chronic adrenocortical insufficiency (Addison disease)
- Secondary adrenocortical insufficiency

Acute adrenal cortical insufficiency can occur in a variety of settings, including

- A *sudden increase in glucocorticoid requirements* in patients with chronic adrenocortical insufficiency.
- *Rapid withdrawal of steroids* from patients with adrenal suppression secondary to long-term glucocorticoid therapy or *failure to increase steroid doses* in adrenalectomized patients during episodes of stress
- *Massive destruction* of the adrenals (e.g., neonatal adrenal hemorrhage, postsurgical disseminated intravascular coagulation, Waterhouse-Friderichsen syndrome)

WATERHOUSE-FRIDERICHSEN SYNDROME (p. 1160)

Waterhouse-Friderichsen syndrome is an uncommon but catastrophic syndrome that is characterized by

- Overwhelming septicemic infection usually caused by *meningococci*, less often by other virulent bacteria (pneumococci, gonococci, staphylococci)
- Rapidly progressive hypotension and shock
- Disseminated intravascular coagulation with purpura
- Massive adrenal hemorrhage with adrenal insufficiency
- Common occurrence in *children* but may occur at any age

Morphologic changes are those of *massive, bilateral adrenal hemorrhage*, which begins in the medulla. The cause of the hemorrhage is unclear but may involve direct bacterial seeding of adrenal vessels, disseminated intravascular coagulation, endotoxin-induced vasculitis, or a hypersensitivity vasculitis. The clinical course can be devastatingly abrupt unless recognition is prompt and appropriate therapy provided.

PRIMARY CHRONIC ADRENOCORTICAL INSUFFICIENCY (ADDISON DISEASE) (p. 1160)

Addison disease, or chronic adrenal insufficiency, is an uncommon condition, occurring most often in adults who suffer destruction of at least 90% of the adrenal cortex. *Causes are multiple,* including the following:

- *Autoimmune adrenalitis* accounts for 60 to 70% of cases of Addison disease. The adrenals may be the sole targets of the reaction, but in the remainder, other autoimmune diseases coexist. Destruction may be part of a *polyglandular syndrome.* Circulating antibodies are present in 50% of cases. The basis of the immune attack is uncertain but may involve genetic mechanisms (increased incidence of HLA-B8 and DR3).
- Infectious processes, particularly tuberculosis and those caused by fungi such as *Histoplasma capsulatum* and *Coccidioides immitis,* may destroy the adrenals.
- *Metastatic neoplasms* are an uncommon cause of adrenal insufficiency. Common primary tumors include carcinomas of the lung and breast.

Morphology

Morphologic features vary, depending on the underlying disease (e.g., metastatic neoplasm, tuberculous granulomas). *Autoimmune adrenalitis* usually produces small glands, lipid depletion of adrenal cortex, and a variable lymphocytic infiltrate in cortex; the medulla is spared.

Clinical Course

Features of Addison disease include weakness, fatigue, anorexia, hypotension, nausea, vomiting, and cutaneous hyperpigmentation. Laboratory values include elevated levels of ACTH, hyperkalemia, and low sodium (hyponatremia), associated with volume depletion and hypotension.

SECONDARY ADRENOCORTICAL INSUFFICIENCY (p. 1161)

Secondary adrenocortical insufficiency may be caused by any disorder of the hypothalamus or pituitary associated with *decreased production of ACTH.* It is distinguished from primary hypoadrenalism by the following:

- Absence of hyperpigmentation (ACTH and precursor peptides with melanocyte-stimulating activity are not elevated in secondary cases).
- Normal or near-normal aldosterone levels (aldosterone production is independent of ACTH; severe hyponatremia and hyperkalemia are *not* features of secondary adrenocortical insufficiency).

ACTH deficiency may be isolated or associated with decreased levels of other pituitary hormones (panhypopituitarism). Morphologically, this condition is characterized by variable degrees of atrophy of the adrenal cortex, with *sparing of the zona glomerulosa and medulla.*

Adrenocortical Neoplasms (p. 1162)

In addition to hyperplasias and neoplasms associated with steroid production, nonfunctional adrenal cortical neoplasms also may occur.

- *Adrenal adenomas* are typically poorly encapsulated, yellow-orange lesions; they may lie within cortex or protrude into medulla or the subcapsular region. Larger lesions may contain areas of hemorrhage, cystic change, and calcification. Adjacent adrenal cortex is of normal thickness (in contrast to atrophic changes seen adjacent to functional adenomas).
- *Adrenal cortical carcinomas* are highly malignant neoplasms, usually of large size at the time of diagnosis. Lesions are predominantly yellow on cut surface but usually contain areas of hemorrhage, cystic change, and necrosis. Histologically, cells range from well differentiated to markedly anaplastic; they may be difficult to differentiate from metastatic cells. The tumors commonly invade vascular channels, with metastases to regional and periaortic lymph nodes and to viscera, especially lung.

ADRENAL MEDULLA (p. 1163)

The adrenal medulla is structurally and functionally distinct from the cortex. Most adrenal medullary disorders are *neoplasms*, the most significant of which are pheochromocytoma, neuroblastoma, and ganglioneuroma. Neuroblastomas and ganglioneuromas are discussed elsewhere.

Pheochromocytoma (p. 1164)

Pheochromocytomas are relatively uncommon neoplasms associated with *catecholamine production* and *hypertension* (account for 0.1 to 0.3% of all cases of hypertension). They may occasionally produce steroids or peptides, with resultant Cushing syndrome or other endocrine disorder. Of lesions, *85% arise within the adrenal medulla*. The remainder of the tumors may occur anywhere within the extra-adrenal paraganglion system; these are chromaffin-negative, extra-adrenal tumors and are often designated *paragangliomas*. Although most occur *sporadically* (90%), some occur in *familial syndromes* (usually autosomal dominant), including

- *von Hippel–Lindau* (visceral cysts, renal cell carcinomas, pheochromocytomas, angiomatosis, cerebellar hemangioblastoma)
- *von Recklinghausen* (neurofibromatosis, café-au-lait spots, schwannomas, meningiomas, gliomas, pheochromocytomas)
- *Sturge-Weber* (cavernous hemangiomas in trigeminal nerve distribution, pheochromocytomas)

Most sporadic lesions occur in adulthood (40 to 60 years) with slight female predominance; familial lesions may arise in childhood, with strong male predominance. Most tumors in the familial syndromes are bilateral (70%), but in the sporadic cases only 10 to 15% are bilateral. Malignancy occurs in 20 to 40% of extra-adrenal tumors and in 2 to 10% of adrenal lesions.

MORPHOLOGY

The tumors vary widely in size (1 gm to 4 kg). The cut surface is usually pale gray or brown and is often associated with hemorrhage, necrosis, or cystic change. Usually the tumors are highly vascular. Fixation of tumor in a dichromate fixative (e.g., Zenker) causes it to turn brown-black because of oxidation of catecholamines (hence the term *chromaffin*). *Microscopically* the tumors are composed of mature polygonal to spindle-shaped medullary-type cells containing basophilic cytoplasmic granules, arrayed in trabeculae or small nests. Cellular and nuclear pleomorphism are common. *There are no reliable histologic predictors of malignancy*: Pleomorphism, mitotic activity, and intravascular neoplastic cells may be seen in benign neoplasms. The only reliable criterion of malignancy is metastasis, most commonly to lymph nodes, liver, lungs, and bones.

CLINICAL FEATURES

The dominant clinical feature in patients with pheochromocytoma is *hypertension*. Classically, this feature is described as an abrupt, precipitous elevation in blood pressure, associated with tachycardia, palpitations, headache, sweating, tremor, and a sense of apprehension. Paroxysmal release of catecholamines may also be associated with episodic headache, anxiety, sweating, tremor, visual disturbances, abdominal pain, and nausea. Sometimes the hypertension is stably elevated. The hypertension may be associated with other organ dysfunction, including congestive heart failure, myocardial infarcts, cardiac arrhythmia, and cerebral hemorrhage. Cardiac complications are attributed to ischemic myocardial damage secondary to catecholamine-induced vasoconstriction *(catecholamine cardiomyopathy)*. Preoperative diagnosis is based on laboratory evaluation, including measurement of urinary catecholamines and their metabolites, plasma catecholamine assays, and radiographic imaging studies (computed tomography, magnetic resonance imaging, or ultrasound).

Tumors of Extra-Adrenal Paraganglia

(p. 1166)

Pheochromocytomas that develop in paraganglia other than the adrenal medulla are often designated *paragangliomas*, although some restrict the term *paraganglioma* to the nonfunctioning tumors. Paragangliomas may arise in any organ that contains paraganglionic tissue. Tumors arising in the carotid body are designated *carotid body* tumors, whereas those originating in the jugulotympanic body are sometimes referred to as *chemodectomas*. The tumors occur most commonly in patients in their teens to twenties and are *multicentric* in 15 to 25% of cases. They are *malignant* in 10 to 40% of cases; 10% of the tumors metastasize widely.

MORPHOLOGY

The tumors are usually firm, 1- to 6-cm lesions, often densely adherent to adjacent tissues. They are composed of well-differentiated neuroendocrine cells arrayed in nests *(Zellballen)* or cords, separated by prominent fibrovascular stroma. Tumors may contain mitotic figures and may exhibit substantial pleomorphism.

MULTIPLE ENDOCRINE NEOPLASIA SYNDROMES (p. 1166)

MEN syndromes are usually *autosomal dominant syndromes* characterized by hyperplasia or tumors of several endocrine glands simultaneously. Variants include

- *MEN I* (parathyroid, pancreatic and pituitary lesions)
- *MEN II or IIa* (pheochromocytomas and adrenal medullary hyperplasia, medullary carcinomas and C-cell hyperplasia of thyroid, parathyroid hyperplasia)
- *MEN IIb or III* (pheochromocytomas and medullary thyroid hyperplasia, medullary carcinomas and C-cell hyperplasia of thyroid, mucosal neuromas, marfanoid features)

Multiple Endocrine Neoplasia I (Wermer) Syndrome (p. 1166)

MEN I is characterized as follows:

- *Parathyroid hyperplasia* or *multiple adenomas* are seen in 90 to 95% of cases, appearing by age 40 to 50.
- *Pancreatic lesions* include islet cell tumors, which may secrete a variety of peptide hormones.
- *Pituitary adenomas* are present in 10 to 15% of cases, frequently a prolactinoma.

Etiology involves mutations in the novel MEN I gene found on chromosome 11q11-13. The dominant clinical manifestations of MEN I are usually defined by the peptide hormones and include such abnormalities as recurrent hypoglycemia in insulinomas and recurrent peptic ulcers in patients with gastrin-secreting neoplasms (Zollinger-Ellison syndrome).

Multiple Endocrine Neoplasia II Syndrome (p. 1166)

MEN II is subclassified into three distinct syndromes:

1. MEN IIa
2. MEN IIb
3. Familial medullary thyroid cancer

MEN IIa or Sipple syndrome is characterized as follows:

- *Medullary thyroid carcinomas* in 100% of patients are usually multifocal. C-cell hyperplasia may also be present. In addition to *calcitonin*, medullary carcinomas may elaborate other biologically active peptides. Most tumors pursue a malignant course.
- *Pheochromocytomas* are present in 50% of patients and are often bilateral and extra-adrenal. Most lesions are clinically benign.
- *Parathyroid hyperplasias* are found in 10 to 20% of cases with evidence of hypercalcemia or renal stones.

MEN II is clinically and genetically distinct from MEN I and has been linked to germ line mutations in the *RET protooncogene* on chromosome 10.

Multiple Endocrine Neoplasia IIb or III (p. 1166–1167)

MEN IIb or III is similar to *MEN IIa*, with additional feature of *neuromas* or *ganglioneuromas* involving lips, oral cavity, eyes, respiratory tract, gastrointestinal tract, urinary bladder, and other sites. Presenting clinical manifestations are often referable to neuromas; mean survival may be shorter than MEN IIa (three to four decades). MEN IIb is genetically distinct and involves a mutation in the *RET* protooncogene that is different from that associated with MEN IIa.

PINEAL GLAND (p. 1168)

Pineal region neoplasms account for less than 1% of brain tumors; they include both *germ cell* tumors and neoplasms of *pineal parenchymal origin*.

Pinealomas (p. 1168)

Pinealomas are classified as *pineoblastomas* or *pineocytomas*, depending on the level of differentiation.

- *Pineoblastomas* occur predominantly in the pediatric population and are composed of *primitive neuroectodermal cells* reminiscent of cerebellar medulloblastoma. They may *invade* local structures and *metastasize* via cerebrospinal fluid pathways. Most patients die within 1 to 2 years.
- *Pineocytomas* are more common in adults and are composed of a variable mixture of *glial* and *neuronal* elements, recapitulating the structure of the mature pineal gland. There is prolonged survival (average 7 years).

Diseases of the Skin

More than just a passive barrier to fluid loss and mechanical injury, skin is composed of interdependent cell types all contributing to its *protective* function:

- *Squamous epithelial cells (keratinocytes)*: Majority of epidermal cells and the major mechanical barrier; also a source of cytokines, which regulate the cutaneous environment
- *Melanocytes*: Produce *melanin* pigment to screen ultraviolet light
- *Langerhans cells*: Dendritic cells that process and present antigen to activate the immune system
- *Neural end organs*: Detect pain and temperature to prevent physical damage
- *Sweat glands*: Permit cooling of the body
- *Hair follicles*: Elaborate the hair shafts and protect repositories of epithelial stem cells

---

DEFINITION OF TERMS

Macroscopic

Macule   Flat, circumscribed area distinguished from surrounding skin by coloration

Papule   Elevated solid area measuring 5 mm or less

Nodule   Elevated solid area measuring greater than 5 mm

Plaque   Elevated flat-topped lesion measuring greater than 5 mm

Vesicle   Elevated fluid-filled lesion measuring 5 mm or less

Bulla   Elevated fluid-filled lesion measuring greater than 5 mm

Blister   Common term for vesicle or bulla

Pustule   Discrete, pus-filled raised area

Wheal   Pruritic, erythematous elevated area resulting from dermal edema

Scale   Dry, platelike excrescence resulting from aberrant cornification

Lichenification   Thick, rough skin with prominent skin markings, often as a result of repeated rubbing

Excoriation   Linear, traumatic lesion resulting in epidermal breakage (i.e., a deep scratch)

Onycholysis   Loss of nail substance

Microscopic

Hyperkeratosis   Stratum corneum thickening, often with aberrant keratinization

Parakeratosis   Abnormal retention of nuclei in stratum corneum

Acanthosis   Epidermal hyperplasia

Dyskeratosis   Abnormal keratinization below the stratum corneum

Acantholysis   Loss of intercellular connections between keratinocytes

Papillomatosis   Elongation or widening of the dermal papillae

Lentiginous   Linear pattern of melanocyte proliferation in the epidermal basal cell layer; may be reactive or neoplastic

Spongiosis   Epidermal intercellular edema

Exocytosis   Inflammatory cells infiltrating the epidermis

Erosion   Focal, incomplete loss of epidermis

Ulceration   Focal complete loss of epidermis; may include dermis and subcutaneous fat

Vacuolization   Vacuoles within or adjacent to cells

DISORDERS OF PIGMENTATION AND MELANOCYTES (p. 1173)

Vitiligo (p. 1173)

Vitiligo is a common disorder presenting as irregular, well-demarcated macules (few to many centimeters) devoid of pigmentation. It occurs in all races but is most apparent in darkly pigmented individuals. It often involves the wrists; axillae; and perioral, periorbital, and anogenital regions.

Pathogenetic theories include

1. Autoimmunity (best supported by the data, including melanocyte autoantibodies and T-cell, macrophage, or Langerhans cell abnormalities)
2. Neurohumoral factors
3. Toxic intermediates in melanin synthesis

Histologically, loss of melanocytes is seen on electron microscopy. This finding contrasts with some forms of *albinism*, in which melanocytes are present but nonfunctional.

Freckle (Ephelis) (p. 1174)

Freckles are common pigmented lesions of childhood: tan-red to brown macules, measuring 1 to 10 mm, occurring after sun exposure, and fading and recurring with subsequent cycles of winter and summer.

Histologically, there is a normal melanocyte number (possibly slight hypertrophy) but increased melanin within basal keratinocytes.

Melasma (p. 1174)

Melasma refers to masklike facial hyperpigmentation, typically seen in hyperestrogenic states such as pregnancy. It presents as blotchy, irregular, ill-defined macules. Sunlight accentuates the pigmentation, which usually fades post partum. Melasma is caused by enhanced melanin transfer from melanocytes to other cell types with subsequent accumulation.

Histologically, melasma is characterized by

- Increased melanin deposition in basal layers (*epidermal type*)
- Papillary dermal macrophage phagocytosis of melanin released from the epidermis (i.e., pigment incontinence [*dermal type*])

Lentigo (p. 1174)

A lentigo (plural, *lentigines*) is a common, benign, hyperpigmented macule (5 to 10 mm) in skin and mucous membranes, most often occurring in infancy and childhood. In contrast to freckles, lentigines do not darken with sun exposure. The cause and pathogenesis are unknown.

Histologically, there is linear basal hyperpigmentation resulting from melanocyte hyperplasia, often with elongation and thinning of rete ridges.

Nevocellular Nevus (Pigmented Nevus, Mole) (p. 1174)

Nevocellular nevus specifically refers to a group of congenital or acquired *melanocyte neoplasms*. Clinically, common acquired nevocellular nevi are well-demarcated, uniformly tan-brown papules measuring 6 mm or less; features of common variants are described in Table 25–1.

NATURAL HISTORY

- Melanocytes of nevocellular nevi derive from basal dendritic cells that have transformed into round-to-oval cells with uniform nuclei and inconspicuous nucleoli.
- Nevi initially form nests along the dermoepidermal junction—*junctional nevi.*
- Eventually, most junctional nevi also extend nests and cords into the underlying dermis—*compound nevi.*
- In mature lesions, the epidermal component may be lost—*dermal nevi.*
- With extension into the dermis, the *nevus cells undergo* maturation, becoming nonpigmented and resembling neural tissue. This is diagnostically important because *melanomas usually show no maturation.*

CLINICAL SIGNIFICANCE

Nevocellular nevi are significant largely as a model of tumor progression and possibly cosmetically.

Dysplastic Nevi (p. 1176)

Dysplastic nevi are found in persons with an autosomal dominant (susceptibility gene on chromosome 1) predisposition to develop many atypical acquired nevi; these may evolve into malig-

Table 25-1. VARIANT FORMS OF NEVOCELLULAR NEVI

Nevus Variant	Diagnostic Architectural Features	Diagnostic Cytologic Features	Clinical Significance
Congenital nevus	Deep dermal and sometimes subcutaneous growth around adnexae, neurovascular bundles, and blood vessel walls	Identical to ordinary acquired nevi	Present at birth; large variants have increased melanoma risk
Blue nevus	Non-nested dermal infiltration, often with associated fibrosis	Highly dendritic, heavily pigmented nevus cells	Black-blue nodule; often confused with melanoma clinically
Spindle and epithelioid cell nevus (Spitz nevus)	Fascicular growth	Large, plump cells with pink-blue cytoplasm; fusiform cells	Common in children; red-pink nodule; often confused with hemangioma clinically
Halo nevus	Lymphocytic infiltration surrounding nevus nests	Identical to ordinary acquired nevi	Host immune response against nevus cells and surrounding normal melanocytes
Dysplastic nevus	Large, coalescent intraepidermal nests	Cytologic atypia	Potential precursor of malignant melanoma

nant melanoma (50% of affected individuals by age 59 years). Dysplastic nevi may also occur as isolated sporadic lesions with a low risk of malignant transformation. Usually, these are larger than typical acquired nevi (>5 mm) and may occur as hundreds of irregular macules or plaques with pigment variegation on both sun-exposed and nonexposed skin (in contrast to typical moles).

Histologically, there is cytologic and architectural atypia, with enlarged and fused epidermal nevus cell nests, lentiginous melanocytic hyperplasia, linear papillary dermal fibrosis, and pigment incontinence.

The risk of developing melanoma *(heritable melanoma syndrome)* is increased for unaffected skin as well as for areas with preexisting nevi. Most dysplastic nevi, however, are clinically stable.

Malignant Melanoma (p. 1177)

Malignant melanoma is a relatively common neoplasm, currently increasing in incidence; sun exposure is an important pathogenic factor, and lightly pigmented individuals are at greater risk than darkly pigmented persons. Hereditary substrates (e.g., dysplastic nevus syndrome) also increase the risk. These are pruritic, variegated, irregular maculopapular lesions most commonly found on skin but occasionally involving the mucosae, conjunctiva, orbit, nail beds, esophagus, and leptomeninges. In contrast to benign nevi, melanomas may be black, brown, red-blue, or gray.

Diagnostically important is a change in coloration. Typically a melanoma initially extends horizontally within the epidermis and superficial dermis *(radial growth phase)* during which it does not metastasize. Specific types of radial growth phase melanomas (e.g., *lentigo maligna* and *superficial spreading*) are defined by architectural and cytologic features and exhibit different biologic behaviors. Eventually a *vertical growth phase* evolves, with extension into the deep dermis, loss of cellular maturation, and development of the capacity to metastasize. The clinical behavior (e.g., *probability of metastasis*) is determined by the characteristics and measured depth of invasion of the vertical growth; prediction of the clinical outcome may be further refined by determination of mitotic rates and the degree of lymphocytic infiltrate.

Histologically, melanoma cells are larger than nevus cells, with irregular nuclei and prominent eosinophilic nucleoli; they grow as loose nests lacking the typical features of melanocyte maturation.

BENIGN EPITHELIAL TUMORS (p. 1179)

Benign epithelial tumors are common, generally biologically inconsequential lesions derived from keratinocytes or skin appendages.

Seborrheic Keratoses (p. 1179)

Seborrheic keratoses are spontaneous lesions, most often occurring in middle-aged and older individuals and most numerous on the trunk (also called *senile keratoses*). Similar smaller facial lesions in nonwhites are called *dermatosis papulosa nigra*. They may occur spontaneously in large numbers as part of a paraneoplastic syndrome *(sign of Leser-Trélat)*, possibly as a result of tumor elaboration of growth factors (e.g., transforming growth factor–α).

Grossly, seborrheic keratoses are uniform, tan-brown, velvety or granular round plaques millimeters to several centimeters in diameter; keratin-filled plugs may be evident.

Histologically, seborrheic keratoses are sharply demarcated, exophytic lesions with hyperplasia of variably pigmented basaloid cells and *hyperkeratosis*; there are occasional keratin-filled *horn cysts.* When irritated and inflamed, the basaloid cells undergo squamous differentiation. When associated with hair follicle epithelium, lesions are endophytic, growing downward *(inverted follicular keratoses).*

Acanthosis Nigricans (p. 1180)

Acanthosis nigricans refers to thickened, hyperpigmented zones, typically in flexural areas (axilla, groin, neck, anogenital region), associated with benign and malignant conditions elsewhere in the body.

- The *benign* type makes up 80% of all cases; it develops gradually, usually arising in childhood through puberty, and occurs
  - As an autosomal dominant trait with variable penetrance
  - In association with obesity or endocrine disorders (especially diabetes and pituitary or pineal tumors)
  - As a component of certain rare congenital disorders
- The *malignant* type arises in middle-aged and older individuals, often in association with an occult adenocarcinoma (possibly tumor elaboration of epidermal growth factors).

Histologically, both types are characterized by hyperkeratosis, with prominent rete ridges and basal hyperpigmentation (without melanocyte hyperplasia).

Fibroepithelial Polyp (p. 1181)

Also called *acrochordon, squamous papilloma,* or *skin tag,* a fibroepithelial polyp is an exceptionally common benign lesion in middle-aged and older individuals, found on the neck, trunk, face, or intertriginous zones. It is a soft, flesh-colored tumor attached by a slender stalk, with a fibrovascular core covered by benign epidermis. It may be associated with pregnancy, diabetes, or intestinal polyposis.

Epithelial Cyst (Wen) (p. 1181)

Epithelial cysts are common lesions presenting as well-circumscribed, firm, subcutaneous nodules, formed by downgrowth and cystic expansion of the epidermal or follicular epithelium.

Histologically, they are subdivided on the basis of the cyst wall characteristics. All are filled with keratin and variable amounts of lipid and debris from sebaceous secretions.

- *Epidermal inclusion cysts:* The wall is almost identical to normal epidermis.
- *Pilar (trichilemmal) cysts:* The wall resembles follicular epithelium (i.e., without a granular cell layer).
- *Dermoid cysts:* The wall is similar to epidermis but with multiple skin appendages, especially hair follicles.
- *Steatocystoma multiplex:* The wall resembles sebaceous gland ductal epithelium with numerous compressed sebaceous lobules (frequently of dominant inheritance).

Keratoacanthoma (p. 1181)

A keratoacanthoma is a self-limited, often *spontaneously resolving*, rapid-growing lesion, typically occurring in sun-exposed skin of whites 50 years of age and older, in men more often than in women. The majority have detectable *p53* oncoprotein (occasionally with mutations), suggesting that these may represent a form of *squamous cell carcinoma* (see later) that regresses because of host-tumor interactions.

Grossly, flesh-colored, dome-shaped nodules are seen, often on the face or hands, measuring 1 cm to several centimeters in diameter, with central keratin-filled craters.

Histologically, cup-shaped epithelial proliferations are seen, often with atypical cells, enclosing a central keratin-filled plug. The pattern of keratinization recapitulates the normal hair follicle (no granular cell layer). Minimal inflammation occurs during the rapid proliferative phase, but as the lesion matures, dermal inflammation and fibrosis supervene, with eventual regression and disappearance.

Adnexal (Appendage) Tumors (p. 1182)

Adnexal tumors are a large family of benign neoplasms (although malignant variants exist, e.g., *sebaceous carcinoma* arising in eyelid meibomian glands). Some have mendelian patterns of inheritance and occur as multiple disfiguring lesions; others may indicate visceral malignancy (e.g., multiple trichilemmomas and breast cancer—*Cowden syndrome*). Most are single or multiple nondescript papules and nodules.

- *Cylindromas* typically occur as multiple coalescing nodules *(turban tumor)* of basaloid cells with apocrine differentiation on the scalp and forehead.
- *Syringomas* usually occur as multiple, small, tan papules near the lower eyelids composed of tadpole-shaped islands of basaloid epithelium with focal eccrine differentiation.
- *Trichoepitheliomas* usually present as multiple flesh-colored papules on the face, scalp, neck, and upper trunk, composed of proliferations of basaloid cells forming hair follicle–like structures.
- *Trichilemmomas* are proliferations of cells resembling the uppermost portion of the hair follicle.
- *Hidradenoma papilliferum* occurs on the face and scalp and is composed of ducts and papillae lined by apocrine-type cells.

PREMALIGNANT AND MALIGNANT EPIDERMAL TUMORS (p. 1184)

Actinic Keratosis (p. 1184)

Actinic keratosis refers to a premalignant dysplastic lesion (not to be confused with seborrheic keratosis) associated with chronic sun exposure, especially in light-skinned individuals. Ionizing radiation, hydrocarbons, and arsenicals may induce similar lesions. Because many undergo malignant transformation, local eradication is indicated.

Grossly, these lesions are usually less than 1 cm, tan-brown, red, or flesh-colored, with a rough consistency. Hyperkeratosis may produce cutaneous horns.

Histologically, there is cytologic atypia in the lower epidermis, frequently with basal cell hyperplasia and dyskeratosis. Intercellular bridges are present. *Hyperkeratosis* and *parakeratosis* may be present, or there may be epidermal atrophy. The dermis contains thickened, blue-gray elastic fibers (*elastosis*), resulting from aberrant synthesis by sun-damaged fibroblasts.

Squamous Cell Carcinoma (p. 1184)

Squamous cell carcinoma is the most common tumor of sun-exposed skin of older individuals; it is more frequent in men than in women with the exception of lower leg lesions. *Sunlight (specifically ultraviolet irradiation)* is the greatest predisposing factor, primarily by directly damaging DNA and causing mutations. Ultraviolet light also causes immunosuppression by injuring antigen-presenting Langerhans cells and augmenting the development of suppressor T lymphocytes. Other predisposing factors include industrial carcinogens (tars), chronic skin ulcers, old burn scars, draining osteomyelitis, ionizing radiation, and (for oral mucosa) tobacco or betel nut chewing. Immunosuppression (as a consequence of chemotherapy or tissue transplantation) and xeroderma pigmentosum (an inherited defect in DNA repair, Chapter 6) increase tumor risk, and human papillomavirus (HPV 36) may also occasionally contribute.

Grossly, in situ squamous cell carcinoma appears as well-demarcated, red, scaling plaques. *Invasive lesions* are nodular, variably hyperkeratotic, and prone to ulceration. Mucosal involvement is manifested as white thickening called *leukoplakia*. Most tumors remain localized, with less than 5% metastasis to regional nodes at the time of resection.

Microscopically, in situ carcinoma has full-thickness epidermal atypia (versus actinic keratosis, which has only basal atypia). *Invasive tumors* vary from well differentiated (with prominent keratinization) to highly anaplastic with necrosis and abortive keratinization.

Basal Cell Carcinoma (p. 1186)

Basal cell carcinoma refers to common, slow-growing tumors, typically in sun-exposed skin; *they rarely metastasize*. Immunosuppression and xeroderma pigmentosum increase the incidence.

Basal cell nevus syndrome is a rare, dominantly inherited disease characterized by multiple basal cell carcinomas beginning in early life, along with bone, nervous system, eye, and reproductive organ anomalies. It is associated with mutations in the PTC tumor-suppressor gene.

Grossly, basal cell carcinomas appear as pearly papules or expanding plaques; some are melanin pigmented. Advanced lesions ulcerate, and there is extensive local invasion, termed *rodent ulcer*.

Microscopically, there is uniform, rather monotonous basal cell proliferation, either as *multifocal superficial growths* over a large area (several centimeters) of skin or as *nodules* extending deeply into the dermis. Anaplasia, mitoses, and tumor giant cells are absent.

Merkel Cell Carcinoma (p. 1187)

Merkel cells are functionally obscure epidermal, neural crest–derived cells (possibly involved in lower animal tactile sensation).

Merkel cell carcinoma is a rare, potentially lethal tumor composed of small, round malignant cells containing neurosecretory-type cytoplasmic granules that closely resemble small cell carcinoma in the lung.

TUMORS OF DERMIS (p. 1187)

Benign Fibrous Histiocytoma (p. 1187)

Benign fibrous histiocytoma refers to a heterogeneous group of benign, indolent neoplasms of dermal fibroblasts and histiocytes. Lesions are usually seen in adults and frequently on the legs of young to middle-aged women. Histogenesis is unknown, although antecedent trauma and aberrant healing are often implicated. Benign fibrous histiocytoma should not be confused with clinically aggressive malignant fibrous histiocytoma, arising in skin and extracutaneous sites.

Grossly, tan-brown, firm papules, sometimes tender, which may achieve several centimeters in diameter, occur. Lateral compression causes them to dimple inward.

Histologically the most common form is the *dermatofibroma,* composed of spindle-shaped fibroblasts in a well-defined, although nonencapsulated mass in the mid-dermis, frequently extending into the subcutaneous fat. Other variants have conspicuous foamy histiocytes with fewer fibroblasts or have numerous blood vessels and hemosiderin deposits *(sclerosing hemangioma).*

Dermatofibrosarcoma Protuberans (p. 1188)

Dermatofibrosarcoma protuberans is a well-differentiated, slow-growing fibrosarcoma of the skin that is locally aggressive but rarely metastasizes.

Grossly, these are firm, solid nodules arising as protuberant, occasionally ulcerated aggregates within an indurated plaque, typically on the trunk.

Microscopically, these are cellular neoplasms composed of radially oriented (storiform) fibroblasts; mitoses are not as numerous as in fibrosarcoma. The overlying epidermis is thinned, and there often is microscopic extension into subcutaneous fat.

Xanthomas (p. 1189)

Xanthomas are not true neoplasms but rather focal accumulations of foamy histiocytes. They may be idiopathic or associated with familial or acquired hyperlipidemias or lymphoproliferative disorders (p. 851). They may be subdivided on the basis of the gross appearance and associated hyperlipidemias:

- *Eruptive xanthoma:* Sudden showers of yellow papules that wax and wane with plasma triglyceride and lipid levels; they occur on the buttocks, posterior thighs, knees, and elbows *(hyperlipidemia types I, IIB, III, IV, and V).*
- *Tuberous xanthoma:* Yellow, flat-to-round nodules over the joints, especially knees and elbows *(types IIA and III).*
- *Tendinous xanthoma:* Yellow nodules over the Achilles tendon and finger extensor tendons *(types IIA and III).*
- *Plane xanthoma:* Linear yellow lesions in skin folds, especially palmar creases *(type III).* Occasionally associated with primary biliary cirrhosis *(type IIA).*

■ *Xanthelasma*: Soft yellow plaques on the eyelids *(types IIA and III, or without lipid abnormality)*.

Microscopically, all lesions are characterized by variably cellular dermal aggregates of macrophages with vacuolated cytoplasm containing cholesterol, phospholipids, and triglycerides.

Dermal Vascular Tumors (p. 1189)

Hemangiomas and malignant vascular tumors, Kaposi sarcoma, and bacillary angiomatosis are discussed in Chapter 12. *Capillary hemangiomas* are the most common form of cutaneous vascular tumors. Occurring throughout life as dark pink papules, the *histologic appearance* is a well-demarcated cluster of endothelium-lined and blood-filled vascular spaces in the dermis.

TUMORS OF CELLULAR IMMIGRANTS TO THE SKIN (p. 1189)

Tumors of cellular immigrants to the skin are proliferative disorders of cells that have arisen elsewhere but that have homed to the skin (e.g., Langerhans cells, T lymphocytes, and mast cells).

Histiocytosis X (p. 1189)

The systemic pattern of histiocytosis is discussed in Chapter 15. The *cutaneous form* may present as solitary or multiple papules or nodules or as scaling erythematous plaques resembling seborrheic dermatitis.

Histologic lesions include variable numbers of eosinophils and diffuse-to-granulomatous dermal infiltrates of round-to-ovoid mononuclear cells with indented, bland nuclei; occasionally the mononuclear cells have foamy, xanthoma-like cytoplasm. Ultrastructural demonstration of Birbeck granules (p. 685) and immunohistochemical documentation of CD1 antigens on the infiltrating cells confirm their derivation from Langerhans cells.

Mycosis Fungoides (Cutaneous T-Cell Lymphoma) (p. 1191)

Mycosis fungoides occurs in various patterns, including

1. A chronic proliferative process—*mycosis fungoides*
2. A nodular eruptive variant—*mycosis fungoides d'emblée*
3. A form with an aggressive course called *adult T-cell leukemia* or *lymphoma* (attributed to human T-cell lymphotropic virus type 1)

Mycosis fungoides arises primarily in the skin and generally remains localized there for many years. *Sézary syndrome* occurs with seeding of the blood by malignant T cells, accompanied by diffuse erythema and scaling *(erythroderma)*; it represents evolution into a more generalized T-cell leukemia or lymphoma.

Grossly, mycosis fungoides initially presents as eczema-like lesions, evolving into scaly, red-brown patches or plaques and eventually into fungating nodules (up to 10 cm) on the trunk, extremities, face, and scalp. Nodular cutaneous growth correlates with deep dermal invasion and the onset of lymph node and visceral involvement.

The *histologic hallmark* of mycosis fungoides is the *Sézary-*

Lutzner cell, a malignant CD4+ (T-helper) cell with a hyperconvoluted or *cerebriform* nucleus. These typically form bandlike dermal infiltrates with invasion by single cells or small clusters into the epidermis *(Pautrier microabscesses)*.

Mastocytosis (p. 1192)

Mastocytosis refers to a family of rare disorders characterized by cutaneous (and occasionally visceral) mast cell proliferation. Symptoms reflect the consequences of mast cell degranulation, with release of histamine (e.g., pruritus, flushing, rhinorrhea, or dermal edema and erythema). The dermal change is called a *wheal* when lesional skin is rubbed (Darier sign) and *dermatographism* when evoked in normal skin. Rarely, epistaxis or gastrointestinal bleeding occurs secondary to heparin release from the mast cells.

Urticaria pigmentosa (50% of all cases) is an exclusively cutaneous form of mastocytosis, with a generally favorable prognosis, occurring mainly in children. Systemic mastocytosis occurs in 10% of patients, usually adults, and carries a much poorer prognosis. The *pathogenesis*, at least in some cases, is due to point mutations of the c-KIT protooncogene, resulting in activation of the KIT tyrosine kinase that directs mast cell growth and differentiation.

Grossly, skin lesions of urticaria pigmentosa and systemic mastocytosis are multiple, round-to-oval, nonscaling, red-brown papules and plaques.

Microscopically, variable dermal fibrosis, edema, eosinophils, and mast cells are visible, the last-mentioned distinguishable by special metachromatic stains.

Disorder of Epidermal Maturation: Ichthyosis (p. 1193)

One of many disorders that impair epidermal maturation, ichthyosis is actually a collection of generally hereditary (autosomal dominant, recessive, or X-linked) clinical entities, presenting at or near birth with marked hyperkeratosis grossly resembling fish scales (hence the name). Acquired variants exist and may be associated with various malignancies. The disorder is clinically grouped according to the mode of inheritance and clinical and histologic features. The primary defect in most forms is increased cell-cell adhesion resulting in abnormal desquamation and consequently scale formation.

Microscopically, ichthyosis is characterized by build-up of compacted stratum corneum, with minimal inflammation and rather subtle changes in epidermal and stratum granulosum thickness.

ACUTE INFLAMMATORY DERMATOSES
(p. 1193)

Acute inflammatory dermatoses constitute an enormous family of conditions, mediated by local or systemic immunologic factors and characterized by short-lived lesions (days to weeks) marked by mononuclear cell infiltrates with associated edema and occasionally local tissue damage.

Urticaria (Hives) (p. 1194)

Urticaria is a common disorder, typically occurring in young adults and marked by focal mast cell degranulation, with histamine-mediated dermal pruritus, edema, and wheal. Individual lesions develop and regress within hours, but sequential lesions may occur for months. *Angioedema* is related but is distinguished by *dermal* and *subcutaneous fat* edema.

Grossly, lesions vary from small, pruritic papules to large edematous plaques. Sites of predilection include any area exposed to pressure, such as the trunk, distal extremities, and ears.

Microscopically, there is a sparse mononuclear perivascular infiltrate associated with edema and occasionally with dermal eosinophils but no evidence of increased mast cell numbers.

Most lesions are mediated by antigen-specific IgE, but *IgE-independent urticaria* can occur by direct chemical-induced mast cell degranulation in sensitive patients or by suppression of prostaglandin synthesis (i.e., with aspirin). Persistent urticaria may reflect an inability to clear the inciting antigen or may announce cryptic collagen vascular disorders or Hodgkin disease.

Hereditary angioneurotic edema consists of recurrent attacks of angioedema with gastrointestinal tract and laryngeal involvement. It is due to deficient C1 esterase inhibitor and unregulated activation of the early complement components.

Acute Eczematous Dermatitis (p. 1194)

Acute eczematous dermatitis refers to a variety of pathogenetically different conditions, all with similar histologic features. Five types, distinguished primarily by their clinical features, are described in Table 25–2. Many forms of *eczema* constitute a cutaneous delayed-type hypersensitivity response, with pathogenesis attributed to cytokine release and nonspecific recruitment of the bulk of the inflammatory cells.

Grossly, all types of acute eczema are pruritic, red, papulovesicular to blistered, oozing, and subsequently crusted lesions (e.g., contact hypersensitivity to poison ivy). With chronic exposure, lesions may evolve into psoriasis-like scaling plaques. Bacterial superinfection produces a yellow crust *(impetiginization).*

Histologically, there is initially *spongiosis*; with progressive fluid accumulation, keratinocytes splay apart, and intraepidermal vesicles form. There is also a dermal perivascular lymphocytic infiltrate with mast cell degranulation and papillary dermal edema. Lesions resulting from drug hypersensitivity may have eosinophils. In chronic lesions, the vesicular phase is replaced with progressive *acanthosis* and *hyperkeratosis.*

Erythema Multiforme (p. 1197)

Erythema multiforme is an uncommon, self-limited hypersensitivity response to certain drugs or infections or to systemic disorders (malignancy or collagen vascular diseases), characterized by extensive epidermal degeneration and necrosis. It is due to CD8 + T cell–mediated cytotoxicity and has similarities to other immunologic cutaneous disorders, such as graft-versus-host disease and skin allograft rejection.

Grossly, lesions are *multiform* and include macules, papules, vesicles, and bullae as well as characteristic *targets* consisting of red maculopapular lesions with central pallor. Symmetric involvement of the extremities is common.

A severe, febrile form typically occurring in children is called *Stevens-Johnson syndrome*; it is marked by erosions and hemorrhagic crusting of the lips, oral mucosa, conjunctiva, urethra, and

Table 25-2. CLASSIFICATION OF ECZEMATOUS DERMATITIS

Type	Cause or Pathogenesis	Histology*	Clinical Features
Contact dermatitis	Topically applied chemicals. Pathogenesis: delayed hypersensitivity	Spongiotic dermatitis	Marked itching, burning, or both; requires antecedent exposure
Atopic dermatitis	Unknown, may be heritable	Spongiotic dermatitis	Erythematous plaques in flexural areas; family history of eczema, hay fever, or asthma
Drug-related eczematous dermatitis	Systemically administered (e.g., penicillin)	Spongiotic dermatitis; eosinophils often present in infiltrate; deeper infiltrate	Eruption occurs with administration of drug; remits when drug is discontinued
Photoeczematous eruption	Ultraviolet light	Spongiotic dermatitis; deeper infiltrate	Occurs on sun-exposed skin; phototesting may help in diagnosis
Primary irritant dermatitis	Repeated trauma (rubbing)	Spongiotic dermatitis in early stages	Localized to site of trauma

*All types, with time, may develop chronic changes.

anogenital regions. Bacterial superinfection may be life-threatening.

Toxic epidermal necrolysis is another variant, characterized by diffuse mucocutaneous epithelial necrosis and sloughing; it is clinically analogous to extensive third-degree burns.

Microscopically, early lesions of erythema multiforme show dermoepidermal junction and superficial perivascular lymphocytic infiltrates with dermal edema and focal basal keratinocyte degeneration and necrosis. *Exocytosis* is associated with epidermal necrosis, blistering, and shallow erosions. *Target lesions* show central epidermal necrosis with associated perivenular inflammation.

CHRONIC INFLAMMATORY DERMATOSES

(p. 1198)

Chronic inflammatory dermatoses are persistent inflammatory disorders (over months to years) characterized by excessive or abnormal scaling and shedding *(desquamation).* These dermatoses are to be distinguished from noninflammatory scaling lesions, such as ichthyosis (described earlier).

Psoriasis (p. 1198)

Psoriasis is a common disorder (1 to 2% of people in the United States). An association with certain human leukocyte antigen (HLA) types suggests a genetic component; the genesis of new lesions at sites of trauma *(Koebner phenomenon)* suggests a role for exogenous stimuli. Nonspecific damage to the stratum corneum may unmask new antigens with subsequent antibody deposition and secondary complement-mediated injury; alternatively, lesions may evolve at sites of abnormally reactive endothelium. Lymphocytes from psoriatic patients also induce dermal angiogenesis and keratinocyte growth, suggesting that the disease may actually be a manifestation of systemic immune dysfunction.

Psoriasis may be associated with other diseases, including myopathies, enteropathies, acquired immunodeficiency syndrome (AIDS), and mild to deforming arthritis (resembling rheumatoid arthritis).

Grossly, findings are as follows:

- Lesions are typically well-demarcated, salmon-pink plaques with silvery scaling; they usually occur on the elbows, knees, scalp, lumbosacral area, intergluteal cleft, and glans penis. *Annular, linear, gyrate,* or *serpiginous* variations occur.
- Psoriasis may also present as total body scaling and erythema—*erythroderma.*
- Nail changes (discoloration, pitting, onycholysis) occur in 30% of patients.
- *Pustular psoriasis* is a rare variant, which, when generalized, may be life-threatening; multiple small pustules form on erythematous plaques.

Microscopically, there is marked acanthosis with rete elongation and mitoses well above the basal layer. The stratum granulosum is thinned or absent, with extensive overlying parakeratosis. Epidermis over the dermal papillae is thinned; dilated vessels in these papillae yield pinpoint bleeds when the overlying scale is removed *(Auspitz sign).*

Aggregates of neutrophils in epidermis occur within small spongiotic foci in the stratum spinosum *(spongiform pustules)* or within the parakeratotic stratum corneum *(Munro microabscesses).* Larger, abscess-like accumulations may also occur in pustular psoriasis.

Lichen Planus (p. 1199)

Lichen planus is a self-limited disease that after 1 to 2 years generally leaves only postinflammatory hyperpigmentation. Oral lesions may persist longer and occasionally become malignant. The *pathogenesis* is unknown, but T-cell infiltrates with Langerhans cell hyperplasia are seen, and cell-mediated immune injury to basal cells is suspected. Koebner phenomenon occurs in lichen planus.

Grossly, lesions are *pruritic, purple, polygonal papules* that may coalesce into plaques; lesions are often highlighted by white dots or lines called *Wickham striae.* Lesions are typically multiple and symmetrically distributed, often on the wrists and elbows and on the glans penis; oral mucosal lesions are generally white and netlike. A form with preferential involvement of hair follicle epithelium is called *lichen planopilaris.*

Histologically, there is a dense, bandlike dermoepidermal junction lymphocytic infiltrate with basal cell degeneration and necrosis and jagged rete *saw-toothing.* Necrotic basal cells may be sloughed into inflamed papillary dermis, forming *colloid* or *Civatte bodies.* Lesions are also typified by chronic changes, including acanthosis, hyperkeratosis, and thickening of the granular cell layer.

Lupus Erythematosus (p. 1200)

Systemic lupus erythematosus (SLE) is detailed elsewhere (Chapter 7). *Discoid lupus erythematosus (DLE) is a localized cutaneous form without systemic manifestations.* Although patients with DLE rarely progress to develop systemic disease, one third of patients with SLE develop DLE-like skin pathology. Thus, evaluation of the cutaneous lesions *alone* does not distinguish the two entities. The *pathogenesis* of DLE involves immune complex–mediated and, to a lesser extent, cell-mediated injury to pigment-containing basal cells (Chapter 7).

Grossly, skin lesions of both SLE and DLE include an ill-defined malar erythema (more characteristic of SLE) or sharply demarcated *discoid* erythematous scaling plaques with zones of irregular pigmentation and small keratotic plugs in hair follicles. Sun exposure exacerbates the lesions.

Microscopically, DLE is marked by dermoepidermal junction, perivascular, and periappendiceal lymphocytic infiltrates. Preferential infiltration of subcutaneous fat is called *lupus profundus.* There are also basal cell vacuolization, epidermal atrophy, and variable hyperkeratosis.

By immunofluorescence, lesions show a *granular* band of immunoglobulin and complement along the dermoepidermal and dermal-follicular junctions *(lupus band test).*

BLISTERING (BULLOUS DISEASES) (p. 1201)

Bullous diseases are primary blistering disorders, as opposed to vesicles and bullae that occur as a secondary phenomenon in a variety of unrelated conditions. The level within the skin where the blister occurs is critical in diagnosis (Fig. 25–1).

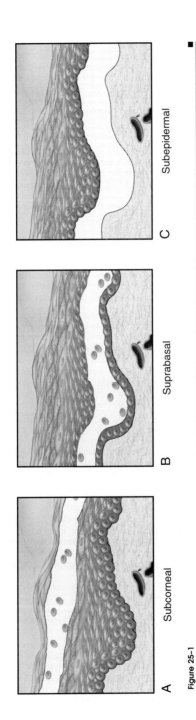

A   B   C

Subcorneal   Suprabasal   Subepidermal

Figure 25–1 ■

Schematic representation of sites of blister formation. *A.* In a subcorneal blister, stratum corneum forms the roof of the bulla (as in impetigo or pemphigus foliaceus). *B.* In a suprabasal blister, a portion of epidermis, including stratum corneum, forms the roof (as in pemphigus vulgaris). *C.* In a subepidermal blister, the entire epidermis separates from the dermis (as in bullous pemphigoid and dermatitis herpetiformis).

587

Pemphigus (p. 1201)

Pemphigus is a rare autoimmune disorder, typically occurring in patients in their thirties to fifties, with no gender predilection. Patients have circulating antibodies to keratinocyte intercellular cement component (desmoglein 3, a component of desmosomes); binding of these antibodies also triggers release of plasminogen activator by keratinocytes.

There are four clinical and pathologic variants:

1. *Pemphigus vulgaris*: Accounts for 80% of pemphigus. This disorder involves the oral mucosa, scalp, face, intertriginous zones, trunk, and pressure points. Lesions are superficial, easily ruptured blisters that leave shallow, crusted erosions. If untreated, it is almost uniformly fatal.

2. *Pemphigus vegetans*: A rare form presenting with large, moist verrucous plaques studded with pustules, typically in flexural and intertriginous zones.

3. *Pemphigus foliaceus*: A more benign form occurring epidemically in South America and sporadically elsewhere. Lesions occur mainly on the face, scalp, and upper trunk. Bullae are extremely superficial, leaving only slight erythema and crusting after rupture.

4. *Pemphigus erythematosus*: A localized, milder variant of pemphigus foliaceus, typically involving only a malar distribution.

Microscopically, all variants are characterized by *acantholysis* with intercellular clefting and eventually broad-based, *intraepithelial* blisters. For pemphigus vulgaris and vegetans, the separation occurs immediately above the basal layer *(suprabasal blister)*, leaving an intact layer of basal cells, described as a row of *tombstones*; in the foliaceus variant, only the stratum granulosum is involved. With anti-immunoglobulin or anticomplement immunofluorescence, netlike *(reticular)* staining may be seen in the epidermis, outlining each keratinocyte.

Bullous Pemphigoid (p. 1203)

Bullous pemphigoid is a relatively common autoimmune blistering disease of skin and mucosa typically affecting elderly individuals. It is caused by antibodies to hemidesmosome proteins responsible for attaching basal cells to the basal membrane; the antibodies cause injury by secondary complement activation and granulocyte recruitment.

Grossly, there are tense bullae containing clear fluid measuring up to 4 to 8 cm in diameter, typically on the inner thigh, forearm flexor surfaces, lower abdomen, and intertriginous zones; oral mucosa is involved in one third of patients. The blisters do not rupture as easily as those in pemphigus and, if uninfected, heal without scarring.

Microscopically, there is a subepidermal nonacantholytic blister with *linear* dermoepidermal junction staining for immunoglobulin and complement. There is a variable, mostly superficial, perivascular infiltrate of lymphocytes, eosinophils, and neutrophils.

Dermatitis Herpetiformis (p. 1204)

Dermatitis herpetiformis is a rare disorder, typically occurring in patients in their twenties to thirties, in men more often than in women. It is associated with specific HLA types and with celiac disease (Chapter 18). Both cutaneous and gastrointestinal lesions respond to a gluten-free diet. Dermatitis herpetiformis is presumably mediated either by immune complex deposition in the skin or by gliadin (a gluten protein) antibodies cross-reacting with junction-anchoring components (e.g., reticulin).

Grossly, intensely pruritic, urticarial plaques and grouped vesicles, characteristically symmetric, involve the extensor surfaces, upper back, and buttocks.

Microscopically, neutrophils and fibrin accumulate in the tips of dermal papillae *(microabscesses)* with overlying basal vacuolization and microscopic blisters coalescing to large subepidermal blisters. Immunofluorescence shows granular immunoglobulin A (IgA) deposits at the dermal papillae tips.

NONINFLAMMATORY BLISTERING DISEASES (p. 1205)

Noninflammatory blistering diseases are primary disorders with vesicles and bullae not mediated by inflammatory mechanisms.

Epidermolysis Bullosa (p. 1205)

Epidermolysis bullosa refers to a pathogenetically unrelated group of disorders that have in common neonatal blistering at pressure sites or trauma. The *junctional type* shows blistering at the lamina lucida in otherwise histologically normal skin. The scarring *dystrophic type* shows blistering beneath the lamina densa that presumably is due to defective anchoring fibrils. The *simplex type* results from epidermal basal cell degeneration.

Porphyria (p. 1206)

Porphyria refers to a group of inborn or acquired disturbances of porphyrin metabolism (there are five major types). Porphyrins are the ring structures that bind the metal ions in hemoglobin, myoglobin, and cytochromes. The pathogenesis is unknown. The cutaneous lesions consist of urticaria and vesicles that are exacerbated by sun exposure and heal without scarring.

Microscopically, there are subepidermal vesicles with associated marked superficial dermal vascular thickening.

DISORDERS OF EPIDERMAL APPENDAGES (p. 1206)

Acne Vulgaris (p. 1206)

Acne vulgaris is a common, chronic, inflammatory dermatosis affecting hair follicles, typically occurring in the middle to late teens, in males more often than in females, presumably secondary to hormonal changes and alterations in hair follicle maturation. It may be induced or exacerbated by sex hormones, corticosteroids, occupational exposure (coal tars), or occlusive conditions (heavy clothes). There may be a heritable component.

The *pathogenesis* is speculative but may involve bacterial *(Propionibacterium acnes)* lipase degradation of sebaceous oils to form highly irritating fatty acids. Antibiotics (e.g., tetracyclines) may be effective by inhibiting the lipase activity. The vitamin A derivative 13-*cis*-retinoic acid has also shown efficacy.

Grossly, noninflammatory acne is characterized by *open comedones* (follicular papules with central black keratin plugs) and *closed comedones* (follicular papules with central plugs trapped beneath the epidermis and therefore not visible). The latter may rupture with inflammation. *Inflammatory acne* shows erythematous papules, nodules, and pustules.

Histologically, comedones are composed of expanding masses of lipid and keratin at the midportion of hair follicles, with follicular dilation and epithelial and sebaceous gland atrophy. There is a variable lymphohistiocytic infiltrate, but with rupture there is extensive acute and chronic inflammation, occasionally with ensuing scar formation.

Panniculitis: Erythema Nodosum and Erythema Induratum (p. 1207)

Panniculitis is inflammation of subcutaneous fat. A rare form of panniculitis, *Weber-Christian disease* (*relapsing febrile nodular panniculitis*) occurs as crops of erythematous plaques or nodules, mainly on the legs, associated with deep lymphohistiocytic infiltrates and occasional giant cells.

Factitial panniculitis (from self-administered foreign substances), deep mycotic infections in immunocompromised hosts, and occasionally disorders such as SLE may mimic the clinical and histologic appearance of primary panniculitis. More common forms of panniculitis may affect

1. Connective tissue septa (*erythema nodosum*)
2. Fat lobules (*erythema induratum*)

Panniculitis may be acute or chronic. It commonly involves the lower extremities.

- *Erythema nodosum* is more common than erythema induratum. It typically has an acute onset and may be idiopathic or occur in association with specific drugs, infections, sarcoidosis, inflammatory bowel disease, or visceral malignancy. It presents with ill-defined, exquisitely tender erythematous nodules, occasionally with fever and malaise. With time, old lesions flatten and become ecchymotic without scarring, while new lesions develop. Deep wedge biopsy shows distinctive early septal widening (edema, fibrin deposition, and neutrophil infiltration) and lymphohistiocytic infiltration (occasionally with giant cells and eosinophils) without vasculitis.

- *Erythema induratum* is an uncommon form of panniculitis, typically affecting adolescents and menopausal women. It may represent a primary vasculitis of subcutaneous fat with subsequent inflammation and necrosis of adipose tissue. It presents as an erythematous, slightly tender nodule that eventually ulcerates and scars. Early lesions show necrotizing vasculitis in small- to medium-sized vessels in deep dermis and subcutis. Eventually the fat lobules develop granulomatous inflammation and necrosis.

INFECTION AND INFESTATION (p. 1208)

A representative sampling follows of common entities with primary clinical manifestations in the skin. Other infections, with secondary cutaneous involvement, are discussed in Chapter 9.

Verrucae (Warts) (p. 1208)

Verrucae are common, spontaneously regressing (in 6 months to 2 years) lesions, typically in children and adolescents. They are caused by papillomaviruses, transmitted by direct contact.

Verrucae are subdivided on the basis of clinical morphology and anatomic location. Certain lesions are typically caused by particular papillomavirus types. For example, types 6, 11, 16, and 18 are associated with anogenital warts. Type 16 is associated with anogenital wart dysplasia and in situ squamous cell carcinoma of the genitalia.

- *Verruca vulgaris*: The most common type of wart, most frequently on the dorsum of the hand. Grossly, they are gray-white to tan, flat to convex, 0.1- to 1-cm papules with a rough pebbly surface.
- *Verruca plana (flat wart)*: Usually on the face or dorsum of the hand. Grossly, they are flat, smooth, tan papules smaller than those of verruca vulgaris.
- *Verruca plantaris (soles) or palmaris (palms)*: Rough, scaly lesions 1 to 2 cm in diameter that may coalesce and be confused with calluses.
- *Condyloma acuminatum (anogenital and venereal warts)*: Soft, tan, cauliflower-like masses measuring up to many centimeters in diameter.

Microscopically, all variants have undulant *(verrucous)* epidermal hyperplasia and superficial keratinocyte perinuclear vacuolization *(koilocytosis)*. Electron microscopy reveals numerous viral particles within nuclei.

Molluscum Contagiosum (p. 1209)

Molluscum contagiosum is a common, self-limited disease caused by a poxvirus, transmitted by direct contact.

Grossly, firm, pruritic, pink to skin-colored, umbilicated papules 0.2 to 2 cm are seen typically on the trunk or anogenital regions. Cheesy material containing diagnostic molluscum bodies can be expressed from the central umbilications.

Microscopically, there is cuplike verrucous epidermal hyperplasia with pathognomonic *molluscum bodies*—large (up to 35 mm) eosinophilic cytoplasmic inclusions in the stratum granulosum or stratum corneum containing numerous virions.

Impetigo (p. 1210 and Chapter 9)

Impetigo refers to streptococcal or staphylococcal skin infection seen in normal children or sick adults, especially on the face and hands. It begins as an erythematous macule that progresses to small pustules and eventually to a shallow erosion with a honey-colored crust.

Microscopically, there are subcorneal pustules filled with neutrophils and gram-positive cocci, with accompanying dermal inflammation. Pustule rupture releases serum and necrotic debris to form the characteristic crust.

Superficial Fungal Infections (p. 1210)

Superficial fungal infections are typically caused by dermatophytes (fungi growing in soil and on animals) and *confined to the nonviable stratum corneum*.

- *Tinea capitis*: Typically noted in children. This involves the scalp, causing asymptomatic hairless patches, associated with mild erythema, crusting, and scale.

- *Tinea barbae:* Uncommon dermatophytosis of the beard area in adult men.
- *Tinea corporis:* Common superficial dermatophytosis of the body, especially in children. Predisposing factors are excessive heat or humidity, exposure to infected animals, or chronic dermatophytosis of the feet or nails. This typically presents with an expanding erythematous plaque with an elevated scaling border (*ringworm*).
- *Tinea cruris:* Typically in the inguinal areas of obese men during warm weather. It occurs as moist red patches with raised scaling borders.
- *Tinea pedis (athlete's foot):* Characterized by erythema and scaling, beginning in the webbed spaces. It affects up to 40% of individuals at some time in their lives. Most of the inflammation is due to secondary bacterial superinfection.
- *Tinea versicolor:* Due to *Malassezia furfur* and typically found on the upper trunk. This displays characteristic groups of various-sized hyperpigmented or hypopigmented macules with a peripheral scale.
- *Onychomycosis:* Nail dermatophytosis characterized by discoloration, thickening, and deformity of the nail plate.

There is histologic variability, but, basically, there are reactive epidermal changes similar to a mild eczematous dermatitis. Fungal cell walls are revealed by special stains. *The organisms are present in the stratum corneum*, and identification and cultures may be obtained by superficial scraping of affected areas.

Arthropod-Associated Lesions (p. 1210)

Arthropod-associated lesions are bites, stings, and infestations associated with arachnids (spiders, scorpions, ticks, mites), insects (lice, bees, fleas, flies, and mosquitos), and chilopods (centipedes). Reactions range from minimal to fatal. Gross bites range from urticarial lesions and inflamed papules or nodules to expanding, erythematous plaques (e.g., *erythema migrans* in the case of the bite from the tick vector for Lyme disease). Arthropod-associated pathologies include the following:

- *A direct irritant effect* of insect parts or secretions.
- Immediate (IgE-mediated, including anaphylaxis) or delayed (cell-mediated) *hypersensitivity responses* to body parts or secretions.
- *Specific effects of venom*:
  - Black widow spider venom causes pain and cramping.
  - Brown recluse spider venom produces significant tissue necrosis, often requiring radical surgical excision of involved areas.
- Lesions associated with *secondary invaders* (bacteria, rickettsiae, parasites).

SCABIES (p. 1212)

Scabies refers to a pruritic dermatosis caused by the mite *Sarcoptes scabiei*. The female burrows beneath the stratum corneum, producing linear, poorly defined furrows on the interdigital skin, palms, and wrists and on the periareolar skin in women and in the scrotal folds in men.

PEDICULOSIS (p. 1211)

Pediculosis is a pruritic dermatosis caused by the head, body, or crab louse. The insect or its eggs can usually be seen attached to hair shafts. Scalp pediculosis is complicated by impetigo and cervical lymphadenopathy, especially in children. Body lice may be accompanied by excoriations and hyperpigmentation.

Although arthropod bites have a variable histologic pattern, there is classically a *wedge-shaped dermal perivascular lympho-histiocytic and eosinophilic infiltrate*. There may be a highly focal central zone of epidermal necrosis with birefringent insect mouth parts delineating the bite site.

In some lesions, there is an urticaria-like response. In others there is a florid inflammatory infiltrate or spongiosis resulting in intraepidermal blisters.

Diseases of the Skeletal System and Soft Tissue Tumors

BONES (p. 1216)

Developmental Abnormalities (p. 1220)

MALFORMATIONS (p. 1220)

Achondroplasia (p. 1220)

Achondroplasia is a genetic derangement in epiphyseal cartilaginous growth resulting in dwarfism. Some cases are familial, but most are acquired mutations.

- Anatomically, there is retarded endochondral bone formation, which results in abnormally short long bones, but because appositional growth is not affected, they are of normal width. The spine is of normal length, and the skull appears large.
- Heterozygotes have normal longevity with easily recognizable disease because head and body are too large for the markedly shortened extremities. Mental, sexual, and reproductive development are normal.
- Homozygous disease with its constricted thoracic cage causes death soon after birth.

Diseases Associated With Abnormal Matrix (p. 1221)

OSTEOGENESIS IMPERFECTA OR BRITTLE BONES (p. 1221)

Osteogenesis imperfecta refers to a group of closely related genetic disorders caused by qualitative or quantitative abnormal synthesis of type I collagen (constitutes about 90% of the matrix of bone).

- Based on specific biosynthetic abnormality, four major subsets of osteogenesis imperfecta have been segregated; some have well-defined modes of inheritance and phenotypic changes, and others are less well characterized.
- Syndromes range from one variant (type II) that is uniformly fatal in the perinatal period (from multiple bone fractures) to other variants marked by increased predisposition to fracture but compatible with survival.

■ *Morphologically the basic change in all is osteopenia (too little bone), with marked thinning of the cortices and rarefaction of the trabeculae.*

MUCOPOLYSACCHARIDOSES (p. 1222)

Mucopolysaccharidoses are a group of lysosomal storage diseases caused by deficiencies in enzymes that degrade the various mucopolysaccharides (e.g., dermatan sulfate, heparan sulfate, others). Chondrocytes play a role in metabolism of mucopolysaccharides, and therefore in these disorders there are abnormalities in hyaline cartilage, including growth plates, costal cartilages, and articular surfaces. Patients are frequently of short stature and have malformed bones as well as other cartilage abnormalities.

OSTEOPOROSIS (p. 1222)

Osteoporosis refers to a reduction in bone mass owing to small but incremental losses incurred in the constant turnover of bone. This common condition is seen most often in the elderly of both sexes but is more pronounced in postmenopausal women. Osteoporosis may occur as a primary disorder of obscure origin or as a secondary complication of a large variety of diseases (Table 26–1). Osteoporosis becomes clinically significant when it induces vertebral instability with back pain and increased vulnerability to fractures of hips, wrists, and vertebral bodies.

Morphology

In postmenopausal and senile osteoporosis, the entire skeleton is involved, but patients may have localized disease with immobilization or paralysis of an extremity.

Table 26–1. CATEGORIES OF GENERALIZED OSTEOPOROSIS

Primary	
Postmenopausal	Idiopathic juvenile
Senile	Idiopathic middle adulthood

Secondary	
Endocrine disorders	Rheumatologic disease
Hyperparathyroidism	Drugs
Hyperthyroidism	Anticoagulants
Hypothyroidism	Chemotherapy
Hypogonadism	Corticosteroids
Acromegaly	Anticonvulsants
Cushing syndrome	Lithium
Prolactinoma	Alcohol
Diabetes, type I	Miscellaneous
Addison disease	Osteogenesis imperfecta
Neoplasia	Immobilization
Multiple myeloma	Pulmonary disease
Carcinomatosis	Chronic obstructive pulmonary disease
Mast cell disease	Homocystinuria
Gastrointestinal	Gaucher disease
Malnutrition	Anemia
Malabsorption	
Subtotal gastrectomy	
Hepatic insufficiency	
Vitamin C, D deficiencies	

- Cortex and trabeculae are thinned, and haversian systems are widened.
- Such bone as remains is of normal composition.

Pathogenesis

The cause of osteoporosis is largely unknown, but many factors probably contribute to slow loss of bone mass (Fig. 26–1). In essence, it is proposed that genetic factors determine the size of the bone mass achieved in young adulthood. Thereafter, aging-related slowing of osteoblastic function and increased osteoclastic activity induced by endocrine influences, particularly decreased serum estrogen levels, perhaps acting through interleukin-1 (IL-1), result in a net negative balance in the continued turnover of bone. Accumulating evidence indicates that estrogen replacement therapy coupled with calcium supplementation, when begun during or soon after the onset of the menopause, can slow or prevent the abnormal loss of bone.

Clinical Features

Osteoporosis causes bone pain owing to microfractures; results in loss in height and stability of the vertebral column; and particularly predisposes to fractures of femoral necks, wrists, and vertebrae. The condition is difficult to diagnose for the following reasons:

- It remains asymptomatic until skeletal fragility is well advanced.
- There is no easy way to determine the severity of the bone loss (radiographs are unreliable with <30 to 40% bone loss); most reliable are absorptiometry and quantitive computed tomography.
- Osteoporosis is only one of a group of osteopenic disorders, which are difficult to differentiate from each other (e.g., osteomalacia, osteogenesis imperfecta, and osteitis fibrosa [hyperparathyroidism]).

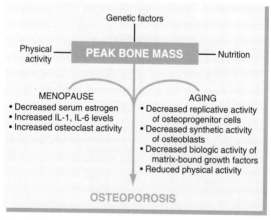

Figure 26–1 ■

Pathophysiology of postmenopausal and senile osteoporosis.

Diseases Caused by Osteoclast Dysfunction
(p. 1224)

OSTEOPETROSIS (p. 1224)

Osteopetrosis refers to a group of rare hereditary diseases characterized by overgrowth and sclerosis of bone, with marked thickening of the cortex and narrowing or filling of the medullary cavity (impairs hematopoiesis). Despite *too much bone*, it is brittle and fractures like chalk.

- The autosomal recessive form is evident at birth, with anemia, neutropenia, infections, and eventual death.
- The autosomal dominant form is benign but predisposes to fractures.
- *Common to all forms is a hereditary defect in osteoclast function resulting in reduced bone resorption and enhanced net bone overgrowth.*
- The nature of the genetic defect is unknown but may involve osteoclast bone–solubilizing enzymes.

PAGET DISEASE (OSTEITIS DEFORMANS)
(p. 1225)

Paget disease is monostotic in about 15% of cases and polyostotic in the remainder, with variation in the stage of the process from one site to another. Paget disease can be divided into the following stages:

1. An initial *osteolytic stage*, followed by
2. A mixed *osteolytic-osteoblastic stage*, evolving ultimately into
3. A burnt-out, *quiescent osteosclerotic stage*

Pathogenesis

The cause of Paget disease is currently considered to be a slow viral infection of osteoblasts and then osteoclasts by paramyxovirus. The virus has been identified in osteoclasts by in situ hybridization but cannot be isolated.

Morphology

Morphologic findings are as follows:

- The *osteolytic phase* is marked by resorption by numerous, overly large osteoclasts (some containing >100 nuclei).
- The *mixed phase* shows, in addition, disordered neo-osteogenesis of predominantly woven bone (but some lamellar) with areas of new bone formation producing *a tilelike or mosaic pattern pathognomonic of Paget disease.* Adjacent marrow is fibrotic.
- Eventually, after many years, there is the *burnt-out phase*, marked predominantly by bone formation and osteosclerosis.
- Because the new bone formation in active disease is disordered and poorly mineralized, it is soft and porous, lacks structural stability, and is vulnerable to fracture or deformation under stress.

Clinical Features

Clinical features include the following:

- Patients may demonstrate fractures, nerve compression, osteoarthritis, and skeletal deformities (e.g., tibial bowing, skull enlargement).

- Any bone can be involved, and coarsening of the facial bones *may produce* leontiasis ossea (lionlike facies). Less commonly, the vascularity of polyostotic lesions can cause high-output heart failure, and sometimes secondary sarcoma develops (in about 1% of patients).

Diseases Associated With Abnormal Mineral Homeostasis (p. 1227)

RICKETS AND OSTEOMALACIA (p. 1227)

Rickets in growing children and osteomalacia in adults are *caused by either vitamin D deficiency or phosphate depletion* resulting in defective matrix mineralization. The causes of vitamin D deficiency include

1. Dietary deficiency
2. Inadequate exposure to sunlight
3. Malabsorption of vitamin D, calcium, or phosphate
4. Derangements in conversion of vitamin D to active metabolites (e.g., in renal disease)
5. End-organ resistance
6. Rare hereditary or acquired disorders of vitamin D metabolism

Morphology

The fundamental defect in osteomalacia or rickets is failure in bone mineralization, resulting in excess unmineralized matrix and abnormally wide osteoid seams.

Clinical Features

In the growing child, the skeleton is weak with bowing of legs and deformities of ribs, skull, and other bones. In adults after bone growth has ceased, it causes no skeletal deformities—only osteopenic osteomalacia.

HYPERPARATHYROIDISM (p. 1228)

Hyperparathyroidism, either primary or secondary (as occurs with renal failure), leads to the following:

1. Demineralization first occurs.
2. In time, increased osteoclastic activity with resorption of bone and peritrabecular fibrosis (osteitis fibrosa) follows.
3. Marrow fibrosis and more marked resorption evolve, with formation of cysts within the marrow cavity (osteitis fibrosa cystica or *von Recklinghausen disease of bone*). This condition is now rare because parathyroid hyperfunction is detected earlier and controlled.

- Bone loss is particularly evident by x-ray as *moth-eaten*, rarefied bones of the distal phalanges and clavicles and loss of the lamina dura about the tooth sockets.
- So-called brown tumors (resembling reparative giant cell granulomas) also can occur within the bones, and, paradoxically, soft tissue metastatic calcifications sometimes appear. The bone changes completely regress after control of hyperparathyroidism.

RENAL OSTEODYSTROPHY (p. 1229)

Renal osteodystrophy refers to a complex set of bone changes appearing in most patients with chronic renal failure. Included are features of osteitis fibrosa cystica admixed with osteomalacia and sometimes, less prominently, areas of osteosclerosis.

- With protracted skeletal disease, metastatic calcifications may develop in the skin, eyes, and arterial walls and around joints.
- The pathogenesis is reviewed on p. 1229 (see also Chapter 26, p. 1150).
- Other factors that may contribute to the bone changes are metabolic acidosis and iron and aluminum deposition in bone (derived from dialysate, which interferes with mineralization of matrix).

Fractures (p. 1229)

Speed of healing and perfection of fracture repair depend on the type of fracture and whether the break has occurred in normal bone or in previously diseased bone (i.e., *pathologic fracture*).

- *Incomplete* (greenstick) and *closed* (intact skin) fractures when aligned heal most rapidly, with potentially complete reconstitution of the preexisting architecture.
- *Comminuted* (splintered bone) and *compound* (open skin wound) fractures heal much more slowly, with poorer end results.

MORPHOLOGY

Morphologic findings are as follows:

- Fracture healing is a continuous process that proceeds through three distinct stages:
  1. *Organization of hematoma* at the site, leading to a soft, organizing, weak *procallus*
  2. Conversion of the procallus to a *fibrocartilaginous callus*
  3. Replacement of the latter by an *osseous callus*, which is eventually remodeled along lines of weight bearing to complete the repair
- If the fracture has been well aligned and the original weight-bearing strains are restored, almost perfect repair is accomplished.
- Imperfect results are seen when there is malalignment, comminution, inadequate immobilization of fracture site, infection, and superimposed systemic abnormality (e.g., atherosclerosis, avitaminosis, dietary deficiency, osteoporosis).

Osteonecrosis (Avascular Necrosis) (p. 1231)

Infarction of bone and marrow is relatively common and can occur in the medullary cavity of the metaphysis or diaphysis and the subchondral region of the epiphysis. The mechanisms leading to the local ischemia include

- Vascular interruption (fracture)
- Thrombosis and embolism (caisson disease)
- Vessel injury (vasculitis, radiation therapy)
- Vascular compression (possibly steroid-induced necrosis)
- Venous hypertension

Among the aforementioned mechanisms, steroid-induced necrosis is most common.

MORPHOLOGY

A local geographic area of pale yellow infarction is seen in marrow (cortex usually not affected because of its collateral blood flow). The focus is marked by death of osteocytes, empty lacunae, and necrotic fat cells. Creeping substitution occurs from margin. In subchondral infarcts, the articular cartilage may collapse into the softened necrotic bone.

CLINICAL FEATURES

Patients may be asymptomatic, but subchondral lesions often cause joint pain and predispose to osteoarthritis later.

Infections (p. 1232)
PYOGENIC OSTEOMYELITIS (p. 1232)

Pyogenic osteomyelitis results from bacterial seeding of bone by

1. Hematogenous spread
2. Extension from a contiguous infection
3. Open fracture or surgical procedure

- Blood-borne infections are most common in developing countries, where *Staphylococcus aureus* (often penicillin resistant) is most often implicated (other pathogens may be involved). Patients with sickle cell anemia are prone, for obscure reasons, to *Salmonella* infection.
- Extension of infection or traumatic inoculation is more common in developed countries, where mixed infections, anaerobes, or both are most often responsible.

  Basically the suppurative reaction is associated with ischemic necrosis, fibrosis, and bony repair.

- Necrosis of a bone segment may produce a *sequestrum.*
- Subperiosteal new bone produces an *involucrum* that encloses and envelops the inflammatory focus.
- If new bone formation continues, the focus becomes sclerotic—*Garré sclerosing osteomyelitis.*
- Chronic cases may lead to bone deformity, sinus tracts, and secondary amyloidosis, but less severe cases may heal or be localized and walled off to create a *Brodie abscess* (sometimes sterile).

  Clinically, pyogenic osteomyelitis is an acute febrile illness with pain, tenderness, and heat referable to local lesion. Subtle lesions, however, may present as unexplained fever in infants or localized pain without fever in adults. During the first 10 days, x-ray changes may be minimal, but radionuclide studies often show localized uptake of tracers. Complications include fracture, amyloidosis, bacteremia with endocarditis, and development of squamous cell carcinoma in sinus tract.

TUBERCULOUS OSTEOMYELITIS (p. 1233)

Tuberculous osteomyelitis is rare in developed countries but more common in developing nations where pulmonary and gastrointestinal tuberculosis is still common.

- Arises as a blood-borne insidious infection, much more destructive and resistant to control than suppurative diseases
- In the spine, known as *Pott disease*
- Produces typical granulomatous reaction

SYPHILIS (p. 1233)

Although rare in the United States, syphilitic bone disease can occur in either congenital or acquired forms.

- *Congenital* syphilis appears at birth and is marked by periostitis. On x-ray, a *crew haircut–like* appearance of new bone formation on cortex is produced. *Saber shin* results when the tibia is involved.
- *Acquired* syphilis appears in the tertiary stage of disease. It may be manifested as periostitis but more often by gummas in bone.

Bone Tumors and Tumor-like Lesions (p. 1233)

There is a great diversity of benign and malignant tumors of bone (Table 26–2). Certain tumors tend to occur within certain age groups and at particular locations; thus, in the diagnosis of bone tumors, the frequency of various lesions, the patient's age, the location of the neoplasm, and its radiologic appearance are all important.

BONE-FORMING TUMORS (p. 1234)

Osteoma (p. 1235)

An osteoma is a bosselated, sessile tumor attached to a bone surface composed of densely sclerotic, well-formed bone (there-

Table 26–2. CLASSIFICATIONS OF PRIMARY TUMORS INVOLVING BONES

Histologic Type	Benign	Malignant
Hematopoietic (40%)		■ Myeloma Malignant lymphoma
Chondrogenic (22%)	■ Osteochondroma Chondroma Chondroblastoma Chondromyxoid fibroma	■ Chondrosarcoma Dedifferentiated chondrosarcoma Mesenchymal chondrosarcoma
Osteogenic (19%)	■ Osteoid osteoma Osteoblastoma	■ Osteosarcoma
Unknown origin (10%)	■ Giant cell tumor	■ Ewing tumor Giant cell tumor Adamantinoma
Histiocytic origin	■ Fibrous histiocytoma	■ Malignant fibrous histiocytoma
Fibrogenic	■ Metaphyseal fibrous defect (fibroma)	■ Desmoplastic fibroma Fibrosarcoma
Notochordal		■ Chordoma
Vascular	■ Hemangioma	■ Hemangio-endothelioma Hemangiopericytoma
Lipogenic	■ Lipoma	■ Liposarcoma
Neurogenic	■ Neurilemmoma	

Data on percentage of each type from Unni KK: Dahlin's Bone Tumors, 5th ed. Philadelphia, Lippincott-Raven, 1996, p 4; by permission of Mayo Foundation.

fore an *osteoblastic tumor* because it makes an osteoid matrix that may become mineralized).

- Osteomas protrude from cortical surfaces, most often the skull and facial bones.
- Of little clinical significance unless their location (e.g., the inner table of the skull) compromises local organ function, they are disturbing cosmetically, or they may be associated with *Gardner syndrome* (p. 831).

Osteoid Osteoma and Osteoblastoma (p. 1235)

Osteoid osteoma is a small, benign neoplasm without malignant potential.

- Of cases, 90% occur between the teens and twenties, are usually about 1 cm in diameter, and are most often located near the ends of the tibia and femur (although all bones have been involved).
- They are painful and appear on x-ray as a small radiolucent nidus within cortex surrounded by densely sclerotic bone.
- *Histologically the radiolucent nidus consists of delicate trabeculae of woven bone rimmed by numerous osteoblasts and surrounded by highly vascular, spindled stroma, in turn enclosed by dense bone.*

The closely related *osteoblastoma* (giant osteoid osteoma) is usually a lytic tumor having the same histologic appearance as osteoma but without the surrounding sclerotic rim.

- Larger than osteoma (>2 cm), osteoblastoma tends to be located in the vertebrae or long bones and does not cause much pain. Although it is considered benign, there are aggressive forms associated with repeated local recurrences; rarely, some transform to osteosarcoma.

Osteosarcoma (Osteogenic Sarcoma) (p. 1236)

Osteosarcoma is best defined as a tumor in which malignant cells directly form osteoid, bone, or both, *resulting in incorporation of anaplastic tumor cells within the lacunae of the osteoid matrix.*

- Excluding multiple myeloma, osteosarcoma is the most common form of primary bone cancer.
- Primary cases arise in the apparent absence of underlying bone disease, mostly in persons younger than 20 years old in the metaphyseal regions of long bones before the epiphyses have closed.
- Secondary osteosarcoma occurs mostly in older people, in both flat and long bones, against a background of preexisting bone pathology (e.g., Paget disease, enchondromas, exostoses, osteomyelitis, fibrous dysplasia, infarcts, fractures) or exposure to oncogenic influences (previous irradiation).

Pathogenesis. Genetic, constitutional, and environmental influences are important.

- Patients with *familial retinoblastoma* have a greatly increased risk of osteosarcomas and have a *hereditary mutation* of the suppressor *Rb* gene on chromosome 13. Patients who survive hereditary retinoblastoma have continued risk of developing osteosarcoma, often in an irradiated area. Sporadic osteosarcomas are not associated with the *Rb* gene but often have mutations of the *p53* suppressor gene on chromosome 17 (Li-Fraumeni syndrome).

■ *Constitutional influences* include the fact that it is during active bone growth that osteosarcoma develops, and favored locations are sites of greatest bone growth (e.g., at base of femoral growth plate).
■ *Irradiation* is the one *environmental factor* known to predispose to secondary osteosarcoma.

Morphology. Of osteosarcomas, 80 to 90% arise in the medullary cavity of the metaphyseal ends of long bones (proximal tibia, distal or proximal femur, and proximal humerus), but any bone can be involved. After 25 years of age, the incidence in flat bones (jaws and pelvis) equals that in long bones and usually is superimposed on underlying bone disease.

■ Osteosarcomas present as gray-white, invasive, and destructive masses showing focal hemorrhages and necrosis and are composed of anaplastic mesenchymal cells.
■ Some are largely fibroblastic, others largely osteoblastic, some chondroid, and others highly vascular (telangiectatic). *All form osteoid-incorporating or bone-incorporating malignant cells.*
■ Cortical penetration of tumor with periosteal elevation causes *Codman triangle,* an x-ray finding in some patients. Tumor rarely penetrates the epiphyseal plate.
■ Extraskeletal osteosarcoma also can occur.

Clinical Features. Osteosarcomas metastasize widely, usually to lung first but also to other organs and bones (lymph node metastases are rare).

■ Osteosarcomas present with local pain, tenderness, and swelling.
■ Surgery alone results in 20% 5-year survivals, but surgery, radiation, and chemotherapy yield 60% 5-year survivals.
■ Osteosarcomas of the jaw and the low-grade variants, parosteal (juxtacortical) and *intraosseous low-grade* osteosarcoma, have a better prognosis than does classic osteosarcoma.

CARTILAGE-FORMING TUMORS (p. 1237)

Osteochondroma (p. 1237)

Osteochondroma is also known as an *exostosis* and may occur as solitary sporadic lesions or in profusion in the autosomal dominant *multiple hereditary exostosis.* Osteochondromas are believed to result from displacement of the lateral portion of the growth plate, which then proliferates in a direction diagonal to the long axis of the bone and away from the nearby joint. The male-female ratio is 3:1.

■ Osteochondromas occur most frequently on metaphysis of long bones. Occasionally the pelvis, scapula, and ribs are involved (rarely the small bones of the hands and feet).
■ *Morphologically, osteochondromas are mushroom-shaped lateral protrusions, capped by hyaline cartilage, with outer, well-formed cortices and medullary cavities in continuity with the underlying marrow cavity.*
■ Exostoses are usually discovered in late childhood or adolescence, often as chance x-ray findings.
■ They are benign lesions, but, rarely in the hereditary condition, chondrosarcomas may arise from one or more.

Chondroma (p. 1238)

Chondromas are benign tumors composed of mature hyaline cartilage.

- Those within the bone are called *enchondromas*, and, similar to exostoses, they are thought to arise from remnants of epiphyseal cartilage left behind.
- Chondromas may be single or multiple. A nonfamilial multiple form is known as *enchondromatosis* or *Ollier disease*, and a familial form with multiple chondromas associated with hemangiomas is known as *Maffucci syndrome*.
- Sarcomatous transformation of solitary sporadic chondromas is rare, but with the multiple tumors in the systemic syndromes, sarcomatous transformation (usually chondrosarcoma) is frequent.
- Chondromas are usually asymptomatic but may cause bone deformity, pain, and fracture. Lesions of the hands and feet are almost always innocuous but may recur when incompletely removed. Those in long bones raise the differential diagnosis of well-differentiated chondrosarcoma.

Chondroblastoma (p. 1239)

Chondroblastoma refers to an uncommon benign tumor almost invariably found in epiphyses of skeletally immature individuals (not to be confused with giant cell tumor or clear cell chondrosarcoma, both occurring in the same location but usually in older patients).

- Resembling embryonic chondroblasts, tumor cells are polygonal, arranged in sheets, and sometimes surrounded by a lace-like pattern of hyaline cartilage. Their nuclei are often deeply indented or longitudinally grooved.
- Multinucleated, osteoclast-like giant cells may be present and abundant enough to suggest giant cell tumor of bone.
- The great majority are benign.

Chondromyxoid Fibroma (p. 1240)

Chondromyxoid fibroma is an uncommon benign tumor composed of chondroid, fibrous, and myxoid tissues.

- Chondromyxoid fibroma occurs in the metaphyses of the long bones about the knee, but any bone can be involved.
- There is a male preponderance, and most occur in the teens and twenties.
- X-ray images show circumscribed lucency with scattered calcifications.
- Because focal atypia can be marked, these tumors can be misconstrued as sarcomas.
- They are adequately treated by curettage and, despite possible recurrence, pose no threat.

Chondrosarcoma (p. 1240)

Chondrosarcoma occurs about half as often as osteosarcoma.

- Of chondrosarcomas, 75% arise de novo (primary); the remaining (secondary) chondrosarcomas arise from enchondromas, osteochondromas, and rarely chondroblastomas.
- Most occur in middle to later life, the primary lesions being in

the central skeleton (ribs, shoulder, and pelvic girdle) and around the knee. Lesions are rare beyond the ankles and wrists.

■ *When transected, they appear as lobulated translucent tumors. Necrosis and spotty calcification may be present.*

■ Distinction from enchondroma may be difficult in grade I (well-differentiated) tumors. Hyperchromatic nuclei, two or more cells per lacuna, multinucleate cells, and anaplasia point toward chondrosarcoma.

■ Equally difficult may be the differentiation of chondrosarcoma with ossification from osteosarcoma with chondroid differentiation. In chondrosarcomas, bone formation occurs within cartilage; osteosarcomas show bone arising out of a background of anaplastic, osteoblastic-fibroblastic cells.

■ *X-ray images may be diagnostic. Classically, there is a localized area of bone destruction punctuated by mottled densities from calcification or ossification.*

■ All tumors require total removal, and 5-year survival rates for grades I, II, and III (increasing cytologic anaplasia) are 90, 81, and 43%. None of the grade I lesions and 70% of the grade III lesions disseminate.

FIBROUS AND FIBRO-OSSEOUS TUMORS
(p. 1242)

Fibrous Cortical Defect (Nonossifying Fibroma)
(p. 1242)

A fibrous cortical defect is a non-neoplastic developmental lesion (sharply defined, radiolucent lesions of the metaphyseal cortex) in the femur, tibia, and fibula.

■ Single (50%) or multiple and bilateral (50%)
■ Does not transform to malignancy
■ Generally asymptomatic but may (when large) lead to fracture
■ Extremely common (reported in one third of normal children)
■ Disappears spontaneously

Fibrous Dysplasia (p. 1242)

Fibrous dysplasia refers to a localized, benign, progressive replacement of bone by a fibrous proliferation intermixed with poorly formed, haphazardly arranged trabeculae of woven bone. The latter are present in variable amounts, are not lined by osteoblasts, and form configurations likened to *Chinese figures*. There are three, somewhat overlapping, presentations:

1. Involvement of a single bone *(monostotic)*—70%.
2. Involvement of several or many bones *(polyostotic)*—25%.
3. *Polyostotic disease associated with various endocrinopathies*—3 to 5%. When accompanied by irregular *(coast of Maine)* skin pigmentation and precocious sexual development, it is termed *McCune-Albright syndrome.*
   ❏ The monostotic form is often asymptomatic, whereas the polyostotic form is frequently associated with deformities and fractures, especially of the craniofacial bones.
   ❏ The clinical course of the polyostotic forms is unpredictable.
   ❏ Rarely, secondary sarcoma develops, sometimes after irradiation.

*Fibrosarcoma and Malignant Fibrous
Histiocytoma* (p. 1243)

Fibrosarcoma and malignant fibrous histiocytoma have overlapping clinical, radiographic, and pathologic features. Some deny the existence of malignant fibrous histiocytoma and reassign lesions.

- Malignant fibrous histiocytoma is more common in men, but fibrosarcoma is equally common in both sexes. Both present as gray-white, infiltrative masses.
- Lesions usually arise de novo but some arise on a background of Paget disease, bone infarcts, and prior radiation.
- Fibrosarcoma is composed of malignant fibroblasts in a herringbone pattern. More often, fibroblasts are moderately well differentiated but may be anaplastic.
- Malignant fibrous histiocytoma is composed of spindled fibroblasts in a storiform (so-called) or starry pattern admixed with bizarre multinucleated giant cells and neoplastic-appearing histiocytes (actually fibroblasts).
- Malignant fibrous histiocytoma is generally a high-grade pleomorphic tumor.
- These conditions may arise in soft tissues as well as in the metaphyses of long bones and pelvis.

Prognosis depends on cytologic grade; anaplastic lesions yield a 20% 5-year survival.

MISCELLANEOUS TUMORS (p. 1244)

*Ewing Sarcoma and Primitive Neuroectodermal
Tumor* (p. 1244)

Ewing sarcoma and primitive neuroectodermal tumor are composed of malignant small round cells, and both are closely related, having an identical 11;22 chromosomal translocation. The major difference is Ewing sarcoma is more undifferentiated, and neuroectodermal tumor often reveals neural differentiation, but the term *Ewing sarcoma* is used here to represent both neoplasms. The undifferentiated small round tumor cells are of probable neural origin.

- Ewing sarcoma arises most often in children 10 to 15 years old, and 80% are younger than 20 years.
- Boys are affected more often than girls; blacks are rarely affected.
- Ewing sarcoma is the second most common bone sarcoma in childhood.
- Ewing sarcoma arises in the medullary cavity in the diaphysis of long tubular bones, especially femur and flat bones of the pelvis.
- Ewing sarcoma usually invades cortex and penetrates the periosteum to produce a soft tissue mass.
- Ewing sarcoma is composed of sheets of uniform small round cells that occasionally produce Homer-Wright pseudorosettes (tumor cells arrayed in a circle about a central fibrillary space).
- Cells have scant cytoplasm, which often contains glycogen.
- Generally, there is little fibrous stroma but prominent necrosis in regions remote from vessels.
- Ewing sarcoma may metastasize to other bones or elsewhere.

Clinically, Ewing sarcoma presents as a painful, enlarging mass often tender, warm, and swollen, suggesting an infection. The periosteal reaction produces layers of reactive bone deposited in an onion-skin fashion. With combined radiation, chemotherapy, and surgery, there is now a 75% 5-year survival rate.

Giant Cell Tumor of Bone (p. 1244)

Giant cell tumor of bone is a locally aggressive neoplasm found most often in the epiphyseal ends of long bones in adults between 20 and 55 years of age. More than half occur about the knees, but virtually any bone can be involved. Giant cell tumor of bone is *rare in skeletally immature people and infrequent in the elderly.*

Morphology. Morphologic findings include the following:

- The histologic pattern is one of uniformly distributed, osteoclast-like, multinucleated giant cells in a plump spindle cell background.
- *The neoplastic cell is the spindled stromal cell; the multinucleated cells are thought to arise from fusion of the spindle cells.*
- There may be foci of necrosis, hemorrhage, hemosiderin, or osteoid.

Clinical Features. X-ray images are distinctive (not pathognomonic), revealing large, lytic, soap-bubble lesions. Absent are stippling and calcifications.

- Histologic features do not allow prediction of which tumors will recur or metastasize. A rare lesion is overtly malignant from the outset.
- This biologic unpredictability complicates clinical management.
  - Majority of tumors are localized and can be eradicated by curettage or conservative resections.
  - 40 to 60% recur locally.
  - 1 to 2% develop deceptively benign-looking metastases to the lungs.
  - About 10% develop obviously anaplastic metastases.

Metastatic Tumors to the Skeleton (p. 1245)

In adults, more than half of skeletal metastases originate from cancers of the prostate, breast, kidney, and lung. In children, there is secondary involvement of skeleton, most commonly from neuroblastoma, Wilms tumor, osteosarcoma, Ewing sarcoma, and rhabdomyosarcoma. Most metastases to bone are lytic. The tumor cells elaborate prostaglandins, interleukins, and parathyroid hormone–related protein that stimulate osteoclastic bone resorption. Osteosclerotic responses are most often induced by prostate and breast cancer by stimulating osteoblastic activity.

JOINTS (p. 1246)

Osteoarthritis or Degenerative Joint Disease
(p. 1246)

Osteoarthritis or degenerative joint disease (DJD) is characterized by progressive deterioration and breakdown of articular cartilage, mainly in weight-bearing joints, leading to subchondral bony thickening and bony overgrowths—osteophytes (*spurs*)—about the joint margins. DJD also causes the bony, knobby protrusions at the margins of the distal interphalangeal joints, creating nontender, subcutaneous *Heberden nodes.* The cause is unknown but is most likely related to metabolic and biochemical alterations.

DJD occurs in two clinical patterns:

1. *Primary DJD*: Occurs de novo, mostly in men in midlife, somewhat later in women. Frequency increases with age to about 80% of those older than 70 years. Association between osteoarthritis and aging is nonlinear, the prevalence increasing exponentially beyond the age of 50 years.

2. *Secondary DJD*: Appears at any age in a previously damaged or congenitally abnormal joint.

The relationship between age and previous injury suggests that *wear and tear* contributes to the genesis of this disease. Shoulder and elbow are often involved in baseball players and knees in basketball players. Usually knees and hands are more common in women and hips in men.

MORPHOLOGY

Morphologic findings include the following:

- Involvement usually is oligoarticular.
- Earliest changes are loss of proteoglycans and decreased metachromasia of the articular cartilage, associated with focal loss of chondrocytes alternating with areas of chondrocyte proliferation (*cloning*) and increased matrix basophilia.
- Next, fissuring, pitting, and flaking of the cartilage develop, followed by vertical clefts down to the subchondral bone.
- Flaking of the cartilage exposes underlying bone, which appears ivory-like (eburnation) as continued joint motion polishes the surface.
- Subchondral microcysts and fractures may develop.
- Synovium shows a mild chronic inflammatory infiltrate (nonspecific synovitis) and can develop osteocartilaginous metaplasia, fragments of which create osteocartilaginous loose bodies (*joint mice*) within the joint space.

PATHOGENESIS

Pathogenesis remains unknown but is clearly related to aging and injury. The cause may well be multifactorial.

- With aging, capacity of chondrocytes to maintain cartilaginous matrix slows.
- Age-related changes include alterations in the proteoglycans and collagen within articular cartilage, which decrease resilience and increase vulnerability to injury.
- Under stresses of injury, chondrocytes elaborate IL-1, which initiates matrix breakdown.
- Secondary mediators, such as tumor necrosis factor-α (TNF-α) and transforming growth factor-β, enhance release of lytic enzymes from chondrocytes, while inhibiting matrix synthesis.
- Precise signals inducing release of cytokines and enzymes are still unknown.

CLINICAL FEATURES

Although DJD may be asymptomatic, most patients experience morning stiffness in affected joints. There is usually no local heat or tenderness, but affected joints often show restricted range of motion, small effusions, and crepitus. Progressive reduction in mobility and increased painfulness with joint motion occur, but progression to bony ankylosis does not occur. Bone spurs and joint narrowing are apparent on x-rays. *There is no known way of preventing or arresting DJD.*

Rheumatoid Arthritis (p. 1248)

Rheumatoid arthritis is basically a severe form of chronic synovitis that can lead to destruction and ankylosis of affected joints. Blood vessels, skin, heart, lungs, nerves, and eyes may also be affected.

- About 1% of the world population suffers from rheumatoid arthritis.
- Women are affected three times more often than men.
- Peak prevalence is in the twenties to thirties.
- There is a familial association and a link with HLA-DR4 or DR1 or both.

MORPHOLOGY

Rheumatoid arthritis generally first affects small, proximal joints of the hands and feet but then may involve, usually symmetrically, the wrists, elbows, ankles, and knees.

- Well-developed lesions show villous hypertrophy of the synovium, synoviocytic hyperplasia, and an intense lymphoplasmacytic and histiocytic synovial infiltrate. Exuberant synovium is known as a *pannus*, which eventually fills the joint space, encroaching on the articular surfaces.
- Release of destructive enzymes (proteases and collagenases) and cytokines (particularly IL-1 and TNF-α) and pannus formation destroy cartilage, leading to changes reminiscent of DJD but with fibrous and bony ankylosis. Neutrophils (rheumatoid arthritis cells) can be present in synovial fluid.
- Other features include rheumatoid nodules in subcutaneous tissues (areas of necrosis surrounded by palisade of fibroblasts and white cells at pressure points such as elbows); acute vasculitis; and nonspecific, fibrosing inflammatory lesions of lungs, pleura, pericardium, myocardium, peripheral nerves, and eyes.

PATHOGENESIS

Although much remains uncertain, the best hypothesis regarding pathogenesis is: *Rheumatoid arthritis is initiated by an arthritogenic microbial agent in an immunogenetically susceptible host. After initial injury, a continuing autoimmune reaction ensues, in which T cells (CD4 +) release cytokines and inflammatory mediators that ultimately destroy the joint.*

- Linkage to HLA-DR4 points to genetic susceptibility.
- Microbial trigger is unknown, but Epstein-Barr virus is a prime suspect. Other agents, such as retroviruses, mycobacteria, *Borrelia*, and *Mycoplasma*, are also suspected.
- Once an inflammatory synovitis is initiated, an autoimmune reaction ensues; CD4 + cells are activated with release of many cytokines, particularly IL-1 and TNF-α. These cells within joints mediate lysis of articular cartilage and initiate the inflammatory synovitis.
- Autoantibodies are produced, some against autologous immunoglobulin G (IgG).
- Autoantibody against the Fc portion of autologous IgG is called

rheumatoid factor (is usually IgM, but sometimes IgG, IgA, or IgE).

■ Rheumatoid factor does not contribute to pathogenesis because about 20% of patients are rheumatoid factor negative, but it may contribute to an Arthus-like reaction in blood vessels (acute vasculitis) and to the production of subcutaneous rheumatoid nodules and other extra-articular lesions.

CLINICAL FEATURES

Clinical features are variable. Most patients experience a prodrome of malaise, fever, fatigue, and musculoskeletal pain before joint mobility is reduced.

■ The lucky patient experiences mild transient disease without sequelae, but most have fluctuating disease with the greatest progression during the initial 4 to 5 years. In a minority, the onset is acute, with rapidly progressive limitation of motion and development of joint deformities.

■ Characteristic deformities are radial deviation of the wrist with ulnar deviation of the fingers.

■ Extra-articular manifestations (mentioned previously), although infrequent, are rarely the presenting features of the disease and tend to develop in patients with high rheumatoid factor titers (possibly related to deposition of circulating immune complexes).

■ Some of the total morbidity of rheumatoid arthritis is caused by gastrointestinal bleeding from long-term aspirin therapy, infections from steroid use, or amyloidosis in long-term severe disease.

■ Variants of rheumatoid arthritis include juvenile-onset rheumatoid arthritis, Felty syndrome (features rheumatoid arthritis, splenomegaly, and neutropenia), arthritis associated with ulcerative colitis, and arthritis associated with Sjögren syndrome.

SERONEGATIVE SPONDYLOARTHROPATHIES
(p. 1252)

Seronegative spondyloarthropathies include ankylosing spondylitis, Reiter syndrome, psoriatic arthritis, and enteropathic arthritis. All have similar clinical features, and many are associated with HLA-B27, but all lack rheumatoid factor (hence seronegative).

■ *Ankylosing spondylarthritis (Marie-Strümpell disease)* is a chronic inflammatory joint disease of vertebrae and sacroiliac joints that usually occurs in males. It begins in adolescence after an infection and is suspected to be of immunogenetic origin, with autoantibodies directed at joint elements. It follows a chronic progressive course, with extension to hips, knees, and shoulders in one third of patients and sometimes uveitis, aortitis, and amyloidosis.

■ Reiter syndrome comprises a triad of arthritis, nongonococcal urethritis or cervicitis, and conjunctivitis. Men are most often affected in their twenties to thirties, and most are positive for HLA-B27. Evidence suggests that disease is caused by an autoimmune reaction initiated by prior infection, usually gastrointestinal or genitourinary. Ankles, knees, and feet may be affected, but in chronic disease, the spine is affected as well, indistinguishable from ankylosing spondylitis. Extra-articular involvements include skin, eyes, heart, tendons, and muscles.

- *Psoriatic arthritis* appears in about 5% of patients with the skin disease. The arthritis usually affects small joints of the hands and feet but may also extend to ankles, knees, hips, and wrists. Spinal disease occurs in about one quarter of the patients. Psoriatic arthritis is not as severe as rheumatoid arthritis. There is less joint destruction.
- *Enteropathic arthritis* appears in 10 to 20% of patients with inflammatory bowel disease as a migratory oligoarthritis of the large joints and spine. It may resemble ankylosing spondylitis but is generally less severe and remits spontaneously in a year or so.

Infectious Arthritis (p. 1253)

Infectious arthritis is uncommon but can rapidly destroy a joint to produce permanent loss of motion. Any of a great variety of microorganisms can seed the joint hematogenously or, more rarely, by direct inoculation or spread from a nearby focus of infection.

- *Suppurative arthritis* is most commonly caused by gonococcus, staphylococcus, streptococcus, *Haemophilus influenzae*, and gram-negative coliforms. Individuals with sickle cell disease are prone to infection with salmonella. *H. influenzae* predominates in children younger than 2 years of age; *S. aureus* in older children and adults; and gonococcus in late adolescence and young adult life. In most instances, a single joint is affected, usually the knee, followed in frequency by hip, shoulder, elbow, wrist, and sternoclavicular joint. Gonococcal arthritis is mostly oligoarticular and often associated with a skin rash and a genetic deficiency of C5, C6, or C7.
- *Tuberculous arthritis* is an insidious chronic arthritis from hematogenous spread or nearby tuberculous osteomyelitis. The most common site is the spine (Pott disease) followed in frequency by hip, knee, elbow, wrist, ankle, and sacroiliac joints. It tends to be a more destructive process than suppurative arthritis.
- *Lyme arthritis* (Chapter 9) follows several days or weeks after the initial skin infection. The arthritis tends to be remitting and migratory and primarily involves large joints, especially the knees, shoulders, elbows, and ankles. The articular involvement morphologically resembles rheumatoid arthritis; in most cases, it clears spontaneously or with therapy, but in about 10% of patients, it results in permanent deformities.

Crystal Arthropathies (p. 1253)

GOUT AND GOUTY ARTHRITIS (p. 1253)

Gout and gouty arthritis refer to a group of conditions that share

1. Hyperuricemia
2. Attacks of acute arthritis triggered by crystallization of urates in joints
3. Asymptomatic intervals
4. Eventual development of chronic tophaceous gout and arthritis

Hyperuricemia is necessary for gout, but only a small fraction of hyperuricemic individuals develop gout. Most cases occur in men (after the twenties); women are almost never affected before menopause.

Pathogenesis

Primary and secondary forms exist:

1. *Primary (90% of all cases)*: The overwhelming majority are idiopathic (>95%), are of multifactorial inheritance, and are associated with overproduction of uric acid with normal or increased excretion or normal production of uric acid with underexcretion. Alcohol use and obesity predispose. A small percentage of primary cases are associated with specific enzyme defects (e.g., X-linked, partial deficiency of hypoxanthine-guanine phosphoribosyltransferase [HGPRT]).

2. *Secondary (10% of all cases)*: Most are associated with increased nucleic acid turnover, which occurs with chronic hemolysis, polycythemia, leukemia, and lymphoma. Less commonly, drugs (especially diuretics, aspirin, nicotinic acid, and ethanol) or chronic renal disease leads to symptomatic hyperuricemia. Lead intoxication may induce *saturnine gout*. Rarely the specific enzyme defects causing von Gierke disease (glycogen storage disease type I) and the Lesch-Nyhan syndrome (with a total lack of HGPRT seen only in men and associated with neurologic deficits) lead to gouty symptoms.

Morphology

Acute arthritis represents an acute oligoarticular or monoarticular inflammatory synovitis initiated by urate crystal formation within joints.

- Needle-shaped crystals are birefringent with polarized light.
- The crystals activate Hageman factor, with the production of chemoattractants (e.g., C3a and 5a) and inflammatory mediators. Neutrophils and macrophages accumulate in joints and phagocytose crystals, leading to release of lysosomal enzymes, toxic free radicals, IL-1, IL-6, IL-8, TNF-α, prostaglandins, and leukotrienes, which collectively produce acute synovitis.
- Chronic arthritis evolves from the progressive precipitation of urates into the synovial linings of joints after recurrent attacks of acute arthritis.
- *The tophus is the pathognomonic lesion of gout*—a mass of urates, crystalline or amorphous, surrounded by an intense inflammatory reaction, composed of macrophages, lymphocytes, fibroblasts, and foreign body giant cells. Tophi tend to occur on the ear, in the olecranon and patellar bursae, and in periarticular ligaments and connective tissue.
- Three types of renal disease result:
  1. Acute uric acid nephropathy (intratubular urate deposition)
  2. Nephrolithiasis
  3. Chronic urate nephropathy (interstitial urate deposition)

Clinical Correlation

About 50% of the initial attacks of acute gouty arthritis involve the great toe or, less frequently, the instep, ankle, or heel.

- Sometimes physical or emotional fatigue, an alcoholic spree, or dietary overindulgence precedes an attack.
- The initial attack subsides spontaneously or with therapy, usually recurring within several months to a few years.

- Other joints become involved, and multiple recurrences lead to chronic gouty arthritis.
- About 90% of patients with chronic arthritis develop some renal impairment.
- Uricosuric therapy is effective in controlling gout.

CALCIUM PYROPHOSPHATE (p. 1257)

Crystal Deposition Disease (p. 1257)

Crystal deposition disease refers to acute or chronic arthritis secondary to deposition of calcium pyrophosphate (chondrocalcinosis or pseudogout). *Many of the clinicopathologic features of this disease are similar to those of gout.*

Pseudogout can be hereditary, sporadic, or associated with trauma or surgery. Calcium pyrophosphate crystals are frequently present in joint specimens from patients with DJD and in intervertebral disc material removed from patients with herniation of disc.

- The deposits appear as circular aggregates (pools) of basophilic-staining rhomboid crystals. Whether these deposits are causing the joint disease or are a secondary phenomenon is unclear.
- In pseudogout, almost any combination of joints as well as the intervertebral disks can be involved, but the knee is most frequently affected.
- Joint involvement may be transient, but about half the patients suffer significant joint damage.

INFLAMMATORY AND TUMOROUS INVOLVEMENT OF JOINTS AND RELATED STRUCTURES (p. 1257)

Ganglion and Synovial Cyst (p. 1258)

A ganglion is a small (1- to 1.5-cm) multiloculated, cavitated (*cystic*) lesion found in connective tissues of joint capsules or tendon sheaths.

- It arises from a focus of myxoid degeneration and softening of connective tissues. The cavities are not lined by epithelium, and they do not communicate with joint cavities.
- Favored location is the small joints of the wrist, where ganglions are palpated as a firm but yielding, pea-sized subcutaneous nodule.
- The lesions are easily treatable by surgical removal; occasionally, they may erode underlying bone.
- *Herniations of a joint space may occur, particularly into the popliteal space from the knee joint when there is a marked increase of intra-articular fluid or exudate, as in rheumatoid or suppurative arthritis. The herniations of the knee joints are known as synovial or Baker cysts.*
- The anatomic changes are those of the underlying articular disease.

Villonodular Synovitis (p. 1258)

Villonodular synovitis is the term for a group of closely related lesions involving synovial membranes and tendons, usually of peripheral joints.

- *Morphologically,* synovial lesions are made up of fibroblasts, histiocytoid cells, and fibrohistiocytoid cells, often admixed with multinucleated, osteoclast-like cells; xanthoma cells; and pigmented macrophages.

- When the process is sharply localized, it is referred to as *nodular tenosynovitis* (or *giant cell tumor of tendons*); when it more diffusely involves the intra-articular synovial membrane (often with hemosiderin pigment), it is called *pigmented villo-nodular synovitis.*
- It is unclear whether these lesions are neoplasms (variants of benign fibrous histiocytoma) or reactive, inflammatory conditions (synovitis).
- They can recur, especially the poorly localized forms, and cause destruction of underlying bone.

SOFT TISSUE TUMORS AND TUMOR-LIKE LESIONS (p. 1259)

Soft tissue tumors are "mesenchymal proliferations that arise in the extraskeletal nonepithelial tissue of the body, exclusive of the viscera, coverings of the brain, and lymphoreticular system." Tumors may arise in any location, although about 40% occur in the lower extremity, especially thighs, 20% in the upper extremity, 10% in the head and neck, and 30% in the trunk and retroperitoneum. Critical to their clinical management are the following parameters:

- Size—the larger the mass, the poorer the outlook.
- Accurate histologic classification and grading (I through III based largely on the degree of differentiation) and an estimate of the rate of growth based on mitoses and extent of necrosis.
- Staging.
- Location of tumor—the more superficial, the better the prognosis.

Fatty Tumors (p. 1260)

LIPOMA AND LIPOSARCOMA (p. 1260)

Lipomas are the most frequent soft tissue tumors, arising in subcutaneous regions at any site but most commonly on the back, shoulder, and neck. They can also arise in the mediastinum, retroperitoneum, or bowel wall.

- Lipomas are delicately encapsulated, usually small tumors recapitulating normal, mature adipose tissue. Uncommonly, atypical examples occur in subcutaneous locations, where they should not be mistaken for liposarcoma.
- *Liposarcomas are much less common and tend to be bulky. They arise from primitive mesenchymal cells, some bearing lipid vacuoles that are requisite in at least some cells for the diagnosis of liposarcoma. Liposarcomas appear virtually anywhere in the body without regard to adipose tissue. Most arise in deep soft tissues and pursue a course closely dependent on their cytologic features.*
- Well-differentiated (lipoma-like) liposarcoma and myxoid liposarcoma (with a nonspecific myxoid background) tend to be low-grade tumors, which are stubbornly recurrent, follow a more protracted course, and metastasize late.
- In contrast, round cell liposarcoma and pleomorphic liposar-

coma are high-grade, aggressive sarcomas (85 to 90% metastasize).
- The myxoid variant (but not the others) has a characteristic balanced 12:16 translocation.

Fibrous Tumors and Tumor-like Lesions
(p. 1261)

REACTIVE PSEUDOSARCOMATOUS PROLIFERATIONS (p. 1261)

Nodular Fasciitis (p. 1261)

Nodular fasciitis refers to a reactive, benign, fibroproliferative lesion, also known as *pseudosarcomatous fasciitis, that is more commonly mistaken for a neoplasm than any other non-neoplastic condition.*

- The lesions appear as palpable nodules or small masses, most often in the extremities (but possibly elsewhere), in young and middle-aged adults of either sex.
- After a period of rapid growth, the tumors tend to plateau in size, indicating progressive maturation.
- *Morphologically, they are composed of spindled fibroblasts and myofibroblasts in a loose myxoid background resembling cultured fibroblasts. Some of the more active cells are enlarged and have prominent nuclei and nucleoli; mitoses may be present.*
- Recurrence after excision, even incomplete excision, is exceedingly rare and should lead to a reappraisal of the original diagnosis.

Myositis Ossificans (p. 1262)

Myositis ossificans is a variant of fasciitis, sometimes preceded by trauma, occurring most often in skeletal muscle but sometimes in subcutaneous fat.

- Favored locations are the extremities, particularly the quadriceps or brachialis muscle.
- *Morphologically, the lesions are circumscribed but unencapsulated masses composed of fibroblasts and myofibroblasts in a myxoid stroma, but, in addition, the periphery has a rim of woven, often mineralized bone. They should not be confused with osteogenic sarcoma.*
- Mature lesions are completely ossified.

Palmar, Plantar, and Penile Fibromatosis (p. 1262)

The *fibromatoses* encompass a group of fibroproliferative lesions with similar histopathologic features but variable clinical presentations.

- When on the palm, the process is known as *palmar fibromatosis (Dupuytren contracture).*
- When on the foot, the process is known as *plantar fibromatosis.*
- When involving the penis, the process is known as *penile fibromatosis (Peyronie disease).*
- These lesions may recur after excision or spontaneously resolve in about 25% of patients.

Desmoid (Aggressive Fibromatosis) (p. 1263)

Desmoids lie in the histologic interface between exuberant fibroproliferative lesions and low-grade fibrosarcomas.

- They present as infiltrative masses in abdominal (affecting mothers in the perinatal period), extra-abdominal (affecting men and women equally), and intra-abdominal (Gardner syndrome) locations.
- They are composed of banal, *tame-looking* fibroblasts (actually myofibroblasts by electron microscopy) that do not metastasize.
- *Although curable by adequate excision, they stubbornly recur in the local site when incompletely removed.*

FIBROMA AND FIBROSARCOMA (p. 1263)

Fibromas are most common in the ovary but may occur around the teeth and at other body sites. They are well-defined, usually small, gray-white tumors composed of sparse mature fibroblasts and collagenous tissue.

Fibrosarcomas occur in deep soft tissue and are gray, soft, *fish-flesh* masses with increased fibroblastic cellularity, anaplasia, high nuclear-cytoplasmic ratios, abundant mitotic figures, and *spindled growth in a herringbone pattern.*

- Fibrosarcomas often are large masses that appear deceptively encapsulated but are nonetheless infiltrative.
- Overall, 60 to 80% of patients survive 5 years with present methods of treatment.

FIBROHISTIOCYTIC TUMORS (p. 1264)

Benign Fibrous Histiocytoma (p. 1264)

Benign fibrous histiocytomas are distinctive unencapsulated but demarcated neoplasms composed of a mixture of cells resembling fibroblasts, myofibroblasts, histiocytes, primitive mesenchymal cells, and cells having intermediate or mixed features (fibrohistio-cytoid cells).

- Benign giant cells and fat-laden foamy cells can also be found.
- Benign lesions predominantly occur in the skin and are most frequently referred to as *dermatofibromas*.
- Other variants may be vascular—*sclerosing hemangioma*.

Tumors of Skeletal Muscle (p. 1265)

RHABDOMYOSARCOMA (p. 1265)

Cardiac rhabdomyomas (probably hamartomas) occur mostly in the setting of tuberous sclerosis. Extracardiac rhabdomyomas are divided into adult and fetal types based on the differentiation of cells (the degree to which they resemble myocytes). Extracardiac rhabdomyomas are too rare for further description.

Rhabdomyosarcoma is more common, especially in children, in the head and neck and urogenital regions. Rhabdomyosarcomas are subdivided into four types based on morphologic features:

1. Embryonal
2. Botryoid
3. Alveolar
4. Pleomorphic

The botryoid pattern is basically a morphologic variant of the embryonal pattern, which in submucosal locations projects into a cavity (e.g., vagina, bladder, as grapelike masses [hence botryoid]).

- The pleomorphic type (rare) occurs in patients older than 45 years; the other three types in about 90% of cases occur before age 20 years. The pleomorphic variant has large, atypical tumor cells, some showing abundant cytoplasm with cross-striations characteristic of skeletal muscle differentiation.

- The other three variants are basically primitive, poorly differentiated tumors of small blue cells that have focal skeletal muscle differentiation (rhabdomyoblasts with abundant eosinophilic cytoplasm or cross-striations).
- Rhabdomyoblastic differentiation may be apparent only with electron microscopic or immunohistochemical techniques (ribosomal-myosin complexes or desmin/myoglobin immunoperoxidase positivity). The alveolar variant is characterized by a 2:13 chromosomal translocation.
- The embryonal, alveolar, and botryoid variants respond to surgery combined with radiation and chemotherapy (3-year median survivals). The pleomorphic variant has a poorer prognosis.

Tumors of Smooth Muscle (p. 1266)

LEIOMYOMA AND LEIOMYOSARCOMA
(p. 1266)

Benign smooth muscle tumors occur predominantly in the female genital tract, particularly the uterus (p. 1266), but they may also occur at other body sites where smooth muscle is well represented (e.g., scrotum, nipple, bowel wall).

- Leiomyosarcomas are uncommon; they occur more frequently in women than in men.
- Most develop in skin and deep soft tissue.
- They are usually large, soft, gray masses of spindle cells with *cigar-shaped* nuclei.
- Variants may be myxoid or epithelioid.
- Superficial lesions often can be excised; deep tumors are invasive and rarely excisable.

Synovial Sarcoma (p. 1266)

These tumors occur around joints (but not in joint spaces), in the parapharyngeal region, in the abdominal wall, and less commonly at other body sites.

- *The highly distinctive feature of these infiltrative sarcomas (shared only by mesotheliomas and carcinosarcomas) is their biphasic pattern of cell growth: distinct epithelial components forming glands and papillary patterns, admixed with well-defined spindle cell components.*
- They range in behavior from aggressive lesions causing death within a few months to extremely indolent tumors permitting cure or long-term survival (5-year survivals are about 50%).
- Most have a reciprocal translocation between chromosomes X and 18 (p11.2;q11.2).

Diseases of Peripheral Nerves and Muscle

MOTOR UNIT (p. 1269)

Normal Structure (p. 1270)

A *motor unit* consists of

1. A spinal anterior horn *lower motor neuron*
2. The *axon* of that neuron
3. The *muscle fibers* it innervates

Peripheral nerves are composed of intermingled *myelinated* (2 to 15 μm) and *unmyelinated* (0.2 to 3 μm) *axons* and their investing Schwann cells grouped into fascicles by connective tissue sheaths:

Epineurium—encloses the entire nerve
Perineurium—encircles each fascicle
Endoneurium—surrounds nerve fibers

Single Schwann cells myelinate axonal segments (internodes) separated by nodes of Ranvier. Protein synthesis does not occur in the axon, and axoplasmic flow delivers proteins and other substances synthesized in the perikaryon down the axon; a retrograde transport system serves as a feedback to the cell body. The *perineurial barrier* is formed by the tight junctions between the perineurial cells. Endoneurial capillaries establish the *blood-nerve barrier*.

Skeletal muscles (muscle fibers) are syncytial cells with multiple nuclei beneath the plasma membrane *(sarcolemma)* and contain identical repeating units *(sarcomeres)* of actin and myosin contractile proteins delimited by perpendicularly disposed Z bands (primarily α-actinin). In normal human muscle, there are two types of fibers with different functional characteristics and staining patterns (Table 27–1). All fibers of a motor unit are of the same type; they are randomly distributed across the cross-section of a muscle, giving a checkerboard pattern with special stains.

Reactions to Injury (p. 1273)

NERVE (p. 1274)

- *Segmental demyelination*: Loss of myelin occurs along discrete regions of axons from dysfunction of the Schwann cell or damage to the myelin sheath; no primary abnormality of the axon is present. With sequential episodes of demyelination

Table 27-1. MUSCLE FIBER TYPES

Characteristic	Type 1	Type 2
Action	Sustained force, weight bearing	Sudden movements, purposeful motion
Enzyme content	NADH: *dark staining*	NADH: *light staining*
	ATPase pH 4.2: *dark staining*	ATPase pH 4.2: *light staining*
	ATPase pH 9.4: *light staining*	ATPase pH 9.4: *dark staining*
Lipids	Abundant	Scant
Glycogen	Scant	Abundant
Ultrastructure	Many mitochondria	Few mitochondria
	Wide Z band	Narrow Z band
Physiology	Slow twitch	Fast twitch
Color	Red	White
Prototype	Soleus (pigeon)	Pectoral (pigeon)

NADH, nicotinamide-adenine dinucleotide (reduced form); ATPase, adenosine triphosphatase.

and remyelination, tiers of Schwann cell processes accumulate around the axon *(onion bulbs).*

■ *Axonal degeneration*: Primary destruction of the axon occurs, with secondary disintegration of its myelin sheath. In the slowly evolving neuronopathies or axonopathies, evidence of myelin breakdown is scant because only a few fibers degenerate at a time. *Wallerian degeneration* is the acute reaction distal to a cut axon and consists of axonal and myelin breakdown with phagocytosis by macrophages.

■ *Axonal regeneration*: Proximal stumps of degenerated axons can regrow guided by Schwann cells vacated by degenerated axons. Regeneration occurs at a rate on the order of 2 mm/day and shows multiple, closely aggregated, thinly myelinated small-caliber axons *(regenerating cluster)*. This regrowth of axons is a slow process, apparently limited by the rate of the slow component of axonal transport and the movement of tubulin, actin, and intermediate filaments.

MUSCLE (p. 1275)

■ *Denervation atrophy*: Down-regulation of myosin and actin synthesis and shrinkage of fibers to small, angulated shapes occur as a result of loss of innervation.

■ *Reinnervation*: This occurs after nerve regeneration or, more commonly, when surviving axons sprout around denervated muscle cells and incorporate the fibers into their motor unit, imparting the same histochemical type to a group of contiguous fibers—*type grouping*.

■ *Group atrophy*: This occurs when a type group becomes denervated.

■ *Myopathic changes*: Varied patterns occur, including segmental necrosis (destruction of a portion of a myocyte), myophagocytosis, myocyte regeneration via satellite cells (large, internalized nuclei; prominent nucleoli; and the cytoplasm, laden with RNA, basophilic), increased central nuclei, and variation in fiber size.

- *Segmental necrosis*: Destruction of a portion of myocyte may be followed by *myophagocytosis* as macrophages infiltrate the region.
- *Regeneration*: Peripherally located satellite cells proliferate and reconstitute a destroyed portion of the fiber, which shows large internalized nuclei, prominent nucleoli, and basophilic cytoplasm.
- *Hypertrophy*: In response to increased load, large fibers may divide along a segment *(muscle fiber splitting)* so that, in cross-section, a single large fiber contains a cell membrane traversing its diameter, often with adjacent nuclei.

DISEASES OF PERIPHERAL NERVE (p. 1275)

Immune-Mediated Neuropathies (p. 1275)

INFLAMMATORY NEUROPATHIES (p. 1275)

Acute Inflammatory Demyelinating Polyradiculoneuropathy (Guillain-Barré Syndrome) (p. 1275)

- Guillain-Barré syndrome is a life-threatening ascending paralysis, with weakness beginning in the distal limbs but rapidly advancing to affect proximal muscles.
- Annual incidence in the United States is 1:100,000 to 2:100,000.
- Nerve conduction velocity is slowed and cerebrospinal fluid protein is elevated in the absence of increased cells.
- Pathologic features are segmental demyelination and chronic inflammatory cells involving the nerve roots.
- Guillain-Barré syndrome appears to be an immunologically mediated disorder, often following a viral infection.

Chronic Inflammatory Demyelinating Polyradiculoneuropathy (p. 1276)

Chronic inflammatory demyelinating polyradiculoneuropathy is a mixed sensorimotor polyneuropathy similar to Guillain-Barré syndrome, but it follows a subacute or chronic course, usually with relapses and remissions. Peripheral nerves show recurrent demyelination and remyelination and onion bulbs.

INFECTIOUS POLYNEUROPATHIES (p. 1276)

- Direct infections of Schwann cells occur in leprosy (p. 385); the host response can be either limited *(lepromatous leprosy)* or vigorous *(tuberculoid leprosy)*.
- Varicella-zoster virus produces latent infection of neurons in the sensory ganglia of the spinal cord and brain stem after chickenpox, and its reactivation leads to a painful vesicular skin eruption in the distribution of sensory dermatomes *(shingles)*, most frequently thoracic or trigeminal.
- In contrast to these direct infectious processes, diphtheritic neuropathy results from the effects of the diphtheria exotoxin. It begins clinically with paresthesias and weakness and is characterized pathologically by segmental demyelination.

Hereditary Neuropathies (p. 1277)

Both strength and sensation are affected in the *hereditary motor and sensory neuropathies*. In the *hereditary sensory and autonomic neuropathies*, symptoms are usually limited to numbness, pain, and autonomic dysfunction, such as orthostatic hypotension (Table 27–2). Some hereditary neuropathies are notable for the deposition of amyloid within the nerve; these *familial amyloid polyneuropathies* have a clinical presentation similar to that of the hereditary sensory and autonomic neuropathies. Some inborn errors of metabolism cause prominent peripheral nerve manifestations (Table 27–3).

Acquired Metabolic and Toxic Neuropathies (p. 1279)

ADULT-ONSET DIABETES MELLITUS (p. 1279)

Three principal patterns of neuropathy occur:

1. *Distal symmetric sensory or sensorimotor neuropathy* (most commonly a chronic axonal neuropathy with dramatic reduction of small myelinated and unmyelinated fibers).
2. *Autonomic neuropathy* (affects about 20 to 40% of diabetics with distal sensorimotor neuropathy).
3. *Focal or multifocal asymmetric neuropathy* (mononeuropathy or multiple mononeuropathy, e.g., unilateral ocular nerve palsies, with sparing of reflexes).

OTHERS (p. 1279)

Neuropathies are encountered in patients with renal failure (before dialysis), chronic liver disease, chronic respiratory insufficiency, and hypothyroidism. Axonal neuropathies also occur with deficiencies of thiamine, vitamin B_{12} (cobalamin) and vitamin B_6 (pyridoxine), and vitamin E (α-tocopherol).

Neuropathies Associated With Malignancy (p. 1279)

- *Direct effects*: Infiltration or compression of peripheral nerves by tumor may cause a mononeuropathy, brachial plexopathy, cranial nerve palsy, or polyradiculopathy involving the lower extremities when the cauda equina is involved by meningeal carcinomatosis.
- *Paraneoplastic syndromes*:
  - Progressive sensorimotor neuropathy (less often a pure sensory neuropathy) is most pronounced in the lower extremities, particularly with small cell lung carcinoma; results in loss of dorsal root ganglion cells and CD8 + T-cell infiltrates; and results in axonal loss in nerves and in the posterior columns of the spinal cord.
  - Peripheral neuropathy with deposition of light-chain amyloid in peripheral nerves (AL type) occurs in patients with plasma cell dyscrasias. Neuropathy may also be related to the binding of monoclonal immunoglobulin M (IgM) to myelin-associated glycoprotein (MAG) independent of the presence of deposition of amyloid.

Toxic Neuropathies (p. 403)

Peripheral neuropathies may occur after exposure to industrial or environmental chemicals, biologic toxins, heavy metals, or therapeutic drugs. Some examples are listed in Table 27–4.

Text continued on page 626

Table 27-2. HEREDITARY NEUROPATHIES (HMSN AND HSAN)

Disease	Inheritance	Clinical Findings	Pathologic Findings
HMSN 1 (Charcot-Marie-Tooth)— hypertrophic type	Autosomal dominant, gene on chromosome 17, myelin-specific protein gene, PMP-22 (type 1A), less often on chromosome 1, myelin protein zero (type 1B); less common X-linked form (gap junction protein connexin-32)	Onset in childhood or early adulthood; progressive calf muscle atrophy (peroneal muscular atrophy, enlarged nerves, pes cavus)	Some segmental demyelination, nerve fiber loss, and onion bulbs
HMSN II—neuronal type	Autosomal dominant (one locus on chromosome 1)	Similar to HMSN 1, without nerve enlargement	Nerve fiber loss, no onion bulbs, loss of anterior horn cells in spinal cord
HMSN III (Déjérine-Sottas)— infantile type	Autosomal recessive (several separate loci including PMP-22 and myelin protein zero)	Onset in early childhood, progressive upper and lower extremity weakness and muscle atrophy, greatly enlarged palpable nerves	Segmental demyelination, severe nerve fiber loss, and prominent onion bulbs

HSAN I	Autosomal dominant	Predominantly sensory neuropathy, often presenting in young adults, with secondary consequences such as foot ulcers	Axonal degeneration (myelinated fibers affected more than unmyelinated)
HSAN II	Autosomal recessive (some cases are sporadic)	Predominantly sensory neuropathy, presenting in infancy or early childhood	Axonal degeneration (myelinated fibers affected more than unmyelinated); nerve biopsy may reveal complete absence of myelinated fibers
HSAN III (Riley-Day syndrome; familial dysautonomia)	Autosomal recessive (most often in Jewish children, locus on chromosome 9q31–q33)	Predominantly autonomic neuropathy, often presenting in infancy with symptoms such as postural hypotension, absence of tears, and excessive sweating	Axonal degeneration (unmyelinated fibers affected more than myelinated); atrophy and loss of sensory and autonomic ganglion cells

HMSN, hereditary motor and sensory neuropathies; HSAN, hereditary sensory and autonomic neuropathies.

Table 27-3. HEREDITARY NEUROPATHIES WITH KNOWN METABOLIC CAUSE

Disease	Metabolic Defect	Inheritance	Clinical Findings	Pathologic Findings
Adrenoleukodystrophy	Peroxisomal transporter enzyme	X-linked; 4% of female carriers are symptomatic	Mixed motor and sensory neuropathy, adrenal insufficiency, spastic paraplegia; onset between 10–20 years (a genetically distinct neonatal form also exists)	Axonal degeneration (myelinated and unmyelinated); segmental demyelination, with onion bulbs; EM: linear inclusions in Schwann cells
Familial amyloid polyneuropathies	Point mutations in transthyretin; rare pedigrees involve other molecules	Autosomal dominant	Sensory and autonomic dysfunction; age of onset is variable (depending on site of mutation)	Amyloid deposits in vessel walls and connective tissue with axonal degeneration
Porphyria (acute intermittent, coproporphyria, variegate)	Enzymes involved in heme synthesis	Autosomal dominant	Acute episodes of neurologic dysfunction, psychiatric disturbances, abdominal pain, seizures, proximal weakness, autonomic dysfunction; attacks may be precipitated by drugs	Acute and chronic axonal degeneration; regenerating clusters
Refsum disease	Phytanic acid α-hydroxylase (peroxisomal enzyme)	Autosomal recessive	Mixed motor and sensory neuropathy with palpable nerves; ataxia, night blindness, retinitis pigmentosa, ichthyosis; age of onset before 20 years (a genetically distinct infantile form also exists)	Severe onion bulb formation

EM: Electron microscopy

Table 27-4. TOXIC NEUROPATHIES RESULTING FROM ORGANIC COMPOUNDS

Toxic Agent	Source of Exposure	Molecular Basis	Clinical Findings	Pathologic Findings
Ethanol	Alcoholic beverages	Probable superimposed nutritional deficiencies	Slowly progressive distal sensorimotor neuropathy	Axonal degeneration (myelinated and unmyelinated fibers)
Acrylamide	Industry (polymerizing agent used as flocculant and for grouting)	?	Numbness and sweating of hands and feet, progressing to distal sensorimotor neuropathy	Axonal degeneration, most pronounced in distal nerve (large-caliber fibers most affected)
Hexane	Industry (solvent), inhalant abuse (glue sniffing)	Protein alkylation; impaired intermediate filament transport	Distal symmetric sensorimotor polyneuropathy	Enlarged axons filled with neurofilaments; axonal degeneration predominantly affecting large-caliber axons
Organophosphorous esters	Industry and contaminated food products (such as pesticides, petroleum additives, and plasticizers)	Induction of esterase activity (*neurotoxic esterase*); altered protein phosphorylation	Rapidly progressive distal sensorimotor polyneuropathy after latent phase (7–21 days)	Axonal degeneration affecting long axons of the peripheral and central nervous systems
Vinca alkaloids	Therapy (vincristine used in therapy of certain malignancies)	Impaired assembly of microtubules	Diminished ankle jerk earliest sign; subsequent progression to sensorimotor neuropathy	Axonal degeneration; large intravenous doses may cause accumulation of filaments in cell bodies

625

Traumatic Neuropathies (p. 1280)

- *Lacerations*: May follow cutting injuries or bone fractures in which a sharp fragment of bone lacerates the nerve.
- *Avulsions*: Follow application of tension to a nerve, often as the result of a force applied to one of the limbs.
- *Traumatic neuroma*: Tangled nodule of axons and connective tissue from regenerating axonal sprouts of the proximal stump after nerve transection.
- *Compression neuropathy (entrapment neuropathy)*: Most commonly seen with the median nerve at the level of the wrist within the compartment delimited by the transverse carpal ligament (*carpal tunnel syndrome*). This neuropathy is observed with any condition that can cause decreased available space within the carpal tunnel, such as tissue edema, but predisposing factors include pregnancy, degenerative joint disease, hypothyroidism, amyloidosis (especially that related to β_2-microglobulin deposition in renal dialysis patients), and excessive usage of the wrist.

Tumors of Peripheral Nerve (p. 1280)

Tumors of peripheral nerve are discussed in association with tumors of the central nervous system (p. 1352 in this volume).

DISEASES OF SKELETAL MUSCLE (p. 1280)
Denervation Atrophy (p. 1280)

Denervation atrophy refers to atrophy caused by any process that affects the anterior horn cell or its processes in the peripheral nervous system.

SPINAL MUSCULAR ATROPHY (INFANTILE MOTOR NEURON DISEASE) (p. 1281)

Spinal muscular atrophy (SMA) refers to a group of syngeneic autosomal recessive motor neuron diseases beginning in childhood or adolescence, with a locus on chromosome 5 (5q12.2-13.3). Histologic findings are large numbers of extremely atrophic fibers, often involving an entire fascicle of a muscle. The most common form (Werdnig-Hoffmann disease, SMA type 1) has onset at birth or within the first 4 months, with death within the first 3 years. SMA 2 and SMA 3 present at later ages, with shorter survival in the earlier-onset form (SMA 2).

Muscular Dystrophies (p. 1281)

The muscular dystrophies are a heterogeneous group of inherited disorders, often beginning in childhood and characterized clinically by progressive muscular weakness and wasting.

X-LINKED MUSCULAR DYSTROPHY (p. 1281)

- *Duchenne muscular dystrophy*: Duchenne muscular dystrophy is the most common dystrophy (incidence about 1:10,000 males); X-linked boys are normal at birth but become weak by age 5 leading to wheelchair dependence by 10 to 12 years of age. The disease progresses relentlessly until death by the early twenties. Weakness begins in the pelvic girdle muscles, then extends to the shoulder girdle. Pathology is also found in the heart, and cognitive impairment appears to be a component of the disease. Histopathologic abnormalities common to Duchenne muscular dystrophy and Becker muscular dystrophy include

1. *Variation in fiber size* (diameter), owing to the presence of both small and giant fibers, sometimes with fiber splitting
2. *Increased numbers of internalized nuclei* (beyond the normal range of 3 to 5%)
3. *Degeneration, necrosis, and phagocytosis of muscle fibers*
4. *Regeneration of muscle fibers*
5. *Proliferation of endomysial connective tissue*

Gene is at Xp21 region and encodes a 427-kD protein (*dystrophin*). Deletions represent a large proportion of mutations, with frameshift and point mutations accounting for the rest. Muscle biopsy specimens from patients with Duchenne muscular dystrophy show minimal evidence of dystrophin by both staining and direct measurements.

- *Becker muscular dystrophy*: Becker muscular dystrophy involves the same genetic locus as Duchenne muscular dystrophy but is less common and much less severe, with onset occurring later in childhood or in adolescence and having a slower, more variable rate of progression. Muscle biopsy specimens from Becker muscular dystrophy patients have diminished amounts of dystrophin, usually of an abnormal molecular weight, reflecting mutations that allow synthesis of some protein.
- *Other X-linked muscular dystrophies*: These disorders, such as Emery-Dreyfuss muscular dystrophy, are associated with mutations distinct from the dystrophin gene.

AUTOSOMAL MUSCULAR DYSTROPHIES
(p. 1282)

Some autosomal muscular dystrophies affect specific muscle groups, and the specific diagnosis is based largely on the pattern of clinical muscle weakness (Table 27–5). A group of the autosomal muscular dystrophies are similar to the X-linked muscular dystrophies and are termed *limb girdle muscular dystrophies* (LGMDs).

Limb Girdle Muscular Dystrophies (p. 1282)

LGMDs affect the proximal musculature of the trunk and limbs with either an autosomal dominant (LGMD 1) or a recessive (LGMD 2) inheritance. Mutations of proteins that interact with dystrophin have been identified in some of the recessive LGMDs.

MYOTONIC DYSTROPHY (p. 1283)

Myotonic dystrophy is an autosomal dominant disease that tends to increase in severity and appear at a younger age in succeeding generations. Myotonic dystrophy presents with abnormalities in gait secondary to weakness of foot dorsiflexors; weakness progresses with atrophy of muscles of the face, and ptosis ensues. Other associated findings include cataracts, frontal balding, gonadal atrophy, cardiomyopathy, smooth muscle involvement, decreased plasma IgG, and an abnormal glucose tolerance test. *Myotonia*, the sustained involuntary contraction of a group of muscles, is the cardinal neuromuscular symptom in this disease. Muscle may show features of a dystrophy (similar to Duchenne muscular

Table 27-5. OTHER MUSCULAR DYSTROPHIES

Disease	Inheritance	Clinical Findings	Pathologic Findings
Fascioscapulohumeral/ muscular dystrophy	Autosomal dominant (gene localized to 4q35)	Variable age at onset (most commonly 10–30 years); weakness of muscles of face, neck, and shoulder girdle	Dystrophic myopathy, but also often including inflammatory infiltrate of muscle
Oculopharyngeal muscular dystrophy	Autosomal dominant (gene localized to 14q11–q13)	Onset in midadult life; ptosis and weakness of extraocular muscles; difficulty in swallowing	Dystrophic myopathy, but often including rimmed vacuoles in type I fibers
Emery-Dreifuss muscular dystrophy	X-linked	Variable onset (most commonly 10–20 years); prominent contractures, especially of elbows and ankles	Mild myopathic changes
Congenital muscular dystrophy	Autosomal recessive	Neonatal hypotonia, respiratory insufficiency, delayed motor milestones. Two subtypes: merosin-negative (mutations in merosin/laminin αII gene) and merosin-positive (gene not yet identified)	Variable fiber size and endomysial fibrosis

dystrophy) as well as a striking increase in the number of internal nuclei and *ring fibers*, with a subsarcolemmal band of cytoplasm that appears distinct from the center of the fiber. Myotonic dystrophy is the only dystrophy that shows pathologic changes in muscle spindles, with fiber splitting, necrosis, and regeneration.

The gene (19q13.2-13.3, *myotonin-protein kinase*) contains a trinucleotide repeat—disease is caused by expansion of the repeat (in normals, <30 repeats are present, whereas in severely affected individuals, several thousand repeats may be present).

Ion Channel Myopathies (Channelopathies) (p. 1285)

- *Hypokalemic, hyperkalemic, and normokalemic periodic paralysis*: Relapsing episodes of hypotonic paralysis are associated with various levels of serum potassium. Hyperkalemic periodic paralysis is caused by mutations in a muscle sodium channel (chromosome 17); periodic acid–Schiff (PAS)–positive vacuoles, especially evident during episodes of acute weakness, correspond to dilation of the sarcoplasmic reticulum.
- *Myotonia congenita*: This is a nonprogressive myotonic disorder, with exacerbations caused by fatigue or stress; it is linked to the skeletal muscle chloride channel (chromosome 7).
- *Paramyotonia congenita*: This is a childhood disorder with myotonia and periods of hypotonia during exercise and exposure to cold. Mutations are in the same sodium channel as hyperkalemic periodic paralysis.
- *Malignant hyperpyrexia (malignant hyperthermia)*: This is an autosomal dominant syndrome of a dramatic hypermetabolic state (tachycardia, tachypnea, muscle spasms, and later hyperpyrexia) triggered by the induction of anesthesia, ordinarily halogenated inhaled agents, and succinylcholine.

Congenital Myopathies (p. 1285)

The congenital myopathies are a group of muscle diseases characterized by onset in early life, nonprogressive or slowly progressive course, proximal or generalized muscle weakness, and hypotonia *(floppy babies)* or severe joint contractures *(arthrogryposis)* (Table 27–6).

Myopathies Associated With Inborn Errors of Metabolism (p. 1286)

Myopathies are often associated with disorders of glycogen synthesis and degradation (Chapter 6) and can also result from disorders of mitochondrial function.

LIPID MYOPATHIES (p. 1286)

The principal morphologic characteristic of lipid myopathies is accumulation of lipid within myocytes in vacuoles, predominantly in type 1 fibers. Fatty acids are metabolized in mitochondria after transport following conjugation with carnitine—myopathies are caused by an abnormal carnitine transport system or deficiencies of the mitochondrial dehydrogenase enzyme systems.

- *Carnitine deficiency* may be limited to muscle (myopathic carnitine deficiency) or secondary to diminished systemic levels

Table 27-6. CONGENITAL AND METABOLIC MYOPATHIES

Disease	Inheritance	Clinical Findings	Pathologic Findings
Central core disease	Autosomal dominant	Early-onset hypotonia and nonprogressive weakness; associated skeletal deformities; may develop malignant hyperthermia	Cytoplasmic cores are lightly eosinophilic and distinct from surrounding sarcoplasm; only found in type 1 fibers, which usually predominate
Nemaline myopathy	Variable	Weakness, hypotonia, and delayed motor development in childhood; may also be seen in adults; usually nonprogressive; involves proximal limb muscle most severely; skeletal abnormalities may be present	Aggregates of subsarcolemmal spindle-shaped particles (*nemaline rods*); occur predominantly in type 1 fibers; derived from Z-band material (α-actinin)
Centronuclear myopathy	Autosomal recessive; rarer severe X-linked recessive; later-onset autosomal dominant; sporadic	Presents in infancy or early childhood with prominent involvement of extraocular and facial muscles; hypotonia, and slowly progressive limb muscle weakness	Abundance of centrally located nuclei involving the majority of muscle fibers; central nuclei are usually confined to type 1 fibers, which are small in diameter, but can occur in both fiber types

(systemic carnitine deficiency). The major symptom is weakness; age at onset is variable.

- *Carnitine palmitoyl transferase deficiency* may result in episodic acute myonecrosis *(rhabdomyolysis)* after prolonged exercise, with appearance of myoglobin in the urine. Renal failure can occur after massive episodes of rhabdomyolysis.

MITOCHONDRIAL MYOPATHIES (OXIDATIVE PHOSPHORYLATION DISEASES) (p. 1287)

Mitochondrial genome (mtDNA) encodes some of the proteins involved in mitochondrial oxidative phosphorylation as well as tRNA and rRNA. Diseases that involve mtDNA show maternal inheritance because the oocyte contributes the mitochondria to the embryo and may present in young adulthood and manifest with proximal muscle weakness, sometimes with severe involvement of the muscles that move the eyes (external ophthalmoplegia). Weakness may be accompanied by other neurologic symptoms, lactic acidosis, and cardiomyopathy. Pathologic findings include aggregates of abnormal mitochondria, causing irregular muscle fiber contour *(ragged red fibers* on Trichrome stains). There are increased numbers of, and abnormalities in the shape and size of, mitochondria, some of which contain paracrystalline *(parking lot)* inclusions or alterations in the structure of cristae.

- Class I mutations involve the genes for mitochondrial protein encoded by nuclear DNA and show autosomal dominant or recessive inheritance.
- Class II mutations involve *point mutations* in mtDNA and include many mitochondrial encephalomyopathies.
- Class III mutations involve *deletions* of mtDNA; many of these disorders show prominent involvement of extraocular muscles *(chronic progressive external ophthalmoplegia, Kearns-Sayre syndrome).*

Toxic Myopathies (p. 1287)

- *Thyrotoxic myopathy*: Acute or chronic, proximal muscle weakness sometimes presents before clinical thyroid dysfunction. In thyrotoxic periodic paralysis, there is weakness and hypokalemia.
- *Alcohol*: *Binge* drinking can produce an acute toxic syndrome of rhabdomyolysis with accompanying myoglobinuria; it may lead to renal failure.
- *Steroids*: Proximal muscle weakness and atrophy may occur in Cushing syndrome or during therapeutic administration of steroids. The severity of clinical disability is variable and not directly related to the steroid level or the therapeutic regimen.

Inflammatory Myopathies (p. 1287)

There are three subgroups of inflammatory muscle diseases:

1. Infectious myositis (p. 394)
2. Noninfectious inflammatory muscle disease, including polymyositis, dermatomyositis, and inclusion body myositis (p. 229)
3. Systemic inflammatory diseases that involve muscle along with other organs (p. 211)

Disorders of the Neuromuscular Junction
(p. 1289)

- *Myasthenia gravis*: This is an autoimmune disease characterized clinically by easy fatigability, ptosis, and diplopia resulting from an immune-mediated injury, which causes a decrease in the number of muscle acetylcholine receptors (AChRs).
  - Morphologically, light microscopic examination of muscle is ordinarily unremarkable or may show disuse type 2 atrophy (rarely, aggregates of lymphocytes—lymphorrhages); ultrastructurally, junctional folds are greatly reduced or abolished at the neuromuscular junction.
  - Antibodies to AChR are present in the serum of 85 to 90% of patients. These antibodies accelerate degradation of the AChR. Plasmapheresis can be effective treatment.
  - About 15% of patients have other autoimmune diseases, including autoimmune thyroid disease, rheumatoid arthritis, pernicious anemia, systemic lupus erythematosus, and other collagen vascular disorders.
  - Thymic hyperplasia is seen in about 65 to 75% of patients, and a thymoma is found in 15%. Resection of thymoma can improve symptoms.
- *Lambert-Eaton myasthenic syndrome*: This is a paraneoplastic disorder of the neuromuscular junction, most commonly with small cell carcinoma of the lung (60% of cases); it differs from myasthenia gravis in having increased contractions with repeated stimuli.

Tumors of Skeletal Muscle (p. 1265)

Tumors of skeletal muscle are discussed with soft tissue tumors.

Diseases of the Central Nervous System

Aspects of the central nervous system (CNS) that are important for understanding pathologic processes include the following:

- Localization of specific neurologic functions to distinct (often spatially clustered) groups of neurons—thus loss of these neurons produces clinical changes that may not be corrected by other neurons.
- Inability to regenerate neurons (so that focal destructive lesions can give rise to permanent clinical deficits).
- Selective vulnerability of certain neurons to injury based on differences in structure and function.
- Physical restrictions of the skull and spine rendering the brain and spinal cord vulnerable to expansile pressure.
- Cerebrospinal fluid (CSF) circulation, the lack of a lymphatic system, and a blood-brain barrier.
- Unique responses to injury and patterns of wound healing.

NORMAL CELLS AND THEIR REACTIONS TO INJURY (p. 1294)

Neurons (p. 1294)

Neurons vary in structure, functional interconnections, and biochemical properties. Pathologic changes are as follows:

- *Axonal reaction*: After an axon is cut or damaged, cytoplasm around the nucleus becomes pale (chromatolysis) and swollen.
- *Acute cell injury (red neuron)*: Intense eosinophilia of perinuclear cytoplasm and pyknosis of the nucleus that follows acute anoxia or ischemia.
- *Atrophy and degeneration*: Loss of neurons without other recognized morphologic change (characteristic of slowly progressive neurologic diseases and system degenerations).
- *Intraneuronal deposits*: Occur in
  - Aging (lipofuscin)
  - Disorders of metabolism (storage material)
  - Viral diseases (inclusion bodies)
  - Degenerative diseases (neurofibrillary tangles in Alzheimer disease and Lewy bodies in Parkinson disease)

Glia (p. 1295)

Glial cells provide supporting functions for neurons and their cellular processes; they also have a primary role in repair, fluid balance, and energy metabolism.

ASTROCYTES (p. 1296)

Astrocytes have a round-to-oval nucleus, finely stippled chromatin, and branching cytoplasmic processes; they contain the intermediate filament glial fibrillary acidic protein. The processes are directed toward capillaries (end feet), neurons, and the subpial and subependymal surfaces. Important functions include

- Structural support, contribute to the blood-brain barrier, and act as metabolic buffers or detoxifiers.
- Principal cells responsible for repair and scar formation in the brain. In damaged brain, they develop conspicuous eosinophilic cytoplasm *(gemistocytic astrocyte)*; later, they form a network of cellular processes, a process referred to as *gliosis*.

Additional pathologic reactions include formation of the following structures:

- *Rosenthal fibers*: Elongated, eosinophilic structures, containing αB-crystallin, within astrocytic processes and found in longstanding gliosis, pilocytic astrocytomas, and Alexander disease.
- *Corpora amylacea*: Lamellated polyglucosan bodies occurring in increasing numbers with advancing age.
- *Alzheimer type II astrocytes*: Glia with an enlarged nucleus and pale chromatin, found in patients with hyperammonemia.

OLIGODENDROCYTES (p. 1297)

Oligodendrocytes have a lymphocyte-sized nucleus with densely packed chromatin and little cytoplasm visible with hematoxylin and eosin stains. They produce and maintain CNS myelin.

EPENDYMA (p. 1297)

Ependyma refers to the single layer of cuboidal cells that lines the ventricular system and rests on subependymal glia. After injury, they do not regenerate, and the underlying subependymal glia proliferate, forming *ependymal granulations*.

MICROGLIA (p. 1297)

Microglia are bone marrow–derived, CD4 + and CR3 + mononuclear cells; they contain a bean-shaped nucleus, and little cytoplasm is visible with hematoxylin and eosin stains. They respond to injury by developing elongated nuclei (rod cells), forming aggregates about small foci of tissue necrosis (microglial nodules), or congregating around portions of dying neurons (neuronophagia).

COMMON PATHOPHYSIOLOGIC COMPLICATIONS (p. 1297)

Three interrelated pathophysiologic phenomena of great significance are

1. *Herniations*
2. *Cerebral edema*
3. *Hydrocephalus*

Herniations (p. 1298)

The volume of the intracranial contents is fixed by the skull. As a result, the introduction of additional tissue or fluid (as may occur in a space-occupying lesion, cerebral edema, or hydrocephalus) raises intracranial pressure, which may lead to life-threatening herniation of the brain through openings of the dural partitions of the cranial cavity or across openings of the skull. The major herniations are as follows:

- *Subfalcine*: Cingulate gyrus herniates under the falx (may compromise the anterior cerebral artery).
- *Transtentorial*: Medial temporal lobe (uncus) passes over the free edge of the tentorium (may lead to distortion of the adjacent midbrain and pons and tearing of feeding vessels *[Duret hemorrhages]* or compress the posterior cerebral artery).
- *Tonsillar*: Cerebellar tonsils herniate through the foramen magnum (may result in compression of the medulla and compromise cardiorespiratory centers).

Cerebral Edema (p. 1298)

The accumulation of extravascular fluid within the brain may cause life-threatening increased intracranial pressure because lymphatic drainage is essentially absent. The blood-brain barrier closely regulates the movement of fluids and other substances in and out of the brain; tight junctions between brain capillary endothelial cells constitute the cellular barrier.

Three types of edema often occur in combination:

1. *Vasogenic*: Accumulation of fluid outside the vascular compartment secondary to increased vascular permeability; commonly seen with cerebrovascular accidents, trauma, tumors, and infections. The brain is heavy, swollen, and softened; there is tissue vacuolation and preferential involvement of white matter.

2. *Cytotoxic*: Secondary to altered cell regulation of fluid; seen in anoxia or toxic or metabolic disturbances. The fluid is intracellular and tends to involve the gray matter.

3. *Interstitial*: Transudation of fluid from the ventricular system across the ependymal lining (characteristic of increased intraventricular pressure).

Hydrocephalus (p. 1298)

Obstruction of CSF flow leads to enlargement of the ventricles with an associated increase in the volume of CSF. Hydrocephalus is most often caused by congenital malformations and leptomeningeal or intraventricular tumors, hemorrhage, or infections.

There are two principal forms of hydrocephalus:

1. *Noncommunicating hydrocephalus*: Blockage anywhere along the ventricular system, most often the aqueduct or the foramina of Monro.

2. *Communicating hydrocephalus*: Obstruction along the subarachnoid path of CSF flow, including the sites of its resorption.

In infants and children in whom fusion of the cranial bones has not yet occurred, hydrocephalus produces enlargement of the head. In adults, hydrocephalus may lead to increased intracranial pressure.

Normal pressure hydrocephalus is a clinical syndrome typically found in elderly people and characterized by mental slowness, incontinence, and gait disturbances associated with a slowly evolving hydrocephalus. In diseases associated with extensive tissue loss, compensatory expansion of the entire CSF compartment results in *hydrocephalus ex vacuo*.

MALFORMATIONS AND DEVELOPMENTAL DISEASES (p. 1299)

Patterns of malformation and developmental lesions are determined by the gestational age of the fetus at the time of the injury. Etiologic environmental factors include maternal and fetal infections, drugs, anoxia, and ischemia. Major categories of CNS malformations are as follows:

- *Neural tube defects*: Failure of closure or reopening of the caudal portions of the neural tube results in malformation of the vertebral arches *(spina bifida)*, which may be associated with a disorganized segment of spinal cord and an overlying meningeal outpouching (myelomeningocele). Antenatal diagnosis can be made by imaging and maternal screening for α-fetoprotein. Folate deficiency during the initial weeks of gestation is a risk factor. *Anencephaly* is a malformation of the anterior end of the neural tube resulting in failure of development of the cerebrum. *Encephalocele* is a malformed diverticulum of CNS tissue extending through a defect in the cranium.
- *Forebrain abnormalities*: These include megalencephaly and micrencephaly (abnormally large or small brain volume), agyria and polymicrogyria (abnormally formed gyri), neuronal heterotopias (abnormal migration of neurons), holoprosencephaly (incomplete separation of the cerebral hemispheres), and agenesis of the corpus callosum.
- *Posterior fossa abnormalities*: *Chiari II malformation* (Arnold-Chiari malformation) consists of a small posterior fossa, a malformed midline cerebellum with extension of the vermis through the foramen magnum, hydrocephalus, and a lumbar myelomeningocele. *Dandy-Walker malformation* is characterized by an enlarged posterior fossa, absent cerebellar vermis, and large midline cyst.
- *Hydromyelia and syringomyelia*: These terms refer to segmental or continuous expansion of the central canal of the spinal cord or formation of a cleftlike cavity in the cord. Most occur in the cervical region. Symptoms are loss of pain and temperature sensation in the upper extremities, with retention of position sense and absence of motor deficits.

PERINATAL BRAIN INJURY (p. 1302)

Cerebral palsy is a nonprogressive neurologic motor deficit, with onset during the perinatal period, associated with several pathologic entities:

- *Intraparenchymal hemorrhage* occurs within the germinal matrix, near the junction between the thalamus and caudate nucleus, and sometimes extends into the ventricular system.
- *Ischemic* infarcts may occur focally in the periventricular white matter *(periventricular leukomalacia)* or develop throughout the hemispheres *(multicystic encephalopathy)*. Ischemia and hemorrhage are seen in premature newborn infants.
- *Ulegyria* (thin, gliotic gyri) and *status marmoratus* (neuronal

loss and gliosis in the basal ganglia and thalamus associated with aberrant and irregular myelin formation) are also related to ischemic injury. Choreoathetosis and related movement disorders are important clinical sequelae.

TRAUMA (p. 1302)

There are four categories of brain trauma:

1. Skull fractures
2. Parenchymal injuries
3. Traumatic vascular injury
4. Spinal cord injury

Skull Fractures (p. 1302)

Skull fractures may cross sutures. Bone displacement into the cranial cavity (i.e., displaced fracture) sometimes occurs. Their relative incidence among skull bones is related to the pattern of falls and the thickness of the bones.

Parenchymal Injuries (p. 1303)

The types of parenchymal injuries are as follows:

- *Concussion*: A transient neurologic syndrome occurring after trauma, with loss of consciousness, respiratory arrest, and loss of reflexes. Amnesia for the event persists. Concussion is unassociated with permanent structural damage.
- *Contusions*: Bruises of the crests of gyri either at the site of impact *(coup contusion)* or at a point opposite *(contrecoup contusion)*. Microscopically, these are foci of hemorrhagic brain. After resolution, a depressed, yellowish glial scar extends to the pial surface *(plaque jaune)*.
- *Laceration*: A penetrating injury leading to tearing of tissue.
- *White matter injury*: Diffuse axonal injury (axonal swellings) and hemorrhages, in the corpus callosum and brain stem, in about 50% of patients who develop coma after trauma. Mechanical forces, including angular acceleration in the absence of impact, damage the axon.

Traumatic Vascular Injury (p. 1304)

Depending on the anatomic position of the ruptured vessel, trauma-related hemorrhages are *epidural*, *subdural*, *subarachnoid*, and *intraparenchymal*.

- *Epidural hematoma*: Arterial blood, usually from a fracture-related rupture of the middle meningeal artery, collects between the dura and the internal surface of the skull and compresses the brain. Patients are often lucid for several hours after the trauma. The lesion may expand rapidly, may cause increased intracranial pressure or herniation, and requires drainage to prevent coma and death.
- *Subdural hematoma*: Venous blood from torn superficial bridging veins between the convexities and the dural venous sinuses collects in the space between the dura and the outer layer of the arachnoid. Chronic subdural hematomas may occur in older individuals and alcoholics, sometimes after relatively minor trauma. The treatment is surgical drainage acutely and removal

of the associated granulation tissue *(membranes)* in long-standing lesions.

■ *Traumatic subarachnoid hemorrhage and traumatic intraparenchymal hemorrhage*: Contusion of superficial cerebral tissue or, less frequently, cerebellar cortex is associated with disruption of small vessels within both the brain parenchyma and the overlying leptomeninges.

Spinal Cord Injury (p. 1306)

Most injuries that damage the spinal cord are associated with displacement of the spinal column, either rapid and temporary or persistent. In the acute phase, there is hemorrhage, necrosis, and white matter axonal swellings. Later the central necrotic lesion becomes cystic and gliotic, and the damaged ascending and descending white matter tracts undergo secondary degeneration.

CEREBROVASCULAR DISEASE (p. 1306)

Cerebrovascular disease is the most prevalent neurologic disorder in terms of both morbidity and mortality. The major categories are

1. Hypoxia, ischemia, and infarction
2. Intracranial hemorrhage
3. Hypertensive cerebrovascular disease

Hypoxia, Ischemia, and Infarction (p. 1307)

Brain oxygen deprivation causes either generalized *(ischemic or hypoxic encephalopathy)* or focal ischemic necrosis *(cerebral infarction).*

HYPOXIA AND ISCHEMIA (p. 1307)

Generalized hypoxia occurs with reduced blood oxygen content or with reduction of whole-brain cerebral perfusion pressure, as with hypotension. *Watershed* or *border zone infarcts* occur with reduced perfusion in those regions of the brain and spinal cord that lie at the most distal fields of arterial irrigation (i.e., at the border zone between major vascular territories); that between the anterior and middle cerebral artery is most at risk.

Morphology

In the first 12 to 24 hours after ischemia, neurons show ischemic cell injury *(red neurons)* and subsequently die. The most susceptible regions are the pyramidal neurons of the Sommer sector of the hippocampus, the Purkinje cell layer of the cerebellar cortex, and the pyramidal neurons in the neocortex *(pseudolaminar necrosis).* Healing is characterized by gliosis.

INFARCTION (p. 1308)

Cerebral infarction as a result of focal obstruction of blood flow may arise from either thrombotic or, more frequently, embolic arterial occlusion. These events are manifest as the *stroke syndrome*—the sudden onset of a neurologic deficit with clinical manifestations referable to the anatomic location of the lesion.

The deficit evolves over time, and the outcome is either fatal or characterized by some degree of slow improvement over a period of months. Venous infarcts are often hemorrhagic; they occur after thrombotic occlusion of the superior sagittal sinus or other sinuses or occlusion of the deep cerebral veins.

- *Thrombosis* most frequently affects the extracerebral carotid system and the basilar artery and usually is due to atherosclerosis.
- *Embolism* most commonly involves the intracerebral arteries (most often in middle cerebral artery distribution); emboli often originate from cardiac mural thrombi related to myocardial infarcts, valvular disease, and atrial fibrillation. Fragments of thrombotic material also may break off from arterial mural thrombi (most often in the carotid artery) or occur as paradoxical emboli (particularly in children with cardiac anomalies).

Morphology

Nonhemorrhagic infarcts (bland or anemic infarcts) are evident at 48 hours as pale, soft regions of edematous brain. The tissue then liquefies, and a fluid-filled cavity containing macrophages is lined by reactive glia. *Hemorrhagic infarcts*, characteristic of embolic occlusion with reperfusion injury, are manifest by blood extravasation, especially in the cerebral cortex.

Nontraumatic Intracranial Hemorrhage
(p. 1310)

Nontraumatic intracranial hemorrhage may be

1. Intraparenchymal
2. Subarachnoid
3. Mixed, as seen in vascular malformations

INTRAPARENCHYMAL HEMORRHAGE (p. 1310)

Intraparenchymal hemorrhage is the leading cause of death in stroke patients; *hypertension* is a predisposing factor in 80% of cases.

Hypertensive intracerebral hemorrhage is most commonly observed in the putamen, thalamus, pontine tegmentum, and cerebellar hemispheres. Vascular rupture is believed to be due to arteriolar injury with formation of microaneurysms *(Charcot-Bouchard aneurysms)*. *Lobar hemorrhages* involve areas supplied by hemispheric arteries and are due to amyloid angiopathy or hemorrhagic diatheses. In patients who survive, the hematoma is slowly resorbed over a period of months with some restitution of function.

Morphology

Macroscopically, acute hemorrhages are characterized by extravasation of blood with compression of the adjacent parenchyma. *Microscopically*, resolution shows an area of cavitary destruction of brain with a rim of gliotic tissue containing pigment-laden macrophages.

SUBARACHNOID HEMORRHAGE (p. 1310)

Subarachnoid hemorrhage occurs most often with rupture of a *berry aneurysm (saccular aneurysm, congenital aneurysm)*, the most frequent type of intracerebral aneurysm (fusiform atherosclerotic aneurysms and mycotic aneurysms also occur).

- Most berry aneurysms occur in the anterior circulation and are found near arterial branch points; multiplicity is found in 20 to 30% of patients.
- Most occur sporadically, but they also are associated with autosomal dominant polycystic kidney disease (p. 937).
- Hypertension and collagen disorders (Ehlers-Danlos syndrome, pseudoxanthoma elasticum, Marfan syndrome) also predispose to their development.

The probability of rupture increases with the size of the lesion; aneurysms greater than 10 mm have a roughly 50% risk of bleeding per year. Rupture often occurs with acute increases in intracranial pressure, such as with straining at stool or sexual orgasm. Between 25 and 50% of patients die with the first rupture. Rebleeding is common in the survivors, and with each episode of bleeding, the prognosis is more grave. Blood in the subarachnoid space can lead to arterial vasospasm. Eventually, blood resorption may lead to meningeal fibrosis and hydrocephalus.

Morphology

At the neck of the aneurysm, the muscular wall and intimal elastic lamina are usually absent or fragmentary, and the wall of the sac is made up of thickened hyalinized intima. With acutely ruptured aneurysms, blood diffusely fills the subarachnoid spaces.

VASCULAR MALFORMATIONS (p. 1313)

There are several types of vascular malformations.

- *Arteriovenous malformations*: Arteriovenous malformations are tangles of numerous, abnormally tortuous and misshapen vessels, containing arteries and veins without an intervening capillary bed, most often in middle cerebral artery territory. Men are affected twice as frequently as women; the lesion is most often recognized clinically between the ages of 10 and 30 years, presenting as a seizure disorder, intracerebral hemorrhage, or subarachnoid hemorrhage.
- *Cavernous hemangiomas*: Cavernous hemangiomas are greatly distended, loosely organized vascular channels with thin, collagenized walls occurring most often in the cerebellum, pons, and subcortical regions.
- *Capillary telangiectasias*: Capillary telangiectasias are microscopic foci of dilated, thin-walled vascular channels separated by relatively normal brain parenchyma and occurring most frequently in the pons.

Hypertensive Cerebrovascular Disease
(p. 1313)

In addition to hypertensive hemorrhage and arteriosclerosis, other pathologic processes include the following:

- *Lacunes or lacunar state*: Small (<15 mm), often multiple cystic infarcts resulting from arteriolar occlusion are most frequently seen in the lenticular nucleus, thalamus, internal capsule, deep white matter, caudate nucleus, and pons. Clinically, they can be silent or cause serious impairment. Because of the common involvement of basal ganglia, thalamus, and adjacent white matter, a number of stereotypic syndromes have been described.

- *Acute hypertensive encephalopathy*: This clinicopathologic syndrome is characterized by diffuse cerebral dysfunction (headaches, confusion, vomiting, and convulsions, sometimes leading to coma), with increased intracranial pressure arising in a hypertensive patient. Rapid therapeutic intervention is required because the syndrome often does not remit on its own. Postmortem examination may show an edematous brain with petechiae and necrosis of arterioles.

INFECTIONS (p. 1314)

Five basic categories of infection are based on the time course, etiologic agent, and site of involvement:

1. Acute bacterial (pyogenic) or viral (aseptic) infections that involve the leptomeninges and CSF *(meningitis)*
2. Acute bacterial infections of the subdural spaces *(subdural empyema)* or CNS parenchyma *(brain abscess)*
3. Chronic bacterial infections of the brain and meninges *(meningoencephalitis)*
4. Acute, subacute, or chronic viral infection of the brain *(encephalitis)*
5. Fungal and parasitic infections

There are four principal routes of entry of organisms into the nervous system:

1. *Hematogenous spread*—most common, usually arterial
2. *Direct implantation*—usually traumatic
3. *Local extension*—from an established infection in an air sinus
4. *Axonal transport*—certain viruses (e.g., rabies, herpes simplex) travel along peripheral nerves.

Meningitis (p. 1314)

BACTERIAL MENINGITIS (p. 1314)

Pathogens include

- *Escherichia coli* and the group B streptococci in neonates
- *Haemophilus influenzae* in infants and children
- *Neisseria meningitidis* in adolescents and young adults
- *Streptococcus pneumoniae* and *Listeria monocytogenes* in elderly people

Clinical Features

Clinical features include meningeal irritation with headache, photophobia, irritability, clouding of consciousness, and neck stiffness. Lumbar puncture shows cloudy or frankly purulent CSF under increased pressure, elevated protein, and a reduced glucose.

Morphology

CSF is cloudy or purulent with neutrophils and organisms; meningeal vessels are engorged. Blood vessels become inflamed and occluded, and hemorrhagic infarction of the underlying brain ensues. In chronic or untreated cases, leptomeningeal fibrosis and consequent hydrocephalus may occur.

VIRAL MENINGITIS (p. 1315)

Enteroviruses (echovirus, Coxsackie, and polioviruses) are the most commonly isolated pathogens. Viral meningitis is usually self-limited. It is characterized by meningeal irritation and CSF with lymphocytic pleocytosis, moderate protein elevation, and nearly always normal glucose content. Often, there is only a mild to moderate lymphocytic infiltration of leptomeninges.

Brain Abscess and Subdural Empyema
(p. 1315)

Predisposing conditions for brain abscess and subdural empyema include acute bacterial endocarditis, cyanotic congenital heart disease, and chronic pulmonary sepsis. Streptococci and staphylococci are the principal organisms identified. With infection of the subdural space, thrombophlebitis may develop in the veins that cross the subdural space (bridging veins), resulting in venous occlusion and infarction of the brain.

CLINICAL FEATURES

Brain abscess usually presents with progressive focal deficits and signs of raised intracranial pressure. CSF pressure, cell count, and protein are increased; glucose is normal. A systemic or local source of infection may be apparent. The increased intracranial pressure and progressive herniation can be fatal, and abscess rupture can lead to ventriculitis, meningitis, and sagittal sinus thrombosis.

MORPHOLOGY

There is a central region of liquefactive necrosis and a fibrous capsule surrounded by reactive gliosis. Brain abscess is often associated with marked cerebral edema.

Chronic Meningoencephalitis (p. 1316)

TUBERCULOUS MENINGITIS (p. 1316)

Tuberculous meningitis causes headache, malaise, mental confusion, and vomiting. There is moderate CSF pleocytosis of mononuclear cells, sometimes with neutrophils, elevated protein, and moderately reduced or normal glucose. Tuberculous meningitis may cause arachnoid fibrosis, hydrocephalus, and obliterative endarteritis. Infection by *Mycobacterium avium-intracellulare* in patients with acquired immunodeficiency syndrome (AIDS) may cause chronic meningitis, brain abscesses, and rarely diffuse encephalitis or cranial or peripheral neuropathy.

Morphology

The subarachnoid space contains a gelatinous or fibrinous exudate of chronic inflammatory cells, with mixtures of lymphocytes, plasma cells, and macrophages and, rarely, well-formed granulomas, most often at the base of the brain, obliterating the cisternae and encasing cranial nerves. Arteries running through the subarachnoid space may show *obliterative endarteritis*, with inflammatory infiltrates in their walls and marked intimal thickening. Well-circumscribed intraparenchymal mass *(tuberculoma)* may also occur.

NEUROSYPHILIS (p. 1317)

Neurosyphilis represents a tertiary stage of syphilis; it occurs in only about 10% of patients with untreated infections.

- *Meningovascular neurosyphilis* is a chronic meningitis sometimes associated with obliterative endarteritis.
- *Paretic neurosyphilis* is the result of brain invasion by spirochetes, with neuronal loss and proliferation of microglia (rod cells) and insidious but progressive loss of mental and physical functions with mood alterations (including delusions of grandeur), terminating in severe dementia (general paresis of the insane).
- *Tabes dorsalis* is the result of spirochete damage to the sensory nerves in the dorsal roots and loss of axons and myelin in the dorsal roots and dorsal columns; impaired joint position sense, locomotor ataxia, loss of pain sensation leading to skin and joint damage (Charcot joints), and other sensory disturbances are associated.

Patients with human immunodeficiency virus (HIV) infection are at increased risk for neurosyphilis, and the rate of progression and severity of the disease appear to be accelerated, presumably related to the impaired cell-mediated immunity.

LYME DISEASE (p. 1317)

Lyme disease is caused by the spirochete *Borrelia burgdorferi* and is transmitted by various species of the *Ixodes* tick. Lyme disease may cause aseptic meningitis, encephalopathy, and polyneuropathies. There is proliferation of microglial cells in the brain as well as scattered organisms.

Viral Encephalitis (p. 1317)

Viral encephalitis refers to parenchymal brain infections, almost invariably associated with meningeal inflammation, having a wide spectrum of clinical and pathologic expressions. *Characteristic features* include perivascular and parenchymal mononuclear cell infiltrate (lymphocytes, plasma cells, and macrophages), microglial nodules, and neuronophagia. The best characterized forms are as follows:

- *Arthropod-borne viral encephalitis:* This form of encephalitis is the cause of most outbreaks of epidemic viral encephalitis; major types include Eastern Equine, Western Equine, Venezuelan, St. Louis, and California. All have animal hosts and mosquito or tick vectors. The typical clinical manifestations are seizures, confusion, delirium, and stupor or coma.
- *Herpes simplex virus (HSV) type 1 (labialis):* HSV-1 occurs in any age group but is most common in children and young adults; about 10% have a history of prior labial herpes. Common symptoms are alterations in affect, mood, memory, and behavior. Hemorrhagic, necrotizing encephalitis, most severe along the inferior and medial regions of the temporal lobes and the orbitofrontal gyri, occurs. Cowdry intranuclear viral inclusion bodies may be found in both neurons and glia.
- *HSV-2 (genitalis):* HSV-2 causes a generalized, severe *encepha-*

litis in neonates. It occurs in up to 50% of neonates born by vaginal delivery to women with primary HSV-2 infection.

- *Varicella-zoster virus (herpes zoster):* Reactivation of latent infection after chickenpox results in a painful vesicular skin eruption in the distribution of a dermatome *(shingles).* It may cause a granulomatous arteritis or a necrotizing encephalitis in immunosuppressed patients.

- *Cytomegalovirus:* In utero infection leads to periventricular necrosis, microcephaly, and periventricular calcification. In patients with AIDS, cytomegalovirus is the most common opportunistic viral pathogen, affecting the CNS in 15 to 20% of patients; it causes a subacute encephalitis with microglial nodules or a periventricular necrotizing encephalitis with typical cytomegalic inclusions.

- *Poliomyelitis:* The virus attacks lower motor neurons and may cause flaccid paralysis with muscle wasting. Death can occur from paralysis of the respiratory muscles and myocarditis. Inflammatory reaction is usually confined to the anterior horns but may extend into the posterior horns. The postpolio syndrome typically develops 25 to 35 years after the resolution of the initial illness and is characterized by progressive weakness associated with decreased muscle bulk and occasional pain. There is no evidence to date for persistence of poliovirus genomes.

- *Rabies:* Rabies is transmitted by the bite of a rabid animal or exposure to bats even without a bite. The virus ascends to the CNS along the peripheral nerves from the wound site. It causes extraordinary CNS excitability, hydrophobia, and flaccid paralysis; death ensues from respiratory center failure. Widespread neuronal necrosis and inflammation, most severe in the basal ganglia, midbrain, and medulla, are present. *Negri bodies* (intracytoplasmic eosinophilic inclusions) are found in hippocampal pyramidal cells and Purkinje cells, sites usually devoid of inflammation.

- *HIV-1:* Up to 60% of patients with AIDS develop neurologic symptoms, and neuropathologic changes have been observed in 80 to 90%. These fall into three categories: *opportunistic infections* of the CNS (notably cytomegalovirus, toxoplasmosis, polyomavirus, varicella-zoster virus, HSV, and cryptococcosis), *primary CNS lymphoma,* and *direct or indirect effects of HIV-1,* which comprise the following four syndromes:
  1. *HIV-1 aseptic meningitis* occurs within 1 to 2 weeks of seroconversion in about 10% of patients; antibodies to HIV-1 can be demonstrated, and the virus can be isolated from the CSF. Microscopically, there is mild lymphocytic meningitis and some myelin loss in the hemispheres.
  2. *HIV-1 encephalitis* manifests as HIV-related cognitive/motor complex, with insidious mental slowing, memory loss, and mood disturbances, later progressing to motor abnormalities, ataxia, bladder and bowel incontinence, and, rarely, seizures. Features are virus-containing microglial nodules with multinucleated giant cells and myelin damage with gliosis.
  3. *Vacuolar myelopathy,* found in 20 to 30% of patients with AIDS at autopsy, consists of destruction of myelinated fibers and macrophages involving the posterior and lateral columns, resembling subacute combined degeneration, but vitamin B_{12} levels are normal. A disease with some similarities is *tropical spastic paraparesis,* a human T-cell lymphotropic virus (HTLV-1)–related myelopathy.

4. *Cranial and peripheral neuropathies and myopathies* include acute and chronic inflammatory demyelinating polyneuropathies, inflammatory myopathy, and a zidovudine-related acute toxic reversible myopathy with *ragged red* fibers and myoglobulinuria.

In children with congenital AIDS, neurologic dysfunction, evident by the first years of life, includes microcephaly with mental retardation and motor developmental delay with long tract signs.

- *Progressive multifocal leukoencephalopathy*: This is an infection of oligodendrocytes by a polyomavirus (JC virus) occurring in immunosuppressed patients. About 65% of normal asymptomatic people have serologic evidence of exposure to JC virus by the age of 14 years. Patients develop multifocal and progressive neurologic manifestations because of irregular regions of destruction of myelin. Lesions consist of patches of demyelination, greatly enlarged oligodendrocyte nuclei with viral inclusions, and astrocytes with greatly enlarged atypical nuclei.

- *Subacute sclerosing panencephalitis*: This is a progressive syndrome of cognitive decline, spasticity, and seizures that develops months or years after an early-age acute infection with measles. *It represents a persistent but nonproductive infection of the CNS by altered measles virus.* There is widespread gliosis and myelin degeneration; viral inclusions, largely within the nucleus, of oligodendrocytes and neurons; variable inflammation of white and gray matter; and neurofibrillary tangles.

Fungal and Parasitic Infections (p. 1322)

Fungal and parasitic infections are most frequently encountered in immunocompromised patients in the industrialized world. The brain is usually involved only late in the disease, when there is widespread hematogenous dissemination of the fungus, most often *Candida albicans*, Mucor, *Aspergillus fumigatus*, and *Cryptococcus neoformans*. In endemic areas, pathogens such as *Histoplasma capsulatum, Coccidioides immitis*, and *Blastomyces dermatitidis* may involve the CNS after a primary pulmonary or cutaneous infection. There are three basic patterns of infection:

1. *Chronic meningitis*: Most commonly by *Cryptococcus neoformans*; may occur in immunocompetent patients.
2. *Vasculitis*: Most frequently seen with *Mucor* and *Aspergillus*, with invasion of blood vessel walls, thrombosis, and hemorrhagic infarction.
3. *Parenchymal invasion*: With granulomas or abscesses, most commonly encountered with *Candida* and *Cryptococcus*.

Other infectious agents that may involve the CNS include protozoa (malaria, toxoplasmosis, amebiasis, and trypanosomiasis); rickettsia (typhus, Rocky Mountain spotted fever), and metazoa (cysticercosis and echinococcosis).

- *Toxoplasma gondii* is one of the most common causes of neurologic symptoms and morbidity in patients with AIDS. Clinical symptoms are subacute and often focal; computed tomography and magnetic resonance imaging studies show multiple ring-enhancing lesions. Abscesses contain both free tachyzoites and encysted bradyzoites. Primary maternal infection with toxoplasmosis, particularly if it occurs early in pregnancy, may be followed by a cerebritis in the fetus and multifocal necrotizing cerebral lesions, which may calcify.

- Among amoeba species, *Naegleria* species cause a rapidly fatal necrotizing encephalitis. A chronic granulomatous meningoencephalitis has been associated with acanthamoeba.

Transmissible Spongiform Encephalopathies (Prion Diseases) (p. 1323)

Transmissible spongiform encephalopathies are a group of diseases predominantly characterized by *spongiform change* caused by intracellular vacuoles in neural cells and associated with abnormal forms of a specific protein, termed *prion protein* (PrP). Diseases include

- Creutzfeldt-Jakob disease (CJD), Gerstmann-Straussler-Scheinker syndrome, fatal familial insomnia, and kuru in humans
- Scrapie in sheep and goats
- Mink transmissible encephalopathy
- Bovine spongiform encephalopathy *(mad cow disease)*

Diseases may be sporadic, infectious, and transmissible.

PrP is a 30-kD normal cellular protein, and disease occurs when it changes from its normal isoform (PrP^c) to an abnormal isoform, termed either *PrP^{sc}* or *PrP^{pres}*. The infectious nature of PrP^{sc} molecules thus comes from their ability to corrupt the integrity of normal cellular PrP^c.

Accumulation of PrP^{sc} appears to be the cause of the pathology in these diseases, but the pathways by which this material causes the development of cytoplasmic vacuoles and eventual neuronal death are yet to be explored.

- *CJD:* This is a rare cause of rapidly progressive dementia. It is primarily sporadic but may be familial. There are well-established cases of iatrogenic transmission. The disease is uniformly fatal, with an average duration of only 7 months, although a few patients survive for several years.
- *Variant CJD:* This is a CJD-like illness found in a small number of patients, mostly in the United Kingdom, and distinguished by several differences from typical CJD:
  - The disease affected young adults.
  - Behavioral disorders figured prominently in the early stages of the disease.
  - The neurologic syndrome progressed more slowly than what is usually observed in patients with CJD.
  Pathologic findings and molecular features are similar to CJD.
- *Gerstmann-Straussler-Scheinker syndrome:* This is an inherited disease with mutations of the *prion protein gene* (PRNP) gene, which typically begins with a chronic cerebellar ataxia, followed by a progressive dementia. The clinical course is usually slower than that of CJD, with progression to death several years after the onset of symptoms.
- *Fatal familial insomnia:* This disorder is named, in part, for the sleep disturbances that characterize its initial stages. The pathologic finding is a *spongiform* transformation of the cerebral cortex and, often, deep gray matter structures (such as caudate and putamen). In advanced cases, there is severe neuronal loss, reactive gliosis, and sometimes expansion of the vacuolated areas into cystlike spaces *(status spongiosus)*. No inflammatory infiltrate is present. In contrast to other prion diseases, FFI does not show spongiform pathology. Instead the most striking alteration is neuronal loss and reactive gliosis in the anterior

ventral and dorsomedial nuclei of the thalamus; neuronal loss is also prominent in the inferior olivary nuclei.

- *Kuru plaques:* These are deposits of aggregated abnormal PrP, which occur in the cerebellum of patients with Gerstmann-Straussler-Scheinker syndrome; they are present in abundance in the cerebral cortex in cases of variant CJD.

DEMYELINATING DISEASES (p. 1326)

Demyelinating diseases are characterized by a preferential damage to myelin with relative preservation of axons.

Multiple Sclerosis (p. 1326)

Multiple sclerosis is defined clinically as distinct episodes of neurologic deficits, separated in time, attributable to demyelinating white matter lesions that are separated in space. The natural course of multiple sclerosis is variable; often, it begins as a relapsing and remitting illness in which episodes of neurologic deficits develop over short periods of time (days to weeks) and show gradual partial remission. The frequency of relapses tends to decrease over time. In some patients, there is a steady neurologic deterioration. The cellular basis for recovery from symptoms is unknown.

Cellular immunity directed against myelin components is a strong candidate for the underlying mechanism of multiple sclerosis. The rate of multiple sclerosis increases with distance from the equator, and individuals take on the relative risk of the environment in which they spent their first 15 years. Risk is 15-fold higher when the disease is present in a first-degree relative, and the concordance rate for monozygotic twins is approximately 25%.

MORPHOLOGY

Lesions *(plaques)* are sharply defined areas of gray discoloration of white matter occurring especially around the ventricles but potentially located anywhere in the CNS. *Active plaques* have evidence of myelin breakdown, lipid-laden macrophages, and relative preservation of axons. Lymphocytes and mononuclear cells are prominent at the edges of plaques and around venules in and around plaques. *Inactive plaques* lack the inflammatory cell infiltrate and show gliosis; most axons within the lesion persist but remain unmyelinated.

- *Neuromyelitis optica (Devic disease)*: A variant of multiple sclerosis occurring especially in Asians, characterized by bilateral optic neuritis and especially destructive demyelinating lesions in the spinal cord.
- *Acute multiple sclerosis*: Occurs in younger individuals and has a rapid course; the plaques are large, with destruction of myelin and some axonal loss.

Other Demyelinating Diseases (p. 1328)

ACUTE DISSEMINATED ENCEPHALOMYELITIS (p. 1328)

Acute disseminated encephalomyelitis is a monophasic disease (follows viral infection or, rarely, a viral immunization) with headache, lethargy, and coma; other characteristics include poly-morphonuclear leukocytes followed by perivenous demyelination with accumulation of lipid-laden macrophages and a mononuclear infiltrate.

ACUTE HEMORRHAGIC LEUKOENCEPHALITIS
(p. 1328)

Acute hemorrhagic leukoencephalitis is more fulminant than acute disseminated encephalomyelitis and includes hemorrhagic necrosis of white and gray matter. There may be a history of a prior viral syndrome.

CENTRAL PONTINE MYELINOLYSIS (p. 1329)

Central pontine myelinolysis is characterized by selective damage to myelin in the basis pontis and portions of the pontine tegmentum, often leading to spastic paresis and associated with rapid correction of hyponatremia.

DEGENERATIVE DISEASES (p. 1329)

Degenerative diseases are characterized by

- Progressive and selective loss of functional systems of neurons
- Onset without any clear inciting event in a patient without previous neurologic deficits
- Empiric grouping according to regions of brain that are primarily affected

Degenerative Diseases Affecting the Cerebral Cortex (p. 1329)

The principal clinical manifestation of degenerative diseases affecting the cerebral cortex is dementia.

ALZHEIMER DISEASE (p. 1329)

Alzheimer disease usually begins after age 50 years, with insidious impairment of higher intellectual function, and progresses over 5 to 10 years. Most cases are sporadic, although at least 5 to 10% of cases are familial (loci on chromosomes 21, 14, and 1). Many patients with trisomy 21 who survive beyond 45 years develop a decline in cognition and the pathologic features of Alzheimer disease. The ε4 allele of apolipoprotein E (chromosome 19) is associated with increased risk for Alzheimer disease.

Morphology

Gyri are narrowed and the sulci widened, especially in the frontal, temporal, and parietal lobes; hydrocephalus ex vacuo follows loss of tissue. Microscopic changes include the following:

- *Neuritic plaques:* These are spherical, 20- to 200-μm diameter collections of dilated, tortuous, argyrophilic neuritic processes (dystrophic neuritis), with a central amyloid core containing amyloid β-peptide (Aβ), a 40– to 43–amino acid peptide derived from a larger molecule, amyloid precursor protein. Plaques are surrounded by microglia and reactive astrocytes. Neuritic plaques occur most often in the hippocampus, amygdala, and neocortex.

- *Neurofibrillary tangles:* These are bundles of argyrophilic paired helical filaments in neuronal cytoplasm, especially in entorhinal cortex, hippocampus, amygdala, basal forebrain, and the raphe nuclei. Neurofibrillary tangles contain hyperphosphorylated tau, MAP2, ubiquitin, and Aβ.
- *Amyloid angiopathy:* Amyloid angiopathy refers to vascular wall deposition of Aβ, which occurs in intracortical and subarachnoid vessels and is an almost invariable accompaniment of Alzheimer disease.

These changes may also occur in the brains of elderly nondemented individuals, so the diagnosis of Alzheimer disease requires clinicopathologic correlation.

PICK DISEASE (p. 1333)

Pick disease is much rarer than Alzheimer disease; it also causes dementia, often with prominent frontal signs. Brain shows atrophy of frontal and temporal lobes, with sparing of the posterior two thirds of the superior temporal gyrus. Rather than plaques and tangles, there are large ballooned neurons (Pick cells) and smooth argyrophilic inclusions (Pick bodies).

Degenerative Diseases of the Basal Ganglia and Brain Stem (p. 1333)

Degenerative diseases of the basal ganglia and brain stem are associated with movement disorders, tremor, and rigidity.

PARKINSONISM (p. 1333)

Parkinsonism refers to a clinical syndrome characterized by diminished facial expression, stooped posture, slowness of voluntary movement, festinating gait (progressively shortened, accelerated steps), rigidity, and a *pill-rolling tremor*, associated with decreased function of the nigrostriatal system.

- *Idiopathic Parkinson disease:* This progressive parkinsonian syndrome comes on in later life and in some is associated with dementia. There is pallor of the substantia nigra and locus ceruleus with loss of their pigmented, catecholaminergic neurons and gliosis; *Lewy bodies* (intracytoplasmic, eosinophilic inclusions, containing α-synuclein) occur in the remaining neurons. Some familial forms are linked to mutations in a gene encoding α-synuclein.
- *Progressive supranuclear palsy:* This progressive striatal syndrome occurs after age 50 and is characterized by loss of vertical gaze, truncal rigidity, dysequilibrium, loss of facial expression, and sometimes progressive dementia. There is widespread neuronal loss and neurofibrillary tangles in the globus pallidus, subthalamic nucleus, substantia nigra, colliculi, periaqueductal gray matter, and dentate nucleus of the cerebellum.
- *Corticobasal degeneration:* This disease of the elderly is characterized by extrapyramidal rigidity, asymmetric motor disturbances, and sensory cortical dysfunction. Motor, premotor, and anterior parietal cortex show severe loss of neurons, gliosis, and *ballooned* neurons. The substantia nigra and locus ceruleus

show loss of pigmented neurons and argyrophilic inclusions similar to those seen in progressive supranuclear palsy.

- *Multiple system atrophies:* This often overlapping group of disorders shares glial cytoplasmic inclusions and includes the following:
  - *Striatonigral degeneration:* Similar to idiopathic Parkinson disease but resistant to L-dopa therapy; widespread neuronal loss and gliosis of the caudate and putamen as well as involvement of pigmented neurons of the zona compacta of the substantia nigra, without Lewy bodies.
  - *Olivopontocerebellar atrophy:* Mostly autosomal dominant inheritance, with cerebellar ataxia, eye and somatic movement abnormalities, dysarthria, and rigidity. Findings are shrinkage of the basis pontis from loss of the pontine nuclei; widespread loss of Purkinje cells, especially in the lateral portions of the hemispheres; and retrograde degeneration in the inferior olives.
  - *Shy-Drager syndrome:* Parkinsonism and autonomic system failure, with loss of the sympathetic neurons of the intermediolateral column of the spinal cord.

HUNTINGTON DISEASE (p. 1335)

Huntington disease is an autosomal dominant movement disorder that becomes clinically manifest between 20 and 50 years of age. Affected patients develop chorea, characterized by jerky, hyperkinetic, sometimes dystonic movements affecting all parts of the body; they may later develop parkinsonism with bradykinesia, rigidity, and dementia. There is striking atrophy of the caudate nucleus and, to a lesser extent, the putamen, with severe loss of medium-sized, spiny striatal neurons. Neurons that contain nitric oxide synthase and cholinesterase are spared. The disease is associated with expansion of a trinucleotide repeat encoding a polyglutamine tract yielding huntingtin, the protein encoded by the Huntington disease gene on chromosome 4p.

Spinocerebellar Degenerations (p. 1337)

Spinocerebellar degenerations affect primarily, to a variable extent, the cerebellar cortex, spinal cord, and peripheral nerves.

- *Spinocerebellar ataxias (SCA):* This is a group of autosomal dominant diseases involving the cerebellum, brain stem, spinal cord, and peripheral nerves. Some forms (SCA1-3, SCA6, and SCA7) are caused by unstable expansions of CAG repeats, which encode polyglutamine tracts in different proteins.
- *Friedreich ataxia:* Friedreich ataxia is autosomal recessive with a male preponderance. The disease comes on at around 11 years of age, and symptoms of gait ataxia, dysarthria, depressed tendon reflexes, Babinski signs, and sensory loss evolve progressively over about 20 years. Associated findings include pes cavus, kyphoscoliosis, diabetes, cardiac arrhythmias, and myocarditis. Gene on chromosome 9q13 usually has expansion of a GAA repeat. Changes include
  1. Fiber loss and gliosis in the posterior columns and distal corticospinal and spinocerebellar tracts
  2. Neuronal loss in Clark column; VIII, X, and XII cranial nerve nuclei; dentate nucleus; Purkinje cells of the superior vermis; and dorsal root ganglion cells
  3. Peripheral neuropathy

■ *Ataxia-telangiectasia:* This autosomal recessive disease presents in childhood with evidence of cerebellar dysfunction and recurrent infections. Telangiectatic lesions are found especially in the conjunctiva. Findings include loss of Purkinje and granule cells, absence of thymus, hypoplastic gonads, and lymphoid malignancy.

Degenerative Diseases Affecting Motor Neurons (p. 1338)

AMYOTROPHIC LATERAL SCLEROSIS (p. 1338)

Amyotrophic lateral sclerosis is characterized by loss of lower motor neurons (muscular atrophy, fasciculations, weakness) and upper motor neurons (hyperreflexia, spasticity, and a Babinski reflex); it may have predominantly bulbar manifestations (involvement of motor cranial nerves, sparing those that control the extraocular muscles). Degeneration of the upper motor neurons results in loss of myelinated fibers in the corticospinal tracts; occasionally, there is atrophy of the precentral gyrus. The disease is more common in men, usually comes on after age 50, and is relentlessly progressive, with death from respiratory complications. Approximately 10% of cases show autosomal dominant inheritance; a locus on chromosome 21 is the copper/zinc–binding superoxide dismutase gene.

WERDNIG-HOFFMANN DISEASE (INFANTILE PROGRESSIVE SPINAL MUSCULAR ATROPHY) (p. 1281)

Werdnig-Hoffmann disease is a severe autosomal recessive form of lower motor neuron disease, which presents in the neonatal period with hypotonia *(floppy infant).* Death ensues within a few months from respiratory failure or aspiration pneumonia. Spinal muscular atrophy has been linked to a locus on chromosome 5q.

X-LINKED SPINAL MUSCULAR ATROPHY (p. 1338)

In X-linked spinal muscular atrophy, lower motor neuron loss is associated with gynecomastia, testicular atrophy, and oligospermia. It has been linked to amplification of a trinucleotide repeat in the coding sequence of the androgen receptor gene, with severity of the disease related to the number of repeats present.

INBORN ERRORS OF METABOLISM (p. 1338)

There are three main groups of inborn errors of metabolism:

1. Neuronal storage diseases
2. Leukodystrophies (white matter diseases)
3. Mitochondrial encephalomyelopathies

Leukodystrophies (p. 1339)

Examples of leukodystrophies are as follows:

■ *Krabbe disease*: This is an autosomal recessive deficiency of galactocerebroside β-galactosidase, the enzyme required for the catabolism of galactocerebroside to ceramide and galactose, with diffuse myelin and oligodendrocyte loss and the aggregation of macrophages around blood vessels as multinucleated cells (*globoid cells*). These macrophages contain storage material (linear inclusions by electron microscopy).

- *Metachromatic leukodystrophy*: This is an autosomal recessive disease with several clinical subtypes (congenital, late infantile, juvenile, and adult), caused by deficiency of arylsulfatase A with an accumulation of sulfatides, especially cerebroside sulfate. Findings include myelin loss and gliosis, with macrophages containing metachromatic material.

Other leukodystrophies include

- Adrenoleukodystrophy
- Pelizaeus-Merzbacher disease
- Canavan disease

Mitochondrial Encephalomyopathies
(p. 1340)

The following are examples of mitochondrial encephalomyelopathies:

- *Leigh disease:* Leigh disease is usually an autosomal recessive disorder, with onset between 1 and 2 years of age as arrest of psychomotor development, feeding problems, seizures, extraocular palsies, weakness with hypotonia, and lactic acidemia. Various biochemical abnormalities have been found in the mitochondrial pathway for converting pyruvate to adenosine triphosphate (ATP). The brain reveals bilateral regions of destruction with a proliferation of blood vessels, usually symmetrically, involving the periventricular gray matter of the midbrain, tegmentum of the pons, and periventricular regions of the thalamus and hypothalamus.
- Various other disorders are caused by alterations in mitochondrial function. These include:
  - Diseases caused by point mutations in mtDNA-encoded tRNA (e.g., *MERRF [myoclonic epilepsy and ragged red fibers] and MELAS [mitochondrial encephalomyelopathy, lactic acidosis, and stroke-like episodes]*)
  - Diseases caused by point mutations in mtDNA-encoded proteins (e.g., *Leber hereditary optic neuropathy*)
  - Diseases caused by deletions of portions of the mtDNA (e.g., *Kearns-Sayre ophthalmoplegia*)

TOXIC AND ACQUIRED METABOLIC DISEASE (p. 1341)
Vitamin Deficiencies (p. 1341)
THIAMINE (VITAMIN B_1) DEFICIENCY (p. 1341)

Beriberi has been discussed (p. 447). Thiamine deficiency may also lead to sudden onset of psychosis (*Wernicke encephalopathy*), which may be followed by a prolonged and largely irreversible disorder of memory (*Korsakoff syndrome*). The disorder is particularly common with chronic alcoholism but also may follow thiamine deficiency from gastric disease (carcinoma, chronic gastritis, or persistent vomiting). Findings are foci of hemorrhage and necrosis, particularly in the mamillary bodies, but also adjacent to the third and fourth ventricles. Lesions in the medial dorsal nucleus of the thalamus appear to be the best correlate of memory disturbance.

VITAMIN B$_{12}$ DEFICIENCY (p. 1341)

Vitamin B$_{12}$ deficiency causes nervous system symptoms as well as anemia. It usually begins with slight ataxia and numbness and tingling in the lower extremities and may progress rapidly to include spastic weakness of the lower extremities or paraplegia. Recovery from early symptoms may be expected with vitamin replacement; however, if complete paraplegia has developed, recovery is poor. Swelling of myelin layers producing vacuoles affects both ascending and descending tracts (subacute combined degeneration), beginning at the midthoracic spinal cord.

Neurologic Sequelae of Metabolic Disturbances (p. 1341)

The following are examples of neurologic sequelae of metabolic disturbances:

- *Hypoglycemia*: Cellular effects of hypoglycemia are similar to those of oxygen deprivation because the brain requires glucose and oxygen. Neurons that are relatively sensitive to hypoglycemia include large cerebral pyramidal cells, hippocampal pyramidal cells in area CA1, and Purkinje cells. If the level and duration of hypoglycemia are of sufficient severity, there may be a global insult to the neurons of the brain.
- *Hyperglycemia*: Hyperglycemia is most commonly found in the setting of inadequately controlled diabetes mellitus and can be associated with either ketoacidosis or hyperosmolar coma. The patient becomes dehydrated and develops confusion, stupor, and eventually coma. The fluid depletion must be corrected gradually; otherwise, severe cerebral edema may follow.
- *Hepatic encephalopathy (hepatic coma)*: Cellular response in hepatic encephalopathy is predominantly glial, with Alzheimer type II cells in the cortex and basal ganglia and other subcortical gray matter regions.

Toxic Disorders (p. 1342)

Toxic disorders include the following:

- *Carbon monoxide*: Pathology resembles hypoxia, with selective injury of the neurons of layers III and V of cerebral cortex, Sommer sector of the hippocampus, and Purkinje cells. Bilateral necrosis of the globus pallidus may also occur and is more common in carbon monoxide–induced hypoxia than in hypoxia from other causes.
- *Methanol poisoning*: Methanol poisoning may lead to blindness, with degeneration of retinal ganglion cells. Selective bilateral putamenal necrosis also occurs when the exposure is severe. Formate, a major metabolite of methanol, may play a role in the retinal toxicity.
- *Chronic ethanol abuse*: As many as 1% of patients with a history of long-term high intake of ethanol develop a clinical

syndrome of truncal ataxia, unsteady gait, and nystagmus. The early changes are atrophy and loss of granule cells predominantly in the anterior cerebellar vermis. In advanced cases, there are loss of Purkinje cells and a proliferation of the adjacent astrocytes *(Bergmann gliosis)*.

- *Fetal alcohol syndrome:* Alcohol consumption during pregnancy, especially in high amounts, may result in the fetal alcohol syndrome, with growth retardation, facial abnormalities, cardiac septal defects, joint abnormalities, microcephaly, delayed development with mental impairment that may range from mild to severe, and neuronal migration abnormalities.
- *Radiation-induced injury:* Injury may develop months to years after irradiation; it can be synergistic with methotrexate. Radionecrosis is composed of large areas of coagulative necrosis in the white matter with adjacent edema. Adjacent to these areas, proteinaceous spheroids may be identified, and blood vessels have thickened walls with intramural fibrin-like material.

TUMORS (p. 1343)

Important features of brain tumors include the following:

1. *Consequences of location:* The ability to remove the neoplasm surgically may be restricted by functional anatomic considerations. Benign lesions can have lethal consequences because of their location.
2. *Patterns of growth:* Most glial tumors, including many with histologic features of a benign neoplasm, infiltrate entire regions of the brain leading to clinically malignant behavior.
3. *Patterns of spread:* Some types of tumor spread through the CSF; however, even the most frankly malignant gliomas (glioblastoma multiforme) rarely metastasize outside of the CNS.

Tumors of the CNS account for as much as 20% of all cancers of childhood. In this age group, 70% of primary tumors arise in the posterior fossa, whereas in adults, a corresponding proportion arise above the tentorium. Among adults, there is a nearly equal incidence of primary and metastatic tumors.

Gliomas (p. 1343)

ASTROCYTOMAS (p. 1343)

Fibrillary Astrocytomas (p. 1343)

Fibrillary astrocytomas represent about 80% of adult primary brain tumors, usually in cerebral hemispheres, but they may also occur in the cerebellum, brain stem, or spinal cord. All astrocytomas are composed of neoplastic astrocytic nuclei, distributed amid astrocytic processes of varying density; grade is determined histologically.

- Well-differentiated tumors *(astrocytoma)* are poorly defined, gray-white, infiltrative tumors that expand and distort a region of the brain; they show hypercellularity and some nuclear pleomorphism.
- More anaplastic and aggressive tumors *(anaplastic astrocytoma)* reveal increased nuclear anaplasia and the presence of mitoses and vascular cell proliferation.
- Extremely high-grade tumors *(glioblastoma multiforme)* are

composed of a mixture of firm, white areas; softer, yellow foci of necrosis; cystic change; and hemorrhage. Increased nuclear density of the highly anaplastic tumor cells along the edges of the necrotic regions is termed *pseudopalisading*.

Low-grade astrocytomas may remain static or progress only slowly for a number of years. Eventually, however, patients often enter a period of rapid clinical deterioration and rapid tumor growth, correlated with the appearance of anaplastic features. The prognosis for patients with glioblastoma is poor: mean length of survival after diagnosis is only 8 to 10 months.

Brain Stem Gliomas (p. 1346)

Brain stem gliomas occur mostly in the first two decades of life. By the time of autopsy, about 50% have progressed to glioblastomas. With radiotherapy, the 5-year survival rate is between 20 and 40%.

Pilocytic Astrocytomas (p. 1346)

Pilocytic astrocytomas occur in children and young adults, usually in the cerebellum but also in the floor and walls of the third ventricle, the optic nerves, and, occasionally, the cerebral hemispheres. They are often cystic with a mural nodule in the wall of the cyst. The tumor is composed of bipolar cells with long, thin hairlike processes; Rosenthal fibers and microcysts are often present. These tumors are rarely infiltrative and grow slowly.

Pleomorphic Xanthoastrocytomas (p. 1346)

Pleomorphic xanthoastrocytomas occur most often relatively superficially in the temporal lobes of children and young adults with a history of seizures. They contain neoplastic astrocytes, sometimes having lipid with bizarre forms, abundant reticulin deposits, and chronic inflammatory cell infiltrates.

OLIGODENDROGLIOMA (p. 1346)

Oligodendrogliomas constitute about 5 to 15% of gliomas and are most common in middle life in the cerebral white matter. In general, patients with oligodendrogliomas have a better prognosis than patients with astrocytomas. Current therapies have yielded an average survival of 5 to 10 years. Cases of poorly differentiated tumors with necrosis have a worse prognosis.

Oligodendrogliomas are well-circumscribed, gelatinous, gray masses, often with cysts, focal hemorrhage, and calcification. The tumor consists of sheets of regular cells with round nuclei containing finely granular chromatin, often surrounded by a clear halo of cytoplasm sitting in a delicate network of anastomosing capillaries. Calcification, present in up to 90% of cases, ranges from microscopic foci to massive deposits.

EPENDYMOMA (p. 1346)

These tumors arise from the ependymal lining of the ventricular system, including the central canal of the spinal cord. CSF dissemination is a common finding. In the first two decades of life, ependymomas typically occur in the fourth ventricle; in middle life, the spinal cord is the most common location.

The tumor cells have regular, round-to-oval nuclei with abundant granular chromatin; they may form ependymal rosettes (canals) or, more frequently, perivascular pseudorosettes.

- *Myxopapillary ependymomas*: Histologically benign lesions arising in the filum terminale of the spinal cord. Cuboidal cells, sometimes with clear cytoplasm, are arranged around papillary cores containing connective tissue and blood vessels. Myxoid areas contain neutral and acidic mucopolysaccharides.
- *Subependymomas*: Solid, sometimes calcified, slow-growing nodules attached to the ventricular lining and protruding into the ventricle. They have clumps of ependymal-appearing nuclei scattered in a dense, finely fibrillar background.

CHOROID PLEXUS PAPILLOMAS (p. 1347)

Choroid plexus papillomas almost exactly recapitulate the structure of the normal choroid plexus, with papillae of connective tissue stalks covered with a cuboidal or columnar ciliated epithelium. Hydrocephalus is common, as a result of either obstruction of the ventricular system or overproduction of CSF. In children, the lateral ventricles are the most common site; in adults, the fourth ventricle is a more frequent site.

COLLOID CYSTS OF THE THIRD VENTRICLE (p. 1348)

Colloid cysts of the third ventricle are non-neoplastic lesions of young adults; they are located at the foramina of Monro and can result in noncommunicating hydrocephalus, sometimes rapidly fatal. The cyst has a thin, fibrous capsule and a lining of low-to-flat cuboidal epithelium; the cyst contents are gelatinous proteinaceous material.

Neuronal Tumors (p. 1348)

GANGLIOGLIOMA (p. 1348)

Ganglioglioma is a glial neoplasm with admixed ganglion cell component of irregularly clustered neurons with apparently random orientation of neurites and frequent binucleated forms. Most occur in the temporal lobe and are slow growing, but occasionally the glial component becomes frankly anaplastic, and the tumor then assumes a much more aggressive course. Mature-appearing neurons may constitute the entire population of a tumor, then termed *gangliocytoma.*

- *Cerebral neuroblastoma*: Rare, aggressive neoplasm that occurs in the hemispheres in children and resembles peripheral neuroblastomas, with small undifferentiated cells and Homer Wright rosettes (p. 485).
- *Neurocytoma*: Found adjacent to the foramen of Monro; evenly spaced, round, uniform nuclei resembling the oligodendroglioma, but ultrastructural and immunohistochemical studies reveal their neuronal origin.
- *Dysembryoplastic neuroepithelial tumor*: Tumor of childhood often presenting as a seizure disorder, with a relatively good prognosis after resection. Features include intracortical location, cystic changes, nodular growth, *floating neurons* in a pool of

mucopolysaccharide-rich fluid, and surrounding neoplastic glia without anaplastic features.

Poorly Differentiated Neoplasms (p. 1348)

Some tumors, although of neuroectodermal origin, express few, if any, of the phenotypic markers of mature cells of the nervous system and are described as poorly differentiated.

MEDULLOBLASTOMA (p. 1348)

Medulloblastomas comprise 20% of childhood brain tumors; they occur exclusively in the cerebellum. Tumors are located in the midline in children, with lateral locations found more often in adults. Rapid growth may occlude the flow of CSF, leading to hydrocephalus. Often well-circumscribed, gray, and friable, they are usually extremely cellular, with sheets of anaplastic cells with hyperchromatic nuclei and abundant mitoses. The cells have little cytoplasm, and the cytoplasm is often devoid of specific markers of differentiation, although neuronal or glial features may be seen. Extension into the subarachnoid space may elicit a prominent desmoplastic response. Dissemination through the CSF is common.

The tumor is highly malignant, and the prognosis for untreated tumor is dismal; however, it is an exquisitely radiosensitive tumor. With total excision and radiation, the 5-year survival has been reported to be as high as 75%.

Other Parenchymal Tumors (p. 1349)

PRIMARY BRAIN LYMPHOMA (p. 1349)

Primary brain lymphomas comprise approximately 2% of extra-nodal lymphomas. One or more dominant masses occur within brain parenchyma; nodal or bone marrow involvement and involvement outside of the CNS are extremely rare late complications. Within the immunosuppressed population (e.g., AIDS), all the neoplasms appear to be of B-cell origin and to contain Epstein-Barr virus genomes within the transformed B cells. Regardless of clinical context, primary brain lymphoma is an aggressive disease with relatively poor chemotherapeutic responses compared with peripheral lymphomas, although it is initially responsive to radiotherapy and steroids. The morphology of the neoplastic lymphocytes is nearly always of a high-grade type. The malignant cells diffusely involve the parenchyma of the brain and accumulate around blood vessels, with some vessel walls expanded by multiple layers of malignant cells.

GERM CELL TUMORS (p. 1350)

Germ cell tumors occur along the midline in adolescents and young adults, with the pineal and suprasellar regions dominating the distribution. Tumors in the pineal region show a strong male predominance, not seen in suprasellar lesions. The histologic appearances of germ cell tumors and their classification are the same as used for other extragonadal sites (p. 1018).

Meningiomas (p. 1350)

Meningiomas are predominantly benign tumors of adults that arise from the meningothelial cell of the arachnoid. They show a moderate (3:2) female predominance within the cranial vault but a 10:1 ratio within the spinal canal. Loss of heterozygosity of the long arm of chromosome 22 is a common finding associated with mutations in the *NF2* gene.

Meningiomas tend to be rounded masses with well-defined dural bases that compress underlying brain but are easily separated from it. Lesions are usually firm to fibrous and lack evidence of necrosis or extensive hemorrhage. Many histologic patterns exist with comparable prognosis:

- *Syncytial* refers to clusters of cells in tight groups without visible cell membranes.
- *Fibroblastic* refers to elongated cells and abundant collagen deposition.
- *Transitional* refers to features of the syncytial and fibroblastic types.
- *Psammomatous* refers to abundant psammoma bodies.
- *Papillary tumors,* with pleomorphic cells arranged around fibrovascular cores, have a worse prognosis.
- *Malignant meningiomas* are unusual tumors and may be difficult to recognize histologically. Features that support this diagnosis include single cell infiltration of underlying brain and abundant mitoses with atypical forms.
- *Sarcomas* of the meninges are uncommon but can include malignant fibrous histiocytomas and hemangiopericytomas.

Metastatic Lesions (p. 1351)

Among general hospital patients, metastatic lesions, mostly carcinomas, account for approximately half of intracranial tumors. Common primary sites are lung, breast, skin (melanoma), kidney, and gastrointestinal tract. The meninges are also a frequent site for involvement by metastatic disease.

Intraparenchymal metastases are sharply demarcated masses, often at the gray-white junction, usually surrounded by a zone of edema. Meningeal carcinomatosis, with tumor nodules studding the surface of the brain, spinal cord, and intradural nerve roots, is an occasional complication particularly associated with small cell carcinoma, adenocarcinoma of the lung, and carcinoma of the breast.

PARANEOPLASTIC SYNDROMES (p. 1351)

Paraneoplastic syndromes are functional and structural changes of the brain in response to malignancy elsewhere in the body, often small cell carcinoma of the lung. Syndromes may improve with plasmapheresis, immunosuppression, or treatment of the neoplasm.

- *Paraneoplastic cerebellar degeneration* is the most common pattern, with loss of Purkinje cells, gliosis, and a mild inflammatory infiltrate associated with an antibody-mediated injury of Purkinje cells.
- *Limbic encephalitis* is a subacute dementia, usually with a prominent component of memory disturbance. Findings are most striking in the anterior and medial portions of the temporal lobe and resemble an infectious process with perivascular in-

flammatory cuffs, microglial nodules, some neuronal loss, and gliosis.
- *Subacute sensory neuropathy* occurs in association with limbic encephalitis or in isolation, with loss of sensory neurons from dorsal root ganglia, in association with inflammation.

Peripheral Nerve Sheath Tumors (p. 1352)

A large proportion of tumors occurring within the confines of the dura are derived from cells of peripheral nerve; comparable tumors arise along the peripheral course of nerves.

SCHWANNOMA (p. 1352)

Schwannoma refers to benign tumors of neural crest–derived Schwann cells, most commonly associated with the vestibular branch of the eighth nerve at the cerebellopontine angle (vestibular schwannoma or acoustic neuroma). Spinal tumors mostly arise from dorsal roots; tumor may extend through the vertebral foramen, acquiring a dumbbell configuration. When extradural, schwannomas are most commonly found in association with large nerve trunks. They are well-circumscribed, encapsulated masses, attached to the nerve but separable from it. Axons are excluded from the tumor, although they may become entrapped in the capsule. Tumors show a mixture of two growth patterns:

1. *Antoni A*, elongated cells with cytoplasmic processes arranged in fascicles in areas of moderate-to-high cellularity with little stromal matrix
2. *Antoni B*, less densely cellular tissue with microcysts and myxoid changes

Electron microscopy shows basement membrane deposition encasing single cells and long-spacing collagen. Malignant change is extremely rare.

CUTANEOUS NEUROFIBROMA AND SOLITARY NEUROFIBROMA (p. 1353)

Cutaneous neurofibroma and solitary neurofibroma occur sporadically and in association with neurofibromatosis type 1 (p. 1354). The skin lesions are evident as nodules, sometimes with hyperpigmentation; these lesions may grow quite large and become pedunculated. The risk of malignant transformation from these tumors is extremely small. Present in the dermis and extending to the subcutaneous fat, these are well-delineated but unencapsulated masses composed of spindle cells in a highly collagenized stroma. Lesions within peripheral nerves are histologically similar.

PLEXIFORM NEUROFIBROMA (p. 1353)

Plexiform neurofibromas irregularly expand a nerve as fascicles are infiltrated; in contrast to schwannomas, it is not possible to separate the lesion from the nerve. The lesion has a loose myxoid background with a low cellularity, including Schwann cells, fibroblasts, perineurial cells, and a sprinkling of inflammatory cells, often including mast cells. Axons can be demonstrated within the tumor. A major concern in the care of neurofibromatosis type 1 patients is the difficulty of surgical removal of these tumors from major nerve trunks, combined with their potential for malignant transformation.

MALIGNANT PERIPHERAL NERVE SHEATH TUMOR (MALIGNANT SCHWANNOMA)
(p. 1353)

Malignant peripheral nerve sheath tumor is a highly malignant, locally invasive sarcoma. These tumors do not arise from malignant degeneration of schwannomas; instead, they arise de novo or from transformation of a plexiform neurofibroma. The lesions are poorly defined tumor masses with frequent infiltration along the axis of the parent nerve as well as invasion of adjacent soft tissues. Tumor cells resemble Schwann cells with elongated nuclei and prominent bipolar processes; fascicle formation may be present. Mitoses, necrosis, and nuclear anaplasia are common. Patterns of other sarcoma types may be present.

NEUROCUTANEOUS SYNDROMES (PHACOMATOSES) (p. 1354)

Neurocutaneous syndromes are a group of mostly autosomal dominant disorders characterized by hamartomas located throughout the body, often prominently involving the nervous system and skin. Neoplasms occur with a high incidence in most of the neurocutaneous disorders. These syndromes include the following:

- *Neurofibromatosis type 1*: This autosomal dominant disorder is characterized by neurofibromas (plexiform and cutaneous), optic nerve gliomas, meningiomas, pigmented nodules of the iris *(Lisch nodules)*, and cutaneous hyperpigmented macules *(café-au-lait spots)*. Even in the absence of malignant transformation of neurofibromas, lesions have disfiguring potential and the potential to create spinal deformity, most commonly kyphoscoliosis. Tumors arising in proximity to the spinal cord or brain stem may also have devastating consequences, independent of their histologic grade. The gene, located at 17q11.2, encodes a protein homologous to guanosine triphosphatase (GTPase)–activating proteins and may play a role in regulating signal transduction related to growth control.
- *Neurofibromatosis type 2*: This is a distinct autosomal dominant disorder (chromosome 22) with a propensity to develop bilateral eighth nerve schwannomas or multiple meningiomas. The gene encodes a member of a group of proteins that interact with both the membrane components and the cytoskeleton.
- *Tuberous sclerosis*: Tuberous sclerosis is characterized by angiofibromas, seizures, and mental retardation. Hamartomas within the CNS include *cortical tubers* (areas of haphazardly arranged neurons and large cells that express phenotypes intermediate between glia and neurons) and subependymal hamartomas (large astrocytic and neuronal cell clusters beneath the ventricular surface, which may give rise to a tumor unique to tuberous sclerosis—subependymal giant cell astrocytoma). In addition, renal angiomyolipomas; retinal glial phakomas; pulmonary and cardiac myomas; hepatic, renal, and pancreatic cysts; leathery cutaneous thickenings (shagreen patches); hypopigmented areas (ash leaf patches); and subungual fibromas may occur. There is variable expressivity and penetrance, and at least two distinct loci are known, on chromosomes 9 (hamartin) and 16 (tuberin).

■ *von Hippel–Lindau disease*: This disease is characterized by
  • Capillary hemangioblastomas in the cerebellar hemispheres, retina, and less commonly within the brain stem and spinal cord
  • Cysts involving the pancreas, liver, and kidney (with a strong propensity to develop renal cell carcinoma of the kidney)
  • Paragangliomas

  Hemangioblastomas contain variable proportions of delicate capillary vessels with *stromal* cells of uncertain histogenesis and abundant vacuolated cytoplasm between them. They commonly are cystic lesions with a mural node. Polycythemia is an associated finding in about 10% of cases, related to erythropoietin production by the tumor. The disease locus on chromosome 3 encodes a tumor-suppressor gene that is also associated with clear cell renal cell carcinoma.

Diseases of the Eye

CONJUNCTIVA (p. 1361)

- *Keratomalacia* (p. 1361): Leading cause of blindness in under-developed countries (principally in undernourished children). It is characterized by keratinization of mucous membrane epithelia, night blindness, and bacterial infection and ulceration of the cornea.
- *Pinguecula*: Raised, yellow subepithelial connective tissue in the nasal bulbar conjunctiva associated with sun exposure.
- *Pterygium*: Pinguecula with a winglike projection of vascularized tissue that extends onto the nasal cornea.
- *Trachoma*: A major cause of blindness worldwide.
  - *Stage I*: Consists of conjunctival inflammatory infiltrates, in the form of *follicles* and fibrovascular tissue growth (*pannus*).
  - *Stage II*: Inflammation becomes florid, follicles increase in number and size, epithelium thickens, and corneal pannus becomes severe.
  - *Stage III*: Follicles disappear, scarring ensues, and upper lid inverts.
  - *Stage IV*: Disease spontaneously arrests, but corneal scarring from previous stages results in severe visual loss.
- *Carcinoma* in situ: An opaque, white, shiny, fleshy mass arising from the epithelium of the conjunctiva or cornea. The mass is characteristic of similar squamous epithelial lesions elsewhere histologically; however, the basal membrane of the epithelium remains intact, and the subepithelial tissue is not invaded.
- *Squamous cell carcinoma*: Similar to carcinoma in situ, but tumor cells invade the subepithelial tissue.

CORNEA (p. 1362)

- *Inflammation*: Noninfectious or infectious. Inflammation may respond to topical antibiotics and steroids, but residual scarring may require transplantation. If the stroma completely melts away, a descemetocele (herniation through the posterior limiting membrane of the cornea) results, and perforation leads to hypotony, invasion of infectious organisms into the globe, and often loss of the eye.
- *Stromal (interstitial) keratitis*: Inflammation under an intact corneal epithelium.
- *Ulcer*: Inflammation with absent overlying epithelium. Risk factors include wearing contact lenses, debilitation, and immune deficiency states.
- *Herpetic infections*: Most common cause of central corneal

662

ulcers, which are usually unilateral and can recur many times. In chronic cases, inflammation may take the form of a discoid opacity *(disciform keratitis)*. After resolution of the infection, the cornea may be uninflamed but scarred and vascularized.

- *Dystrophies*: Hereditary corneal disorders that are bilateral, often symmetric, and can cause severe visual loss reparable by corneal transplantation (Table 29–1).

UVEA (CHOROID, CILIARY BODY, IRIS)
(p. 1364)

Granulomatous Uveitis (p. 1364)

- *Infectious causes*:
  - Bacterial (tuberculosis, leprosy, syphilis, tularemia)
  - Viral (cytomegalic inclusion disease, herpes zoster)
  - Fungal (blastomycosis, cryptococcosis, coccidioidomycosis)
  - Parasitic (onchocerciasis, toxoplasmosis)

  The inflammation may extend from the uvea, to the retina, vitreous, and sclera.

- *Sarcoidosis*: In one third of cases, results in granulomatous anterior uveitis, characterized by keratic precipitates. Retinal involvement is frequently associated with central nervous system sarcoidosis and carries a grave prognosis.

- *Sympathetic ophthalmia*: A rare, *bilateral* uveitis associated with penetrating injuries to *one* eye. Initial symptoms are loss of accommodation, blurred vision, photophobia, and appearance of keratic precipitates and choroidal infiltrates in the sympathizing eye. Prompt removal of the injured eye (if blind) appears to result in milder inflammation in the noninjured eye.

Uveal Melanomas (p. 1365)

Uveal melanomas constitute 79% of all *nonskin* melanomas.

MORPHOLOGY

Most melanomas arise in the choroid. They may spread laterally between the sclera and retina or may produce bulbous masses projecting into the vitreous cavity and pushing the retina ahead of them. The morphologic subtypes are shown in Table 29–2.

CLINICAL PRESENTATION

An iris melanoma usually presents as a pigmented mass, somewhat light in color. A choroidal melanoma can cause retinal detachment, macular edema, retinal detachment, or choroidal hemorrhage. A melanoma in any uveal region may extend to the surface of the globe and present as an episcleral mass. Iris melanomas are usually resected only when intraocular spread causes pain or visual loss. Enucleation or radiation is used for ciliary body and choroidal melanomas.

LENS (p. 1367)

Cataracts are opacities in the lens and are a major cause of visual loss throughout the world. The most common type, *senile cataract*, is idiopathic and develops in older patients. *Posterior*

Table 29-1. CORNEAL DYSTROPHIES

Dystrophy	Etiology	Clinical Appearance
Granular	Autosomal dominant disease due to defects in gene encoding β-keratoepithelin	Sharply defined, variably sized, white opacities in the anterior portion of the stroma
Lattice	Same as granular	Linear opacities form a lattice configuration concentrated in the central portion of the anterior stroma
Avellino	Same as granular	Similar to granular and lattice deposits
Reis-Bücklers	Due to another mutation in the same gene	Protein deposits under the corneal epithelium and Bowman layer in the anterior stroma
Macular	Autosomal recessive; responsible genes not yet known. (*Most severe dystrophy*)	Diffuse cloudiness of the anterior stroma with aggregates of gray-white opacities in the axial region. Results in severe impairment of vision by age 30
Fuchs	Dominantly inherited. (*Most common dystrophy*)	Edema of the corneal stroma and epithelium due to loss of endothelial cells

Table 29-2. MORPHOLOGY OF UVEAL MELANOMAS

Classification	Characteristics	Percent of Uveal Melanomas	Percent of Patients Dead 15 Years After Enucleation
Spindle A	Cohesive tumor cells with small, spindle-shaped nuclei containing a nuclear fold. Nucleoli are indistinct, cytoplasm is scant, and cell borders are difficult to identify	5	8
Spindle B	Cohesive cells with distinct, spindle-shaped nuclei with prominent nucleoli. Cells contain cytoplasm, and cell borders are difficult to identify	40	15
Epithelioid	Poorly cohesive, large cells with round nuclei, prominent nucleoli. Abundant eosinophilic cytoplasm, well-demarcated cell borders	3	72
Mixed cell type	Spindle cells (usually B) with many (>5–10%) epithelioid cells	45	60
Necrotic	Cell type obscured by extensive necrosis	7	60

subcapsular cataracts develop anterior to the posterior capsule and spread toward the periphery. A cataractous lens may swell osmotically *(intumescent cataract).* The cortex may liquefy entirely, and the sclerotic nucleus may sink into the cortex *(morgagnian cataract).* Long-standing cataractous lenses shrink, and lenticular debris diffuses into the aqueous humor *(hypermature cataract).*

RETINA (p. 1368)

The retina has a basic three-neuron organization. An electrical impulse generated in the photoreceptor cells is transmitted to cells of the inner nuclear layer, then to the ganglion cell layer. The axons of the ganglion cells extend through the optic nerve and synapse in the brain.

Retinopathy of Prematurity (Retrolental Fibroplasia) (p. 1368)

Retinopathy of prematurity is no longer a leading cause of infant blindness, but the condition still occurs with disturbing frequency (Chapter 11, p. 472). It affects mostly premature infants who have been exposed to oxygen inhalation therapy.

- *Vaso-obliterative phase*: There is functional constriction of the immature retinal blood vessels followed by a structural obliteration. The peripheral retina fails to vascularize.
- *Vasoproliferative phase*: This phase takes place on cessation of exposure to oxygen. There is a proliferation of new blood vessels and fibroblasts into the vitreous.
- *Cicatricial phase*: In about 25% of cases, the fibrovascular component shrinks, and hemorrhages may occur.

Vascular endothelial growth factor (VEGF) plays an important role in the pathogenesis. High oxygen therapy inhibits VEGF production and causes endothelial *apoptosis*, and the subsequent oxygen cessation causes increased VEGF production and neovascularization.

Retinopathy Associated With Diabetes Mellitus (p. 1369)

Approximately 60% of diabetic patients develop retinopathy 15 to 20 years after initial diagnosis. It is a major cause of blindness in the United States and Europe.

- *Background retinopathy*: The thickness of basement membranes varies, pericyte degeneration takes place, and *microaneurysms* and *arteriovenous shunts* develop. Capillary microaneurysms may develop thromboses and become occluded; intraretinal vascular shunts occur in areas of ischemic retina.
- *Proliferative retinopathy*: This occurs in response to severe ischemia and hypoxia of the retina. The new capillaries are incompletely formed and poorly supported; once they extend into the vitreous cavity, bleeding is common. *Neovascularization* and the development of a fibrous component often culminate in retinal detachment.

Hypertensive Retinopathy (p. 1370)

Hypertensive retinopathy is a common complication of hypertension.

- *Grade I* consists of a generalized narrowing of the arterioles.
- *Grade II* is characterized, in addition, by focal arteriolar spasms.
- *Grade III* exhibits flame-shaped hemorrhages, dot-and-blot hemorrhages, cotton-wool spots, and hard waxy exudates.
- *Grade IV*, the most severe, has in addition to grade III changes, optic disc edema.

Retinitis Pigmentosa (p. 1370)

Retinitis pigmentosa refers to a group of hereditary, bilateral, progressive retinopathies in which there is loss of rods and cones associated with proliferation of retinal pigment epithelium and the appearance of pigmented interstitial cells in the sensory retina (pigmentary retinopathy). Night blindness is an early symptom. Retinal pigmentation is distributed in a branching reticulated pattern, the optic disc appears pale, and retinal blood vessels are attenuated. The disorder is inherited as autosomal dominant, recessive, or sex-linked recessive trait or as a maternally inherited (mitochondrial) trait. In a minority of patients, deafness (Usher syndrome) and endocrinologic disturbances (Bardet-Biedl syndrome) occur. Mutations in the genes for a number of photoreceptor (peripherin) and other ocular (opsin) proteins are described.

Macular Degeneration (p. 1371)

Age-related macular degeneration is the most common cause of decreased vision in the elderly. In the *atrophic form*, Bruch membrane thickens generally and focally. The choriocapillaris is often focally obliterated, the pigment epithelium is atrophic and depigmented, and the photoreceptors degenerate. New vessels may grow from the choroid through defects in Bruch membrane. In the *exudative form*, the new vessels produce exudates and hemorrhage under the retina. The end result is a fibrous scar in the macular region with degeneration of the neural retina and permanent loss of central vision.

Retinal Detachment (p. 1371)

- *Rhegmatogenous* retinal detachment arises when a break or tear in the retina allows vitreous fluid beneath the retina.
- *Serous or exudative* retinal detachment occurs when fluid accumulates beneath an intact sensory retina.
- *Traction detachments* develop after fibrous or glial membranes form in the vitreous.

Retinoblastoma (p. 1372)

Retinoblastoma is the most common malignant eye tumor of childhood.

GENETIC ETIOLOGY

Retinoblastomas arise from retinal cells that have an initial germ line or somatic mutation affecting one allele of the retinoblastoma gene *(RB)* and have lost the function of the remaining wild-type *RB* allele. Hereditary retinoblastoma (30 to 40%) is transmitted as a dominant trait and is usually bilateral. Those affected have a 30% risk of developing a second cancer by age 40. In nonhereditary retinoblastoma (60 to 70%), patients have only one tumor and are not at an elevated risk for other cancers.

MORPHOLOGIC AND CLINICAL FEATURES

The tumors are white friable nodules often with satellite seeding. The tumor cells are small, round, and resemble undifferentiated retinoblasts. *Rosettes* are often present.

OPTIC NERVE (p. 1373)

Papilledema (p. 1373)

Edema of the optic disc is usually associated with increased intracranial pressure. The subarachnoid space surrounding the optic nerve is a direct extension of the subarachnoid space around the brain; any increase in intracranial pressure is thus transmitted to the optic nerve. Acutely, there is edema and vascular congestion of the nerve head, obliteration of the optic cup, hemorrhages, and displacement of the adjacent retina leading to retinal and choroidal folds. Chronically, degeneration of nerve fibers, gliosis, and optic atrophy may occur.

Optic Neuritis (Neuropathy) (p. 1374)

Optic neuritis refers to inflammatory or noninflammatory pathologic processes that include demyelinative diseases. It is caused by systemic or ischemic disease, toxic conditions, spread of inflammation, and infection.

Optic Atrophy (p. 1374)

Optic atrophy represents the end stage of many optic nerve diseases; it is characterized by loss of myelin and axons, glial proliferation, thickening of the pial septa, and widening of the subarachnoid space.

Tumors (p. 1374)

Primary tumors are gliomas and meningiomas. Rarely, hemangiomas and hemangiopericytomas occur. Extraocular spread is usually fatal, but most cases in developed countries are diagnosed before this point. Radiation therapy, laser photocoagulation, and cryotherapy are used in eyes with potential for useful vision; enucleation is preferred for large tumors.

GLAUCOMA (p. 1374)

Glaucoma is classically characterized by high intraocular pressure producing ocular damage. The damage includes intracellular and intercellular epithelial edema of the cornea and corneal stromal edema; degenerative pannus formation; corneal scarring; cataracts; necrosis of the iris and the ciliary body stroma; atrophy, hyalinization, and shortening of the ciliary processes; and venous stasis in the retina.

- *Primary angle-closure glaucoma* occurs in anatomically predisposed eyes, such as small, hyperopic eyes.
- *Open-angle glaucoma* is caused by poor transport of aqueous humor out of the eye through the angle.
- *Congenital glaucoma* and *juvenile glaucoma* are usually hereditary, caused by defects in genes encoding several classes of molecules (cytochromes and transcription factors).

Index

Note: Page numbers in *italics* refer to illustrations;
page numbers followed by t refer to tables.

B lymphocytes *(Continued)*
  dyscrasias of, amyloidosis in, 139
  in HIV infection, 133, 134t
  in lymphomas. See *Lymphoma(s)*.
  mature. See *Plasma cell(s)*.
  precursor, neoplasms of, 334t, 336, 337t, 338
  proliferation of, in Epstein-Barr virus infections, 165–166
Babesia microti, 197
Bacillary angiomatosis, 273–274
Bacteremia, endocarditis in, 288
  osteomyelitis in, 600
Bacteria, airborne, as air pollutants, 216
  characteristics of, 173
  gastrointestinal infections due to, 180t, 181–182
  gram-positive, 184–186
  immune evasion by, 175
  normal populations of, 173
  pyogenic, inflammatory response to, 176
  respiratory infections due to, 377–378
  virulence factors of, 175, 185
Bacteriophages, 173
Baker cyst, 613
Balanoposthitis, 501
Balloon angioplasty, vascular complications of, 276
Ballooned neurons, in corticobasal degeneration, 649
Barbiturates, abuse of, 209
Bardet-Biedl syndrome, retinitis pigmentosa in, 667
Barrett esophagus, 400–401
  malignant transformation of, 403–404
Bartholin cyst, 516
Bartonella henselae, in bacillary angiomatosis, 273–274
Basal cell(s), necrosis of, in lichen planus, 586
Basal cell carcinoma, 579
Basal cell nevus syndrome, 579
Basal ganglia, degenerative diseases of, 649–650
Basophil(s), in hypersensitivity reactions, 111
Basophilia, in polycythemia vera, 361
Basophilic cells, in pituitary adenoma, 546
Basophilic leukocytosis, 331
Bathing suit distribution, of erythema marginatum, in rheumatic heart disease, 286
bax gene and product, in apoptosis, 156
bcl-2 genes and products, in apoptosis, 12, 13, *13*, 157
BCR-ABL fusion gene, in chronic myelogenous leukemia, 359–360
Beard region, tinea infections of, 592
Becker muscular dystrophy, 627
Beckwith-Wiedemann syndrome, 256
Becquerel, as radiation unit, 222
Beef tapeworm, 199
Behavior, inflammation effects on, 57
Bence Jones protein, 139, 343
  in urine, 489
Bends, the, gas embolism in, 83–84, 229
Benign fibrous histiocytoma, of skin, 580
  of soft tissue, 616
Benign prostatic hyperplasia, 512–513
Benign tumors. See *Tumor(s), benign*; specific tumors.
Benzene, health effects of, 216
Benzo[a]pyrene, health effects of, 216
  metabolism of, 206
Berger disease, 481–482
Bergmann gliosis, 654
Beriberi, 238
Bernard-Soulier syndrome, 323
Berry aneurysm(s), congenital, 258, 473
  rupture of, 639–640
Berylliosis, granulomatous inflammation in, 56t
Beryllium, health effects of, 218t
Beta cells, antibodies to, 465
  in diabetes mellitus, absence of, 464
    destruction of, 464–465, 467
    dysfunction of, 466
  tumors of, 468–469
Beta particles, injury due to, 222–226, 224t